Principles of Flexible Endoscopy for Surgeons

Jeffrey M. Marks · Brian J. Dunkin
Editors

Principles of Flexible Endoscopy for Surgeons

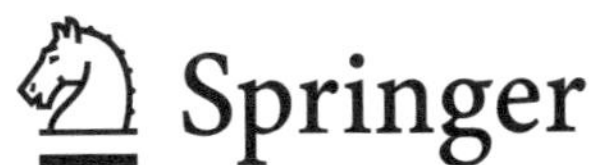 Springer

Editors
Jeffrey M. Marks, M.D., F.A.C.S., F.A.S.G.E
Department of Surgery
Case Medical Center
University Hospitals
Cleveland, OH, USA

Brian J. Dunkin, M.D., F.A.C.S.
The Methodist Institute for Technology,
  Innovation, and Education (MITIE)
The Methodist Hospital
Houston, TX, USA

ISBN 978-1-4939-4206-0   ISBN 978-1-4614-6330-6 (eBook)
DOI 10.1007/978-1-4614-6330-6
Springer New York Heidelberg Dordrecht London

I wish to thank my wife Gayle and children Andrea, Jamie, and Jared for all of their endless support and inspiration in my life and in my work.

Jeffrey M. Marks

I would like to thank my wife Annie and children Joseph and Megan for sharing my dedication to providing exceptional healthcare despite personal sacrifices; and to my mentors—Drs. Jeffrey Ponsky and Jeffrey Marks—for guiding me down the road to a meaningful career.

Brian J. Dunkin

Foreword

Why should there be a book devoted to techniques of flexible endoscopy? There are volumes of books related to this subject. However, most all of these volumes deal with the relationship of endoscopy to the practice of gastroenterology and do not address any special considerations related to the management of surgical problems. Some gastroenterologists question the need for surgeons to perform flexible endoscopy of the gastrointestinal tract at all! These individuals fail to recognize the special questions surgeons must answer regarding the care of their patients and the role of endoscopy in planning surgical intervention as well as treating complications. It is important to note that the majority of endoscopic innovations have been developed by surgeons.

Drs. Marks and Dunkin are highly experienced and respected surgical endoscopists. They have been innovators and pioneers of new methodology and have taught endoscopic skills to hundreds of surgical residents and practicing surgeons throughout the world. In this volume, they have brought together a team of outstanding surgical endoscopists to address basic endoscopic principles and present new and developing technologies that directly impact the care of surgical patients. Issues of management of surgical complications are addressed as well as alternatives to traditional surgical techniques. Surgical endoscopy is a constantly evolving area of practice and it is impossible for a single text to remain current for long. However, the combination of the basic principles presented, along with instructional videos will help prepare the reader for new developments to come. This volume is an important addition to a surgeon's library.

Cleveland, OH, USA   Jeffrey L. Ponsky, M.D., F.A.C.S.

Preface

Flexible endoscopy has become an increasingly integral part of surgery over the past several decades as advancements in therapeutic endoscopic tools have augmented the care of complex surgical patients. Preoperative endoscopic findings can provide information vital to a successful surgery. In addition, intra-operative endoscopy has gained increased popularity to augment laparoscopic techniques that lack the tactile feedback readily available with open surgery. Finally, many postoperative patients can now be managed with flexible endoscopic techniques, avoiding challenging revisional surgery and a possible lengthy and complicated recovery. The appropriate management of these patients, and resultant improved outcomes, requires a keen understanding of recent endoscopic advancements, which are not routinely a core component of surgical training programs.

There are numerous texts on flexible endoscopy, but they are uniformly created by and for gastroenterologists, not surgeons. Surgeons have a unique understanding of the anatomy of the GI tract and have specific needs regarding the information acquired from GI endoscopy in order to plan for surgical interventions. Surgeons also realize the limitations of surgery for managing complex complications and are particularly dedicated to pursuing endoscopic solutions to these difficult problems when warranted. As a result, this text, written entirely by surgical endoscopists, presents a comprehensive overview of past, present, and future flexible endoscopic techniques, with a focus on educating surgeons who may or may not already have the skills to perform flexible endoscopy. In addition to the endoscopic management of surgical issues, the role of surgery in the management of endoscopic complications is described. Basic as well as advanced flexible endoscopic techniques are presented in both a didactic and visual mode with extensive illustration, endoscopic images, and accompanying video clips.

Internet Access to Video Clip

The owner of this text will be able to access these video clips through Springer with the following Internet link: http://www.springerimages.com/videos/978-1-4614-6329-0.

Cleveland, OH, USA Jeffrey M. Marks
Houston, TX, USA Brian J. Dunkin

Acknowledgements

The editors would like to thank the chapter authors for their excellent contribution to this text and for their dedication to surgical endoscopy training.

Contents

Contributors

Sajida Ahad, M.D. Department of Surgery, Southern Illinois University School of Medicine, Springfield, IL, USA

Michael Larone Campbell, M.D. Department of Surgery, University of South Florida, Tampa, FL, USA

Bipan Chand, M.D., F.A.C.S. Associate Professor of Surgery, Minimally Invasive Surgery, Loyola University, Maywood, IL, USA

Conor Delaney, M.D., Ph.D. Division of Colorectal Surgery, University Hospitals Case Medical Center, Cleveland, OH, USA

Brian J. Dunkin, M.D., F.A.C.S. Section of Endoscopic Surgery, MITIE[SM] (The Methodist Institute for Technology, Innovation, and Education), The Methodist Hospital, Houston, TX, USA

Jeffrey L. Eakin, M.D., B.A. Department of General Surgery Center for Minimally Invasive Surgery, The Ohio State University Medical Center, Columbus, OH, USA

Kevin El-Hayek, M.D. Surgical Endoscopy, Department of Bariatric and Metabolic Institute, Cleveland Clinic Hospital, Cleveland, OH, USA

Robert D. Fanelli, M.D., F.A.C.S., F.A.S.G.E. Chief-Minimally Invasive Surgery and Surgical Endoscopy, Department of Surgery, The Guthrie Clinic Ltd., One Guthrie Square, Sayre, PA, USA

Joanne Favuzza, D.O. Division of Colorectal Surgery, University Hospitals Case Medical Center, Cleveland, OH, USA

Andrew K. Hadj, M.D., B.S. Department of Surgery, University of Melbourne, Austin Health, Melbourne, VIC, Australia

David Hardy, M.D. Department of Surgery, Augusta State University and Georgia Health Sciences University, Augusta, GA, USA

Jeffrey W. Hazey, M.D., F.A.C.S. Division of General and Gastrointestinal Surgery, Department of Surgery, The Ohio State University, Columbus, OH, USA

Toshitaka Hoppo, M.D., Ph.D. Department of Surgery, Institute for the Treatment of Esohageal & Thoracic Disease, West Penn Allegheny Health System, Pittsbrugh, PA, USA

Eric Hungness, M.D. Department of Surgery, Northwestern University, Chicago, IL, USA

Samuel Ibrahim, M.D. Department of General Surgery, Cleveland Clinic Foundation, Cleveland, OH, USA

Blair A. Jobe, M.D., F.A.C.S. Department of Surgery, Institute for the Treatment of Esohageal & Thoracic Disease, West Penn Allegheny Health System, Pittsbrugh, PA, USA

Ariel Eric Klevan, M.D., F.R.C.S.C. Department of Surgery, Jackson Memorial Hospital, University of Miami Hospital, Miami, FL, USA

Bruce MacFadyen Jr., M.D. Department of Surgery, Medical College of Georgia, Augusta, GA, USA

Jeffrey M. Marks, M.D., F.A.C.S., F.A.S.G.E. Department of Surgery, University Hospitals, Case Medical Center, Cleveland, OH, USA

Jose Martinez, M.D., F.A.C.S. Department of Surgery, Miller School of Medicine, University of Miami, Miami, FL, USA

John D. Mellinger, M.D., F.A.C.S. Department of Surgery, Southern Illinois University School of Medicine, Springfield, IL, USA

W. Scott Melvin, M.D. Department of General Surgery, The Ohio State University Hospital, Columbus, OH, USA

Dean J. Mikami, M.D., F.A.C.S. Department of Gastrointestinal Surgery, Wexner Medical Center at the Ohio State University, Columbus, OH, USA

Vimal K. Narula, M.D., F.A.C.S. Division of General and Gastrointestinal Surgery, Department of Surgery, The Ohio State University, Columbus, OH, USA

Mehrdad Nikfarjam, M.D., Ph.D., F.R.A.C.S. Department of Surgery, University of Melbourne, Austin Health, Melbourne, Australia

Eric M. Pauli, M.D. Department of Surgery, Penn State Hershey Medical Center, Hershey, PA, USA

Jonathan Pearl, M.D. Department of Surgery, Uniformed Services University, Bethesda, MD, USA

Melissa S. Phillips, M.D. Department of Surgery, University of Tennessee Graduate School of Medicine, Knoxville, TN, USA

Jeffrey L. Ponsky, M.D. Department of Surgery, CWRU, University Hospitals Case Medical Center, Cleveland, OH, USA

Benjamin K. Poulose, M.D., M.P.H. Department of Surgery, Vanderbilt University Medical Center, Nashville, TN, USA

Sowsan Rasheid, M.D. Department of Surgery—Colorectal, University of South Florida, Tampa, FL, USA

Lane Ritter, M.D. Department of Surgery, University of Virginia Health System, Charlottesville, VA, USA

Jaime E. Sanchez, M.D., M.S.P.H. Department of Surgery, Division of Colon and Rectal Surgery, University of South Florida, Tampa, FL, USA

Bruce Schirmer, M.D. Department of Surgery, University of Virginia Health System, Charlottesville, VA, USA

Ahmed Sharata, M.D. Department of General and Minimally Invasive Surgery, Oregon Clinic, Portland, OR, USA

Jacqee M. Stuhldreher, M.D. Department of General Surgery, University Hospitals Case Medical Center, Cleveland, OH, USA

Lee L. Swanstrom, M.D. Division of Gastrointestinal and Minimally Invasive Surgery, The Oregon Clinic, Oregon Health and Sciences University, Portland, OR, USA

Ezra Teitelbaum, M.D. Department of Surgery, Northwestern University, Chicago, IL, USA

Thadeus L. Trus, M.D. Department of Surgery, Dartmouth-Hitchcock Medical Center, Lebanon, NH, USA

Evan K. Tummel, M.D. Division of Colon and Rectal Surgery, University of South Florida, Tampa, FL, USA

Melina C. Vassiliou, M.D., M. Ed. Department of Surgery, Montreal General Hospital, McGill University, Montreal, QC, Canada

Vic Velanovich, M.D. Department of Surgery, University of South Florida, Tampa, FL, USA

Daniel von Renteln, M.D. Department of Interdisciplinary Endoscopy, University Hospital, University Medical Center Hamburg-Eppendorf, Hamburg, Germany

Jeremy Warren, M.D. Department of Surgery, Augusta State University and Georgia Health Sciences University, Augusta, GA, USA

A History of Flexible Gastrointestinal Endoscopy

Eric M. Pauli and Jeffrey L. Ponsky

Background

For millennia, physicians have endeavored to view the interior of the gastrointestinal tract in order to diagnose and treat disease. Greek, Roman, and Egyptian scholars are all known to have created specula with which body orifices were viewed. Early endoscopes of the nineteenth century were rigid instruments with large lumens that lacked lens systems and depended upon light provided by candle or flame. Later rigid instruments employed lens assemblies and small bulbs at the tip of the instrument which generated intense heat. Early in the twentieth century, instruments with semiflexible rubber tips were developed to facilitate passage of the endoscope into the esophagus. In the mid-twentieth century, the development of fiber-optic technology permitted the evolution of flexible endoscopes that transmitted "cold light" from an outside source. Light was carried by a fiber-optic bundle from the external source, through the endoscope, to the interior of the viscus being viewed. As light returned through the endoscope, each fiber carried a parcel of the image.

It was from these early fiber-optic endoscope systems that the modern era of flexible gastrointestinal endoscopy has evolved. Throughout this evolution, surgeons have played an unparalleled role in the development of diagnostic and therapeutic modalities. This chapter provides an overview of the history of flexible gastrointestinal endoscopy with particular emphasis on the role of surgeons (frequently in multidisciplinary collaboration) in the development of the techniques outlined in this text.

E.M. Pauli, M.D.
Department of Surgery, Penn State Hershey Medical Center,
Hershey, PA, USA
e-mail: epauli@hmc.psu.edu

J.L. Ponsky, M.D. (✉)
Department of Surgery, CWRU, University Hospitals Case Medical
Center, Cleveland, OH, USA
e-mail: jeffrey.ponsky@uhhospitals.org

Rigid and Semiflexible Gastrointestinal Endoscopy

The first technically successful attempt at rigid endoscopy was performed by Philipp Bozzini in 1805 when the German physician used his *lichtleiter* (German for "light conductor") to direct candle light into the human body through metal casings (Fig. 1.1a) [1]. Tin tubes of various sizes were developed for the nose, esophagus, bladder, and rectum (Fig. 1.1b). Technical advancement in light sources saw the replacement of a candle with a mixture of turpentine and alcohol (to increase illumination and decrease smoke) and ultimately by wire/filament light sources [2–4]. Maximilian Carl-Friedrich Nitze, a general practitioner with an interest in the urinary bladder, developed a working cystoscope with an internal, filamentous light source and lenses to magnify the image [3, 5]. He later developed a cystoscope capable of holding glass plates with light-sensitive coating capable of producing permanent photographs of the cystoscopic image [6].

In 1880, Johann Mikulicz-Radecki (Fig. 1.2), a Polish-Austrian surgeon working for Theodore Billroth, produced the first gastroscope, which he based off of Nitze's cystoscope. His modifications included mirrors to create a 30° angled field of view and a miniature version of Thomas Edison's electric incandescent globe as a light source [7]. He later added a separate air channel to his 650 mm long, 13 mm diameter instrument. With it, Mikulicz was the first to describe the endoscopic view of a gastric carcinoma and performed the endoscopic removal of a bone obstructing the esophagus by pushing it into the stomach with his instrument [8, 9].

Examination of the lower GI tract occurred along parallel lines. Howard Kelly, professor of Obstetrics and Gynecology, Halsted-trained surgeon and one of the "Founding Four" of Johns Hopkins Hospital, was the first to describe rigid sigmoidoscopy. In 1895, he used his 350 mm long self-designed instrument to view the distal colon and rectum by reflecting electric light from a conventional bulb of a head-mounted mirror (Fig. 1.3).

J.M. Marks and B.J. Dunkin (eds.), *Principles of Flexible Endoscopy for Surgeons*,
DOI 10.1007/978-1-4614-6330-6_1, © Springer Science+Business Media New York 2013

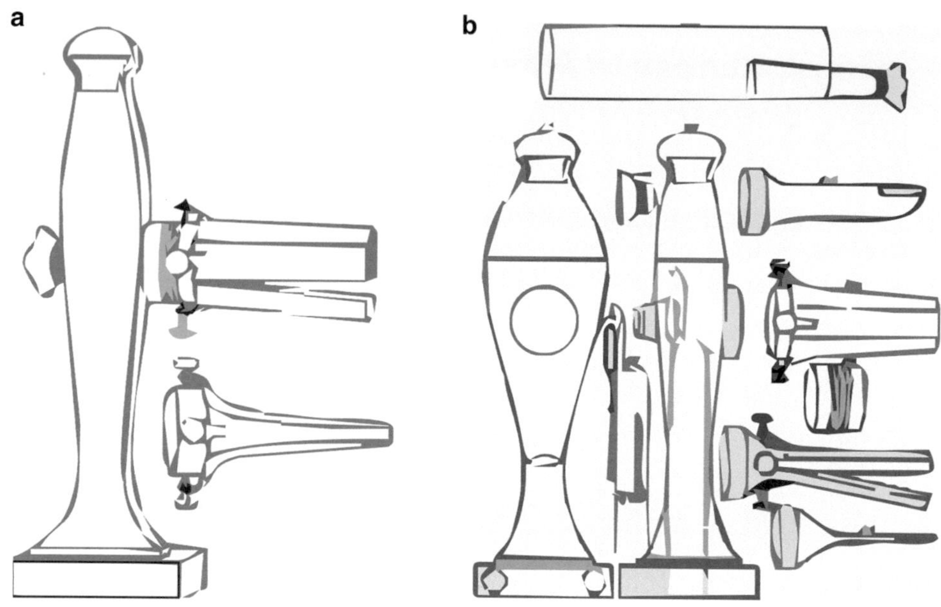

Fig. 1.1 Bozzini's *lichtleiter* (**a**) assembled with speculum attached and (**b**) unassembled, and with a variety of the available specula

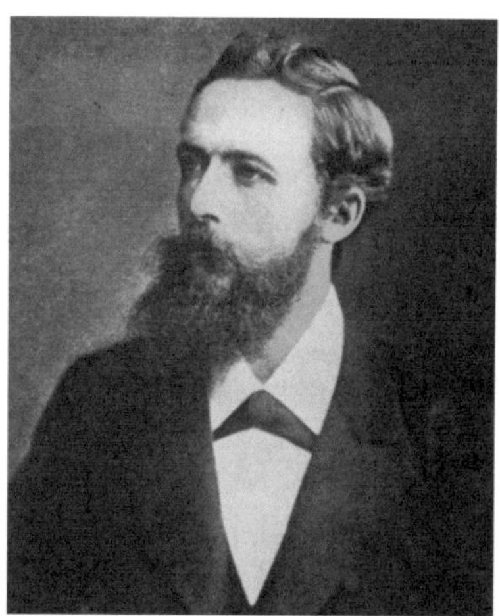

Fig. 1.2 Johann Mikulicz-Radecki (1850–1905) was an innovator in many areas of surgery, including producing the first gastroscope

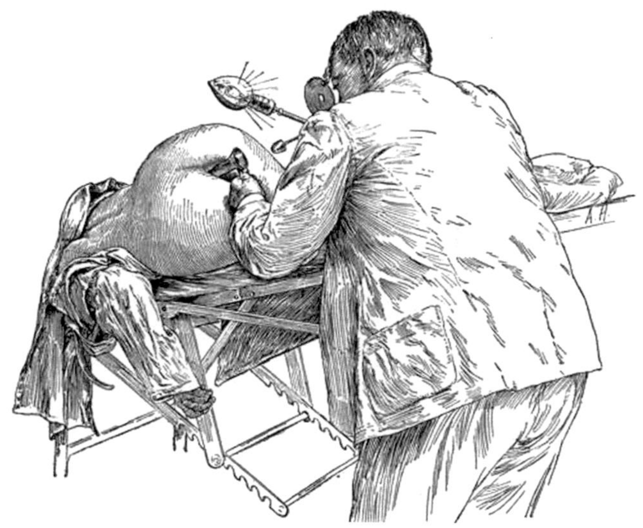

Fig. 1.3 Howard Kelly (1858–1943) performed sigmoidoscopy by reflecting light from a bulb of a head-mounted mirror and down a rigid tube

In 1911, Henry Elsner introduced a two-part gastroscope. The rigid outer cannula allowed passage of the flexible rubber-tipped inner optical component. This two-part system and flexible tip greatly reduced the perforation rate of gastroscopy. It was the Elsner gastroscope with which Rudolph Schindler, a medical gastroenterologist, pathologist, and army surgeon, pioneered the field of gastroscopy, publishing his findings in *Lehrbuch und Atlas der Gasteroskopie* (Textbook and Atlas of Gastroscopy) in 1923 [10]. He later modified the Elsner scope to include a separate channel to flush the lens of secretions and ultimately create, with Wolf, a semiflexible gastroscope [11]. The proximal and distal rigid segments of this device were connected by a passively flexible segment that used a series of prisms to transmit the image through the gentle curve (Fig. 1.4). The maximum bending angle for this endoscope was around 30–34°, after which, image transmission failed [3]. This Wolf–Schindler gastroscope was adopted as the endoscope worldwide due to its greatly improved safety and efficacy.

In April 1933, Edward Benedict, a general surgeon, and Chester Jones, an endoscopist, described the first American trials using the Wolf–Schindler gastroscope at the Massachusetts

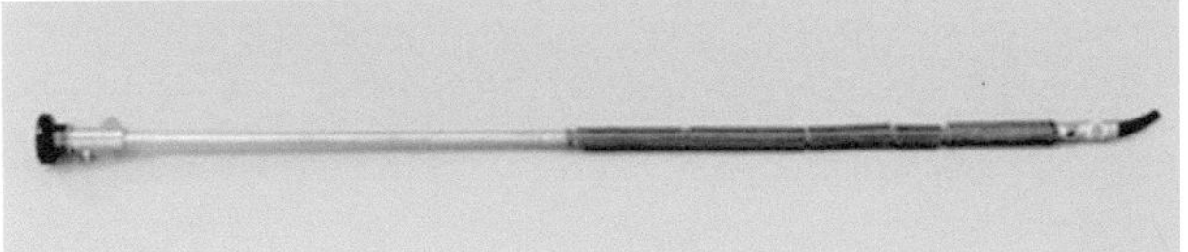

Fig. 1.4 Wolf–Schindler gastroscope with flexible distal segment and rigid proximal segment

General Hospital [12]. So enamored was Benedict by his initial experience with gastroscopy, that he gave up his general surgical practice to focus on laparoscopy and endoscopy. In 1948, Benedict was the first to develop a functional, operative gastroscope, including the development of biopsy forceps [13]. By widening the diameter of the Wolf–Schindler gastroscope from 11 to 14 mm, he was able to add a suction channel that permitted the passage of his biopsy instrument. This permitted direct sampling of endoscopically identified lesions for histological analysis [14].

Despite these progressive improvements, however, the limitations of lens systems, rigid or semirigid instrumentation, internal placement of the light source, as well as high degrees of light loss (more than 90 %) all combined to limit the reach and visual capabilities of these early endoscope systems [15]. While semiflexible instruments with biopsy capabilities were functional for many clinical purposes, the development of totally flexible endoscopic tools would revolutionize the diagnostic and therapeutic capabilities of endoscopists.

Diagnostic Flexible Gastrointestinal Endoscopy

The use of bundled, pure glass (silica) fibers as a conduit for light and optical images for medical purposes was described by Heinrich Lamm, a gynecologist, in late 1930. Lamm demonstrated that the principle of total internal reflection of light allowed image transduction even when the fiber-optic bundles were bent or flexed. Unfortunately, the fibers used by Lamm allow a high degree of light loss and image degradation. It was not until 1954 when Harold Hopkins, a Professor of Applied Physics at Imperial College in London, and his student, Narinder Kapany, developed a flexible fiber-optic system with low light and image loss [16]. The Hopkins system utilized glass rods coated in a reflective cladding as well as two separate fiber bundles [12]. The "coherent" bundle contained fibers whose relative positions in the input and output ends are the same; this permitted pure image transmission (Fig. 1.5). The "incoherent" bundle fibers were randomly arranged but permitted high-intensity light transmission through the length of the bundle.

Utilizing these new fiber-optic bundles, Basil Hirschowitz, a gastroenterologist in fellowship training at the University of Michigan, developed a prototype flexible gastroscope with

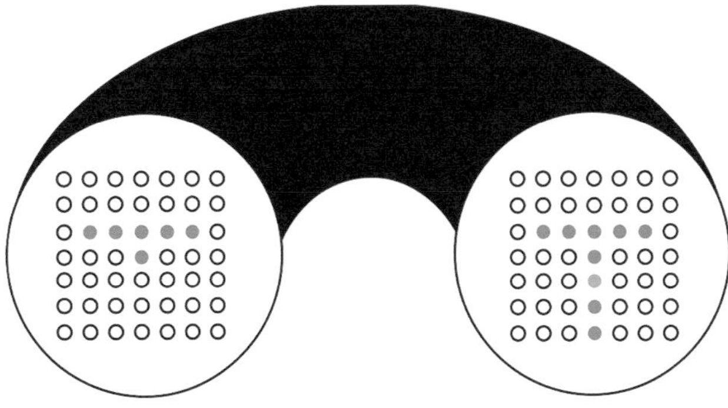

Fig. 1.5 Schematic of a coherent fiber-optic bundle. The preserved relative fiber positions in the input and output ends are the same, permitting pure image transmission

his colleagues in the physics department. In early 1957, Hirschowitz first utilized the gastroscope on himself and several days later performed the first fiber-optic gastroscopy on a patient (Fig. 1.6) [17]. His gastroscope was a 92 cm long, 11 mm wide instrument with coherent fiber-optic bundles that transmitted images illuminated by a light at the distal end. This device was a side-viewing instrument with a single air/suction/irrigation channel and an adjustable lens on the handpiece to allow variable focus. The advantage of the flexible endoscope was almost immediately evident, as in nearly 50 % of patients, the duodenum was successfully examined with the endoscope [18]. The Hirschowitz gastroduodenal fiberscope was introduced to the market in late 1960 by the American Cystoscope Makers, Inc (ACMI) and quickly gained favor [19, 20].

Modifications on the Hirschowitz endoscope occurred rapidly over the next several years as manufacturers developed progressively longer, forward-viewing devices with greater tip control. The addition of a second incoherent fiber-optic bundle allowed light to be transmitted down the endoscope shaft and permitted the use of an external light source.

The idea for this external light source is credited to George Berci, a surgeon working in Los Angeles, California [5]. He discussed the idea with Karl Storz, the German instrument manufacturer who produced the endoscopes in collaboration with Hopkins [21–23]. This new endoscope transmitted the light from an external 150 W light bulb down the shaft of the device to provide internal illumination. While this was a vast improvement over internal light bulbs at the distal instrument tip, the degree of illumination was still considered insufficient. In 1976, Berci introduced the miniature, high-intensity (300 W), explosion-proof xenon arc globe as the light source for an endoscope, the same bulb currently in use by every manufacturer of endoscopic instruments [23, 24].

By 1971, a 105 cm long "panendoscope" was available from both Olympus and ACMI. These end-viewing devices had an external light source, four-way steerable tip control

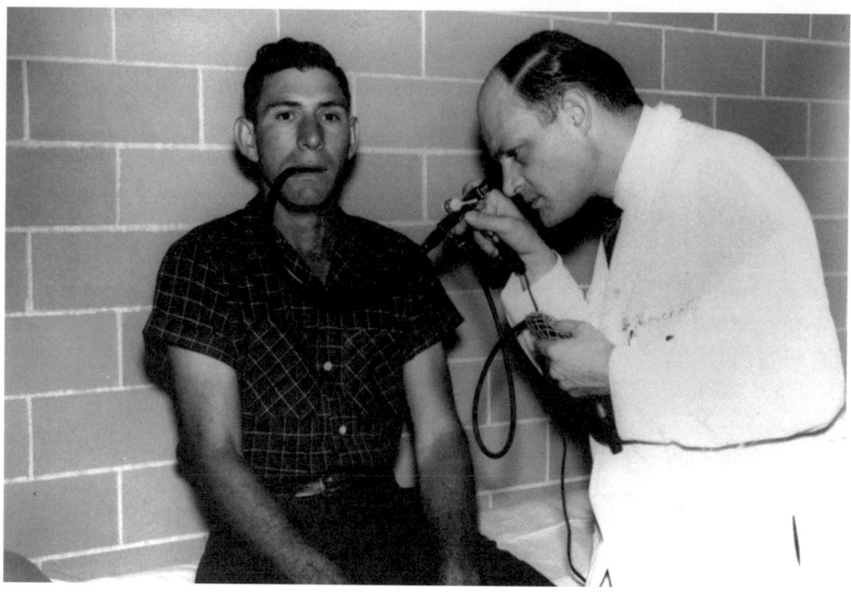

Fig. 1.6 Basil Hirschowitz (1925–2013) performing the first fiber-optic gastroscopy on a patient

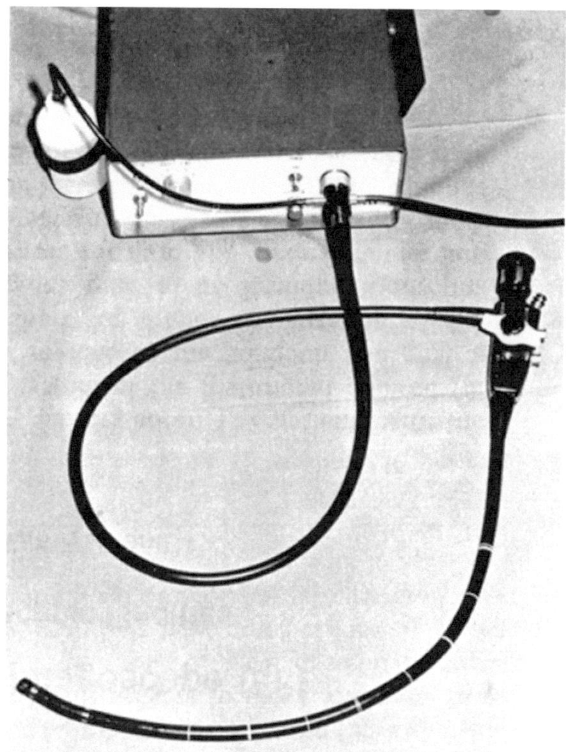

Fig. 1.7 Panendoscope, with external light source, lens irrigation capabilities, four-direction tip control, and suction

capable of 180° retroflexion, lens washing capabilities, and a biopsy channel (Fig. 1.7). These devices made evaluation of the duodenum during upper endoscopy a matter of routine.

Recognizing the opportunity that duodenal access represented, William S. McCune, a surgeon at George Washington University in Washington D.C., performed the first endoscopic retrograde cholangio-pancreatography (ERCP) in 1968 [25]. Utilizing an endoscope with both forward- and side-viewing capabilities, McCune and colleagues nonselectively cannulated the ampulla of Vater with a catheter passed through a guide tube taped onto the shaft of the instrument. Radio-opaque contrast solution was injected, permitting evaluation of the pancreatic and common bile duct.

The Japanese, under the leadership of Itaru Oi, further developed this technique and demonstrated its practicality. Using a Machida fiberduodenoscope (FDS-LB) capable of 60° distal tip rotation, Oi and colleagues visualized the papilla in 94 % of cases and cannulated it in 41 patients [26, 27]. His methods were subsequently popularized and taught to thousands of endoscopists by Drs. Peter Cotton, Steve Silvis, Jack Vennes, and Joseph Geenen [28–34].

Soon after the development of a forward-viewing flexible gastroscope, investigators turned modified versions of the devices to examination of the colon and rectum. Robert Turell, a surgeon at The Mount Sinai Hospital in New York, first described flexible colonoscopy, but ultimately concluded that his instrument was not yet fit for routine clinical application [35, 36]. Further manufacturer developments improved the sigmoidoscope. Bergein Overholt, while a gastroenterology fellow at New York Hospital-Cornell University Medical Center, New York, pursued and popularized flexible diagnostic sigmoidoscopy [37, 38]. He later became instrumental in the development of dedicated colonoscopic length endoscopes.

By 1970, both ACMI and Olympus were producing flexible colonoscopes designed to permit cecal intubation. The primary impediment to this now routine task was a lack

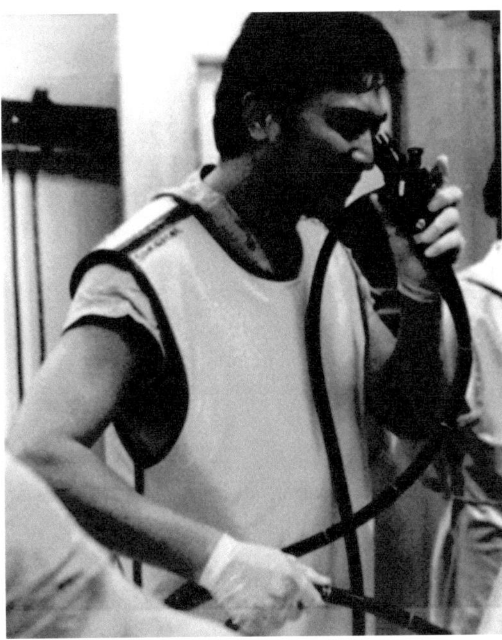

Fig. 1.8 Hiromi Shinya performing colonoscopic exam. Note the lead apron; fluoroscopy was heavily utilized to develop modern methods of navigation through the colon

of standardized technique to advance the endoscope beyond the more distal colon. While many notable physicians contributed to the development of these techniques (including Jerome Wayne, Christopher Williams, and Bergein Overholt), it was Hiromi Shinya, a Japanese born, American trained surgeon, who developed many of the colonoscopic techniques that made the technique popular in the United States (Fig. 1.8) [5]. Shinya, with William Wolff at Beth Israel Medical Center in New York, began his colonoscopy work in 1967 with an Olympus-EF gastroscope. He ultimately transitioned to a dedicated 186 cm long colonoscope (Olympus CF-LB) [39].

With this endoscope and his technical expertise, Shinya and Wolff reported ever-improving cecal intubation rates in their early experience of 241 patients and established the advantage of endoscopy over barium enema [40, 41]. Shinya also adapted the wire loop method of polypectomy to the endoscope. In September 1969 he performed the first colonoscopic snare polypectomy on a 1.5 cm pedunculated proximal sigmoid polyp [42]. Within the next 3 years he and Wolff performed hundreds of snare polypectomies with minimal morbidity and no mortality, sparing patients open surgical resection of these lesions [43, 44].

Therapeutic Flexible Gastrointestinal Endoscopy

Shinya and Wolff ushered in the era of therapeutic colonoscopy by making snare polypectomy the new standard of care. For polyps not amenable to snare resection, marking of

lesions discovered at colonoscopy became necessary and a technique of endoscopic injection of India ink was developed [45]. Jeffrey Ponsky, at the time a surgery resident at University Hospitals of Cleveland, Ohio, and James King, a gastroenterologist in Canton, Ohio, described the use of 1–2 ml of India ink to create a surgically identifiable black mark on the antimesenteric border of the colon near the lesion to be resected. Within short order, additional colonoscopic interventions were described, including foreign body removal, suture excision, and the application of sclerosing agents and electrocautery to bleeding lesions [46].

Many of the techniques used for therapeutic colonoscopy had initially been developed and described for diseases of the upper gastrointestinal tract, most notably control of gastrointestinal hemorrhage. Diagnostic upper endoscopy was already having profound impact on the treatment algorithms and clinical outcomes for upper gastrointestinal bleeding (UGIB). Choichi Sugawa, a surgeon at Wayne State University in Detroit, Michigan, and his colleagues completed upper endoscopy in 41 of 42 patients with UGIB, correctly identifying the source of bleeding in 95 % of these patients [47]. Hellers and Ihre, surgeons working in Stockholm, Sweden, evaluated their UGIB patients in the immediate pre- and post-endoscopy era and saw failure to reach a diagnosis fall from almost 40 to 5–7 % [48]. Operation rates increased (due to more accurate diagnosis of the bleeding site), transfusion requirements decreased, and mortality in both the operated (47 % vs. 11 %) and non-operated (17 % vs. 8 %) population fell dramatically.

Recognizing the potential benefits of endoscopic intervention for UGIB, surgeons and gastroenterologists alike rapidly developed methods to control endoscopically identified hemorrhage. C Roger Youmans, Jr, a surgeon at the University of Texas in Galveston, first described endoscopic management of gastric hemorrhage [49]. Passing a rigid cystoscope through a preexisting gastrostomy site, Youmans utilized the continual flow of irrigation fluid to identify the bleeding site, which was subsequently fulgurated (Fig. 1.9) [50].

Methods of endoscopic cautery through a flexible gastroscope were subsequently described [51, 52]. Sugawa's experience in diagnostic gastroscopy for UGIB transitioned to therapeutic endeavors. In 1975, he reported clinical success in managing six patients with UGIB from a variety of causes by using electrocoagulation with a Cameron-Miller flexible suction coagulator electrode (Fig. 1.10) [53]. John Papp, a gastroenterologist at Michigan State University, and Walter Gaisford, a surgeon at LDS Hospital in Salt Lake City, Utah, subsequently described similarly high success rates (92–95 %) in series of 245 and 160 patients with UGIB, respectively [54–56].

In the following years, additional therapies for UGIB were developed. Working at the University of Hamburg,

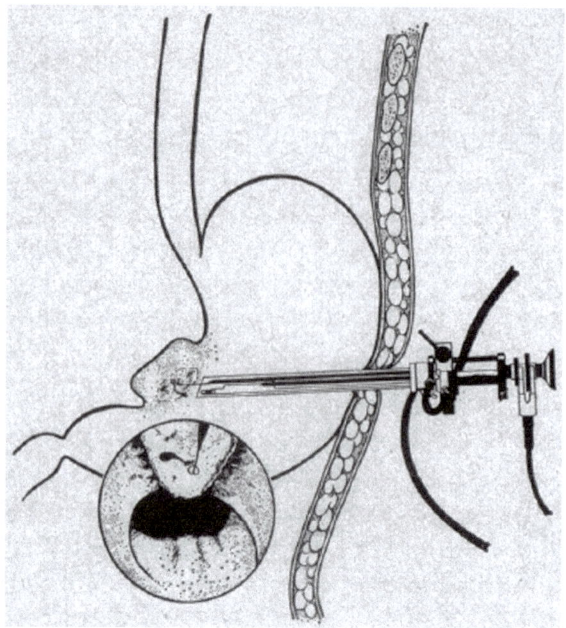

Fig. 1.9 Electrocautery of a bleeding gastric ulcer using a rigid cystoscope passed through a preexisting gastrostomy site. With permission from [49]. Copyright 1970 American Medical Association

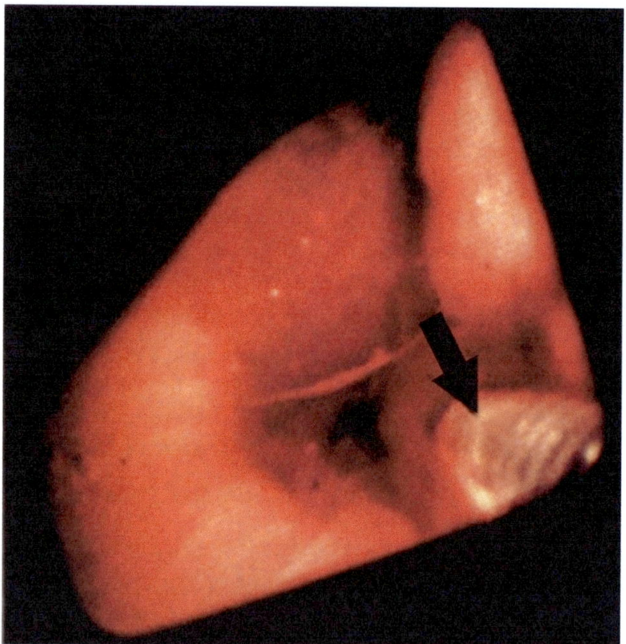

Fig. 1.10 Management of a bleeding gastric ulcer using a Cameron-Miller flexible suction coagulator electrode (*arrow*) passed through a flexible gastroscope. With permission from [53]. Copyright 1975 American Medical Association

German surgeon Nib Soehendra described the use of a sclerosing agent (1.5 % solution of Aethoxysklerol®) to induce hemostasis in bleeding gastric ulcers [57]. Additional sclerosing agents (like 95 % ethanol) and vasoconstrictive agents (dilute epinephrine) were soon applied to bleeding lesions throughout the GI tract [58]. In 1985, Masanori Hirao and his surgical colleagues at Kin-Ikyo Chuo Hospital in Sapporo, Japan, described the endoscopic injection of a mixture of hypertonic saline and dilute epinephrine solution to promote hemostasis and vascular sclerosis [59]. Three years later, Greg van Steigman, a surgeon, and John Goff, a gastroenterologist, at the University of Colorado in Denver, described 132 endoscopic variceal band ligations in 44 patients with no major complications (perforation, secondary bleeding) and no treatment failures [60]. This markedly decreased the need for portal systemic shunting for hemorrhage.

Diagnostic and therapeutic methods for UGIB were soon applied to the lower GI tract and, in similar fashion, polypectomy methods from the colon were applied to the stomach [61–63]. Endoscopic methods continued to replace traditional open surgical procedures. In 1979, Drs. Michael Gauderer and Jeffrey Ponsky performed the first percutaneous endoscopic gastrostomy (PEG) [64]. This was first published and presented in 1980 and soon was the most widely practiced approach for feeding access. This was soon followed by similar approaches to the jejunum for long-term enteral access in patients who could not tolerate gastric feedings [65]. Around the same time frame, descriptions of the use of plastic endoprosthesis for the relief of malignant obstructions and balloon dilation of benign stricture/obstructions were recorded [66–70].

A therapeutic dimension was added to ERCP in 1974 by Drs. Kawai in Japan and Classen in Germany who independently developed methods of endoscopic sphincterotomy to permit extraction of common bile duct stones [71–74]. Soon after, endoscopic biliary stenting for strictures and malignancy was developed by Soehendra [75]. Subsequent advances in ERCP have included expandable metal stenting, cholangioscopy, excision of ampullary masses, pancreatoscopy, and pancreatic duct stenting, all of which were made possible by the methods defined by these early pioneers.

Video Endoscopy and the Era of Advanced Endoscopic Techniques

Conventional rigid and fiber-optic endoscopy limited the practitioner in a number of ways that suppressed further advances in therapeutic techniques. The use of a single optical axis meant that the endoscopist utilized only one eye, which was held close to the controls of the device. This was an uncomfortable position, and one which limited the teaching ability as well as the ability of the assistants to visualize the actual endoscopic procedure (and to subsequently provide actual "assistance" in the procedure). Image documentation of the procedures was also difficult, as the endoscopist could not simultaneously observe the image and capture it on film when the camera was attached to the eye piece of the endoscope. Video technology was the solution to all of these issues.

The first report of video endoscopy occurred in France with 1956 when a regular video camera was attached to the end of a rigid gastroscope to project black and white images onto a television screen. Because of the size and expense of early video equipment, this endeavor required transporting the patient to a video studio. Refinement in video equipment in the 1960s and 1970s made these efforts easier, but clinical enthusiasm was never great [3].

In 1984, Welch Allyn removed the coherent fiber-optic image bundle in a colonoscope and replaced it with electrical wires attached to a charge-coupled device (CCD), a light-sensitive image sensor, at the instrument tip [76]. Images were focused on the CCD chip by a small lens and were converted into digital signals that traveled to an image-processing unit and were converted back to a visual image on a television monitor. These modifications altered virtually none of the other design elements of the endoscope and actually improved instrument flexibility and image quality [3].

Digital endoscopy changed the way in which diagnostic and therapeutic endoscopic procedures were performed. The endoscopist could now view an enlarged image with both eyes from a convenient distance and simultaneously record it [77]. Furthermore, digital signals permitted image enhancement, noise filtering, and video transmission and recording. Equally as important, the surgeon could now stand upright and use both hands to operate in a coordinated fashion with assistants and trainees viewing the same image simultaneously [78].

The coordinated efforts of surgeon and assistant increased the complexity of endoscopic therapeutic interventions. In the early 1990s, techniques for resection of large mucosal lesions via endoscopic mucosal resection (EMR) permitted removal of early GI tract malignancies without a formal surgical resection [79–81]. Even larger areas of neoplasia can be removed via endoscopic submucosal dissection (ESD) in which the endoscope is passed into the submucosal plane beneath the mucosa. More recently, a modified version of esophageal ESD has been utilized for the management of achalasia. This method, per-oral endoscopic myotomy (POEM), grew out of laboratory work performed in the United States and was first performed in humans in Japan [82–84]. It is now being performed clinically throughout the world and by surgeons in a number of centers in the United States [84–86].

Self-expanding metal stents (SEMS) were first introduced in 1989 for the relief of malignant obstruction of the biliary tree [87]. It was quickly recognized that the use of an expandable tubularized metal stent had potential benefit for other malignant and recalcitrant strictures of the GI tract. In 1990, Domschke, a gastroenterologist at the University of Erlangen in Nuremberg, Germany, positioned a stainless steel SEMS across a malignant esophageal stricture under endoscopic guidance [88]. Soon, SEMS were being placed for palliation of malignant gastric outlet and colon obstructions and as a bridge to non-emergent surgery [89–91].

Over the last two decades, SEMS and, more recently, self-expanding plastic stents (SEPS) have gained popularity and shown tremendous therapeutic potential for stricture/obstructions of the esophagus, gastric outlet, and colon. Stents with an external impermeable coating currently have an evolving role in the management of enteric fistulae, perforations, and anastomotic leaks.

The early twenty-first century saw the development of numerous endoscopic therapies for gastro-esophageal reflux disease (GERD) and its complications including endoscopic gastroplasty, application of radiofrequency (RF) energy to the lower esophageal sphincter, injection/implantation of a bioprosthetic into the submucosa of the lower esophagus, and ablation of Barrett's esophagus with dysplasia [92–99].

Within the same time frame, endoscopists began to tackle the growing world epidemic of morbid obesity, developing endoscopic bariatric procedures with improved effectiveness compared with medications, but with a lower risk profile than traditional surgery. Primary procedures for weight loss have included the development of intra-gastric space-occupying devices, barrier-type devices that permit malabsorption, and endoscopic suturing devices to plicate the stomach and restrict calorie intake [100–105]. Such endoscopic suturing platforms have also been utilized as revisional techniques for failed bariatric operations, permitting plication of dilated gastrojejunal anastomosis after Roux-en-Y gastric bypass surgery or shrinkage of a dilated gastric pouch [106, 107].

As endoscopic therapies grew in complexity, it was perhaps inevitable that the realm of minimally invasive laparoscopic surgery and therapeutic flexible endoscopy would merge into a common area of technology and methodology called Natural Orifice Translumenal Endoscopic Surgery (NOTES™) [108]. Introduced in the early 2000s through exciting collaborations between surgeons and gastroenterologists, NOTES involves crossing the lumen of the esophagus, stomach, colon, vagina, or bladder with an endoscope to perform a surgical procedure in the intra-abdominal space. The technique was first reported in 2000 by Anthony Kalloo, a gastroenterologist, and colleagues at the Johns Hopkins Hospital in Baltimore, Maryland (Fig. 1.11) [109–111]. An endoscopic full-thickness gastrotomy was made, pneumoperitoneum created, and endoscopic peritoneoscopy with liver biopsy performed. The resultant gastrotomy was closed with endoscopic clips [110]. Though in its infancy, the concept of translumenal surgery has fired the imagination of the current generation of surgical endoscopists.

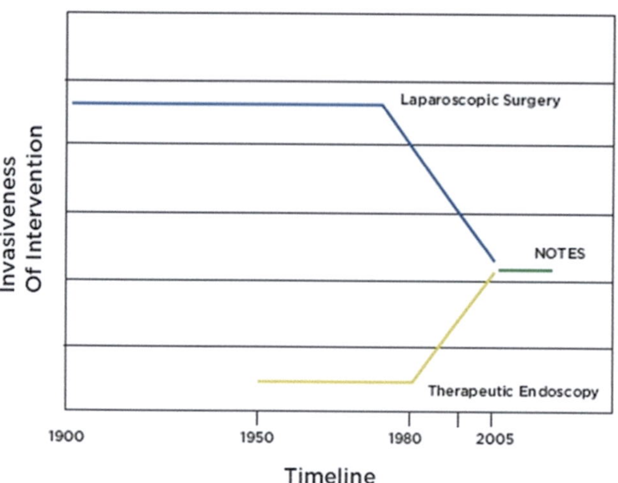

Fig. 1.11 Timeline of the merger of laparoscopic surgery and therapeutic endoscopy. With permission from [111]. Copyright 2007 McMahon Publishers

Conclusion

As this chapter illustrates, surgeons have been pioneers in endoscopy since the beginning and have been instrumental in developing many of the platforms, methods, and equipment described in this chapter, all in an effort to create less invasive alternatives to traditional surgical approaches. The continued evolution of minimally invasive surgery will inevitably require the use of a flexible endoscopic platform and the surgeon who poses skills in flexible endoscopy will be well positioned to embrace new techniques and technology and move the field forward.

References

1. Bozzini PH. Lichtleiter, eine Erfindung zur Anschauung innerer Teile und Krankheiten. J Prak Heilk. 1806;24:107.
2. Lamaro VP. Gynaecological endoscopic surgery—past, present and future. In: St. Vincents Clinic, Proceedings, vol. 12, no. 1; 2004. p. 23–9, see http://www.clinic.stvincents.com.au/about-us/publications.
3. Gross S, Kollenbrandt M. Technical evolution of medical endoscopy. Presented at Proceedings of the 13th International Student Conference on Electrical Engineering; May 21, 2009; Prague, Czech Republic. http://www.lfb.rwth-aachen.de/files/publications/2009/GRO09d.pdf. Accessed Dec 2011.
4. Haubrich WS. Gastrointestinal endoscopy. In: Kirsner JB, editor. The growth of gastroenderologic knowledge during the twentieth century. Philadelphia: Lea and Febiger; 1994. p. 474–90.
5. Morgenthal CB, Richards WO, Dunkin BJ, et al. The role of the surgeon in the evolution of flexible endoscopy. Surg Endosc. 2007; 21:838–53.
6. Prevedello DM, Doglietto F, Jane JA, et al. History of endoscopic skull base surgery: its evolution and current reality. J Neurosurg. 2007;107:206–13.
7. Zajaczkowski T. Johann Anton von Mikulicz-Radecki (1850–1905)—a pioneer of gastroscopy and modern surgery: his credit to urology. World J Urol. 2008;26(1):75–86.
8. Marsh BR. Historic development of bronchoesophagology. Otolaryngol Head Neck Surg. 1996;114:689–716.
9. Kuczkowski J, Stankiewicz C, Kopacz A, et al. Jan Mikulicz-Radecki (1850–1905): pioneer of endoscopy and surgery of the sinuses, throat, and digestive tract. World J Surg. 2004; 28:1063–7.
10. Schindler R. Lehrbuch und Atlas der Gasteroskopie. Munchen: Lehmann; 1923.
11. Schindler R. Gastroscopy with a flexible gastroscope. Am J Dig Dis. 1935;2:656–63.
12. Berci G, Forde KA. History of endoscopy: what lessons have we learned from the past? Surg Endosc. 2000;14:5–15.
13. Benedict EB. An operating gastroscope. Gastroenterology. 1948; 11:281–95.
14. Benedict EB. Gastroscopic biopsy. Gastroenterology. 1959;37:447–8.
15. Modlin IM. A brief history of endoscopy. Milan: Multimed; 2000.
16. Hopkins HH, Kapany NS. A flexible fibrescope, using static scanning. Nature. 1954;173:39–41.
17. Hirschowitz BI, Curtiss LE, Peters CW, Pollard HM. Demonstration of a new gastroscope, the "fiberscope". Gastroenterology. 1958;35: 50–3.
18. Hirschowitz BI, Balint JA, Fulton WF. Gastroduodenal endoscopy with the fiberscope: an analysis of 500 examinations. Surg Clin North Am. 1962;42:1081–90.
19. Weisinger BB, Cramer AB, Zacharis LC. Comparative accuracy of the fiberscope and standard gastroscope in the diagnosis of gastric lesions; preliminary report. Gastroenterology. 1963;44:858A.
20. Cohen NN, Hughes RW, Manfredo HE. Experiences with 1000 fibergastroscopic examinations of the stomach. Am J Dig Dis. 1966;11:943–50.
21. Berci G, Kont LA. A new optical endoscope with special reference to cystoscopy. Br J Urol. 1969;41:564–71.
22. Berci G. A new approach in optics: the Hopkins "rod-lens" system. Proceedings of the 15th American Symposium Society. J Photo-optic Engineers. 1970;3:207.
23. Morgenstern L. George Berci: past, present, and future. Surg Endosc. 2006;20:S410–1.
24. Berci G. More light. Endoscopy. 1975;7:201–9.
25. McCune WS, Schorb PE, Moscovitz H. Endoscopic cannulation of the ampulla of Vater: a preliminary report. Gastrointest Endosc. 1968;34:278–80.
26. Oi I, Takemoto T, Nakayama K. "Fiberduodenoscopy" early diagnosis of cancer of the papilla of vater. Surgery. 1970;67:561–5.
27. Oi I. Fiberduodenoscopy and endoscopic pancreatocholangiography. Gastrointest Endosc. 1970;17:59–62.
28. Blumgart LH, Cotton PB, Burwood R, et al. Endoscopy and retrograde choledochopancreatography in the diagnosis of the jaundiced patient. Lancet. 1972;2:1269–73.
29. Cotton PB, Blumgart LH, Davies GT, et al. Cannulation of papilla of Vater via fiber-duodenoscope: assessment of retrograde cholangiopancreatography in 60 patients. Lancet. 1972;1:53–8.
30. Vennes JA, Silvis SE. Endoscopic visualization of the bile and pancreatic ducts. Gastrointest Endosc. 1972;18:149–52.
31. Cotton PB. ERCP. Gut. 1977;18:316–41.
32. Geenen JE, Rolny P. Endoscopic therapy of acute and chronic pancreatitis. Gastrointest Endosc. 1991;37:377.
33. Schuman B. The development of the endoscope. In: DiMarino Jr AJ, Benjamin SB, editors. Gastrointestinal disease an endoscopic approach, vol. I. Malden, MA: Blackwell Science; 1997. p. 9–24.
34. Sircus W. Milestones in the evolution of endoscopy: a short history. J R Coll Physicians Edinb. 2003;33:124–34.
35. Turell R. Fiber optic coloscope and sigmoidoscope. Preliminary report. Am J Surg. 1963;105(1):133–6.
36. Turell R. Fiber optic sigmoidoscopes; up to date developments. Am J Surg. 1967;113:305–7.

37. Overholt BF. Clinical experience with the fibersigmoidoscope. Gastrointest Endosc. 1968;15(1):27.
38. Overholt BF. Flexible fiberoptic sigmoidoscopes. Cancer. 1969;19:80–4.
39. Shinya H, Wolff WI, Geffen A, Ozoktay S. Colonofiberoscopy: a new and valuable diagnostic modality. Gastroenterology. 1971;60:828A.
40. Wolff WI, Shinya H. Colonofiberoscopy. JAMA. 1971;217(11):1509–12.
41. Wolff WI, Shinya H, Geffen A, Ozaktay SZ. Colonofiberoscopy: a new and valuable diagnostic modality. Am J Surg. 1972;123:180–4.
42. Sivak Jr MV. Polypectomy: looking back. Gastrointest Endosc. 2004;60:977–82.
43. Wolff WI, Shinya H. Polypectomy via the fiberoptic colonoscope: removal of neoplasms beyond the reach of the sigmoidoscope. N Engl J Med. 1973;288:329–32.
44. Wolff WI, Shinya HA. A new approach to colonic polyps. Ann Surg. 1973;178:367–76.
45. Ponsky JL, King J. Endoscopic marking of colonic lesions. Gastrointest Endosc. 1975;22:42–3.
46. Frümorgen P, Zeus J, Demling L. New aspects of therapeutic colonoscopy. Endoscopy. 1975;7:59–63.
47. Sugawa C, Werner MH, Hayes DF, et al. Early endoscopy: a guide to therapy for acute hemorrhage in the upper gastrointestinal tract. Arch Surg. 1973;107:133–7.
48. Hellers G, Ihre T. Impact of change to early diagnosis and surgery in major upper gastrointestinal bleeding. Lancet. 1975;2:1250–1.
49. Youmans Jr CR. Cystoscopic control of gastric hemorrhage. JAMA. 1970;212(11):1962.
50. Youmans Jr CR, Patterson M, McDonald DF, Derrick JR. Cystoscopic control of gastric hemorrhage. Arch Surg. 1970;100:721–3.
51. Blackwood WD, Silvis SE. Electrocoagulation of hemorrhagic gastritis. Gastrointest Endosc. 1971;2:53–5.
52. Katon RM. Experimental control of gastrointestinal hemorrhage via the endoscope: a new era dawns. Gastroenterology. 1976;70:272–7.
53. Sugawa C, Shier M, Lucas CE, Walt AJ. Electrocoagulation of bleeding in the upper part of the gastrointestinal tract: a preliminary experimental clinical report. Arch Surg. 1975;110:975–9.
54. Papp JP. Endoscopic electrocoagulation of upper gastrointestinal hemorrhage. JAMA. 1976;236:2076–9.
55. Gaisford WD. Endoscopic electrohemostasis of active upper gastrointestinal bleeding. Am J Surg. 1979;137(1):47–53.
56. Papp JP. Endoscopic electrocoagulation in the management of upper gastrointestinal tract bleeding. Surg Clin North Am. 1982;62:797–806.
57. Soehendra N, Werner B. Ner technique for endoscopic treatment of bleeding gastric ulder. Endoscopy. 1976;8:85–7.
58. Tatsuka T, Otani T, Kanamaru K, Okuda S. Submucosal injection of ethanol under direct vision for the treatment of gastric protuberant lesion. Gastroent Endosc. 1974;16:572–9.
59. Hirao M, Kobayashi T, Masuda K, et al. Endoscopic local injection of hypertonic saline-epinephrine solution to arrest hemorrhage from the upper gastrointestinal tract. Gastrointest Endosc. 1985;31:313–7.
60. Van Stiegmann G, Goff JS. Endoscopic esophageal varix ligation: preliminary clinical experience. Gastrointest Endosc. 1988;34:113–7.
61. Tedesco FJ, Waye JD, Raskin JB, et al. Colonoscopic evaluation of rectal bleeding: a study of 304 patients. Ann Intern Med. 1978;89:907–9.
62. Seifert E. Endoscopic polypectomy. J Gastroenterol. 1973;8(3):103–9.
63. Brandt L, Frankel A, Waye JD. Endoscopic nonoperative gastric polypectomy. Dig Dis. 1973;18:1087–90.
64. Gauderer MWL, Ponsky JL, Izant RJ. Gastrosotmy without laparotomy: a percutaneous endoscopic technique. J Pediatr Surg. 1980;15:872–5.
65. Ponsky JL, Aszodi A. Percutaneous endoscopic jejunostomy. Am J Gastroenterol. 1984;79:113–6.
66. Tytgat GN, den Hartog Jager FCA. Non-surgical treatment of cardio-esophageal obstruction: role of endoscopy. Endoscopy. 1977;9:211–5.
67. den Hartog Jager FCA, Bartelsman JFWM, Tytgat GN. Palliative treatment of obstructing esophagogastric malignancy by endoscopic positioning of a plastic prosthesis. Gastroenterology. 1979;77:1008–14.
68. Benjamin SB, Cattau EL, Glass RL. Balloon dilation of the pylorus: therapy for gastric outlet obstruction. Gastrointest Endosc. 1982;28:253–4.
69. Brower RA, Freeman LD. Balloon catheter dilation of a rectal stricture. Gastrointest Endosc. 1984;30:95–7.
70. Merrell N, McCray RS. Balloon catheter dilation of a severe esophageal stricture. Gastrointest Endosc. 1982;28:254–5.
71. Kawai K, Akasaka Y, Hashimoto Y, Nakajima M. Preliminary report on endoscopic papillotomy. J Kyoto Pref Univ Med. 1973;82:353.
72. Kawai K, Akasaka Y, Murakami K, et al. Endoscopic sphincterotomy of the ampulla of Vater. Gastrointest Endosc. 1974;20:148–51.
73. Classen M, Demling L. Endoskopische Sphinkterotomie der Papilla Vateri und Steinextraktion aus dem Ductus choledochus. Dtsch Med Wochenschr. 1974;99(11):496–7.
74. Classen M, Safrany L. Endoscopic papillotomy and removal of gallstones. BMJ. 1975;4:371–4.
75. Soehendra N, Reynders-Frederix V. Palliative bile duct drainage: a new endoscopic method of introducing a transpapillary drain. Endoscopy. 1980;12:8–11.
76. Sivak Jr MV, Fleischer DE. Colonoscopy with a videoendoscope: preliminary experience. Gastrointest Endosc. 1984;30:1–5.
77. Litynski GS. Endoscopic surgery: the history, the pioneers. World J Surg. 1999;23:745–53.
78. Berci G, Paz-Partlow M. Electronic imaging in endoscopy. Surg Endosc. 1988;2:227–33.
79. Inoue H, Endo M, Takeshita K, et al. Endoscopic resection of carcinoma in situ of the esophagus accompanied by esophageal varices. Surg Endosc. 1991;5:182–4.
80. Makuuchi H, Machimura T, Soh Y, et al. Endoscopic mucosectomy for mucosal carcinomas in the esophagus. Jpn J Gastroenterol Surg. 1991;24:2599–603.
81. Tada M, Murata M, Murakami F, et al. Development of the strip-off biopsy. Gastroenterol Endosc. 1984;26:833–9.
82. Pasricha PJ, Hawari R, Ahmed I, et al. Submucosal endoscopic esophageal myotomy: a novelexperimental approach for the treatment of achalasia. Endoscopy. 2007;39(9):761–4.
83. Pauli EM, Mathew A, Haluck RS, et al. Technique for transesophageal endoscopic cardiomyotomy (Heller myotomy): video presentation at the Society of American Gastrointestinal and Endoscopic Surgeons (SAGES) 2008, Philadelphia, PA. Surg Endosc. 2008;22(10):2279–80.
84. Inoue H, Minami H, Kobayashi Y, et al. Peroral endoscopic myotomy (POEM) for esophageal achalasia. Endoscopy. 2010;42(4):265–71.
85. Inoue H, Kudo SE. Per-oral endoscopic myotomy (POEM) for 43 consecutive cases of esophageal achalasia. Nihon Rinsho. 2010;68(9):1749–52.
86. von Renteln D, Inoue H, Minami H. Peroral endoscopic myotomy for the treatment of achalasia: a prospective single center study. Am J Gastroenterol. 2012;107(3):411–7.
87. Huibregtse K, Cheng J, Coene PP, et al. Endoscopic placement of expandable metal stents for biliary strictures—a preliminary

report on experience with 33 patients. Endoscopy. 1989;21(6): 280–2.

88. Domschke W, Foerster EC, Matek W, Rödl W. Selfexpanding mesh stent for esophageal cancer stenosis. Endoscopy. 1990;22: 134–6.

89. Itabashi M, Hamano K, Kameoka S, Asahina K. Self expanding stainless steel stent application in rectosigmoid stricture. Dis Colon Rectum. 1993;36:508–11.

90. Truong S, Bohndorf Geller VH, et al. Self-expanding metal stents for palliation of malignant gastric outlet obstruction. Endoscopy. 1992;24:433–5.

91. Tamim WZ, Ghellai A, Counihan TC, et al. Experience with endoluminal colonic wall stents for the management of large bowel obstruction for benign and malignant disease. Arch Surg. 2000;135:434–8.

92. Swain P, Park PO, Kjellin T, et al. Endoscopic gastroplasty for gastroesophageal reflux disease. Gastrointest Endosc. 2000;51:AB144.

93. Filipi CJ, Lehman GA, Rothstein RI, et al. Transoral, flexible endoscopic suturing for treatment of GERD: a multicenter trial. Gastrointest Endosc. 2001;53:416–22.

94. Pleskow D, Rothstein R, Lo S, et al. Endoscopic full-thickness plication for the treatment of GERD: a multicenter trial. Gastrointest Endosc. 2004;59:163–71.

95. Pleskow D, Rothstein R, Lo S, et al. Endoscopic full-thickness plication for the treatment of GERD: 12-month follow-up for the North American open-label trial. Gastrointest Endosc. 2005;61:643–7.

96. Triadafilopoulos G, DiBaise JK, Nostrant TT, et al. The Stretta procedure for the treatment of GERD: 6 and 12 month follow-up of the U.S. open label trial. Gastrointest Endosc. 2002;55:149–56.

97. Rothstein RI, Dukowicz AC. Endoscopic therapy for gastroesophageal reflux disease. Surg Clin North Am. 2005;85:949–65.

98. Fockens P, Bruno MJ, Hirsch DP. Endoscopic augmentation of the lower esophageal sphincter: pilot study of the gatekeeper reflux repair system in patients with GERD. Gastrointest Endosc. 2002;55:AB257.

99. Shaheen NJ, Sharma P, Overholt BF, et al. Radiofrequency ablation in Barrett's esophagus with dysplasia. N Engl J Med. 2009;360:2277–88.

100. Mathus-Vliegen EM, Tytgat GN. Intragastric balloon for treatment-resistant obesity: safety, tolerance, and efficacy of 1-year balloon treatment followed by a 1-year balloon-free follow-up. Gastrointest Endosc. 2005;61(1):19–27.

101. Hashiba K, Brasil HA, Wada AM, et al. Experimental study an alternative endoscopic method for the treatment of obesity: the butterfly technique. Gastrointest Endosc. 2001;53:AB112.

102. Gersin K, Keller J, Stefanidis D, et al. Duodenal-jejunal bypass sleeve: a totally endoscopic device for the treatment of morbid obesity. Surg Innov. 2007;14(4):275–8.

103. Kelleher B, Stone C, Burns M, Gaskill H. The butterfly procedure for endoluminal treatment of obesity. Gastrointest Endosc. 2003;57:AB186.

104. Swain CP, Park P-O, Savides T, et al. In vivo evaluation of the butterfly endoluminal gastroplasty procedure for obesity. Gastrointest Endosc. 2003;57:AB83.

105. Fogel R, De La Fuente R, Bonilla Y. Endoscopic vertical gastroplasty: a novel technique for treatment of obesity: a preliminary report. Gastrointest Endosc. 2005;61:AB106.

106. Thompson CC. Per-oral endoscopic reduction of dilated gastrojejunal anastomosis following Roux-en-Y gastric bypass: a possible new option for patients with weight regain. Surg Obes Relat Dis. 2005;1:223.

107. Schweitzer M. Endoscopic intraluminal suture plication of the gastric pouch and stoma in postoperative Roux-en-Y gastric bypass patients. J Laparoendosc Adv Surg Tech A. 2004;14:223–6.

108. Pearl JP, Ponsky JL. Natural orifice translumenal endoscopic surgery: a critical review. J Gastrointest Surg. 2007;12(7): 1293–300.

109. Kalloo AN, Kantsevoy SV, Singh VK, et al. Flexible transgastric peritoneoscopy: a novel approach to diagnostic and therapeutic interventions in the peritoneal cavity. Gastroenterology. 2000;118:A1039.

110. Kalloo AN, Singh VK, Jagannath SB, et al. Flexible transgastric peritoneoscopy: a novel approach to diagnostic and therapeutic interventions in the peritoneal cavity. Gastrointest Endosc. 2004;60:114–7.

111. Kalloo A, Giday SA. Natural orifice transluminal endoscopic surgery: a clinical review. Gastroenterol Endosc News. 2007;7:1–6.

Basic Components of Flexible Endoscopes

Benjamin K. Poulose

Technical Characteristics and Components of Flexible Endoscopic Equipment

Modern flexible endoscopic systems represent a technologic convergence of endoscopic instrumentation and image processing techniques. Optimal utilization of modern flexible endoscopes requires a basic understanding of these technologies to provide effective diagnosis and therapeutics. Figure 2.1 shows the basic schematic of a modern endoscopic system. Overall, the design has not changed for over 50 years. The target tissue is illuminated by light transmitted to the tip of the endoscope via a fiber-optic bundle. The image is then transmitted back to a video processor on the endoscopic tower. Conversion to standard analog or digital output occurs by the imageprocessor for viewing on a video monitor. Advances in technology have supplemented this basic setup with light-emitting diode illumination and charge-coupled device (CCD)-acquired images electronically transmitted back to the video processor. The image can now be transmitted to a flat panel monitor in high-definition (HD) format. In addition to light and video transmission, flexible endoscopes have a working channel through which instrumentation is passed, and channels for irrigation and insufflation. A thorough understanding of the particular endoscope and system available to the endoscopist will facilitate timely performance of the procedure and a working basis for troubleshooting problems.

Scope Sizes, Channel Sizes, Viewing Directions

A variety of endoscopes are available to the proceduralist for performance of diagnostic and therapeutic tasks. The basic components of a modern flexible endoscope are outlined in Fig. 2.2a, b and Video 2.1. Usually the endoscopist holds the control handle in the left hand and the insertion tube in the right. The fingers of the left hand are free to manipulate the deflection wheels, brakes, and buttons of the control handle. It is most efficient if the endoscopist's left-hand fingers can manipulate all components of the control handle so that right-hand passage of the insertion tube through the gastrointestinal tract is not interrupted to manipulate the control wheels. Figure 2.3 shows the basic schematic of an endoscope tip. In general, scope selection is guided by the orifice of insertion and by the particular task requiring endoscopic intervention. From a physical standpoint, modern flexible endoscopes vary in insertion tube length, insertion tube diameter, tip diameter, field of view, direction of view, degree of tip deflection, and instrument channel characteristics. Certain principles of endoscope mechanics are worth noting. Most endoscopes combine the working channel and suction channel, often limiting one's ability to suction while an instrument is present within the working channel. Newer endoscopes may have a separate irrigation channel managed by foot pedal, which can facilitate visualization. The endoscopist should also have some familiarity with scope care. The optics, electronics, and controls of the endoscope can be easily damaged with misuse and lack of equipment familiarity. Special care should be taken to ensure that integrity of the insertion tube casing is maintained to prevent potential harm to the patient and costly repairs. These issues can be minimized with a thorough understanding of the endoscope used and with proper endoscopic technique. A practical approach to common equipment problems encountered during endoscopy is outlined in Table 2.1. The following discussion is limited to flexible endoscopes used to visualize the gastrointestinal tract.

This chapter contains a video segment that can be found by accessing the following link: http://www.springerimages.com/videos/978-1-4614-6329-0.

B.K. Poulose, M.D., M.P.H. (✉)
Department of Surgery, Vanderbilt University Medical Center, Nashville, TN, USA
e-mail: benjamin.poulose@Vanderbilt.Edu

J.M. Marks and B.J. Dunkin (eds.), *Principles of Flexible Endoscopy for Surgeons*, DOI 10.1007/978-1-4614-6330-6_2, © Springer Science+Business Media New York 2013

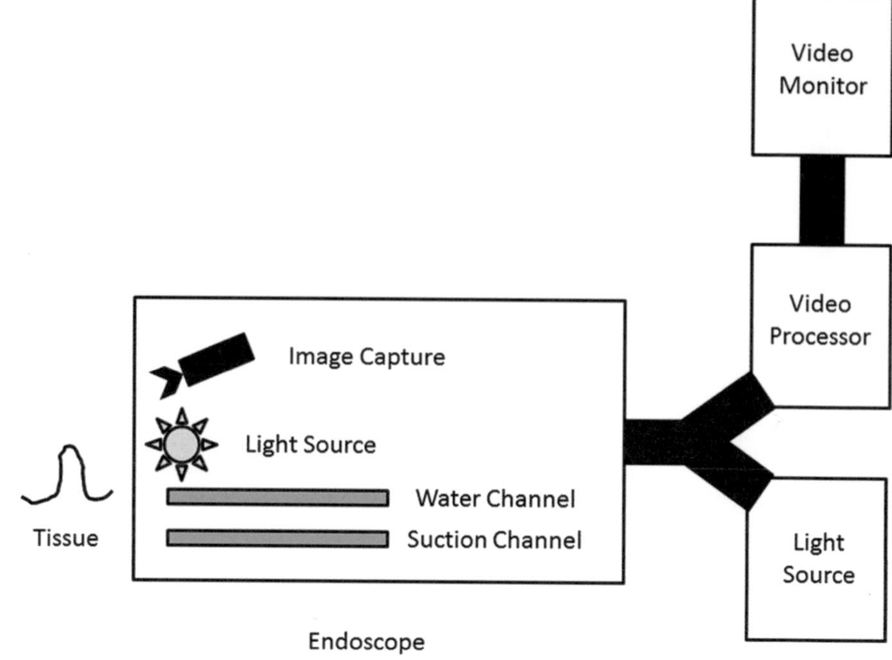

Fig. 2.1 Shows the basic schematic of a modern endoscopic system

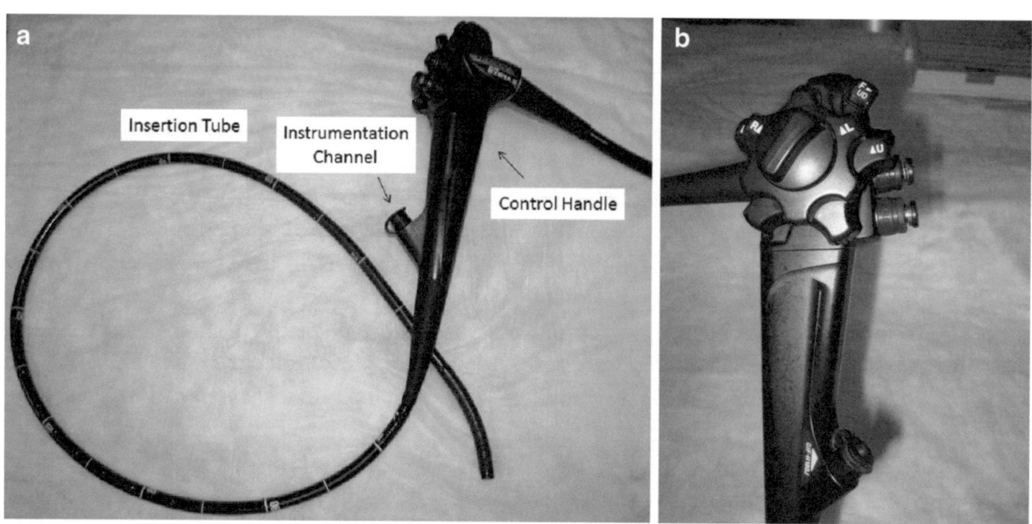

Fig. 2.2 The basic components of a modern flexible endoscope

Gastroscopes

Flexible gastroscopes are used to visualize the posterior oropharynx, esophagus, stomach, and proximal duodenum. Three basic types of forward-viewing gastroscopes exist: diagnostic, therapeutic, and slim scopes. Diagnostic gastroscopes serve as the "workhorse" of upper endoscopic evaluations and usually have a tip diameter between 9 and 10 mm with a single instrument working channel of 2.8 mm. This endoscope serves well for nearly all diagnostic applications and several therapeutic ones. The latter typically includes resection of mucosal lesions, treatment of upper gastrointestinal bleeding, and placement of a percutaneous endoscopic gastrostomy tube. Therapeutic gastroscopes usually are larger than their diagnostic counterparts with tip diameters of 10–12 mm depending on the presence of one or two instrument channels. These endoscopes can be useful when a larger instrument channel is needed (up to 4.2 mm) for suction and tissue resection or when traction/counter-traction maneuvers are necessary. Slim gastroscopes have reduced diameter insertion tubes and tips (5–6 mm) to enable traversal of strictures and narrow lumenal openings; these scopes can sometimes be used without intravenous sedation (usually via transnasal insertion, see Chap. 18 on Unsedated Endoscopy).

Fig. 2.3 Shows the basic schematic of an endoscope tip

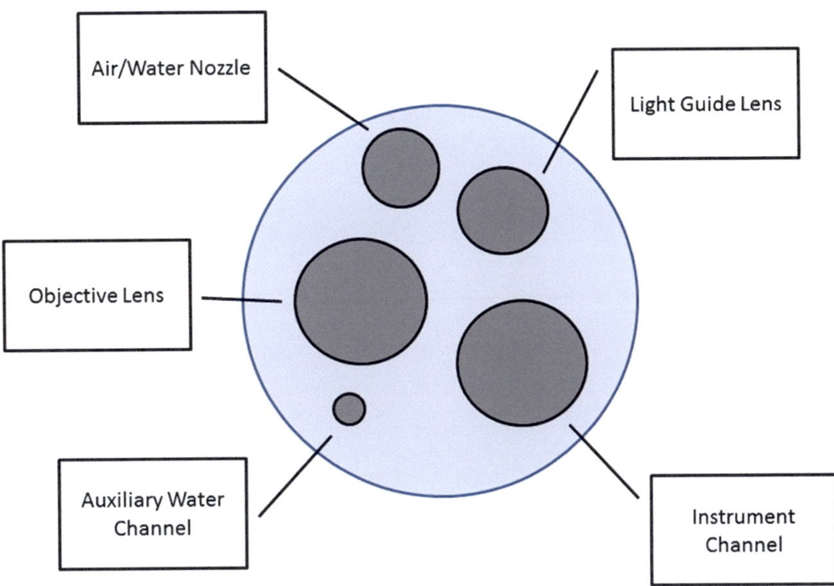

Table 2.1 Troubleshooting common endoscopic equipment problems

Problem	Potential solution
No endoscopic image	Ensure power to all components, ensure that mechanical and video couplings are well seated in appropriate position
Poor-quality image	Check scope tip free of lubricant, ensure functioning light source, white balance endoscope
Inadequate insufflation	Increase insufflation flow setting, ensure endoscope coupling well seated, ensure adequate gas supply if using CO_2
Inadequate suction	Check suction canister and tubing for correct setup or obstruction, check adequate suction from vacuum supply, remove instrument from working channel of endoscope

Table 2.2 Characteristics of gastroscopes[a]

	Tip diameter (mm)	Maximum angulation (°)	Number of instrument channels	Instrument channel diameter (mm)
Slim scope	5.5	210	1	2.0
Diagnostic	9.9	210	1	2.8
Single therapeutic	12.9	200	1	4.2–6.0
Double therapeutic	12.2	210	2	2.8/3.7

[a]*Source*: Olympus, USA (http://www.olympusamerica.com/msg_section/msg_endoscopy.asp#)

Due to the smaller size, they often cannot insufflate or suction with the same degree of efficacy as larger scopes and the endoscopic view is somewhat more limited. Table 2.2 summarizes features for typical gastroscopes. It should be noted for all gastroscopes that "up" deflection affords the greatest angulation; this is an important consideration when attempting to visualize difficult areas (i.e., gastroesophageal junction or fundus of stomach in retroflexed view).

Colonoscopes and Sigmoidoscopes

Colonoscopy remains one of the most challenging procedures for the endoscopist. Performance of high-quality colonoscopy is facilitated by selection of the correct scope for a particular patient. Compared to a diagnostic gastroscope, colonoscopes have an increased tip diameter, longer insertion tube length, and variable stiffness control mecha-

nism to help passage of the scope into the proximal colon (Fig. 2.4). Most colonoscopes have tip diameters of 11–13 mm with somewhat more uniform angulation capability compared to the diagnostic gastroscope. Specifically, colonoscopes have more equal deflection in the up–down axis compared to gastroscopes, which have more deflection in the "up" direction. Small-diameter pediatric colonoscopes are used routinely by some endoscopists to improve comfort, and can be particularly useful during difficult colonoscopies with angulated anatomy or strictures. They can also be used for push enteroscopy to visualize the proximal jejunum. Flexible sigmoidoscopes generally have similar characteristics to colonoscopes but with shorter insertion tube lengths and the lack of variable stiffness mechanisms. Table 2.3 summarizes working characteristics of common colonoscopes and flexible sigmoidoscopes. In lieu of a dedicated lower flexible endoscope, a diagnostic gastroscope can often be used to evaluate the rectum and sigmoid colon. This is especially useful information during operative cases where a quick evaluation of rectosigmoid mucosa is warranted but a dedicated lower endoscope is unavailable.

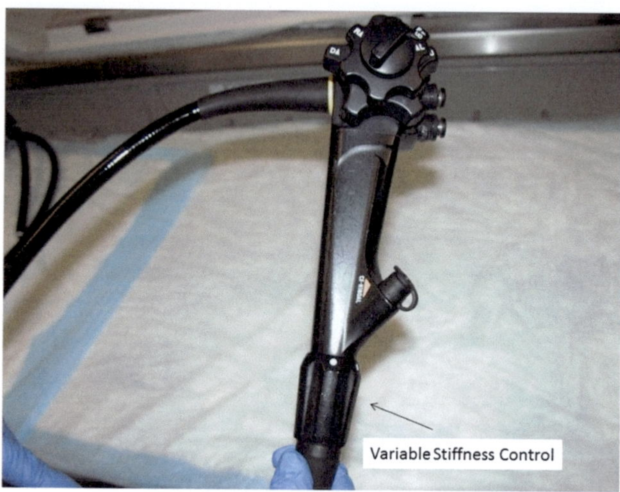

Fig. 2.4 Colonoscopes usually have an increased tip diameter, longer insertion tube length, and variable stiffness control mechanism to help passage of the scope into the proximal colon

Table 2.3 Characteristics of colonoscopes[a]

	Tip diameter (mm)	Working length (mm)	Maximum angulation (°)	Number of instrument channels	Instrument channel diameter (mm)
Flexible sigmoido-scope	13.2	730	180	1	3.7
Pediatric intermediate	11.3	1,330	180	1	3.2
Adult intermediate	13.2	1,330	180	1	3.7
Adult long	13.2	1,680	180	1	3.7

[a]*Source*: Olympus, USA (http://www.olympusamerica.com/msg_section/msg_endoscopy.asp#)

Specialty Endoscopes

A wide array of specialty endoscopes exists to perform complex diagnostic and therapeutic maneuvers. Figure 2.5 shows the more common specialty scopes in use in most endoscopic suites. Duodenoscopes, used for endoscopic retrograde cholangiopancreatography (ERCP), require training for efficient and safe usage. The angle of view is 90° in relation to the insertion tube axis, affording excellent view of the ampulla of Vater. In addition to the performance of ERCP, this endoscope is invaluable for the diagnosis and treatment of periampullary diseases and can help with viewing posterior duodenal bulb ulcers. The successful performance of endoscopic ultrasound (EUS) also requires specialty endoscopic training. Typically two types of echoendoscopes are used: linear and radial scanning scopes. Initially designed as a primarily diagnostic modality, more experienced interventional endoscopists are utilizing EUS for therapeutic maneuvers including pseudocyst drainage, trans-enteric biliary access, and placement of radiation seeds.

Operative choledochoscopes have gained resurgence in popularity with the increased performance of laparoscopic common bile duct exploration. In general, these endoscopes have only one-way deflection, utilize a fiber-optic transmitted image, and range from 3 to 5 mm in tip diameter. A small 1.9 mm diameter working channel is provided for retrieval baskets and lithotripsy probes. Figure 2.6 shows a typical choledochoscope and Table 2.4 summarizes characteristics of these endoscopes. The thinner diameter version works well in laparoscopic transcystic applications via a standard 5 mm port but requires great care to protect the insertion tube from damage by laparoscopic port valve mechanisms and instruments. The larger diameter version affords an improved view but usually needs to be introduced via direct choledochotomy. If dedicated choledochoscopes are not readily available in the operating room, ureteroscopes and cystoscopes can often substitute well for this purpose. Intra-ductal choledochoscopy can be one of the more difficult endoscopic procedures to perform given the smaller endoscopes and smaller diameter of the targeted lumen. Optimal visualization is afforded by saline infusion of the bile duct via the choledochoscope itself. In addition, a twisting motion is often necessary to compensate for lack of a second-axis deflection.

Per oral choledochoscopy can also be accomplished with special equipment. Usually, this requires a "mother–daughter" scope system by which a separate endoscope ("daughter") is introduced into the bile duct via the "mother" endoscope (usually a duodenoscope). The advantage of this system is endoscopic access of the biliary tree for diagnosis and therapeutic maneuvers. A drawback of this setup is the requirement of two endoscopists at the time of the procedure. Single-operator systems (Boston Scientific Spyglass system) do afford direct endoscopic access to the biliary tree and can be performed via duodenoscope.

Imaging Techniques

Optimization of the Endoscopic Image

Similar to laparoscopy, GI endoscopy relies on video imaging for successful diagnosis and treatment. Several simple maneuvers can be used to maximize endoscopic visualization. The simple act of smearing lubricant on the endoscope tip can obscure the image enough to interfere with the procedure. This can be avoided by applying lubricant gel to the insertion tube and not to the tip of the scope itself. Appropriately white balancing the image can also facilitate production of a true color image. Most endoscopic light sources are equipped with a "Manual/Auto" switch to control light intensity. This should be left in the "Auto" position to avoid images that are too dark or too bright. Liberal washing of the lens with the irrigation button and attention to overall good endoscopic technique are critical to successful endoscopic visualization.

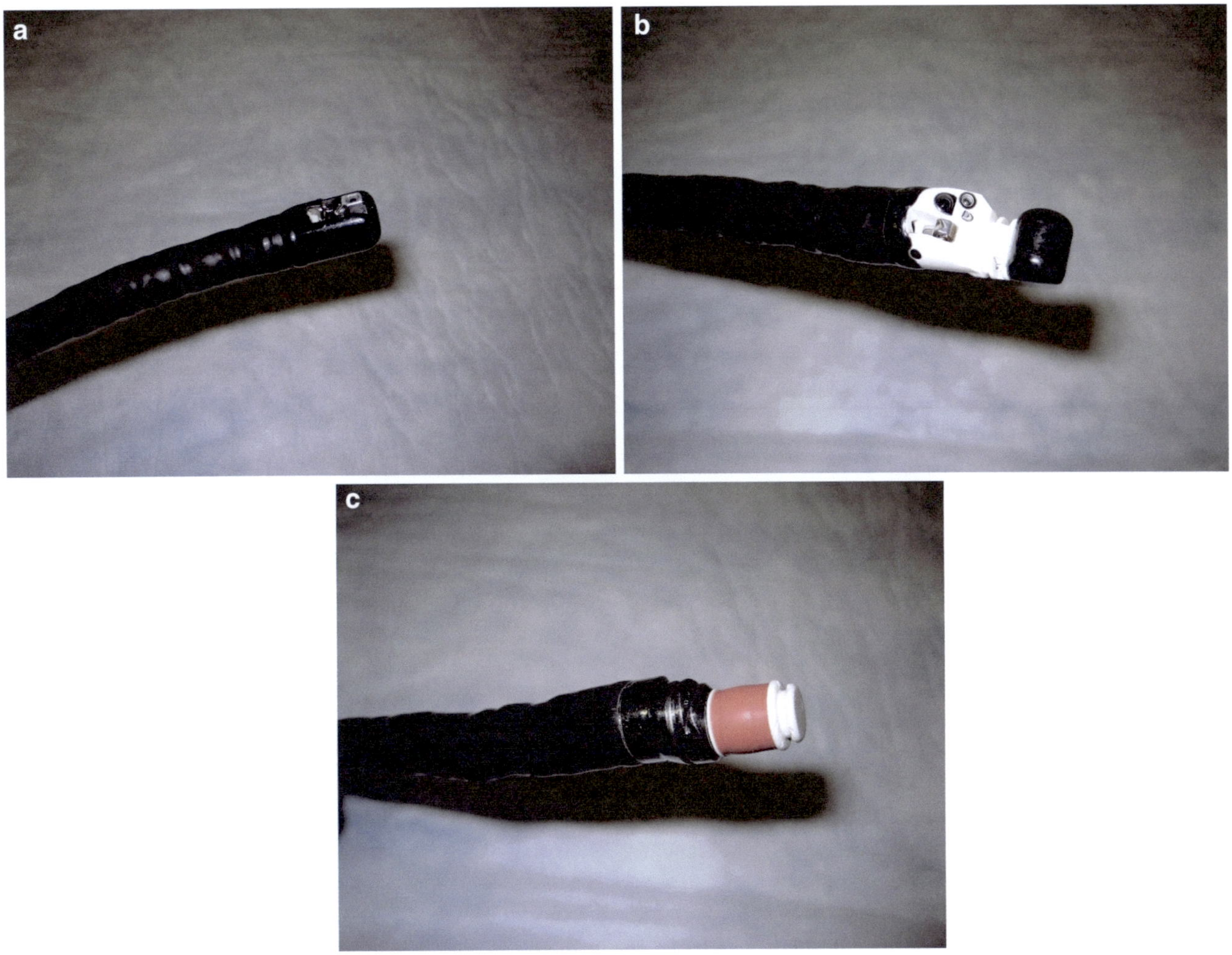

Fig. 2.5 The more common specialty scopes in use in most endoscopic suites. (**a**) Duodenoscope. (**b**) Linear echo. (**c**) Radial echo

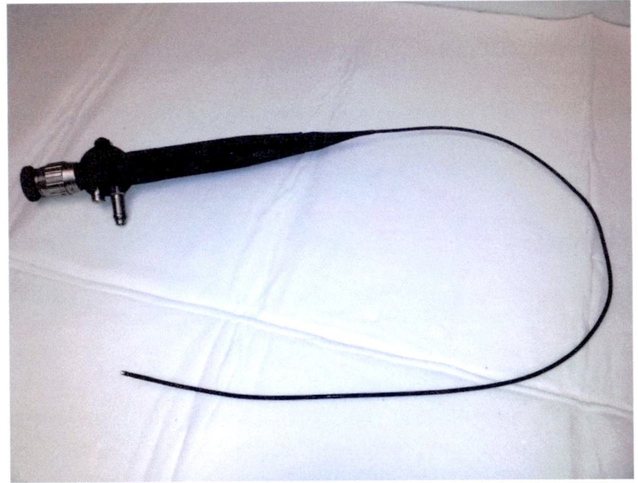

Fig. 2.6 A typical choledochoscope

Table 2.4 Characteristics of choledochoscopes[a]

	Tip diameter (mm)	Maximum angulation (°)	Number of instrument channels	Instrument channel diameter (mm)
Laparoscopic choledochoscope	2.8	160	1	1.2
Standard choledochoscope	5.3	180	1	2.3

[a]*Source*: Karl Storz, USA

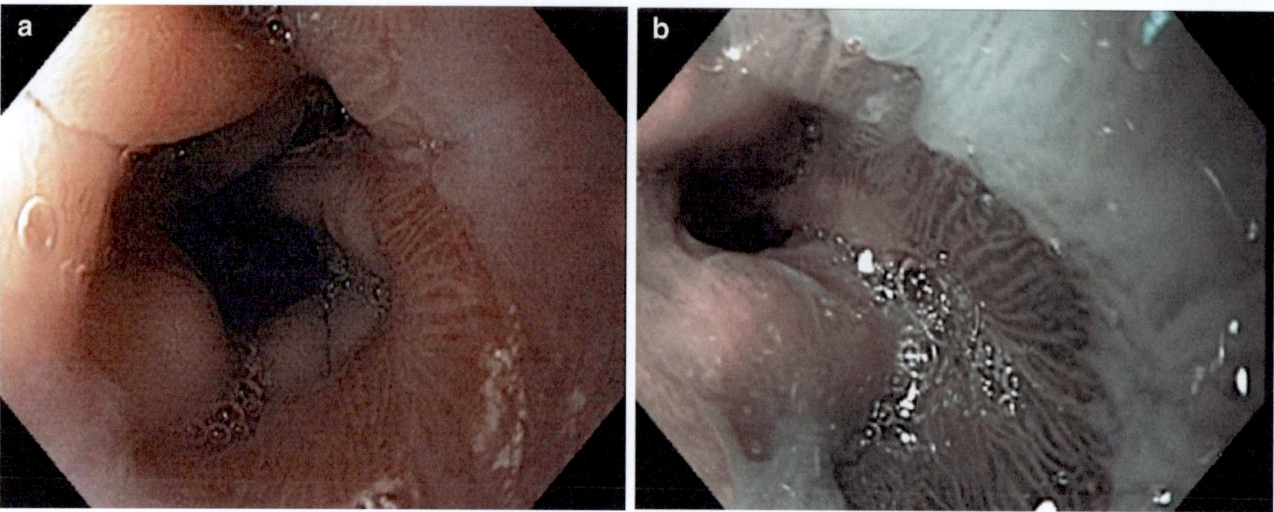

Fig. 2.7 Narrow band imaging (NBI) is most commonly used to evaluate areas of Barrett's esophagus for dysplastic epithelium

Advances in video technology have also resulted in improved resolution with endoscopic systems. Standard-definition (SD) endoscopy typically affords a 4:3 aspect ratio with 640×480 pixel resolution. High-definition systems change the aspect ratio to 16:9 typically with typical resolutions of either $1,280 \times 720$ pixels or $1,920 \times 1,080$ pixels. Both the endoscope and video equipment need to be rated for the proper resolution to gain a higher resolution image [1]. Although HD technology offers a subjectively larger and higher resolution image, the impact on clinical outcomes is unclear.

Narrow Band Imaging

Several emerging techniques are being developed to supplement the traditional image obtained through "white light" videoendoscopy. Most of these imaging techniques are designed to enhance mucosal detail and to separate normal from abnormal tissue. One of the more popular image processing techniques is narrow band imaging (NBI). NBI is most commonly used to evaluate areas of Barrett's esophagus for dysplastic epithelium (Fig. 2.7a, b) [2]. This is accomplished by usage of light filters that increase the relative contribution of blue light, enhancing mucosal detail. One of the main advantages of NBI is that it is a purely image processing-based modality without the need for physical staining of tissue.

Confocal Microscopy

Confocal microscopy (CM) potentially affords the endoscopist with the ability to evaluate gastrointestinal tissue at the microscopic level for "real-time" diagnostic capability. The basic CM system requires that the objective lens be placed directly onto the target tissue for analysis. Images comparable to pathologic slides can be produced (Fig. 2.8a, b) [3].

Optical Coherence Tomography

Optical coherence tomography (OCT) is a light-based imaging processing technique used to produce high-resolution cross-sectional images by analyzing reflected infrared light [4, 5]. Typically, images are produced to a depth of 1–3 mm (Fig. 2.9). OCT is gaining some popularity in the differentiation of dysplastic epithelium in the setting of Barrett's esophagus.

Summary

Modern flexible endoscopy represents a culmination of technologic and procedural advancements that enable endoscopists to diagnose and treat a multitude of gastrointestinal problems in a minimally invasive fashion. Knowledge of available variations in endoscopic equipment and in supporting technologies improves the efficiency of endoscopic procedures.

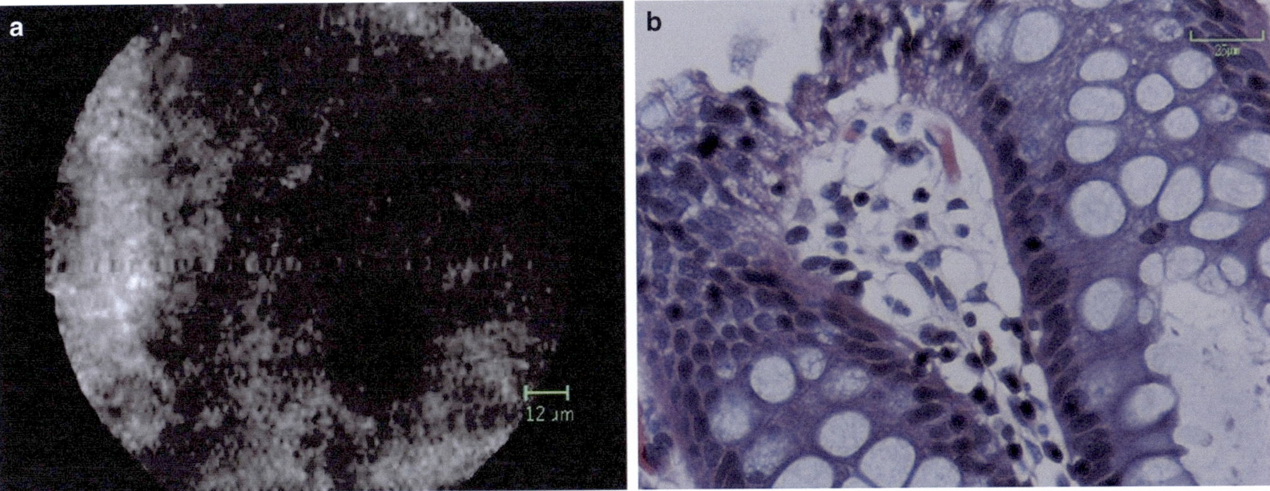

Fig. 2.8 Confocal microscopy enables the endoscopist to visualize gastrointestinal tissue at the microscopic level in real time. Here, normal colonic mucosa is seen in (**a**), while a representative pathologic section is shown in (**b**)

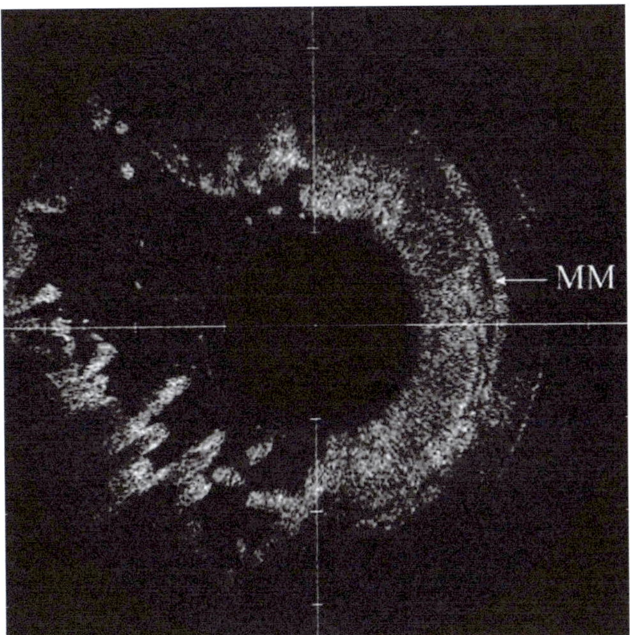

Fig. 2.9 Optical coherence tomography reveals cross-sectional imaging of the gastrointestinal tract. The normal duodenal wall is visualized in this image

References

1. Technology Status Evaluation Report. High resolution and high-magnification endoscopy. Gastrointest Endosc. 2000;52(6):864–6.
2. Curvers WL, van Vilsteren FG, Baak LC, et al. Endoscopic tri-modal imaging versus standard video endoscopy for detection of early Barrett's neoplasia: a multicenter, randomized, crossover study in general practice. Gastrointest Endosc. 2011;73(2):195–203.
3. Yoshida S, Tanaka S, Hirata M, et al. Optical biopsy of GI lesions by reflectance-type laser-scanning confocal microscopy. Gastrointest Endosc. 2007;66(1):144–9.
4. Sivak Jr MV, Kobayashi K, Izatt JA, et al. High-resolution endoscopic imaging of the GI tract using optical coherence tomography. Gastrointest Endosc. 2000;51(4):474–9.
5. Peery AF, Shaheen NJ. Optical coherence tomography in Barrett's esophagus: the road to clinical utility. Gastrointest Endosc. 2010;71(2):231–4.

Setup and Care of Endoscopes

3

Ariel Eric Klevan and Jose Martinez

Introduction

The introduction of a flexible endoscope to mainstream clinical practice has revolutionized the diagnosis and treatment of gastrointestinal, urologic, and pulmonary illnesses. The flexibility of these scopes has far surpassed the limitations of the traditional rigid endoscope, allowing the endoscopist to reach and treat anatomical areas never thought to be amenable to this kind of treatment. These scopes and their associated tools allow endoscopists to diagnose and treat disease processes that traditionally required invasive surgery. These procedures are now done in a truly minimally invasive fashion, often on an outpatient basis. Two types of endoscopes are commonly used: fiber-optic and videoendoscopes [1, 2].

The fiber-optic scope uses an array of thousands of glass fibers in a tightly packed manner to allow for visualization of the field of interest [2]. The glass fiber bundles are designed to transmit light from an outside light source into the lumen being examined. Another set of these glass fiber bundles transmit the image from the organ of interest back to the eyepiece of the scope. Fiber-optic scopes are not commonly used in gastrointestinal (GI) endoscopy today except in specialized very-small-diameter scopes. Currently, the most commonly seen fiber-optic scopes are laryngoscopes, bronchoscopes, choledochoscopes, and ureteroscopes.

The more modern videoendoscope uses a combination of traditional fiber-optic technology combined with digital video imaging. Light is still transmitted to the end of the instrument via a fiber-optic bundle, but the image is acquired via a charge-coupled device (CCD) placed under a lens at the distal tip of the scope [1, 2]. This CCD functions similar to a video camera in that the image is transmitted digitally back to a video processor while maintaining a non-degraded image quality. Digital endoscopes have largely replaced fiber-optic ones because of the significant improvement in image definition.

An understanding of the setup and care of endoscopes is important for the endoscopist to have as optimal imaging and procedure performance are only possible with proper endoscope setup. Prior to using any scope, the endoscopist must be certain it has gone through proper cleaning and sterilization. He or she should also be aware of common pitfalls that require a calculated approach to resolve, and understand that flexible endoscopes are quite fragile and expensive and require appropriate care to maintain their high-quality visual images on a long-term basis.

Setting Up the Endoscope and Tower

Performing any endoscopic procedure requires some setup. Most of this has already been performed by the time the endoscopist enters the procedure room but a thorough understanding is crucial to minimize scope damage and prevent pitfalls. The main components are the endoscopy tower, monitors, flexible endoscopes, and lastly all the necessary attachments. The endoscopy tower usually contains a light source with built-in air insufflator, image processor, and a monitor. Image-capturing devices, energy sources, as well as power irrigation systems are often added to more robust endoscopy towers. The connections between each of these can be quite complex and are often done at the time of initial purchase and setup of the tower. Although these connections do not have to be performed on a daily basis,

This chapter contains a video segment that can be found by accessing the following link: http://www.springerimages.com/videos/978-1-4614-6329-0.

A.E. Klevan, M.D., F.R.C.S.C.
Department of Surgery, Jackson Memorial Hospital,
University of Miami Hospital, Miami, FL, USA

J. Martinez, M.D., F.A.C.S. (✉)
Department of Surgery, Miller School of Medicine,
University of Miami, Miami, FL, USA
e-mail: JMartinez4@med.miami.edu

J.M. Marks and B.J. Dunkin (eds.), *Principles of Flexible Endoscopy for Surgeons*,
DOI 10.1007/978-1-4614-6330-6_3, © Springer Science+Business Media New York 2013

Table 3.1 Troubleshooting

Problems	Possible reasons
No irrigation	Water bottle not connected
	Water level too low or high
	Water bottle lid not closed tightly
	Gasket missing on water bottle
	Irrigation valve is stuck or broken
No insufflation	Power is off
	Light guide plug not fully inserted
	Insufflation valve stuck or broken
	Biopsy channel cap missing
No suction	Suction is not connected
	Debris clogged in biopsy channel
	Instrument in biopsy channel
Abnormal colors	White balance not performed
	Monitor requires color adjustment
	Improper video cable setup
No light from scope	Power is off
	Light guide plug not fully inserted
	Lamp on standby
	Light bulb burned out
Unable to advance instrument into biopsy channel	Damaged channel
	Scope angulation too severe
	Instrument larger than biopsy channel

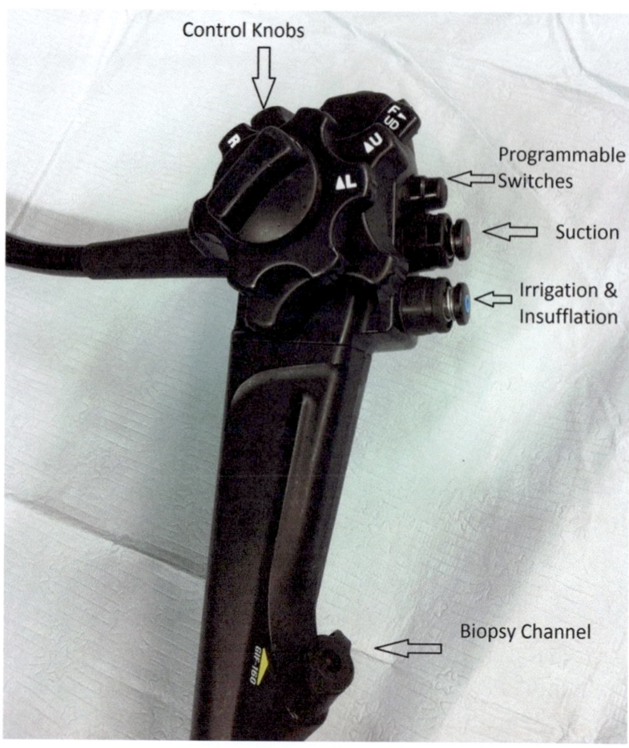

Fig. 3.1 Endoscope control section

a basic understanding of audiovisual connections should be a must for the endoscopist. One video cable inadvertently pulled loose from the back of the tower can be the source of complete image blackout. A complete understanding of the numerous problems that can be encountered and appropriate solutions should be well known to the endoscopist and are summarized in Table 3.1.

Flexible endoscopes come in many diameters and lengths. There are forward- as well as side-viewing scopes. During room setup the appropriate scope for the intended procedure should be carefully selected as well as a backup scope in case a different one is needed. Examples include a pediatric scope if difficulty is encountered advancing an adult colonoscope along a sharp angulation or changing to a neonatal gastroscope to traverse an esophageal stricture. These pre-procedure setups minimize wasted time when a problem is encountered, as well as give the rest of the endoscopy team an expected game plan for the upcoming procedure.

The required setup of the endoscope prior to being connected is to verify that the appropriate level of sterilization was performed for the intended procedure. Many endoscopy suites have employed a system to label the endoscope with a tag when it completes the required sterilization process. The tag is broken at the beginning of the next procedure. One must also verify the suction, irrigation/insufflation, and working channel buttons/caps have been properly placed. A common channel introduces air and water into the lumen by depressing a blue trumpetlike valve on the scope. If a finger is placed over this irrigation/insufflation button, the air exits the tip of the scope while fully pressing the button will result in releasing a jet of water across the CCD lens.

Pressing the adjacent red button results in suctioning of air or luminal fluid/debris. The endoscopist should test the suction, irrigation, and insufflation features of the endoscope prior to every use (Fig. 3.1).

Step by Step: Connecting the Endoscope

The tower should be connected to power but the light source and image processor powered off. The appropriate endoscope is chosen for the intended procedure (Fig. 3.2).

The umbilical cable of the scope is inserted into the light source on the tower. The video processor cable is connected from the image processor to the umbilical cable of the scope (Fig. 3.3).

The water bottle, filled to the appropriate mark (do not overfill) with sterile water, is connected to the umbilical cable. Power irrigation can also be connected at this time if the scope has that capability.

Suction is connected to the umbilical cord. Ensure that it is set to constant and maximum suction and minimize tubing length to maximize suction power.

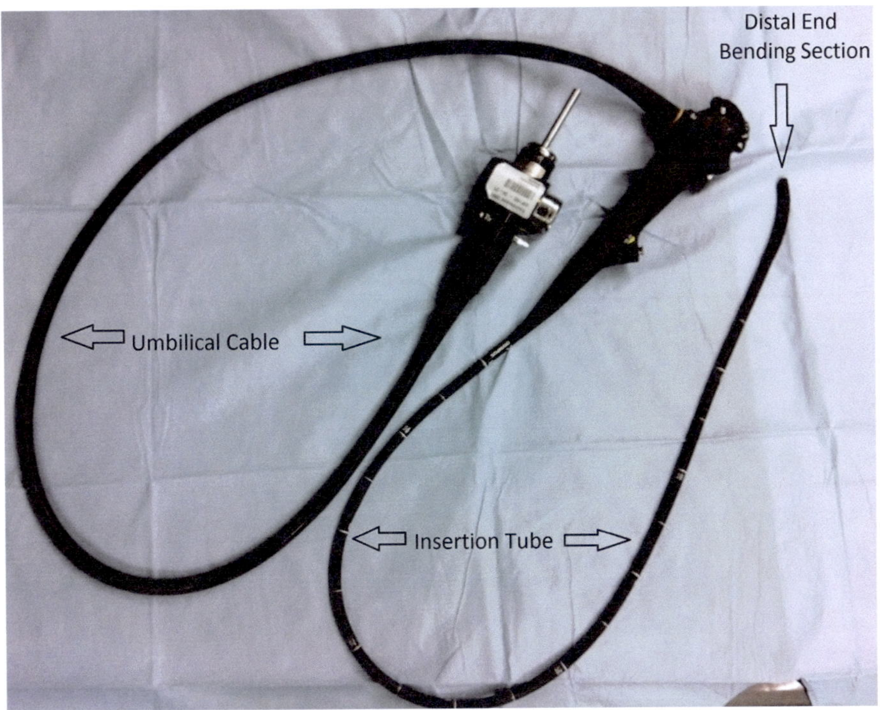

Fig. 3.2 Endoscope umbilical cable

Proceed to power up the image processor, light source, and any other attached devices.

Ensure that all functions of the scope are working properly. The suction, irrigation, and insufflation buttons are tested with a water basin. The power irrigation system is tested if connected. Ensure that all wheels and knobs are properly turning. Connections should be rechecked if any functions are not working properly.

The light source lamp ignition button is identified and turned on. This step should be done as close to initiation of procedure as possible to minimize unwanted lamp usage. If the procedure is delayed, the lamp should be switched to "off" or "standby" depending on the system being used.

Next perform a white balance. The lamp needs to be on for this to be done correctly. Point the tip of the endoscope on a white object and press the "white balance" button on the image processor until white balance confirmation is given on the video screen.

A sharp image should now be obtained on any available object. Test image-capturing device if connected to one.

Ensure that proper adjunctive items such as biopsy forceps and polypectomy snares are available.

Finally, to avoid bite damage to the endoscope, dentures are removed and/or a bite block is placed prior to initiating procedural sedation (Video 3.1).

Setup for a mobile procedure (i.e., in the ICU or ER) is somewhat different than procedures in the endoscopy suite as one typically only has access to one monitor. The tower and monitor are typically positioned opposite to the endoscopist. If the mobile tower allows, separate the monitor from the rest of the tower and position it across the patient to maximize ergonomic comfort for the endoscopist.

Equipment Care and Cleaning

Storage and Transfer

Flexible endoscopes are commonly stored in well-ventilated vertical cabinets (Fig. 3.4). These cabinets allow for the scopes to vertically hang from the handle of the scope with the umbilicus and the distal scope suspended freely. These cabinets and the vertical racks promote drying, as well as minimize twist or kinks from developing over time. One should not store endoscopes in poorly ventilated spaces or racks that hold the umbilical cable upright as this will allow moisture to pool at the dependent part of the tube, leading to bacterial and fungal overgrowth [4]. The cabinets also provide protection from physical impact. In addition, endoscopes should be stored without removable parts to allow ongoing drying of channel and channel openings and the deflection wheels should be unlocked [3, 4].

The endoscopes are handled carefully in between procedures. The transfer to the endoscopy suite or travel cart must be performed carefully by holding the head, tip, and umbilical cord as the optics can be easily damaged if the

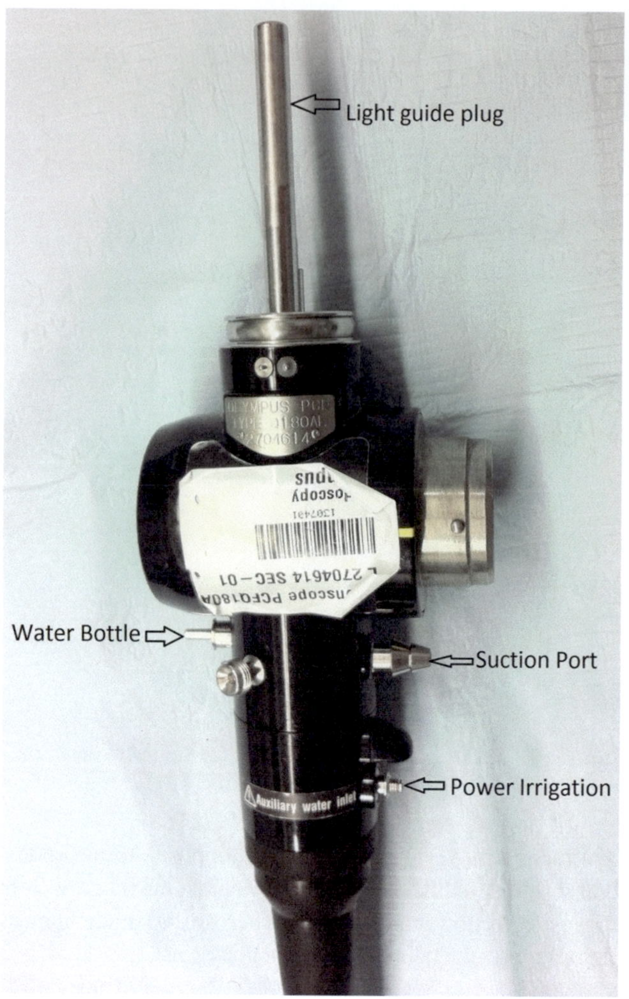

Fig. 3.3 Light guide plug

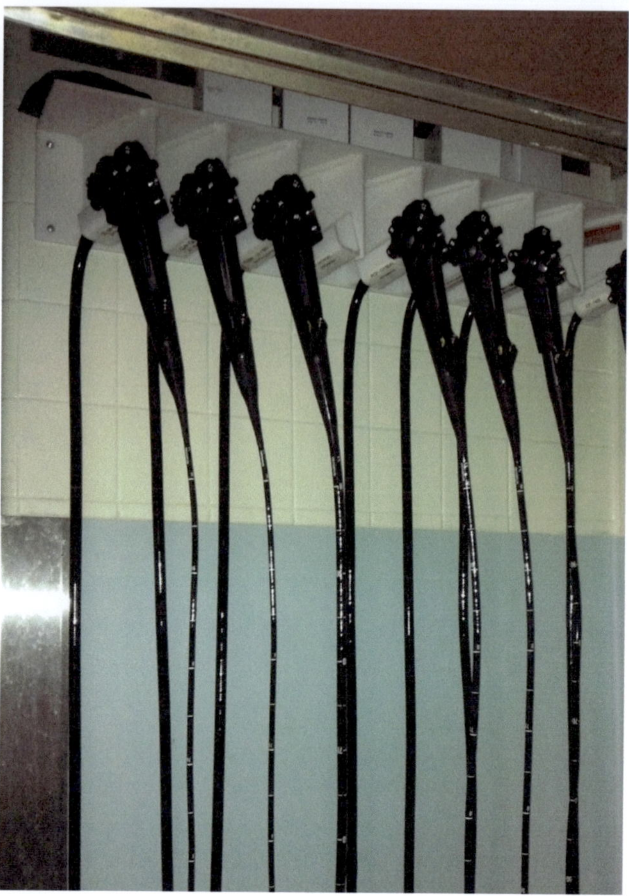

Fig. 3.4 Endoscope cabinet

scope hits another firm surface [2]. An endoscope should never travel while connected to its light source on the travel cart as this risks catching the umbilicus on an object while the cart is rolling.

Cleaning and Disinfection

The cleaning and disinfecting of endoscopes is a major component of their daily maintenance. All used endoscopes should be regarded as potential carriers of infectious pathogens and universal precautions should be adopted. Local formal infection control protocols should be written with the aid of experts, equipment manufacturers, and relevant national advisory bodies [2]. All unit staff should then be proficient with the locally adopted guidelines. Cleaning and disinfection should take place in a specialized allocated area within or in close proximity to the endoscopy unit. This area should include clearly defined and discrete clean and dirty areas, multiple workstations, double sinks, and a separate hand washbasin [2]. The endoscope processing area should have disinfector units, ultrasound cleaners, and adequate ventilation [2].

The disinfection of medical devices is divided into three levels, based on the risk of infection transmission associated with their use: sterilization, high-level disinfection, and low-level disinfection [2, 3]. The level of disinfection corresponds to whether an item is labeled "critical," "semicritical," or "noncritical." Critical reusable accessories penetrate blood vessels or sterile tissue (mucus membranes or body cavities). Examples of devices used in endoscopy that are categorized as "critical" and must be sterilized prior to use include biopsy forceps, sclerotherapy needles, and sphincterotomes [3]. Reusable items are autoclaved or gas sterilized, while disposable items are presterilized. Endoscopes and dilators are considered semicritical as they come in contact with, but do not typically penetrate, mucus membranes [3]. Such devices must undergo at least high-level disinfection. This is typically accomplished by processing the endoscope on a disinfection machine (Fig. 3.5). Once processed, these endoscopes are handled with clean hands and gloves and stored in a drying cabinet. Finally, noncritical accessories, such as cameras and the endoscopic cart, do not come in contact with the patient

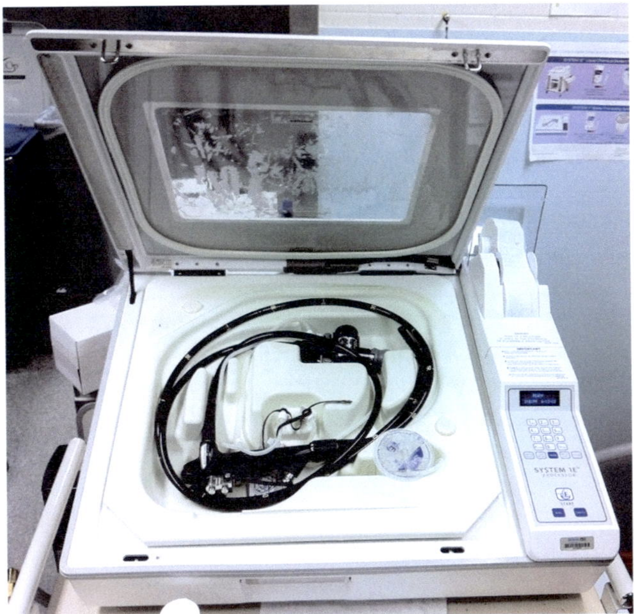

Fig. 3.5 Automated endoscope reprocessor

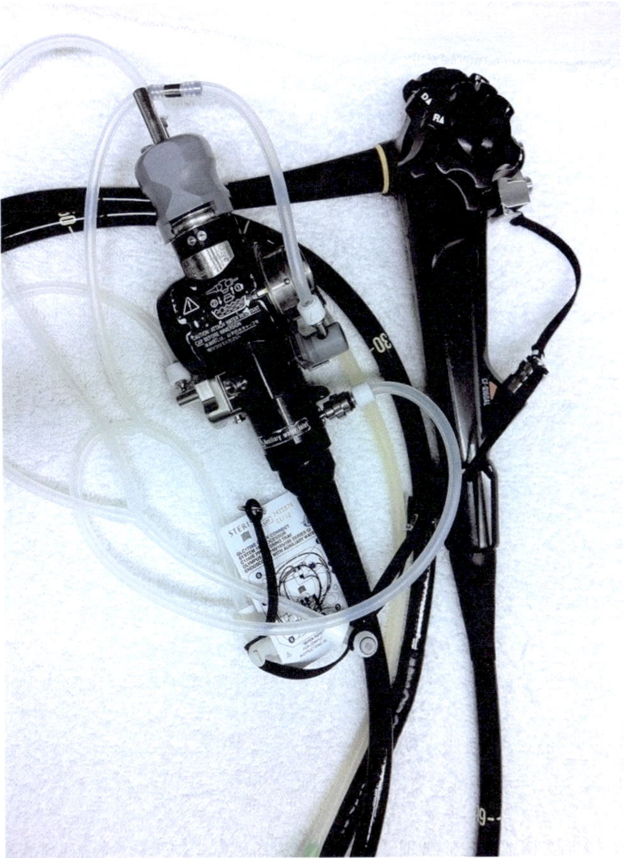

Fig. 3.6 AER adaptor on power irrigation scope

or only touch intact skin. These devices undergo low-level disinfection between cases via surface wipe down with a disinfectant [3].

The initial part of disinfection, also known as "precleaning," occurs immediately following the procedure and involves mechanically cleaning all bodily fluids and debris from the endoscope and its channels, as disinfectant fluid does not penetrate organic material [3]. The endoscopist can facilitate this process by dunking the tip of the scope in a clean basin directly after withdrawal from the patient and suctioning a cleaning solution while the endoscope is still attached to its power source. One should use a prepared basin of enzymatic cleaning solution as per the original manufacturer's instructions. The suction button is held down until the fluid in the tubing is clear.

Subsequently, the endoscope may be cleaned in a fashion similar to the following: [2, 3].

The umbilical connections are capped and the scope is transferred (in protective covering if outside of the endoscopy suite) to a designated cleaning area.

The endoscope is wiped down with a cloth soaked in enzymatic detergent.

Water and enzymatic solution are suctioned (again) to ensure that the solution is visibly clean.

The air/water channel is flushed with the manufacturer's flushing device.

The scope is tested for leaks with a pressurizing leak-testing device prior to reprocessing, as per manufacturer guidelines. The bending section at the distal end of the endoscope is especially prone to leaks (Video 3.2).

All valves and biopsy caps are removed.

The scope is completely immersed in a solution of warm water and neutral detergent. It is then washed with a soft cloth.

The distal end of the scope is brushed with a soft brush (i.e., toothbrush), focusing on removing any debris or tissue around the air/water channel outlet and any bridge/elevator if present.

A brush to clean the biopsy channel and suction port is provided by the manufacturer. The brush is passed through the suction channel at least three times, until it emerges clean. The brush itself is also cleaned before each reinsertion. The suction button is removed and the brush is passed through the suction channel opening, down the shaft of the scope until it emerges from the distal end, at least three times. The brush is then passed in the opposite direction at least three times. The process is repeated for all channels.

The scope is subsequently placed in an automated endoscope reprocessor (AER) for further cleaning and disinfection. One should ensure model-specific compatibility between the AER and endoscope. Some of the newer AER eliminate the need for manual brushing of the individual scope. Scopes with power irrigation must also have the appropriate adaptor connected when placed in the AER (Fig. 3.6).

Endoscopic accessories such as channel valves, water bottles, and cleaning brushes should be cleaned with similar attention using enzymatic detergents.

Disinfection

Following the cleaning exercise outlined above, the AER cleaning adapter is attached to the suction, biopsy, and air/water channels [2]. Each channel is flushed with detergent until it is visualized in the opposite end [2]. Air must be expelled from all channels and the scope is bathed in a disinfectant, such as 2 % glutaraldehyde [2]. This agent is the most commonly used disinfectant and is supported by multiple scientific studies and professional organizations [3]. Glutaraldehyde is noncorrosive to metals, rubbers, and plastics, and destroys viruses and bacteria within 4 min [2]. It is recommended that endoscopes and accessories are soaked for 20 min at 20 °C with adequate precleaning [3]. Other agents have been used for disinfection, including alcohol, peracetic acid, chlorine dioxide, and Sterox [2]. Regardless of the agent chosen, one should choose a high-level disinfectant cleared by the FDA (or equivalent local authority) for this purpose, as well as one that is compatible with the particular endoscope in use.

The incidence of pathogen transmission from endoscopes is estimated to be 1 in 1.8 million procedures [3]. When transmissions have been detected, they were most commonly caused from lapses in accepted cleaning and disinfection guidelines. Endoscopes and their associated devices and accessories have been reported to cause transmission of pathogens such as hepatitis C virus, *Escherichia coli*, *Pseudomonas*, and *Salmonella* [3, 4]. Transmission of *Clostridium difficile* and *Helicobacter pylori* may also be possible [4].

While high-level disinfection is adequate for most endoscopic procedures, some cases require complete sterilization of the endoscope which cannot be done in an AER or standard autoclave. Sterilization of a flexible endoscope is most commonly done using ethylene oxide gas. However, the process is lengthy, often requiring an overnight sterilization cycle [1]. One must also ensure that this type of sterilization is compatible with the manufacturer's recommendations. This mode of scope sterilization is often requested when the endoscope will be used in the sterile field intraoperatively such as in enteroscopy or laparoscopically guided trans-abdominal ERCP in post Roux-en-Y gastric bypass patients.

Transmission of hospital-acquired infections can be further minimized by using sterile or filtered water for scope reprocessing. Tap water may contain bacteria such as Pseudomonas and Mycobacterium species, which can multiply in the static moist environment of the drying scope [4]. If tap water is used, one can subsequently rinse the scope channels with 70 % alcohol [4].

Reprocessors subsequently rinse the endoscopes using the all-channel irrigator to remove traces of disinfectant fluid. The channels are washed with 70–90 % ethyl or isopropyl alcohol and dried with forced air [3]. If a reprocessor is not used then this is done manually. Once the instruments are entirely dry, they are hung vertically in a well-ventilated cabinet [3, 4]. Detailed records of each endoscopic disinfection should be kept. The endoscopes are labeled (or a seal placed) after the completion of the cleaning process to be differentiated from the dirty scopes. When the scope is used, the seal or label is removed. Finally, endoscopes and automatic reprocessors should undergo routine surveillance for the presence of infectious bacteria.

Endoscopes gradually become contaminated during storage [3]. Although there has been some debate over the length of safe "shelf time" of clean endoscopes prior to requiring repeat disinfection, current evidence suggests that intervals of 5–14 days are safe [3]. Contamination during this interval is negligible and seems to involve only common skin organisms as opposed to pathological organisms. The frequencies for replacing clean water bottles and air/irrigation tubing as well as waste vacuum and suction tubing/canisters have not been determined. Scopes and accessories that have been stored for longer intervals than advised in the local institutional protocol should be reprocessed and decontaminated. Recent guidelines do not directly endorse or reject quality control surveillance such as routine microbiological testing of reprocessed endoscopes for pathogens. However, such programs should use standard microbiological techniques if performed.

Occupational Exposure

All staffs involved with handling soiled endoscopes are at risk of exposure to infectious bodily fluids and universal precautions should be employed. Gowns, gloves, and eye protection should be worn and local infection control guidelines should be followed [3]. These may include prompt disposal of sharps and hazardous waste into appropriate containers as well as placing soiled endoscopes directly into a designated "contaminated sink" or container.

The occupational risks involved with glutaraldehyde use include irritation to the skin, eyes, throat, and lungs and can lead to sensitization reactions such as dermatitis, sinusitis, or asthma [2]. Furthermore, chemical colitis, pancreatitis, and mucosal damage have been described in patients [4]. Glutaraldehyde should be used in well-ventilated areas following OSHA guidelines [5]. If not available, a ductless ventilation device containing filters to absorb glutaraldehyde vapors should be used [4]. Cleaning staffs can protect themselves from exposure with the use of fluid resistance gowns, heavy domestic rubber gloves (regular medical rubber gloves are permeable to it), as well as facial and eye protection [2].

Maintenance

The surveillance and maintenance of endoscopes should occur on a daily basis. Scopes should be tested for appropriate function with each cleaning, prior to storage. Common problems identified from routine use include loosening of the wheel locks, stretching of the control wires with decreased tip deflexion from manufacture specification, and tear of the bending portion at the tip of the endoscope. Although the endoscope should still be functional, it is recommended that the scope be sent for repair prior to worsening of these problems leading to higher costs. Endoscope repairs have been classified into three types: minor, major, and refurbishment level [6]. Minor repairs require minimal scope disassembly, parts, and labor. The common repairs that fall onto this category are distal tip cover replacement, control knob repair, and air/water O-ring/valve replacement. Major repairs involve replacing of one or more major components of the endoscope, such as the biopsy/suction channel and elevator repair. Refurbishment-level repairs require the replacement of all critical components and all patient contact components, such as when damage is made to the CCD. These repairs are also known as complete overhaul.

The video processor and light source rarely need any maintenance except for light bulb replacement. Most modern light sources demonstrate "life of bulb used" or "remaining." When the critical point is reached, the bulb should be replaced to maintain best visualization and image quality.

Endoscope repair and refurbishment can be completed by one of the two types of organizations. The first, original equipment manufacturers (OEMs), such as Olympus America Inc., Melville, NY; Pentax Precision Instrument Corp., Orangeburg, NY; and Fujinon Inc., Wayne, NJ, all provide their own repair services and were initially the exclusive repair providers for their instruments [6]. OEMs use proprietary parts, adhesives, lubricant specifications, and repair manuals and must comply with the FDA's Quality System Regulations (QSR), which require the repair to return the scope to its specifications. Third-party repair providers or independent service organizations (ISOs) have more recently become available and can also be used for repair and maintenance [6]. ISOs are considered "refurbishers" and are not regulated by the FDA. Some ISOs have established relationships with OEMs (i.e., Pentax and Fujinon) as "certified/authorized" repair providers. These ISOs have access to the OEM's proprietary parts, adhesives, training, and repair manuals. Even though "unauthorized" ISOs are not under the same regulatory scrutiny, it remains exceedingly difficult to prove that their use for endoscopic maintenance compromises patient safety.

References

1. Chand B, Ponsky JL, Scott-Conner CEH. Flexible endoscopes: characteristics, troubleshooting, and equipment care. In: Scott-Conner CEH, editor. The SAGES manual fundamentals of laparoscopy, thoracoscopy, and GI endoscopy. 2nd ed. New York: Springer; 2006.
2. Cotton PB, Williams CB. Practical gastrointestinal endoscopy the fundamentals. 5th ed. Oxford: Blackwell Publishing; 2003.
3. Multisociety guideline on reprocessing flexible gastrointestinal endoscopes: 2011. Gastrointest Endosc 2011;73:1075–84.
4. Shumway R, Broussard JD. Maintenance of gastrointestinal endoscopes. Clin Tech Small Anim Pract. 2003;18:254–61.
5. Best practices for the safe use of glutaraldehyde in health care. Occupational Safety and Health Administration 2006. Report No.:OSHA 3258-08N 2006.
6. ASGE Technology Status Evaluation Report. Endoscope repair by original equipment manufacturers and independent service organizations January 2003. Gastrointest Endoscosc. 2003;57:639–42.

Michael Larone Campbell, Jaime E. Sanchez,
Sowsan Rasheid, Evan K. Tummel, and Vic Velanovich

Introduction

Prior to performing endoscopic procedures it is imperative that the physician be knowledgeable of the many aspects of patient care in all phases of the encounter. This chapter focuses on the pre-procedural phase. Care must be taken to address patient risk factors as well as the procedure-associated risks that could potentially affect outcome. Co-morbid conditions must be taken into consideration and risk modification employed such as administration of pre-procedural antibiotics when indicated and discontinuation of anticoagulants when necessary. By being prepared to meet the challenging complexities related to a patient's overall health the physician should be able to minimize procedural complications and improve patient safety and outcomes.

History

The encounter between the endoscopy patient and the endoscopist must begin with an adequate and thorough history. This is imperative given the fact that many endoscopy patients go to an "open" endoscopy suite and are likely being seen by the endoscopist for the first time.

Appropriate gastric emptying is critical in patients undergoing elective procedures, and as such these patients should abstain from oral intake of clear liquids for 2 h, and for at least 6 h after a light meal [1]. Patients with any pathology that results in delayed gastric emptying should fast for a longer period of time to allow appropriate gastric clearance. Examples include diabetic patients, pregnant patients, or those with any obstructing gastric pathology.

To increase the diagnostic accuracy and therapeutic safety of colonoscopy, the quality of bowel preparation should be taken into account. Ideally all fecal matter should be emptied from the colon to optimize visibility of the entire colonic mucosa. However, care should be taken to limit patient discomfort and to prevent significant changes in fluid and electrolyte balance. Standard polyethylene glycol (PeG) solutions and sodium phosphate (NaP) based compounds are the most commonly used preparations. NaP compounds however should be avoided in patients at risk of severe electrolyte and/or fluid disturbances. These patients include the elderly, patients with congestive heart failure, renal or hepatic insufficiency, or patients taking medications such as angiotensin receptor blockers, ACE inhibitors, or diuretics [2]. Older PeG solutions may result in poor patient compliance owing to the low palatability and the high volume of liquid required. Newer PeG formulations however have better palatability and require ingestion of a lower volume of liquid.

Management of Co-morbid Diseases

The management of comorbidities in the peri-endoscopic period should be considered an adjunct to the pre-procedural risk assessment performed for complicated patients. Although most endoscopies are performed using either minimal or moderate sedation (formerly "conscious sedation"), some similar risk categories such as those associated with general anesthesia should be considered. These include arrhythmias, hypotension, myocardial infarction, and thromboembolic events. Understanding the various depths of sedation is

M.L. Campbell, M.D.
Department of Surgery, University of South Florida, Tampa, FL, USA

J.E. Sanchez, M.D., M.S.P.H. • E.K. Tummel, M.D.
Department of Surgery, Division of Colon and Rectal Surgery,
University of South Florida, Tampa, FL, USA

S. Rasheid, M.D.
Department of Surgery—Colorectal, University of South Florida,
Tampa, FL, USA

V. Velanovich, M.D. (✉)
Department of Surgery, University of South Florida, Tampa, FL, USA
e-mail: vvelano1@hfhs.org

J.M. Marks and B.J. Dunkin (eds.), *Principles of Flexible Endoscopy for Surgeons*,
DOI 10.1007/978-1-4614-6330-6_4, © Springer Science+Business Media New York 2013

essential to provide safe and effective procedural anesthesia. A typical patient with minimal sedation has unaffected respiratory and cardiovascular functions. Moderate sedation usually involves adequate spontaneous ventilation as well as unaltered cardiovascular function in the young, healthy patient (for more details see Chap. 5). In those with advanced age or compromised cardiopulmonary function certain precautions should be taken. Patients with chronic obstructive pulmonary disease, coronary artery disease, advanced age, and valvular heart disease appear to be at highest risk of complications [3]. Patients with a history of snoring have been shown to independently predict difficulty with bag-mask ventilation, and intubation [4]. Past and current renal, or hepatic diseases should also be identified, and neurotoxic agents such as meperidine should be avoided in these patients owing to the possibility of mental status changes such as seizures and delirium (further discussed in Chap. 5) [5]. Patients with prior seizure disorder should be identified and sedatives, which lower the seizure threshold, avoided. In addition, the endoscopist should assess for patient drug allergies, prior adverse reactions to anesthetics, sedation requirements during prior procedures, smoking and alcohol history, and drug or opioid tolerance. Patients with a prior history of opioid or other substance use will invariably require more sedative, and the endoscopist should prepare accordingly. Women of childbearing age should also be asked about the possibility of pregnancy as certain medications are contraindicated.

Pre-procedural medication administration should be undertaken and include beta blockade and bronchodilators as deemed appropriate. Anticoagulation is a significant topic and is discussed in depth later in the chapter. Of all the risks associated with endoscopic procedures, the cardiopulmonary sequelae are the ones most focused upon, and seem to occur at an average rate of 0.27 % overall [6]. Thus far, no pre-procedural intervention, such as pre-oxygenation or administration of a beta blocker or bronchodilator, has been definitively shown to minimize these risks during endoscopy. Modern literature suggests that arrhythmias and hypoxemia may be observed during endoscopic procedures as frequently as 50 % or more of the time [7–9]. Hypoxemia is often vaguely defined, but its reported incidence is associated with upper endoscopy (more frequently than lower endoscopy), deeper sedation, and compression of the airway or laryngospasm from or during esophagogastroduodenoscopy (EGD). There seem to be few clinically significant episodes of hypoxia—such as those necessitating endotracheal intubation—with a reported incidence of 0.001 % [10]. Furthermore, there is little evidence to suggest that the utilization of supplemental oxygen actually changes the incidence of adverse events and some propose that it is associated with a higher rate of unplanned events [11–13]. Arrhythmias during endoscopy are of unclear etiology, and they appear to most frequently be either sinus bradycardia or tachycardia, or supraventricular tachyarrhythmias. Hemodynamically significant arrhythmias are infrequently encountered and may be a sign of impending or active ischemia. Typically arrhythmias are of short duration and are self-limiting. Proposed mechanisms include parasympathetic or sympathetic stimulation, or even hypoxemia. They have been associated with patients who have previous evidence of cardiac disease [6].

Administration of beta blockers seems to reduce the frequency of arrhythmias and prevent tachycardia in some cases [14]. Myocardial ischemic events during endoscopy are infrequent, and less likely to occur during lower endoscopy than upper endoscopy [15]. Upper endoscopy has been shown to be associated with hypoxemia, suggesting that oxygen supplementation during the procedure could act as a preventive measure [16]. Alternatively, others suggest that tachycardia is more to blame than hypoxemia, and thus might be thwarted with peri-procedural beta blockade [17, 18]. The risks of thromboembolic and cerebrovascular events are discussed later in the chapter and have been found to be exceedingly low especially in those whom anticoagulation is not discontinued temporarily [19]. Endoscopy is globally viewed as a relatively low-risk procedure as described by the American Heart Association Guidelines, but should still be viewed as a formidable entity whose risks and benefits must be weighed and expressed to the patient [20].

Assessment of Risk Status for Gastrointestinal Endoscopy

There are several factors that influence the risk of endoscopic procedures and the adverse events that may result. These include the actual procedure being done, as well as the experience and skill of the endoscopic team (physician, nurses, technicians, anesthesia staff, etc.). The patient's physiological and anatomical status is also a major contributing factor. Complications or adverse events (AEs) that could result following endoscopic interventions may be broadly divided into cardiopulmonary adverse events (CP AEs) and noncardiopulmonary adverse events (nCP AEs).

Cardiopulmonary Adverse Events

A retrospective review of the Clinical Outcomes Research Initiative, the largest multicenter endoscopic database, found that cardiopulmonary AEs during moderate sedation constitute a major proportion of endoscopic associated complications. Of the 324,737 endoscopic procedures reviewed, adverse events occurred in 1.4 %, of which 0.9 % were CP AEs [13]. One useful definition of what constitutes a CP AE is that defined by Gangi et al. as any arrhythmia, hypotension, chest pain (or angina equivalent), or myocardial infarction (MI) wherein the event required intervention and occurred within 2 days of the procedure [21]. Factors associated with a higher incidence of CP AEs include the following: patient age, higher American Society of Anesthesiologists (ASA) classification grade, inpatient status, trainee involvement, and nonuniversity hospitals [22]. Cardiopulmonary disease and recent MI may also predict complications.

In a single center study of 233 patients undergoing routine outpatient endoscopic procedures, it was found that there was no significant difference in the rates of transient hypoxia between patients at high and low risk of obstructive sleep apnea (OSA) [23]. This suggests that the majority of patients with no diagnosis of OSA can undergo moderate sedation for routine endoscopic procedures with standard monitoring practices. The risk of AEs with deep sedation or with general anesthesia without endotracheal intubation in patients with OSA is, in contrast, more pronounced.

Non-cardiopulmonary Adverse Events

Non-cardiopulmonary adverse events (nCP AEs) are also of importance in endoscopy. In contrast to CP AEs, which may be dependent on patient co-morbidities, the nCP AEs are more procedure dependent.

Colonoscopy and Predictors of nCP AEs (See Chap. 17)

Non-cardiopulmonary adverse events as sequelae to colonoscopic procedures are very rare. Certain interventions undertaken during colonoscopy are known to increase the possibility of incurring complications such as bleeding and perforation. Patients older than 65 years have a higher propensity for both bleeding and perforation compared to their younger counterparts. Rarely, splenic injury has been reported as an adverse event and is related to a difficult procedure in which significant scope manipulation in the area of the splenic flexure is necessary for completion. Polypectomy is one of the most important predictors of clinically significant bleeding, which occurs in ~1 % of cases. If no polypectomy is performed, bleeding occurs in approximately 1.6/1,000 cases [24–28]. As would be expected, polypectomy also increases the risk of perforation (up to 0.5 %), whereas it is exceedingly rare if polypectomy is not performed (~0.1 %) [24, 25, 28–31]. Although polyp size has been shown to increase the risk of bleeding, neither polyp morphology nor technique employed for resection has been conclusively demonstrated to influence risk for bleeding or perforation [25, 32, 33]. The risk of infection is extremely low from either diagnostic or therapeutic colonoscopy.

However, post-polypectomy syndrome may occur, wherein patients develop fever, abdominal pain, leukocytosis, and peritoneal inflammation after polypectomy is performed. There is no frank perforation, by definition, but the electrical current applied at the time of polypectomy extends beyond the mucosa into the muscularis propria and serosa, thus causing peritoneal inflammation. This is also a very uncommon occurrence, with an incidence ranging from 0 to 1.2 % in four studies [34–37]. Post-polypectomy syndrome occurs most often after the removal of large (>2 cm) sessile polyps, as these polyps usually necessitate large amounts of electrosurgical energy applied for long periods of time [37]. Table 4.1 summarizes the nCP AEs associated with colonoscopy.

Esophagogastroduodenoscopy and Predictors of nCP AEs (See Chap. 14)

Diagnostic upper endoscopy carries some risk that is primarily associated with sedation. In addition, as summarized in Table 4.2, therapeutic interventions done during EGD are associated with some of the same risks seen in colonoscopy, including bleeding, perforation, and infection. Studies have revealed several factors, which may increase the risk of perforation. These include polypectomy, endoscopic mucosal resection (EMR), dilation (achalasia more than nonachalasia), variceal therapy, hemostatic procedures, stenting, and foreign body removal [38–49]. Stricture formation is another adverse event which increases with EMR, variceal therapy, and ablative procedures [38, 43, 47, 50, 51]. While infection is a very rare occurrence, peristomal infection after percutaneous endoscopic gastrostomy (PEG) tubes seem to be increased if peri-procedural antibiotics are not administered [52].

Endoscopic Retrograde Cholangiopancreatography and Predictors of nCP AEs (See Chap. 19)

Endoscopic retrograde cholangiopancreatography (ERCP) has much of the same adverse events as EGD and colonoscopy, including bleeding, perforation, and infection. Pancreatitis is also a significant adverse event associated with ERCP. Table 4.3 documents the adverse events associated with ERCP. Infections are more frequent with ERCP than with EGD or colonoscopy though still an uncommon occurrence. Jaundiced patients and liver transplant patients are at increased risk of infection (OR 1.4 and 5.2, respectively) [53, 54].

The risk of bleeding is affected by several factors particularly if a therapeutic procedure is performed (sphincterotomy OR 4.7) [55]. There has not been a demonstrably increased risk with antiplatelet agents, but restarting anticoagulants within 3 days has been shown to increase the risk of bleeding [56]. Patients with coagulopathy or cholangitis are also at increased risk of bleeding [56].

Table 4.1 Colonoscopy and predictors of non-cardiopulmonary adverse events

Adverse event	Modifying factor	Risk magnitude (OR)	Comments
Infection			Very rare
Bleeding[a]	Polypectomy (vs. no polypectomy)	10.3	Very rare (1.6/1,000) without polypectomy; uncommon with polypectomy (<1 %); one study found higher risk with biopsy alone but may have included self-limited bleeding
	Age	1.4 (>65 years); 1.6 (>60 years); 1.03 per year	
	Year/era	1.7/5 year period in past	Bleeding seems to be decreasing with time
	Male sex	1.2–9.2	Unexplained, and possibly due to uncorrected confounders
	Nonscreening/nonsurveillance indication	1.3	May have included minor self-limited bleeding
	Polyp size	2.4–28 for >10 mm; 1.1/1 mm increase; 12 f or 5–10 mm vs. 5 mm	
	Polyp number	1.1–1.3	
	Anticoagulation after polypectomy	3.7–13.4 (current), 5.2 (resumed within 1 week)	One study showed greater relative risk increase with small polyps
	Antiplatelets	3.7 for clopidogrel plus aspirin or NSAID	No increase risk with aspirin or clopidogrel alone, but the combination increases bleeding
	Cardiovascular disease[b]	2.1	Hypertension, ischemic or valvular heart disease for >6 months, an arrhythmia requiring medication, or cerebrovascular disease
	Renal disease[b]	3.3	Serum creatinine level of >3 mg/dL for >6 months
	Polyp morphology[b]	1.4 for sessile in one study; 1.5 for peduncular in another study	Sessile, semipedunculated, or lateral spreading vs. others; other studies did not see a difference
	Pure cutting current[b]	7.0	Also inadvertent cold polypectomy had higher risk (OR 7.2); pure coagulation current may trade off a decrease in immediate for an increase in delayed bleeding
	Poor bowel prep[b]	1.5	Adequate or poor higher risk than good or excellent
Perforation	Polypectomy	2.3–3.0	Rare (~0.1 %) without polypectomy, uncommon (0.5 %) after polypectomy
	Age	2.1(>60 years)	
	Comorbidities	3.0	Deyo score of ≥3 based on Charlson index
	Renal failure, on dialysis	19.2	
Splenic injury	Female sex	–	Very, very rare (0.001 %); predictors reported based on literature review
	Difficult procedure	–	

Modified from [32]. Used with permission from the Copyright Clearance Center. License Number: 2747710078744

NSAID nonsteroidal anti-inflammatory drug, *OR* odds ratio

[a]Apart from polypectomy, other risk factors for bleeding are only within the postpolypectomy group and do not necessarily apply to cases without polypectomy; the odds ratios for these other factors are with respect to the lower risk category of polyps, not vs. no polypectomy at all

[b]Many of these factors were not found by other studies, and this study was mainly of immediate bleeding (4 % bleeding rate, most stopping within 60 s) rather than clinically important delayed bleeding

Patients with postsurgical anatomy are also at a higher risk of perforation (discussed later in chapter) [53, 55]. Other modifying factors which increase the risk of perforation include intramural contrast injection and sphincterotomy [53].

Endoscopic Ultrasound (EUS) and predictors of nCP AEs (See Chap. 19)

The risk of infection after EUS is increased if a fine needle aspiration (FNA) of a pancreatic cyst is performed [57]. Transrectal and transcolonic FNAs also increase the risk of infection [58, 59]. The literature is limited with regard to post EUS bleeding, but this is a rare event. Perforation is similarly rare, although cervical esophageal perforation (particularly in older patients who have previously had a difficult intubation) has been reported [60].

Pneumoperitoneum may occur as an iatrogenic complication of nontraumatic diagnostic upper gastrointestinal endoscopy and ERCP [61, 62]. This is an uncommon occurrence and usually implies bowel perforation. Pneumoperitoneum complicating EUS-FNA followed by ERCP has been reported and is more common than pneumoperitoneum occurring

Table 4.2 Esophagogastroduodenoscopy and predictors of noncardiopulmonary adverse events

Adverse event	Modifying factor	Comments
Infection		Very rare
Bleeding (delayed)	Polypectomy	Very rare without polypectomy; 5–15 % with polypectomy; OR 8.1 if immediate bleeding at gastric EMR
	Variceal therapy	Sclerotherapy (25 %) greater than banding (6 %)
	Hemostasis (nonvariceal)	
Perforation	Polypectomy	Rare [~0.5 % of EMR; higher (about 5–10 %) with ESD]
	Dilation (of achalasia)	2–3 % in meta-analyses of pneumatic dilation
	Dilation (nonachalasia)	Higher with Maloney, 10 % perforation in anastomotic strictures in children, 5 % anastomotic strictures in adults, 15–20 % post-caustic ingestion, 2 % radiation stricture
	EGD in eosinophilic esophagitis (with or without dilation)	Can occur even with passage of an endoscope, but mucosal tears are much more common than true perforations, which seem rare
	Variceal therapy	Sclerotherapy, 2 %
	Foreign body	No perforation in 2 series of food impactions
	Stent	Review, 7–15 %
	Hemostasis (nonvariceal)	Low risk (<1 %) unless sclerosants used; very rare with nonsclerosant monotherapy
	Ablation	20 % after photodynamic therapy (n = 102)
Stricture	Variceal therapy	Sclerotherapy, 26 %; much greater than banding 2 %
	EMR	5–25 % of esophageal EMR (especially if circumferential resection, ≤70 %); 3 % for peripyloric

Modified from [32]. Used with permission from the Copyright Clearance Center. License Number: 2747710078744
EGD esophagogastroduodenoscopy, *EMR* endoscopic mucosal resection

after EUS-FNA alone, which has just a single case report [63, 64]. Proposed mechanisms for this complication include air dissecting interstitially through perineural or perivascular sheaths that are subjected to high intraluminal pressures [65]. Other postulations include air entering the peritoneum through an ulcer base or some other mucosal break [65]. Retroduodenal perforation is also rare after EUS but may occur as a complication after ERCP. This may occur from a sphincterotomy extending beyond the intramural portion of the bile duct or pancreatic duct [63]. The incidence of retroduodenal perforation after sphincterotomy ranges from 0.3 to 1.4 % [66, 67].

When ERCP and EUS/FNA are being performed under the same sedation for complementary diagnostic information and to reduce overall procedure time and cost, some propose ERCP to precede EUS/FNA to reduce to these risks [63]. Presentation may vary from asymptomatic to abdominal discomfort and distension, nausea, vomiting, leukocytosis, fever, and frank peritonitis. Conservative management with extremely close observation, as opposed to laparotomy, is often successful for the treatment of pneumoperitoneum or retroperitoneal air seen in these patients [63, 68, 69]. This includes making the patient nil per os (NPO) and starting IV fluids and antibiotics. Decompression via computed tomography guided drainage with a transabdominal catheter into the pneumoperitoneum has also been shown to be an effec-

tive treatment [69]. However, as peritonitis may be indicative of a life threatening process, close observation by a surgeon and early operative intervention must always be considered.

As with ERCP, patients with surgically altered anatomy may be at increased risk of perforation, particularly if the endoscopist is unfamiliar with these alterations [60]. Pancreatitis is very rare after EUS, particularly if an FNA is not performed [70–72]. Bile leak, though rare, may be increased in patients who have a gallbladder FNA performed [73]. Table 4.4 summarizes these adverse events and associated modifying factors.

It is not uncommon for patients with surgically altered anatomy to required endoscopic procedures. Understanding the underlying anatomy is essential to accurately interpret the endoscopic findings in these patients. The following points may aide in the successful completion of endoscopic procedures in patients with surgically altered gastrointestinal anatomy:

1. Review the patient's surgical report, paying particular attention to the extent of anatomic resection, the length of surgically created limbs of bowel, the type of reconstruction (e.g., Billroth I or Billroth II) and anastomosis (e.g., end to side vs. side to side)
2. Review any postoperative imaging studies available
3. Select an appropriate endoscope and accessories depending on the patients anatomy

Table 4.3 ERCP and predictors of noncardiopulmonary adverse events

Adverse event	Modifying factor	Risk magnitude (OR)	Comment(s)
Infection	Liver transplant	5.2	Very rare (0.25–0.5 %) (risk decreasing with time: OR 0.9 per year)
	Fistulae, nondrainable ducts (e.g., hilar, intrahepatic strictures)		
	Ductoscopy		
	Jaundice	1.4	
	Small center	1.4	
Bleeding (delayed)	Sphincterotomy	4.7	Very rare; can also occur with large balloon sphincteroplasty; no increased risk with antiplatelet agents
	Small center	1.1	
	Intraprocedure bleeding	1.7	
	Coagulopathy	3.3	
	Anticoagulation within 3 days[a]	5.1	
	Cholangitis[a]	2.6	
	Small-volume endoscopist[a]	2.2 (>1/week) 53	Defined as >2 s prothrombin time, hemodialysis or platelet count >80,000/mm^3
Perforation	Postsurgical anatomy	2.5	
	Precut sphincterotomy	2.0	
	Intramural contrast	1.9	
	Sphincterotomy		Rare
Pancreatitis[b]	Suspected SOD	1.9–9.7	Biliary sphincterotomy is not a risk factor
	Female	1.8–3.5	
	Post-ERCP pancreatitis (prior)	5.4	
	Younger age	1.1/5-year decrease; 1.1 (age <70 years); 1.6 (age <60 years)	
	Normal bile dect	1.05	
	Normal bilirubin	1.9	
	No chronic pancreatitis	1.9	
	Nonuniversity center	2.0	
	Difficult cannulation	1.8–9.4	Early precut sphincterotomy may reduce risk vs. persistence
	Pancreatic sphincterotomy	1.5–3.8	
	Pancreatic injection	1.04–1.5	Most studies define as any injection
	No pancreatic stenting	1.4–3.2	Significant in high-risk ERCP, especially SOD
	Trainee involvement	1.5	
	Balloon sphincteroplasty	2.0	For stone disease, heterogeneous studies

Modified from [32]. Used with permission from the Copyright Clearance Center. License Number: 2747710078744

OR odds ratio, *SOD* sphincter of Oddi dysfunction, *ERCP* endoscopic retrograde cholangiopancreatography

[a]These risk factors were determined only in sphincterotomy subgroup and do not necessarily predict bleeding in all ERCPs.

[b]As is evident in this section, some factors have more consensus than others on their role as a risk factor for post-ERCP pancreatitis; factors only found significant in one of many studies may or may not be true risk factors

Some of the more common types of prior foregut surgical operations that patients presenting to the endoscopist have undergone include the following:

- Billroth I gastrectomy
- Billroth II gastrectomy
- Total gastrectomy with esophagojejunostomy
- Roux-en-Y gastrojejunostomy
- Gastric bypass for obesity
- Roux-en-Y hepaticojejunostomy
- Whipple operation (pancreaticoduodenectomy)
  - Classic
  - Pylorus-preserving
- Choledochoduodenostomy
- Antireflux operations
- Myotomy for achalasia
- Esophagectomy

Endoscopic considerations regarding each of these are discussed in later chapters. Similar consideration should be

Table 4.4 EUS and predictors of noncardiopulmonary adverse events

Adverse event	Modifying factor[a]	Comments
Infection	FNA	Very rare with FNA
	Pancreatic cysts	Rare (0.2 %), especially with antibiotic prophylaxis; risk factors thought to include incomplete drainage, multiple punctures
	Mediastinal cysts	Common and can be severe; FNA best avoided
	Transrectal/colonic FNA	Uncommon (4 %); good prep critical
	Celiac block	Rare
Bleeding (delayed)	FNA	Very rare (1–4 %), mostly intraluminal
Perforation	Age, difficult intubation, inexperience	0.03 % cervical esophageal perforation (older patient, history of difficult esophageal intubation, inexperienced operator)
Pancreatitis	FNA	Very rare
	FNA of pancreas mass	Very rare without FNA, rare with FNA (1–2 %); placement of fiducials can be associated with pancreatitis
	FNA for nonfocal chronic pancreatitis	Seems much higher than for masses, especially if Trucut is used (13 %); intracystic brushing may increase risk
Bile leak	Gallbladder FNA	High risk (>50 %), not recommended
Pneumothorax	Lung mass FNA	Very rare

Modified from [32]. Used with permission from the Copyright Clearance Center. License Number: 2747710078744

FNA fine needle aspiration

[a]Adjusted odds ratios not clear for any of these risk factors as they have not been subject to multivariate analysis

given to patients with surgically altered large bowel anatomy who require colonoscopy and who may require unique equipment (e.g., double balloon-assisted colonoscopies). Several studies show that colonoscopies are technically more difficult to perform in women than men, especially in women who have undergone abdominal and gynecological operations. This is likely due to post-surgical pelvic adhesions. While hysterectomy makes traversing the sigmoid colon with the colonoscope more painful and difficult, it does not significantly diminish the cecal intubation rate, alter procedure discomfort, or sedative dose required. Furthermore, hysterectomized women who have also had a sigmoid resection appear to more easily complete colonoscopy [74, 75].

Patients should also be asked about any smoking, drug or alcohol history. Allergies to anesthetics as well as sedation requirements during prior procedures should also be ascertained. Patients with increased opioid or alcohol tolerance will likely require more sedative.

Other considerations that need to be addressed by the endoscopist include the management of patients with implanted medical devices such as cardiac pacemakers and implanted cardioverter-defibrillators and patients who require anticoagulation for prior medical conditions. These along with the management and use of antibiotic prophylaxis are addressed later in the chapter.

Physical Exam

An assessment of the mental status of the patient initiates the physical exam. Patients who have no mental status deficiencies, minimal anxiety, and consent to participate in the procedure require minimal to no sedation. General anesthesia may be required for patients with high levels of anxiety, mental retardation, or any neurologic condition that may limit the ability of the patient to actively participate in the procedure.

Examination of the patient's oral and neck anatomy as well as overall body habitus should then be performed. Mallampati classification (see Fig. 5.1) helps guide management of patients in whom bag-mask ventilation and/or intubation may be difficult [76, 77]. This is done by placing the patient in the sitting position. Next the patient is asked to open his/her mouth and protrude the tongue. An assessment of the visualization of the posterior pharynx is then performed. A Mallampati classification of III predicts difficulty with bag-mask ventilation, and Mallampati classification of IV predicts difficulty with both bag-mask ventilation and intubation [76]. The body habitus of a patient is also important when assessing for sedation risks, as obesity also predicts difficulty with intubation [4].

The cardiopulmonary examination should focus on the presence of any underlying dysrhythmias, murmurs, or respiratory findings. Examination of the abdomen is also important. Pre-procedural findings such as tenderness and distention should be noted and not mistaken for post-procedural onset. The presence of any previous surgical scars or hernias should also be noted. Oral and nasal piercing is of particular concern because of the risks of swallowing and aspiration. Consequently, patients should be advised to remove piercing before anesthesia [78]. Emergency situations are especially risky and anesthesiologists should be aware of the piercing removal techniques. In case of piercing loss, endoscopy of the upper airway and digestive tract

Table 4.5 American Society of Anesthesiologists (ASA) physical status classification

ASA classification	Definition	Example
I	A normal healthy patient	28-year-old male with no past medical history, present for screening colonoscopy due to first degree relative with early colorectal cancer
II	Mild systemic disease	50-year-old female with controlled type-2 diabetes mellitus and hypertension
III	Severe systemic disease	65-year-old male with chronic obstructive pulmonary disease and history of a cerebrovascular accident
IV	Severe systemic disease that is a constant threat to life	45-year-old female with end stage renal disease due to lupus nephropathy
V	Moribund and not expected to survive without the operation	75-year-old male who suffered a stroke, now with multisystem organ failure, and acute onset lower gastrointestinal bleed

should be performed to eliminate aspiration or swallowing of the foreign body.

Using the data from the history and physical examination, the patient is then risk stratified for the procedure using then American Society of Anesthesiologists (ASA) physical status classification. Explanations of the ASA classifications, with patient examples, are seen in Table 4.5. Increasing ASA classification correlates with increased incidence of adverse outcomes following sedation administration [79].

Informed Consent

After the appropriate workup has been completed, informed consent must be obtained prior to proceeding with the endoscopic procedure. The risks and benefits of the specific procedure should be explained. These risks, summarized in Tables 4.1–4.4, include the following:
1. Colonoscopy: Bleeding, infection, colonic perforation, splenic injury.
2. EGD: Bleeding, infection, perforation, strictures.
3. ERCP: Bleeding, infection, perforation, pancreatitis.
4. EUS: Bleeding, infection, perforation, pancreatitis, bile leak, pneumothorax.

Beyond these risks, patients taking anticoagulation medication should also be counseled regarding the risk of bleeding or thromboembolism depending on the underlying condition requiring the anticoagulation and whether or not the anticoagulant is continued or stopped. These risks are discussed later in the chapter.

Management of Patients with Cardiac Pacemakers and Implanted Cardioverter-Defibrillators

Patients with implanted electronic devices (IEDs) are often encountered in the endoscopy suite. Among the more common devices encountered are cardiac pacemakers and implantable cardioverter-defibrillators. Given that electrosurgical energy is often necessary during endoscopy, it is critical for the endoscopist to be aware of interference with IEDs and the potential injury to patients that may occur.

Understanding the differences between unipolar and bipolar/multipolar electrocautery is also key. In unipolar cautery, current flows from the electrosurgical device (ED) through the patient then to the dispersive electrode (aka "grounding pad") before terminating back at the generator. The grounding pad serves as the return electrode. In bipolar/multipolar electrocautery however, current flows from one or more electrodes on the ED, through the patient's tissues in the immediate vicinity of the ED, and then back to one or more electrodes on the ED. The electromagnetic field (EMF) generated in bipolar and multipolar cautery is subsequently often negligible.

Some of the more common applications of monopolar cautery include the following:
1. Performing endoscopic polypectomy (mainly in the stomach or colon).
2. Endoscopic sphincterotomy of the pancreatic or biliary sphincters.
3. "Hot biopsy"—in which the base of small polyps are simultaneously coagulated and ablated
4. Argon plasma coagulation used in ablating mucosal lesions or for hemostasis.

Bipolar electrocautery however is more often used in cases of vascular lesions or hemorrhaging ulcers where local control of hemorrhage is desired or in mucosal ablation.

Implanted electronic devices can be affected by either a conducted EMF (e.g., electrosurgery) or a radiated EMF (such as in magnetic resonance imaging). This effect is called electromagnetic interference (EMI). The amount of EMI that occurs depends on both the sensitivity of the implanted device and also on properties of ED [80]. These variables are noted in Table 4.6 [80–83].

Applied electrosurgical currents in patients with IEDs could, in theory, be manifested in the following ways [80, 82].
1. The output of the IED may be inhibited or triggered, depending on whether the EMI is interpreted as physiologic or pathophysiologic. ICDs could discharge if the EMI is interpreted as ventricular fibrillation, and similarly pacemakers may be inhibited if the EMI is interpreted as intrinsic cardiac activity.

Table 4.6 The amount of EMI that occurs depends on both the sensitivity of the implanted device and also on properties of ED

Variables that determine the sensitivity of an IED to an EMF [79]	Properties of the ED that affects the EMI [79]
Distance between the anode and cathode of the implanted device	Intensity of the generated EMF
Programmed sensitivity of the IED to electrical signals	Cutting current > coagulation current [80]
Number of leads, if any	Waveform of the generated signal
Implanted devices programmed to use bipolar sensing are less likely to experience EMI	Frequency of the generated signal
	Distance between the site being cauterized and the leads of the IED

EMI electromagnetic interference, *ED* electrosurgical device, *EMF* electromagnetic field, *IED* implanted electronic devices

2. The IED may reset to any of several preset manufacturer modes if the signal is interpreted as noise.
3. The tissue immediately adjacent to the implanted device could be damaged if sufficient current passes through the implanted leads.
4. Conduction of a continuous series of electric impulses may occur down the implanted leads, resulting in stimulation of the target tissue (e.g., ventricular or atrial fibrillation with CPs or ICDs).
5. The IED and/or its battery may be permanently damaged with very high levels of current.

Most of the above theoretical situations, in particular 3, 4, and 5, are improbable in the setting of gastrointestinal endoscopy as the current source is not in sufficiently close proximity to the pulse generator or implanted leads [80, 82].

Current guidelines from the American Society for Gastrointestinal Endoscopy are as follows: [80, 82]

1. Determine the type of IED present
2. Determine patient's physiologic indication for the device prior to endoscopy (e.g., The patient's underlying cardiac rhythm and the degree of pacemaker dependence)
3. When possible, use endoscopic techniques/devices that produce limited or no EMF. Examples include bipolar/multipolar current, sutures, clips etc.
4. Apply electrosurgical energy for the shortest duration necessary, and use as low a power setting as possible.
5. Place the grounding pad far away from the pulse generator and leads in a manner that does not place the IED and leads between the grounding pad and the cautery source.
6. Avoid applying electrosurgical energy cautery within 15 cm of the IED
7. Use continuous pulse oximetry and EKG monitoring during the procedure
8. Have appropriate equipment available should there be an adverse event directly related to device malfunction/interference. This should include equipment for resuscitation and cardioversion-defibrillation.
9. Most patients with CPs may undergo routine gastrointestinal endoscopic electrosurgery without changes in management.
10. When prolonged electrosurgery is anticipated in patients with CPs, consider placing a magnet over the pulse generator during the use of electrocautery. This causes the CP to work in asynchronous mode.
11. Consultation with a cardiologist is recommended when patients with an ICD is scheduled to undergo any electrosurgery. Consider deactivating the ICD and if so, continuous rhythm monitoring should be done. ICDs should be reprogrammed as soon as the procedure is completed but not before discontinuing rhythm monitoring.
12. In the case where a patient has both an ICD and a CP and the CP cannot be reprogrammed to an asynchronous mode, use bipolar energyor a device with no EMF whenever possible.

Since the publication of these guidelines, one prospective study evaluating patients with ICDs undergoing endoscopic procedures found that no EMI or arrhythmic events were triggered during endoscopic procedures in patients with pectorally implanted transvenous ICDs [83]. This suggests that the current routine practice of reprogramming ICDs for gastrointestinal endoscopy may not be necessary. Of note, only monopolar electrosurgery was used in that study.

Anticoagulation in the Peri-endoscopic Period

Management of patients on anticoagulation in the peri-endoscopic period requires weighing the risk of thromboembolism from discontinuation of the drugs against the risk of procedure-related bleeding. Depending on the risk involved, it should be determined if active reversal with or without bridging therapy is required. Additionally, the timing of restarting anticoagulation after the procedure needs to be ascertained. The risk of bleeding associated with endoscopic procedures can be grouped into low and high-risk procedures, <1 % and >1 % risk, respectively (Table 4.7). Furthermore, the risk of thromboembolism for which patients are anticoagulated is similarly categorized into low and high-risk conditions (Table 4.8).

Risk of Thromboembolism Related to Patient Co-morbidity

Atrial Fibrillation

Atrial Fibrillation (AF) is among the more common reasons for a patient to be anticoagulated. The lifetime risk of thromboembolism from AF without anticoagulation in patients over the age of 40 years is ~0.25 %. This increases to 1.3 %

Table 4.7 Risk of bleeding from procedures [84–86, 93]

Low risk (<1 %)	High risk (>1 %)
Diagnostic endoscopy with or without biopsy – EGD – Flexible sigmoidoscopy – Colonoscopy	Polypectomy – Gastric – Duodenal/ampullary – Colonic
ERCP without dilation or sphincterotomy	PEG
Biliary/pancreatic stenting without sphincterotomy	Mucosectomy
EUS without FNA	Esophageal stenting
Push enteroscopy	FNA by EUS
ERCP without dilation or sphincterotomy	Laser ablation and coagulation Endoscopic sphincterotomy Ampullectomy Pneumatic or bougie dilation Variceal treatment

EGD esophagogastroduodenoscopy, *EUS* endoscopic ultrasound, *FNA* fine need aspiration, *ERCP* endoscopic retrograde cholangiopancreatography, *PEG* polyethylene glycol

Table 4.8 Condition risk for thromboembolism [84–86, 93]

Low risk	High risk
>3 months after DVT	0–3 months after DVT
Nonvalvular atrial fibrillation without risk factors	Atrial fibrillation with some risk factors
Mechanic valve in the aortic position	Mechanical valve in the mitral position
	Prosthetic heart valves in two positions
	Mechanical valve and prior thromboembolic event
	First generation heart valves (caged-ball or disk valves)
	Recent acute coronary event (<6 weeks)
	Severe left ventricular dysfunction

DVT deep vein thrombosis

per patient-year for patients aged 50–59 and 5.1 % for patients between ages 80–89 years [84]. Warfarin is the most commonly used drug for AF and in one large retrospective study was shown to reduce the risk of systemic embolism by 71 % when compared to placebo, and 50 % when compared to antiplatelet therapy alone. Compared to placebo however, there is a statistically increased risk of bleeding (OR 3.1) for patients placed on warfarin therapy, while there is no significant increased bleeding risk when compared to antiplatelet therapy. For anticoagulated patients undergoing endoscopy, the 30-day stroke risk is 1.17 % per procedure should there be adjustments in their anticoagulation. The risk ranged from 0.31 % for otherwise healthy patients to 2.93 % in patients with multiple co-morbidities. There were no strokes in patients whose anticoagulation was not altered or discontinued [19].

Cardiovascular Disease and Coronary Stents

Patients who are anticoagulated for underlying cardiovascular disease are also at increased risk of adverse events should their anticoagulation be held. This risk is highest in patients with acute myocardial infarction (MI) and lowest in those on antiplatelet therapy for primary prevention of cardiovascular events. In a meta-analysis of 135,000 patients, antiplatelet therapy reduced the occurrence of vascular events by 25 %, nonfatal MI by one-third, nonfatal stroke by one-quarter, and vascular mortality by one-sixth. Furthermore, clopidogrel reduced serious vascular events by 10 % compared with aspirin [87].

Patients with coronary stents also require anticoagulation as stent thrombosis carries a very high risk of severe morbidity and mortality. Patients with angiographic evidence of stent thrombosis in one study had a 64.4 % incidence of death or myocardial infarction at the time of stent thrombosis and an 8.9 % 6-month mortality [88]. Guidelines for patients with bare metal stents recommend using antiplatelet therapy with high dose aspirin and clopidogrel for a minimum of 6 weeks after percutaneous coronary intervention. After this these patients require the use of low dose aspirin. Because re-endothelialization of bare metal stents is incomplete during the first month, an interruption of antiplatelet therapy during this time presumably carries a high risk of stent thrombosis. In drug eluting stents, there is an even more pronounced delay in re-endothelialization and guidelines recommend patients continue on dual antiplatelet therapy for 1 year [89].

Prosthetic Valves

Current guidelines recommend that all patients with mechanical valves be anticoagulated with warfarin. The risk of major systemic embolization in patients with mechanical valves is 4 per 100 patient years without anticoagulation, 2.2 per 100 patient years with antiplatelet therapy, and 1 per 100 patient years with warfarin [90]. Prosthetic valves in the mitral position confer a higher risk compared to the aortic position (1.3 major embolic events per 100 patient years vs. 0.8, respectively) [90]. Other factors which increase risk include advanced age, persistent AF, multiple valve prostheses, previous thromboembolism and left ventricular dysfunction. Most endoscopists will hold anticoagulation for ≤7 days peri-procedurally. While there have not been any specific studies looking at cessation of anticoagulation in patients with prosthetic valves peri-endoscopically, the aforementioned risk of major systemic embolization (4 per 100 patient years) translates to a 0.08 % risk of thromboembolism in a 7 day period. In one study, none of 159 patients with prosthetic valves undergoing 180 non-cardiac operations, with an average perioperative cessation of 6.6 days had a thromboembolic event [91].

Venous Thromboembolism

The risk of recurrence of venous thromboembolism (VTE) in patients who have their anticoagulation temporarily stopped for endoscopic procedures has not been well studied. Patients with symptomatic proximal deep venous thrombosis (DVT) or pulmonary embolus (PE) who are not anticoagulated are at greatest risk of recurrence during the first month (~50 %). Warfarin reduces the 1-month risk to roughly 10 %, and 3 months of treatment reduces the risk to 5 %. If ceasing anticoagulation is necessary for a high-risk endoscopic procedure within the first 2 weeks after VTE, then consideration should be given to placement of a vena cava filter. Current guidelines from the American College of Chest Physicians recommend an anticoagulation period of 3 months in VTE in the context of a risk factor, a minimum of 3 months in the first episode of unprovoked VTE, and indefinite therapy for second/recurrent VTE [84, 92].

Drug-Related Bleeding Risk in Periendoscopic Period

Warfarin

Warfarin inhibits vitamin K-dependent coagulation factor synthesis (II, VII, IX, X, proteins C and S) and has a half-life of between 20 and 60 h depending on the rate of clotting factor catabolism. Should the common target INR of 1.5 be desired, it will take approximately 4 days in most patients for the INR to fall to 1.5 from 2.0 to 3.0, or 5 days if starting from an INR of ~2.5–3.5 [93]. One study that retrospectively reviewed 1,657 patients who underwent colonoscopic polypectomy on either anticoagulation or antiplatelet agents found that warfarin use was an independent risk factor for bleeding (OR: 13.37) [94].

Aspirin and Non-steroidal Anti-inflammatory Drugs

Aspirin and non-steroidal anti-inflammatory drugs (NSAIDs) inhibit platelet cyclooxygenase which reduces prostaglandin and thromboxane synthesis. Thromboxane promotes platelet aggregation and as such aspirin and NSAIDs irreversibly render platelets non-functional for the 7–10 days of its lifespan. Selective COX-2 inhibitors such as celecoxib do not alter platelet functionality. In vivo studies have shown that aspirin, but not NSAIDs, may prolong colonic mucosal bleeding times. However, how this translates clinically is not certain. No difference in post-polypectomy bleeding was found in one case-controlled study with patients on aspirin/ NSAIDs with matched controls [84]. This corroborates findings from other studies [95]. The effect of aspirin/ NSAIDs on post-sphincterotomy bleeding is less clear.

Clopidogrel

Clopidogrel is a thienopyridine and it inhibits adenosine diphosphate-induced platelet aggregation. Other less commonly used thienopyridines are prasugrel and ticlopidine. Prasugrel is newer and has a more potent antiplatelet activity but also has a significantly higher risk of bleeding compared to clopidogrel, particularly in stroke patients and the elderly. Ticlopidine is also not frequently used due to its increased risk of thrombotic thrombocytopenic purpura and neutropenia [84].

Clopidogrel and Aspirin have recently been studied in a prospective randomized study to evaluate their bleeding risk in patients undergoing gastroduodenal biopsies. Of the total 630 patients (350 patients taking clopidogrel and 280 taking aspirin), there were no clinical bleeding events in either group, and only one patient (from the aspirin group) experienced an endoscopic bleeding event [96]. The risk of bleeding is increased when both aspirin and clopidogrel are used in combination. In the Management of Atherothrombosis with Clopidogrel in High Risk Patients (MATCH) study, the rate of life threatening GI-bleeding was 0.6 % in the clopidogrel group, compared to 1.4 % in the combined aspirin and clopidogrel groups. Also, major GI bleeding occurred at a rate of 0.9 % in the clopidogrel group compared to 1.12 % in the combined group [97].

Glycoprotein IIA/IIIB Inhibitors

These antiplatelet agents are primarily used in acute coronary syndromes and coronary stent implantation. They include abciximab, tirofiban, and eptifibatide. The antiplatelet effects can be partially reversed by platelet infusion or by DDAVP but should only be stopped when there is a life-threatening hemorrhage.

Dipyridamole

Dipyridamole is also an antiplatelet agent and is mainly used in combination with aspirin for secondary prevention of TIAs and ischemic strokes. It does not seem to increase the risk of GI bleeding on its own or further increase the bleeding risk of aspirin when used in combination with aspirin. The ASGE guidelines propose that endoscopic procedures may be performed without cessation of the drug when used at standard doses for non-high-risk procedures [98].

Fondaparinux

Fondaparinux indirectly inhibits factor Xa by inducing a conformational change in antithrombin III. It is not a LMWH, but is FDA approved for perioperative VTE prophylaxis and for initial DVT and PE treatment. It is not ideal as bridging therapy owing to its extremely long half-life (17–21 h).

Bridging Therapy

Unfractionated Heparin and Low Molecular Weight Heparin

Patients who will require temporary cessation of anticoagulation may also require bridging therapy. This is generally achieved with unfractionated heparin (UFH) or with LMWH. The LMWHs are clotting factor Xa inhibitors but have less effect on thrombin in comparison to UFH. Because they are renally excreted, caution should be taken in patients with renal insufficiency. They can be administered subcutaneously owing to their longer half-life as compared to UFH (4.5–7 h vs. 1.5–2 h). This allows for outpatient administration, which provides a cost benefit, as opposed to UFH, which is administered IV and requires hospitalization. LMWH has also been observed to have a similar safety profile in comparison to UFH and is usually preferred when bridging is required [99].

Reversal Agents

Several anticoagulant reversal agents are available should a risk–benefit analyses determine that reversal is advisable. Warfarin is fully reversed with oral or intravenous (IV) vitamin K. Vitamin K has a slow onset, however, with effects not starting until approximately 6 h after administration, and full effect not reached until 24 h. The IV route has a faster onset of action compared to oral, but is associated with more side effects including anaphylactic reactions. While awaiting the effects of Vitamin K, fresh frozen plasma (FFP) or prothrombin complex may be administered. FFP requires blood type ABO compatibility, however, and as with any blood product has a side effect profile that includes transfusion reactions and transmission of infections. Heparin, and to a lesser extent Low Molecular Weight Heparin (LMWH), can be reversed with protamine sulfate. However, given their relatively short half-lives, reversal prior to endoscopy is often unnecessary as cessation of the drug will usually suffice. Fondaparinux which is often used for DVT prophylaxis in heparin induced thrombocytopenia (HIT) positive patients has a longer half-life and can be reversed with activated factor VII. Reversal of antiplatelet agents such as aspirin and NSAIDs is often done with platelet transfusion and/or DDAVP, although the utility of platelet transfusion is not evidence based. Furthermore,

Table 4.9 Warfarin management based on procedure risk and patient risk [84, 93]

	Low-risk procedure	High-risk procedure
Low-risk patient	No change in warfarinization. Delay elective procedures if INR supratherapeutic	Hold warfarin 3–5 days before procedure. Consider giving vitamin K 1 day prior to procedure if INR >1.5 (or FFP immediately before the procedure)
High-risk patient	No change in warfarinization. Delay elective procedures if INR supratherapeutic	Hold Warfarin 3–5 days before procedure and bridge with LMWH[a]/UFH[b]

INR international normalized ratio, *FFP* fresh frozen plasma, *LMWH* low molecular weight heparin

[a]The last dose of LMWH should be given at either half-dose 24 h pre-procedure (for patients receiving once-daily dosing) or the morning dose the day of the procedure (for patients receiving twice-daily dosing)

[b]UFH may be held 4–6 h before the procedure

the side effect profile of platelet transfusion should be considered. Clopidogrel and the glycoprotein Iia/IIIb inhibitors (e.g., Abciximab, eptifibatide, and tirofiban) may also be reversed with platelet infusion and DDAVP.

Summary for Holding, Bridging, Reversal, and Reinstitution

While specific guidelines for management of anticoagulation during endoscopic procedures are not widely available or clear, one is able to coordinate anticoagulation in a manner similar to other interventional procedures. One must take into consideration the risk status of both the patient and the planned procedure. As Tables 4.9 and 4.10 summarize, patients who are low or high risk and are undergoing low-risk procedures may be considered for not having anticoagulation stopped. Similarly, single clopidogrel or aspirin antiplatelet therapy may be continued in the pre-procedural period. Combination therapy of both aspirin and clopidogrel predisposes to higher risk of bleeding and consideration should be given to discontinuing one of these agents. However, if a high-risk procedure is planned, anticoagulation should be withheld for 3–5 days and thought should be given to the possible use of reversal agents. Conversely, high-risk patients who will be undergoing high-risk procedures should be bridged with either LMWH. Single agent antiplatelet therapy may be continued if the risk of discontinuation outweighs the benefit to the patient. Similarly, the restarting of anticoagulation or antiplatelet agents following the completion of endoscopic procedures must take into consideration the agent to be restarted and the type of procedure or intervention done. Table 4.11 summarizes the timing of reinstitution of the most commonly used agents after gastrointestinal endoscopy. It is important to note that reinstituting these agents should be delayed for a period of time if the procedure performed confers a higher risk for post-procedure bleeding.

Table 4.10 Pre-procedural antiplatelet management [92, 93]

Indication/antiplatelet therapy	Recommended duration of therapy
Bare metal stent	Continue antiplatelet therapy + aspirin if endoscopy is scheduled during the first 6 weeks of stent placement
	Continue low dose aspirin after the first 6 weeks of stent placement but antiplatelet therapy may be stopped
Drug-eluting stent	1 year of dual antiplatelet therapy. Do not hold therapy for endoscopy within this first year
Primary prevention of MI or stroke	Hold aspirin 7–10 days prior to high-risk procedures and patients at high risk (such as those with underlying bleeding disorders). May continue aspirin for low-risk procedures
Patients on NSAIDs	Short half-life NSAIDs (e.g., Ibuprofen, diclofenac, ketoprofen, indomethacin): Stop drug on the day of therapy for high-risk procedures. Continue therapy for low-risk procedures
	Intermediate half-life NSAIDs (naproxen, celecoxib, diflunisal, sulindac): Stop drug 2–3 days prior to high-risk procedures. Continue for low-risk procedures
	Long half-life NSAIDs (meloxicam, nabumetone, piroxicam): Hold 10 days prior to high-risk procedures. May continue for low-risk procedures
Patients on ticlopidine and dipyridamole	Limited data suggest therapy does not need to be held for low-risk procedures. For high-risk procedures and patients on dual dipyridamole + aspirin, consider holding for 7–10 days

NSAIDs nonsteroidal anti-inflammatory drugs

Table 4.11 Restarting anticoagulation/antiplatelet agents after gastrointestinal endoscopy [84, 93]

Drug	Timing of reinstitution	Comments
Warfarin	Same night post procedure	For high-risk procedures, wait 72 h
Heparin	2–6 h post-procedure	
LMWH	24 h post-procedure (if adequate hemostasis achieved)	Resume at a lower dose for high-risk procedures and consider waiting for 48–72 h
Aspirin/NSAIDs	Next day	
Clopidogrel	Next day	Delay further for high-risk procedures

NSAIDs nonsteroidal anti-inflammatory drugs, *LMWH* low molecular weight heparin

Antibiotic Prophylaxis in Flexible Gastrointestinal Endoscopy

Several serious and possibly fatal conditions may result directly from bacterial translocation that occurs at the time gastrointestinal endoscopy. Although rates of transient bacteremia from endoscopy are reported to be low overall, and the usefulness of antibiotic prophylaxis controversial, certain specific situations and at risk populations may warrant peri-procedural antibiotics due to the likely catastrophic risks associated with infection. Transient bacteremia related to endoscopy has been well documented for decades with rates for both upper and lower endoscopy ranging from 0 to 5 % on average, but reported to be as high as 13 % [100–107]. This appears to be equally true when ERCP is performed in a non-obstructed biliary system or during polypectomy and fulguration in lower endoscopy (although procedures involving dilation, sclerotherapy, or stenting of the esophagus carry higher rates of transient bacteremia) [101, 102, 108, 112, 113]. In comparison, transient bacteremia has been described from common daily activates such as food chewing, tooth brushing, and flossing, at rates higher than from diagnostic endoscopy [102, 109]. In fact, even a simple rectal exam is associated with bacteremia in about 4 % of patients [110]. The microbiological profile of bacteremia following endoscopy typically results from either the normal flora of the organ being instrumented, infection at the site of the procedure (such as in cholangitis at the time of ERCP for biliary obstruction), or a contaminate organism. In upper gastrointestinal endoscopy, bacteria that reside in the mouth or other contaminate such as *Staphylococcus* and *Streptococcus* (especially *Streptococcus viridians*) are the most common [100, 111]. Others include *Bacillus*, *Propionibacterium* and *Serratia marcescens* [100]. Colonoscopy usually results in bacteremia from gut flora such as *Enterococcus*, *Bacteroides* or *Escherichia coli* [101]. However, evidence that endoscopy directly leads to complications from transient bacteremia is deeply lacking. Sequelae such as infective endocarditis or infections of orthopedic prostheses, vascular grafts, pacemakers and other implanted materials appear to be exceedingly rare [112–116]. In addition, there are no conclusive data that demonstrate efficacy in preventing most of these perceived complications with the use of antibiotics prior to endoscopy. Indeed, the risk of local infection would be too low to even warrant the widespread use of antibiotics for prophylaxis when considering the risks of allergy, microbial resistance, and the possible development of pseudomembranous colitis caused by their use [112–116]. Nonetheless, there are times in which the use of antibiotic prophylaxis has been established in reducing infection and mortality. This is most noteworthy in cases of cirrhosis with acute GI bleeding, PEG tube placement, and when instrumenting cystic lesions [112–114].

Current guidelines for antibiotic prophylaxis in gastrointestinal endoscopy have evolved greatly within the last few years as data are more rigorously scrutinized. Most notably, the American Heart Association (AHA) dramatically changed their stance on the need for antibiotic prophylaxis in their 2007 guidelines for the prevention of endocarditis [109]. Other prominent organizations such as the American Society of Gastrointestinal Endoscopy (ASGE) and the British Society of Gastroenterology (BSG) have since concurred in their latest guidelines [112, 113]. Current recommendations derived from these organizations are presented below.

Antibiotic Prophylaxis Guidelines

Prevention of Infective Endocarditis

- *Not recommended* in diagnostic or therapeutic gastrointestinal endoscopy, including patients with cardiac risk factors (valvular heart disease, valve replacement, shunts, etc.). However, patients exhibiting signs or symptoms that may be related to endocarditis should be promptly evaluated and treated accordingly [109, 112, 113].

Cirrhosis and Upper Gastrointestinal Bleeding

- *Recommended* in all patients from the time of admission, as a full course of antibiotics, to prevent infection and reduce mortality. Ceftriaxone or piperacillin/tazobactam is suggested [112, 113].

Prosthetic Joints, Vascular Grafts, and Other Implants

- *Not recommended* for any gastrointestinal endoscopic procedure [112, 113].

Immunocompromise

- *Recommended* only in patients with severe neutropenia ($<0.5 \times 10^9$/L) or profound immunocompromise undergoing endoscopic procedures associated with high risk of bacteremia. Therapy should be guided toward gram-negative bacteria such as *E. coli* with assistance from a hematologist or infectious disease expert [112].

Endoscopic Retrograde Cholangiopancreatography

- *Not recommended* in biliary decompression unless complete drainage is not expected to be achieved. In this case, or when decompression is unsuccessful, a full course of antibiotics rather than a single dose is indicated for the prevention of cholangitis. Gentamicin or a fluoroquinolone such as ciprofloxacin is suggested, though guiding therapy according to culture results is imperative in established cholangitis [74, 75].
- *Recommended* in patients with communicating pancreatic fluid collections or when drainage of a pseudocyst will be performed in order to prevent infection of a sterile cavity. A fluoroquinolone such as ciprofloxacin or gentamicin is suggested [74, 75].
- *Recommended* in patients with a history of liver transplantation to prevent cholangitis. In this case, gentamicin with the addition of amoxicillin or a fluoroquinolone such as ciprofloxacin is suggested. Vancomycin may be considered as an alternative [74, 75].

EUS and FNA

- *Not recommended* for diagnostic EUS without FNA [74, 75].
- *Not recommended* for EUS with FNA of solid lesions in the upper GI tract. No current recommendation for solid lesion in the lower GI tract due to insufficient data [74, 75].
- *Recommended* for EUS with FNA of cystic lesions of the GI tract to prevent infection of a sterile cavity. Amoxicillin/clavulanic acid or a fluoroquinolone such as ciprofloxacin is suggested [74, 75].

PEG

- *Recommended* for prevention of peristomal infection. Amoxicillin/clavulanic acid or other antibiotic that cover skin flora such as the cefazolin or cefuroxime is suggested [74, 75].

Natural Orifice Transluminal Endoscopic Surgery

- *Reasonable* to use antibiotic prophylaxis, as is the standard of care in other intraperitoneal operations, although data are limited [75].

Esophageal Dilation

The rates of bacteremia after esophageal bougienage range from 12 to 22 %, the highest rate among all gastrointestinal endoscopic procedures along with sclerotherapy [111, 117, 118]. The rate of bacteremia is higher when malignant strictures are dilated (as opposed to benign strictures), and also higher when multiple dilations are performed (as opposed to a single dilation) [117]. The organisms cultured are usually mouth flora and not from the actual dilator, with the most common by far being *S. viridians* [111, 117].

Despite the relatively high incidence of bacteremia with esophageal dilation, routine peri-procedural prophylaxis is not currently recommended [119, 120]. Previous guidelines recommended prophylaxis in high-risk patients such as those with any cardiac condition, synthetic vascular grafts, or prosthetic joints [120]. More recent guidelines however have dropped these recommendations [113]. In immunocompromised patients however, such as those with neutropenia or advanced hematologic malignancy, antibiotic prophylaxis is recommended [112]. The prophylactic antibiotic of choice for these patients is ampicillin or amoxicillin.

Conclusion

As the physician is being presented with more complex and high-risk patients it has become increasingly essential to be able to manage them in manner that would optimize their final outcome and recovery. This is particularly true with endoscopic procedures, which have long been viewed as simple and low risk in nature. In having appropriate pre-procedural preparation the patient's care is improved and complications minimized.

References

1. American Society of Anesthesiologists Task Force on Sedation and Analgesia by Non-Anesthesiologists. Practice guidelines for sedation and analgesia by non-anesthesiologists. Anesthesiology. 2002;96(4):1004–17.
2. Parente F, Marino B, Crosta C. Bowel preparation before colonoscopy in the era of mass screening for colo-rectal cancer: a practical approach. Dig Liver Dis. 2009;41(2):87–95.
3. Hart R, Classen M. Complications of diagnostic gastrointestinal endoscopy. Endoscopy. 1990;22(5):229–33.
4. Kheterpal S et al. Incidence and predictors of difficult and impossible mask ventilation. Anesthesiology. 2006;105(5):885–91.
5. Stock SL, Catalano G, Catalano MC. Meperidine associated mental status changes in a patient with chronic renal failure. J Fla Med Assoc. 1996;83(5):315–9.
6. Cohen LB. Patient monitoring during gastrointestinal endoscopy: why, when, and how? Gastrointest Endosc Clin N Am. 2008;18:651–63.
7. McAlpine JK, Martin BJ, Devine BL. Cardiac arrhythmias associated with upper gastrointestinal endoscopy in elderly subjects. Scott Med J. 1990;35(4):102–4.
8. Bailey PL, Pace NL, Ashburn MA, et al. Frequent hypoxemia and apnea after sedation with midazolam and fentanyl. Anesthesiology. 1990;73(5):826–30.
9. Froehlich F, Thorens J, Schwizer W, et al. Sedation and analgesia for colonoscopy: patient tolerance, pain, and cardiorespiratory parameters. Gastrointest Endosc. 1997;45(1):1–9.
10. Sieg A, Hachmoeller-Eisenbach U, Eisenbach T. Prospective evaluation of complications in outpatient GI endoscopy: a survey among German gastroenterologists. Gastrointest Endosc. 2001;53(6):620–7.
11. Patterson KW, Noonan N, Keeling NW, et al. Hypoxemia during outpatient gastrointestinal endoscopy: the effects of sedation and supplemental oxygen. J Clin Anesth. 1995;7(2):136–40.
12. Holm C, Rosenberg J. Pulse oximetry and supplemental oxygen during gastrointestinal endoscopy: a critical review. Endoscopy. 1996;28:703–11.
13. Sharma VK, Nguyen CC, Crowell MD, et al. A national study of cardiopulmonary unplanned events after GI endoscopy. Gastrointest Endosc. 2007;66(1):27–34.
14. Oei-Lim VL, Kalkman CJ, Bartelsman JF, et al. Cardiovascular responses, arterial oxygen saturation and plasma catecholamine concentration during upper gastrointestinal endoscopy using conscious sedation with midazolam or propofol. Eur J Anaesthesiol. 1998;15(5):535–43.
15. Holm C, Christensen M, Rasmussen V, Schulze S, Rosenberg J. Hypoxaemia and myocardial ischaemia during colonoscopy. Scand J Gastroenterol. 1998;33(7):769–72.
16. Murray AW, Morran CG, Kenny GNC, et al. Examination of cardiorespiratory changes during upper gastrointestinal endoscopy. Anaesthesia. 1991;46:181–4.
17. Rosenberg J, Jørgensen L, Rasmussen V, Vibits H, Hansen PE. Hypoxaemia and myocardial ischaemia during and after endoscopic cholangiopancreatography: call for further studies. Scand J Gastroenterol. 1992;8:717–20.
18. Rosenberg J, Overgaard H, et al. Double blind randomised controlled trial of effect of metoprolol on myocardial ischaemia during endoscopic cholangiopancreatography. BMJ. 1996;313(7052):258.
19. Blacker DJ, Wijdicks EFM, McClelland RL. Stroke risk in anticoagulated patients with atrial fibrillation undergoing endoscopy. Neurology. 2003;61:964–8.
20. Eagle K et al. ACC/AHA guideline update for perioperative cardiovascular evaluation for noncardiac surgery—executive summary. A report of the American College of Cardiology/American Heart Association Task Force on Practice Guidelines (Committee to update the 1996 guidelines on perioperative cardiovascular evaluation for noncardiac surgery). Circulation. 2002;105:1257–67.
21. Gangi S, Saidi F, Patel K, et al. Cardiovascular complications after GI endoscopy: occurrence and risks in a large hospital system. Gastrointest Endosc. 2004;60:679–85.
22. Romagnuolo J, Cotton PB, Eisen G, et al. Identifying and reporting risk factors for adverse events in endoscopy. Part I: cardiopulmonary events. Gastrointest Endosc. 2011;73:579–85.
23. Khiani VS, Salah W, et al. Sedation during endoscopy for patients at risk of obstructive sleep apnea. Gastrointest Endosc. 2009;70(6):1116–20.
24. Rabeneck L, Paszat LF, Hilsden RJ, et al. Bleeding and perforation after outpatient colonoscopy and their risk factors in usual clinical practice. Gastroenterology. 2008;135:1899–906. 1906 e1.
25. Crispin A, Birkner B, Munte A, et al. Process quality and incidence of acute complications in a series of more than 230,000 outpatient colonoscopies. Endoscopy. 2009;41:1018–25.
26. Paspatis GA, Vardas E, Theodoropoulou A, et al. Complications of colonoscopy in a large public county hospital in Greece. A 10-year study. Dig Liver Dis. 2008;40:951–7.
27. Shiffman ML, Farrel MT, Yee YS. Risk of bleeding after endoscopic biopsy or polypectomy in patients taking aspirin or other NSAIDS. Gastrointest Endosc. 1994;40:458–62.
28. Macrae FA, Tan KG, Williams CB. Towards safer colonoscopy: a report on the complications of 5000 diagnostic or therapeutic colonoscopies. Gut. 1983;24:376–83.
29. Ko CW, Riffle S, Michaels L, et al. Serious complications within 30 days of screening and surveillance colonoscopy are uncommon. Clin Gastroenterol Hepatol. 2010;8:166–73.
30. Misra T, Lalor E, Fedorak RN. Endoscopic perforation rates at a Canadian university teaching hospital. Can J Gastroenterol. 2004;18:221–6.
31. Mai CM, Wen CC, Wen SH, et al. Iatrogenic colonic perforation by colonoscopy: a fatal complication for patients with a high anesthetic risk. Int J Colorectal Dis. 2010;25:449–54.
32. Romagnuolo J, Cotton PB, Eisen G, et al. Identifying and reporting risk factors for adverse events in endoscopy. Part II: noncardiopulmonary events. Gastrointest Endosc. 2011;73:586–97.
33. Kim HS, Kim TI, Kim WH, et al. Risk factors for immediate postpolypectomy bleeding of the colon: a multicenter study. Am J Gastroenterol. 2006;101:1333–41.
34. Levin TR, Zhao W, Conell C, et al. Complications of colonoscopy in an integrated health care delivery system. Ann Intern Med. 2006;145:880.
35. Waye JD, Lewis BS, Yessayan S. Colonoscopy: a prospective report of complications. J Clin Gastroenterol. 1992;15:347.
36. Waye JD, Kahn O, Auerbach ME. Complications of colonoscopy and flexible sigmoidoscopy. Gastrointest Endosc Clin N Am. 1996;6:343.
37. Christie JP, Marrazzo 3rd J. "Mini-perforation" of the colon—not all postpolypectomy perforations require laparotomy. Dis Colon Rectum. 1991;34:132.
38. Kantsevoy SV, Adler DG, Conway JD, et al. Endoscopic mucosal resection and endoscopic submucosal dissection. Gastrointest Endosc. 2008;68:11–8.
39. Gotoda T, Yamamoto H, Soetikno RM. Endoscopic submucosal dissection of early gastric cancer. J Gastroenterol. 2006;41:929–42.
40. Singer M, Busse R, Seib HJ, et al. Endoscopic polypectomy of the upper gastro-intestinal tract: results and clinical features (author's translation) [German]. Dtsch Med Wochenschr. 1975;100:2313–6.

41. Spinelli P, Cerrai FG, Casella G, et al. Endoscopic treatment of polyps in the resected stomach. Minerva Chir. 1994;49:393–6.

42. Alexander S, Bourke MJ, Williams SJ, et al. EMR of large, sessile, sporadic nonampullary duodenal adenomas: technical aspects and long-term outcome (with videos). Gastrointest Endosc. 2009;69:66–73.

43. Schmitz RJ, Sharma P, Badr AS, et al. Incidence and management of esophageal stricture formation, ulcer bleeding, perforation, and massive hematoma formation from sclerotherapy versus band ligation. Am J Gastroenterol. 2001;96:437–41.

44. Chung SC, Leung JW, Sung JY, et al. Injection or heat probe for bleeding ulcer. Gastroenterology. 1991;100:33–7.

45. Gevers AM, De Goede E, Simoens M, et al. A randomized trial comparing injection therapy with hemoclip and with injection combined with hemoclip for bleeding ulcers. Gastrointest Endosc. 2002;55:466–9.

46. Marmo R, Rotondano G, Piscopo R, et al. Dual therapy versus monotherapy in the endoscopic treatment of high-risk bleeding ulcers: a meta-analysis of controlled trials. Am J Gastroenterol. 2007;102:279–89; quiz 469.

47. Newcomer MK, Brazer SR. Complications of upper gastrointestinal endoscopy and their management. Gastrointest Endosc Clin N Am. 1994;4:551–70.

48. Vicari JJ, Johanson JF, Frakes JT. Outcomes of acute esophageal food impaction: success of the push technique. Gastrointest Endosc. 2001;53:178–81.

49. Weinstock LB, Shatz BA, Thyssen SE. Esophageal food bolus obstruction: evaluation of extraction and modified push techniques in 75 cases. Endoscopy. 1999;31:421–5.

50. Seewald S, Ang TL, Gotoda T, et al. Total endoscopic resection of Barrett esophagus. Endoscopy. 2008;40:1016–20.

51. Guynn TP, Eckhauser FE, Knol JA, et al. Injection sclerotherapy-induced esophageal strictures. Risk factors and prognosis. Am Surg. 1991;57:567–71; discussion 571–2.

52. Lipp A, Lusardi G. Systemic antimicrobial prophylaxis for percutaneous endoscopic gastrostomy. Cochrane Database Syst Rev. 2006;(4): CD005571.

53. Loperfido S, Angelini G, Benedetti G, et al. Major early complications from diagnostic and therapeutic ERCP: a prospective multicenter study comment. Gastrointest Endosc. 1998;48:1–10.

54. Cotton PB, Connor P, Rawls E, et al. Infection after ERCP, and antibiotic prophylaxis: a sequential quality-improvement approach over 11 years. Gastrointest Endosc. 2008;67:471–5.

55. Cotton PB, Garrow DA, Gallagher J, et al. Risk factors for complications after ERCP: a multivariate analysis of 11,497 procedures over 12 years. Gastrointest Endosc. 2009;70:80–8.

56. Freeman ML, Nelson DB, Sherman S, et al. Complications of endoscopic biliary sphincterotomy. N Engl J Med. 1996; 335:909–18.

57. Lee LS, Saltzman JR, Bounds BC, et al. EUS-guided fine needle aspiration of pancreatic cysts: a retrospective analysis of complications and their predictors. Clin Gastroenterol Hepatol. 2005;3:231–6.

58. Fais S, Kaplan R, Hawes RH, et al. Role of endoscopic ultrasound with guided fine needle aspiration (EUS-FNA) in the diagnosis of pelvic masses [abstract]. Gastrointest Endosc. 2005;61:AB276.

59. Schwartz DA, Harewood GC, Wiersema MJ. EUS for rectal disease. Gastrointest Endosc. 2002;56:100–9.

60. Das A, Sivak Jr MV, Chak A. Cervical esophageal perforation during EUS: a national survey. Gastrointest Endosc. 2001;53: 599–602.

61. Taub SJ, Nagurka C, Raskin JB. Tension pneumoperitoneum as a nontraumatic complication of upper gastrointestinal endoscopy. Gastrointest Endosc. 1980;26:153–4.

62. Bar-Meir S, Lang A, Shemesh E, et al. Pneumoperitoneum after insertion of endoscopic biliary stent for post-cholecystectomy bile leak. Gastrointest Endosc. 1993;39:818–20.

63. Mergener K, Jowell PS, Branch MS, et al. Pneumoperitoneum complicating ERCP performed immediately after EUS-guided fine needle aspiration. Gastrointest Endosc. 1998;47:541–2.

64. Andrews AH, Horwhat JD. Massive pneumoperitoneum after EUS-FNA aspiration of the pancreas. Gastrointest Endosc. 2006;63(6):876–7.

65. Katz D, Cano R, Antonelle M. Benign air dissection of the esophagus and stomach at fiberesophagoscopy. Gastrointest Endosc. 1972;19:72–4.

66. Aliperti G. Complications related to diagnostic and therapeutic endoscopic retrograde cholangiopancreatography. Gastrointest Endosc Clin N Am. 1996;6:379–407.

67. Freeman ML, Nelson DB, Sherman S, Haber GB, Herman ME, Dorsher PJ, et al. Complications of endoscopic biliary sphincterotomy. N Engl J Med. 1996;335:909–18.

68. Prochazka Zárate R, Vidales Mostajo G, Villa-Gómez Roig G, et al. Tension pneumoperitoneum as a complication of endoscopic ultrasound guided transgastric drainage of pancreatic pseudocyst: case report and review of the literature. Rev Gastroenterol Peru. 2012;32(1):88–93.

69. Patel S, Chang GL, Messersmith R, Chi KD. Conservative treatment of nonresolving pneumoperitoneum after endoscopic procedures, by computed tomography (CT)-guided needle decompression. Endoscopy. 2007;39 Suppl 1:E170.

70. Bournet B, Migueres I, Delacroix M, et al. Early morbidity of endoscopic ultrasound: 13 years' experience at a referral center. Endoscopy. 2006;38:349–54.

71. Eloubeidi MA, Tamhane A, Varadarajulu S, et al. Frequency of major complications after EUS-guided FNA of solid pancreatic masses: a prospective evaluation. Gastrointest Endosc. 2006;63:622–9.

72. Tournoy KG, Burgers SA, Annema JT, et al. Transesophageal endoscopic ultrasound with fine needle aspiration in the preoperative staging of malignant pleural mesothelioma. Clin Cancer Res. 2008;14:6259–63.

73. Jacobson BC, Waxman I, Parmar K, et al. Endoscopic ultrasound-guided gallbladder bile aspiration in idiopathic pancreatitis carries a significant risk of bile peritonitis. Pancreatology. 2002;2:26–9.

74. Lacasse M, Dufresne G, Jolicoeur E, Rochon L, Sabbagh C, Deneault J, et al. Effect of hysterectomy on colonoscopy completion rate. Can J Gastroenterol. 2010;24(6):365–8.

75. Garrett KA, Church J. History of hysterectomy: a significant problem for colonoscopists that is not present in patients who have had sigmoid colectomy. Dis Colon Rectum. 2010;53(7):1055–60.

76. Mallampati SR et al. A clinical sign to predict difficult tracheal intubation: a prospective study. Can Anaesth Soc J. 1985;32(4): 429–34.

77. Gottschalk A, Muravchick S, Miller RD. Head and neck surgery. In: Miller RD, Muravchick S (Eds.). Atlas of anesthesia (Vol. 5): Subspecialty Care. Churchill Livingstone: Philadelphia, 1998.

78. Mercier FJ, Bonnet MP. Tattooing and various piercing: anaesthetic considerations. Curr Opin Anaesthesiol. 2009;22(3):436–41.

79. Forrest JB et al. Multicenter study of general anesthesia. III. Predictors of severe perioperative adverse outcomes. Anesthesiology. 1992;76(1):3–15.

80. Petersen BT, Hussain N, Marine JE, et al. Technology status evaluation report: Endoscopy in patients with implanted electronic devices. Gastrointest Endosc. 2007;65(4):561–8.

81. Betra YK, Bali IM. Effect of coagulation current and cutting current on a demand pacemaker during transurethral resection of the prostate. A case report. Can Anaesth Soc J. 1978;25:65–6.

82. Peterson BT. Reducing risk during endoscopy in patients with implanted electronic devices. Techn Gastrointest Endosc. 2007;9:208–12.

83. Guertin A, Osman F, Ling T, et al. Electromagnetic interference (EMI) and arrhythmic events in ICD patients undergoing gastrointestinal procedures. Pacing Clin Electrophysiol. 2007;30:734–9. doi:10.1111/j.1540-8159.2007.00743.x.

84. Kwok A, Faigel DO. Management of anticoagulation before and after gastrointestinal endoscopy. Am J Gastroenterol. 2009;104(12):3085–97; quiz 3098.

85. Eisen GM, Baron TH, Dominitz JA, et al. Guideline on the management of anticoagulation and antiplatelet therapy for endoscopic procedures. Gastrointest Endosc. 2002;55(7):775–9.

86. Wayne J. Colonoscopy 'my way': preparation, anticoagulants, antibiotics and sedation. Can J Gastroenterol. 1999;13:473–6.

87. Antithrombotic Trialists' Collaboration. Collaborative meta-analysis of randomized trials of antiplatelet therapy for prevention of death, myocardial infarction, and stroke in high risk patients. BMJ. 2002;324:71–86.

88. Cutlip DE, Baim DS, Ho KK, et al. Stent thrombosis in the modern era: a pooled analysis of multicenter coronary stent clinical trials. Circulation. 2001;103:1967–71.

89. Douketis JD, Berger PB, Dunn AS, Jaffer AK, Spyropoulos AC, Becker RC, et al. The perioperative management of antithrombotic therapy: American College of Chest Physicians Evidence-Based Clinical Practice Guidelines (8th Edition). Chest. 2008;133(6 Suppl):299S–339.

90. Cannegieter SC, Rosendaal FR, Briet E. Thromboembolic and bleeding complications in patients with mechanical heart valve prostheses. Circulation. 1994;89:635–41.

91. Tinker JH, Tarhan S. Discontinuing anticoagulant therapy in surgical patients with cardiac valve prostheses. Observations in 180 operations. JAMA. 1978;239:738–9.

92. Kearon C, Kahn SR, Agnelli G, et al. Antithrombotic therapy for venous thromboembolic disease: American College of Chest Physicians Evidence-Based Clinical Practice Guidelines (8th edition). Chest. 2008;133:454S–545.

93. Hittelet A, Deviere J. Management of anticoagulants before and after endoscopy. Can J Gastroenterol. 2003;17(5):329–32.

94. Hui AJ, Wong RMY, Ching JYL, et al. Risk of colonoscopic polypectomy bleeding with anticoagulants and antiplatelet agents: analysis of 1657 cases. Gastrointest Endosc. 2004;59:44–8.

95. Yousfi M, Gostout CJ, Baron TH, et al. Postpolypectomy lower gastrointestinal bleeding: potential role of aspirin. Am J Gastroenterol. 2004;99:1785–9.

96. Whitson MJ, Dikman AE, von Althann C, et al. Is gastroduodenal biopsy safe in patients receiving aspirin and clopidogrel? A prospective, randomized study involving 630 biopsies. J Clin Gastroenterol. 2011;45(3):228–33 [0192-0790].

97. Diener HC, Bogousslavsky J, Brass LM, et al. Aspirin and clopidogrel compared with clopidogrel alone after recent ischaemic stroke or transient ischaemic attack in high-risk patients (MATCH): randomization, double-blind, placebo-controlled trial. Lancet. 2004;364:331–7.

98. Diener HC, Cunha L, Forbes C, et al. European Stroke Prevention Study. Dipyridamole and acetylsalicyclic acid in the secondary prevention of stroke. J Neurol Sci. 1996;143:1–13.

99. Constans M, Santamaria A, Mateo J, et al. Low-molecular weight heparin as bridging therapy during interruption of oral anticoagulation in patients undergoing colonoscopy or gastroscopy. Int J Clin Pract. 2007;61:212–7.

100. Sontheimer J, Salm R, Friedrich G, van Wahlert J, Peltz K. Bacteremia following operative endoscopy for the upper gastrointestinal tract. Endoscopy. 1991;23:67–72.

101. Low D, Shoenut P, Kennedy J, et al. Prospective assessment of risk of bacteremia with colonoscopy and polypectomy. Dig Dis Sci. 1987;32:1239–43.

102. Durack DT. Prevention of infective endocarditis. N Engl J Med. 1995;332:38–44.

103. LeFrock JL, Ellis CA, Turchik JB, Weinstein L. Transient bacteremia associated with sigmoidoscopy. N Engl J Med. 1973;289:467–9.

104. Buchman E, Berglund EM. Bacteremia following sigmoidoscopy. Am Heart J. 1960;60:863–6.

105. Everett ED, Hirschmann JV. Transient bacteremia and endocarditis prophylaxis. A review. Medicine (Baltimore). 1977;56:61–77.

106. Kumar S, Abcarian H, Prasad ML, Lakshmanan S. Bacteremia associated with lower gastrointestinal endoscopy: fact or fiction? II. Proctosigmoidoscopy. Dis Colon Rectum. 1983;26:22–4.

107. Nelson DB. Infectious disease complications of GI endoscopy: Part I: endogenous infections. Gastrointest Endosc. 2003;57:546–56.

108. Pelican G, Hentges D, Butt J, Haag T, Rolfe R, Hutcheson D. Bacteremia during colonoscopy. Gastrointest Endosc. 1975;23:33–5.

109. Wilson W, Taubert KA, Gewitz M, et al. Prevention of infective endocarditis: guidelines from the American Heart Association Rheumatic Fever, Endocarditis, and Kawasaki Disease Committee, Council on Cardiovascular Disease in the Young, and the Council on Clinical Cardiology, Council on Cardiovascular Surgery and Anesthesia, and the Quality of Care and Outcomes Research Interdisciplinary Working Group. Circulation. 2007;116:1736–54.

110. Hoffman BI, Kobasa W, Kaye D. Bacteremia after rectal examination. Ann Intern Med. 1978;88:658–9.

111. Zuccaro Jr G, Richter JE, Rice TW, et al. Viridans streptococcal bacteremia after esophageal stricture dilation. Gastrointest Endosc. 1998;48:568–73.

112. Allison MC, Sandoe JA, Tigje R, Simpson IA, et al. Antibiotic prophylaxis in gastrointestinal endoscopy. Gut. 2009;58:869–80.

113. ASGE STANDARDS OF PRACTICE COMMITTEE, Banerjee S, Shen B, Baron TH, Nelson DB, Anderson MA, et al. Antibiotic prophylaxis for GI endoscopy. Gastrointest Endosc. 2008;7:791–8.

114. Rey JR, Axon A, Budzynska A, Kruse A, Nowak A. Guidelines of the European Society of Gastrointestinal Endoscopy (E.S.G.E) antibiotic prophylaxis for gastrointestinal endoscopy. Endoscopy. 1998;30:318–24.

115. Oliver G, Lowry A, Vernaxa A, et al. Practice parameters for antibiotic prophylaxis—supporting documentation. Dis Colon Rectum. 2000;43:1194–200.

116. Banerjee S, Shen B, Baron TH, et al. Antibiotic prophylaxis for GI endoscopy. Gastrointest Endosc. 2008;67:791–8.

117. Nelson DB, Sanderson SJ, Azar MM. Bacteremia with esophageal dilation. Gastrointest Endosc. 1998;48:563–7.

118. Hirota WK, Wortmann GW, Maydonovitch CL, et al. The effect of oral decontamination with clindamycin palmitate on the incidence of bacteremia after esophageal dilation: a prospective trial. Gastrointest Endosc. 1999;50:475–9.

119. Al-Mourgi MA, Bueno R. Chapter 36. Techniques for dilation of benign esophageal stricture. In: Sugarbaker DJ, Bueno R, Krasna MJ, Mentzer SJ, Zellos L, editors. Adult chest surgery. New York: McGraw-Hill; 2009. http://www.accesssurgery.com/content.aspx?aID=5288598. Accessed 25 Apr 2012.

120. Hirota WK, Petersen K, Baron TH, et al. Guidelines for antibiotic prophylaxis for GI endoscopy. Standards of Practice Committee of the American Society for Gastrointestinal Endoscopy. Gastrointest Endosc. 2003;58(4):475–82.

Jacqee M. Stuhldreher and Melissa S. Phillips

Introduction

After a patient has been properly prepared for endoscopy as described in Chap. 4, intraprocedural management focuses on keeping the patient comfortable while safely and successfully performing the procedure. This chapter reviews intraprocedural considerations to accomplish this goal.

Room Setup

Preparation of the layout of the endoscopy area will help eliminate potential difficulties encountered during the procedure. Endoscopy suites are designed around the following basic principles. First, there must be access to necessary endoscopic equipment, including monitors for visualization, designated energy sources, and disposable items. Next, equipment necessary for sedation, monitoring, and airway management must also be easily accessible, and finally, patient positioning must be considered in anticipation of making modifications based on the specific procedure and patient comorbidities.

Each endoscopy suite must contain appropriate endoscopic equipment for the desired procedure. Chapter 2 of this text discusses the technical components of the endoscope that are required. If there is a need for an energy source for the planned procedure, an electrosurgical generator should be included in the available equipment. The surgical endoscopist should be familiar with the equipment needs of each specific procedure to assure that all necessary items are present before the start of the case. Each room must also have equipment for monitoring of patient vitals as well as items needed for airway management, including nasal cannula oxygen, airway adjuncts (e.g., nasal trumpet or oral airway), suction, bag-mask ventilation, and options for endotracheal intubation. In a central area of the endoscopy lab, there should be a cart containing supplies needed for cardiac and respiratory arrest. The location of this cart should be known by all employees working in the endoscopy lab, and the cart should be serviced regularly to ensure it contains needed medications, a working cardiac defibrillator, and devices for airway management.

The equipment within the endoscopy suite must be positioned in a way that each device can reach the patient when needed. It is also important that the endoscopist be able to perform the procedure and have access to the patient in a way that is ergonomical. Visualization of monitors displaying the endoscopic images must be available to both the endoscopist and those assisting in the procedure. We choose to place the endoscopy tower and procedure monitor in a parallel fashion to the patient bed and behind the endoscopist to allow for ergonomic management of the endoscope while maintaining procedure visualization and a working space for the assistants. A secondary procedure monitor is positioned across from the endoscopist and on the opposite side of the patient to optimize visualization. If the patient will be having sedation administered by an anesthesiologist or nurse anesthetist, additional space must be created for their equipment.

J.M. Stuhldreher, M.D.
Department of General Surgery, University Hospitals Case
Medical Center, 11100 Euclid Ave, Cleveland, OH 44106, USA
e-mail: jacqueearagon@yahoo.com

M.S. Phillips, M.D. (✉)
Department of Surgery, University of Tennessee Graduate
School of Medicine, Knoxville, TN, USA
e-mail: phillips.melissa@gmail.com

Required Personnel

Performance of gastrointestinal endoscopy requires at least three well-trained individuals: the endoscopist, a nurse for patient monitoring and medication administration, and a technologist to assist with the technical aspects of the procedure. Each person in the room must be familiar with the planned

J.M. Marks and B.J. Dunkin (eds.), *Principles of Flexible Endoscopy for Surgeons*,
DOI 10.1007/978-1-4614-6330-6_5, © Springer Science+Business Media New York 2013

procedure so that they can anticipate both technical and clinical needs. Physicians and nurses involved in sedation should undergo an initial training in sedation and periodic participation in educational activities to assess competency [1]. If there is involvement of an anesthesiologist or nurse anesthetist in sedation and monitoring, the nurse in the room may be reassigned to assist with the technical aspects of the procedure, potentially eliminating a need for a dedicated technologist, particularly for more routine procedures. Open communication among the individual team members is essential to a successful procedure.

Patient Positioning

Choice of patient position is often dependent on the specific gastrointestinal endoscopic procedure. The goal of patient positioning is to maximize safety while allowing for access to the patient. A majority of endoscopies, such as esophago-gastroduodenoscopy (EGD) or colonoscopy, are performed in the left lateral decubitus position. Despite no published literature to support this method, lateral positioning is used to move intragastric fluid away from the gastroesophageal junction and intuitively minimize the patient's risk for aspiration. Special positioning consideration must be given to patients in whom access to the abdominal wall is required such as patients undergoing endoscopic enteral access (see Chap. 11) or colonoscopy through a stoma in which the supine position is most ideal. Routinely, patients undergoing endoscopic retrograde cholangiopancreatography (ERCP) (see Chap. 19) require prone positioning to aid the endoscopist in maintaining position in the second portion of the duodenum while addressing the papilla.

The endoscopist should never hesitate to use patient positioning to aid in the performance of a complete procedure. Repositioning of the patient will often aid with the ability to traverse a difficult colonic segments, improve visualization [2], or even improve adenoma detection rates [3]. Positioning of the patient in the left lateral position allows distension of the cecum and hepatic flexure, supine the transverse colon, and right lateral the descending colon. The right lateral position straightens the splenic flexure and can improve visualization or traversal of that part of the colon while the supine position can help gain access to the cecum, and the prone position may be useful to decrease loop formation.

Patient Monitoring

Patients should be evaluated in the preprocedural area to assess for any change in clinical condition since they were last evaluated and to confirm the appropriateness of the planned procedure. Baseline vital signs are obtained adequate

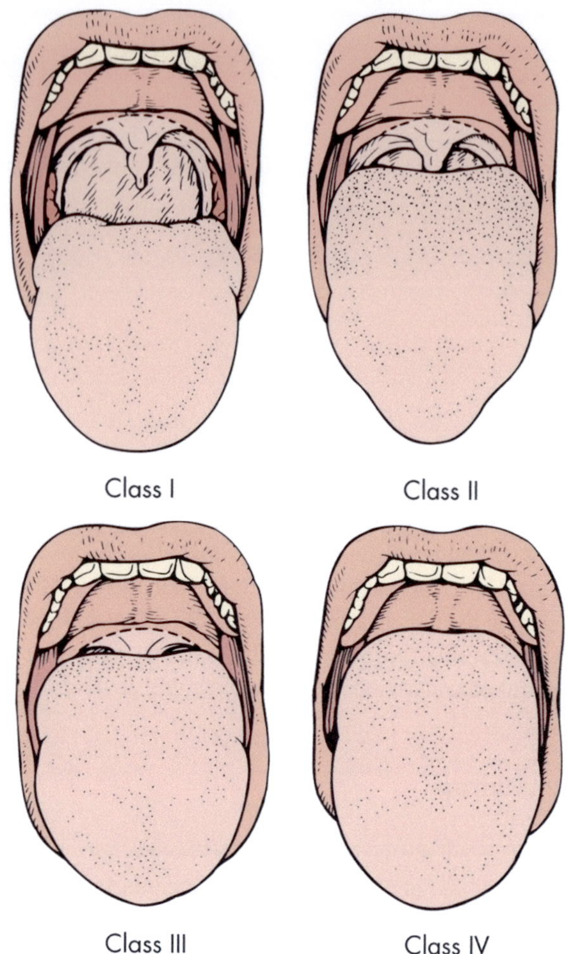

Fig. 5.1 Mallampati airway classification is a system for classifying airways with regard to anticipated difficulty of tracheal intubation and involves visualization of the tonsillar pillars, the uvula, and the soft palate while the patient is sitting up and looking forward. Visualization of all three structures corresponds to class I (no difficulty); visualization of the soft palate and uvula corresponds to class II (minor difficulty); visualization of only the soft palate corresponds to class III (moderate difficulty); and inability to visualize any of these three structures corresponds to class IV (severe difficulty). *Reprinted kind permission from Springer Science + Business Media B.V.*

intravenous access established before the start of the procedure. Mallampati airway classification is a system for classifying airways with regard to anticipated difficulty of tracheal intubation and involves visualization of the tonsillar pillars, the uvula, and the soft palate while the patient is sitting up and looking forward (Fig. 5.1).

The endoscopy suite should be equipped with appropriate monitoring devices including EKG telemetry, blood pressure monitoring, and continuous pulse oximetry [4]. Each room should have a dedicated suction set up for airway management, separate from that used for the endoscope. There should also be ready access to equipment and medications needed for cardiopulmonary resuscitation including a bag-mask ventilation set, emergent airway box with intubation supplies, commonly used resuscitation medications, and a defibrillator. It is recommended that there be at least one other individual assisting with the procedure who can share the responsibility of monitoring the patient and administering medications while the endoscopist is performing the procedure.

The use of noninvasive hemodynamic monitoring is standard practice during endoscopic procedures. Vital signs should be assessed and documented frequently. Level of sedation should also be assessed and documented. Early identification of derangements in consciousness or hemodynamic status is imperative, as prompt intervention may prevent clinically significant event such as hemodynamic collapse or respiratory distress.

Continuous arterial oxygen saturation by means of pulse oximetry with heart rate recording and frequent blood pressure evaluation should be the minimum level of monitoring that occurs in patients undergoing flexible endoscopy. Despite the inability to show reduction in complications, the American Society of Anesthesia (ASA) and the American Society of Gastrointestinal Endoscopy (ASGE) both recommend the use of continuous pulse oximetry during endoscopic procedures [5, 6]. The administration of sedative agents increases the frequency of hypoxic episodes during endoscopy, therefore most units use continuous supplemental oxygen supplied via nasal cannula to decrease the severity of hypoxic events in patients receiving sedatives. Preoxygenation is not necessary and does not change the frequency of hypoxic episodes [7]. Oxygenation is a less sensitive marker for early episodes of hypoventilation or apnea and other methods of ventilation monitoring may be considered in high-risk patients.

One such method is capnography which, when used in the setting of general anesthesia, has been shown to significantly decrease mortality, providing quantitative and continuous data regarding patient ventilation. The use of capnography has been proposed as a method of preventing oversedation and detecting episodes of apnea during endoscopy. The data provided during endoscopy is not quantitative, due to the inability to fully capture both nasal and oral exhaled carbon dioxide; however, it is possible to detect the respiratory pattern of a patient. The current literature describing the use of capnography is not conclusive in the improvement of patient safety for routine endoscopy. It is, however, supported [8] as a useful adjunct in reducing hypoxemic episodes in patients in whom it is difficult to visually assess respirations, such as those who are in the prone position, or those who are undergoing deep sedation, such as in endoscopic ultrasound (EUS) or ERCP.

The benefit of routine electrocardiogram monitoring has not been clearly established for healthy patients. Telemetry monitoring should, however, be used in patients with a higher risk of cardiovascular complications [5], including a history of coronary artery disease, arrhythmias, or pulmonary disease. Additionally, electrocardiogram monitoring should be considered in patients who are undergoing prolonged or more complex procedures.

All patients undergoing gastrointestinal endoscopy should have serial abdominal examinations throughout the procedure. Significant distention should be a warning sign to the endoscopist and requires additional evaluation. It is important to remember that the first manifestation of a perforation may be increasing sedation requirements and a restless patient, even before the development of a distended abdomen. Nurses in the recovery area should continue to follow the patient's abdominal exam prior to discharge.

Despite the lack of medication administration, patients undergoing unsedated endoscopy are also at risk for oxygen desaturation. Those with underlying chronic obstructive pulmonary disease, age >60 years, and smokers are at the highest risk [9]. In addition, when performing unsedated endoscopy, there is the possibility that the patient may ultimately require sedatives, and therefore the monitoring described above should be considered even for patients undergoing unsedated endoscopy.

Options for Endoscopic Sedation

The goal of sedation during flexible endoscopy is to provide an environment in which a safe, comfortable, and successful procedure can be performed. A variety of medications can be used to alleviate patient anxiety and discomfort, decrease conscious memory of the procedure, and improve patient-reported outcomes. Based on patient preferences, existing comorbidities, and type of procedure to be performed, the endoscopist and patient decide together on an appropriate level of sedation to be provided. Specific factors to consider include risk of aspiration, required patient positioning, history of problems with sedation, and history of substance abuse [10].

Unsedated Endoscopy

Performing upper and lower endoscopy without sedation is uncommon in the USA [11]. However, unsedated endoscopy is safe, and with appropriate patient selection does not change the endoscopist's ability to perform the procedure [12]. The lack of sedative allows the patient to resume normal activities immediately following the procedure, which is often of benefit for patients in rural communities who travel several hours to undergo endoscopic evaluation. Predicting which patients will tolerate endoscopy without sedation is multifactorial [13]. Females and patients without a high school level of education are less likely to agree to unsedated endoscopy.

Lack of knowledge regarding the options for sedation seems to be a factor in determining which patients will prefer to undergo endoscopy without sedation, as individuals who have a better understanding of the procedure itself, including gastroenterology nurses, seem to be more willing to forego sedation. Unsedated endoscopy is discussed in further detail in Chap. 18 of this text.

Topical Anesthesia

Topical agents applied to the pharyngeal cavity are used in an attempt to improve patient comfort by attenuating the gag reflex and potentially decrease the amount of systemic sedatives required during upper endoscopy. Topical anesthesia, including lidocaine, benzocaine, and tetracaine, may be administered independently or in combination with intravenous sedation agents. Although there is variability in the literature regarding measurable benefit offered by topical pharyngeal anesthesia [14–16], a single meta-analysis [17] of 53 studies reports increased patient tolerance and improved ease of endoscopy. The use of topical anesthesia for lower endoscopy and/or anoscopy is yet to be established.

Levels of Sedation

Endoscopy can be performed under a broad range of sedation, defined by the ASA in four categories [5]: minimal, moderate, deep, and general anesthesia. Minimal sedation describes a state in which the patient is calm and relaxed, but maintains responsiveness and the ability to control his/her airway. Moderate sedation is a state of relaxation and drowsiness, in which the patient maintains airway control and responds to painful stimuli. For the majority of endoscopic procedures, moderate sedation meets the goals of both the patient and the endoscopist. Deep sedation refers to a state of deep somnolence. The patient requires repeated, painful stimuli in order to demonstrate a response and may have difficulty with airway control. The final level of sedation is that which is seen with general anesthesia, during which the patient is essentially unresponsive and requires airway support.

Upper and lower endoscopic procedures in the USA are most commonly performed with sedation, up to 98 % according to the results of a nationwide survey [11]. Previously referred to as "conscious sedation," moderate sedation is the most common level of sedation provided for patients undergoing endoscopy. This level of sedation will usually alleviate patient anxiety and pain while still allowing him or her to respond to intraluminal distention or pressure. This enables the endoscopist to use patient feedback to adjust the endoscope position, identify loop formation, or desufflate to improve safety and comfort. Diagnostic or therapeutic EGD and colonoscopy are frequently performed with moderate sedation. More advanced procedures, such as ERCP and EUS, may also be performed under moderate sedation, but sometimes require a temporary transition to deep sedation for certain portions of the procedure that cause either more discomfort or require the patient to remain motionless for technical reasons. It has been shown that unintended episodes of deep sedation can occur during endoscopic procedures, and the endoscopist must be continuously aware of the patient's level of consciousness as oversedation may lead to an unexpected loss of airway or cardiopulmonary failure.

General Anesthesia

As mentioned above, patients may require intermittent periods of deep sedation in order to tolerate a given procedure. If the level of sedation needed is not compatible with reliable airway protection in a patient, the endoscopist will need to collaborate with an anesthesiologist or nurse anesthetist who can provide deep sedation or general anesthesia. The determination of who will require deep sedation or general anesthesia is multifactorial. Therapeutic interventions in patients with acute diseases are often performed under general anesthesia. A history of poor tolerance with moderate sedation, and concern for aspiration should lead the endoscopist to consider general anesthesia [10]. One study demonstrated that in patients undergoing EGD or colonoscopy, those who were female or had a body mass index (BMI) >35 kg/m^2 were less likely to tolerate the procedure with moderate sedation only. In addition, it was also shown that a training endoscopist performing the procedure is correlated with decreased patient tolerance [18].

Deep sedation or general anesthesia may also be required because of the planned procedure. Patients with concern for a large volume of upper gastrointestinal contents should be candidates for general anesthesia. Examples of this may include patients with a massive upper gastrointestinal bleed or patients with esophageal strictures in whom the endoscopist fears a large collection of proximal debris. Additionally, patients in whom the endoscopist expects a difficult procedure may benefit from general anesthesia to avoid the potential of exceeding the half-life of the administered sedation medications. This could include a prolonged ERCP, difficult esophageal stent placement/removal, or patients with large and/or multiple foreign bodies requiring endoscopic removal.

Sedative Agents for Flexible Endoscopy

The goal of sedation is to allow successful completion of the procedure while minimizing the associated risks of sedation. Additionally, sedation helps alleviate anxiety, discomfort, or pain associated with flexible endoscopic procedures.

Each method for sedation has advantages and disadvantages and should be tailored to fit the specific needs of the patient and the procedure. The majority of endoscopic procedures in the USA are performed using a combination of a benzodiazepine and an opioid agent. The use of propofol is, however, gaining popularity. An overall knowledge of available options for sedation is important for the endoscopist so that he or she may pick the best sedation plan for the patient.

Topical Anesthetics

Topical anesthetics may be provided independently or in combination with sedation medications. These agents are generally administered as a spray and provide local anesthesia to the oropharynx. Commonly used topical agents include benzocaine, tetracaine, butamben, and lidocaine. The literature is mixed in its support of improved patient tolerance of endoscopy with the use of these medications; some studies show improved patient tolerance [19], while others show no difference when compared to intravenous sedation [20]. These medications primarily work via inhibition of voltage-gated sodium ion channels, diminishing sensory nerve transmission. The onset of action is 30 s with duration of action of 30–60 min. A step-wise application strategy will generally allow access to the most posterior aspects of the oropharynx while inhibiting the gag reflex that could be triggered by the spray itself. When using topical anesthetics in our practice, we typically spray the posterior tongue and soft palate first. After the agent has taken effect, the patient will then tolerate the use of a tongue depressor, which can be used to gain access to the posterior pharynx for additional topical anesthesia application. Adverse effects of topical anesthetics include allergic reaction to ester-type local anesthetics, tinnitus, circumoral and tongue numbness, seizures, hypotension, and methemoglobinemia [21].

Benzodiazepines

Midazolam is the most commonly administered benzodiazepine, due to its effects of sedation, anterograde amnesia, and anxiolysis as well as its rapid onset of action. When compared to diazepam and lorazepam, midazolam possesses favorable properties for use in procedures requiring moderate sedation, including minimal local irritation upon administration and rapid onset of action due to its high lipogenicity [22]. Following administration, the effects of midazolam are apparent in 60 s, and the peak effect occurs at 3–5 min. The effects of a single dose of midazolam will last for 30 min. Most endoscopic procedures are performed using between 2 and 7 mg of midazolam, usually in combination with an opioid. Metabolism is primarily hepatic; however, it has been shown that midazolam is safe when used in patients with cirrhosis. Care should be taken when administering benzodiazepines to the elderly or those with renal failure, as the duration of action may be prolonged. Midazolam will induce a decreased physiologic response to hypoxia and hypercarbia, which contributes to the respiratory depression that can occur with higher doses. The respiratory depression effects seen with midazolam are augmented when used in conjunction with opioids.

Opioids

Opioids are mu receptor agonists, facilitating analgesia, sedation, and a state of euphoria. The two most frequently administered opioids in the setting of endoscopic sedation are fentanyl and meperidine [11]. Both provide similar analgesia during endoscopic procedures; however, recovery time is often faster with fentanyl when compared to meperidine [23]. All opioids are associated with respiratory depression and thus, careful monitoring should be performed when these medications are administered. Opioids are synergistic with benzodiazepines, thus concomitant administration can decrease the effective doses of both medications for sedation as well as increase the respiratory depression that can occur if careful monitoring is not performed.

Fentanyl is a synthetic opioid that is 100 times more potent than morphine. The general dose of fentanyl for endoscopic procedures is between 50 and 200 µg. The onset of action [24] when administered intravenously is 30 s, and the effects may persist for up to 1 h. Fentanyl undergoes hepatic metabolism, and the resultant inactive metabolites are renally excreted. For this reason, fentanyl is safe in patients with renal and/or hepatic failure. Furthermore, fentanyl has minimal effect on the cardiovascular system and, due to the lack of histamine release, fentanyl is not generally associated with hypotension, which may be seen with other opioids.

Meperidine is another synthetic opioid commonly used for sedation purposes. Dosing for endoscopic procedures generally ranges from 50 to 200 mg. Onset of action may be seen within 1 min, and effects will persist for 1–2 h. Metabolism is primarily hepatic; however, active metabolites of meperidine are excreted renally. Specifically, the metabolite normeperidine may accumulate in patients with renal failure and, at high levels, may cause seizures. For this reason, meperidine administration is contraindicated in patients with renal disease. Patients who have taken monoamine oxidase inhibitors within 14 days of meperidine administration are also at risk for accumulation of normeperidine and subsequent seizure activity. Finally, in addition to mu agonist properties, meperidine also demonstrates antimuscarinic agonism, which may lead to tachycardia [25].

Propofol

The use of propofol in sedation for flexible endoscopy is becoming more common around the country and worldwide. A recent survey [11] revealed that 25 % of endoscopists use propofol as their preferred sedative agent when performing endoscopy. Propofol is purely a sedative agent with no analgesic properties. The mechanism of action [26] is primarily via activation of the GABA-A receptor and concurrent inhibition of the *N*-methyl-D-aspartic acid (NMDA) receptor, leading to subsequent depression of central nervous system neuronal transmission. Metabolism occurs mainly in the liver; however, extrahepatic metabolism also occurs, and inactive metabolites are excreted renally.

The onset of propofol is rapid, usually less than 1 min. In the setting of procedural sedation, it is usually administered as a continuous infusion. Patients are usually provided an initial bolus dose of 30–40 µg, followed by an infusion of 10–15 µg/kg min. After discontinuation of the infusion, time to awakening ranges from 5 to 10 min. Patients report less nausea and less drowsiness following sedation with propofol than with opioids and benzodiazepines [27], making it a suitable sedative agent.

Propofol is formulated as a lipid emulsion, consisting of approximately lipids, glycerol, egg phosphatide, and ethylenediaminetetraacetic acid (EDTA). Patients with egg allergies should not receive propofol. Respiratory depression occurs by a mechanism similar to opioids and benzodiazepines, decreasing brainstem sensitivity to elevations in serum carbon dioxide. Hypotension is also commonly seen in patients following propofol administration, particularly in patients who are hypovolemic. This usually resolves with intravenous fluid bolus. In addition, pain and discomfort at the site of injection are also common in the awake patient.

Current joint recommendations [28] from the American College of Gastroenterology (ACG), the American Gastroenterological Association (AGA), and ASGE regarding the use of propofol for endoscopic procedures do not mandate the involvement of an anesthesiologist or certified nurse anesthetist. A recent survey [11] shows, however, that 60 % of endoscopists using propofol reported working with an anesthesiologist and/or a certified nurse anesthetist. If administering this medication, it is mandatory that the endoscopist undergo training for airway management and have immediate access to the resources to provide airway and/or cardiopulmonary support in the event of hemodynamic collapse.

Alternative Sedatives

In the USA, most procedures are performed either with the use of a benzodiazepine and narcotic combination or with the use of propofol. Other medications, including ketamine, nitrous oxide, and remifentanyl have been used in flexible endoscopy, but have not shown a risk-to-benefit profile that warrants replacing the above detailed sedation medications. Additionally, the use of patient-controlled sedation, similar to patient-controlled analgesia pumps for postoperative pain control, has been reported to have increased patient satisfaction, but have not come into common use in most endoscopy suites.

Reversal Agents

Naloxone is an opioid antagonist, which has a high affinity for the mu receptor. When given intravenously, naloxone, with a standard dose of 0.4 mg, will reverse the effects of opioid agents within 2 min. Clinically, this is evidenced by resolution of opioid-induced respiratory depression, analgesia, and sedation. The effects, however, are short acting with a half-life of 30–60 min [29]. Patients who are treated with naloxone must be closely monitored for signs and symptoms of recurrent sedation as the effects of a longer-acting opioid agent may continue to be in effect after the naloxone is metabolized. If this is the case, the patient may require additional doses of naloxone until the opioid effect has fully resolved. No formal recommendations exist regarding the required length of post-reversal agent monitoring, but the authors would recommend a minimum of 3 h to assure full clearance of the naloxone without return of sedation. Adverse effects of naloxone include tachycardia, hypertension, and pain.

Flumazenil is a competitive antagonist of the GABA-A receptor, and although infrequently needed, may be used in the endoscopy suite to temporarily reverse the sedation and respiratory depression caused by benzodiazepine overdose. Flumazenil facilitates return of upper airway muscle tone and protective reflexes, which are dampened with benzodiazepines [30]. The standard dose is 0.1 mg given intravenously, and following administration, the effects are observed almost immediately. The duration of effect, however, is approximately 1 h. Similar to naloxone, the cardiopulmonary status of a patient with benzodiazepine overdose must be monitored closely, as the effects of the benzodiazepine often outlast the reversal effects of flumazenil. Patients may require multiple doses, if a long-acting benzodiazepine has been used. With flumazenil, adverse hemodynamic effects occur infrequently; however, patients may more commonly experience anxiety, shivering, and nausea.

As opioids and benzodiazepines have synergy in their sedation, the administration of a single reversal agent, either naloxone or flumazenil, may be adequate to correct the physiologic abnormality present. There is no contraindication to administering both medications simultaneously, but the endoscopist should be aware of the dramatic patient response that may accompany such a reversal.

Identification and Treatment of Peri-procedural Complications

Flexible endoscopy, in general, is safe and well tolerated with an estimated mortality rate of 0.02 % [31]. Despite this overall low-risk profile, complications can and do occur. The majority of complications, if recognized early and treated appropriately, will not have a negative impact on the patient. If the initial warning signs of a complication are not appreciated; however, significant problems may develop and progress to adverse patient outcomes. Surgeons should be familiar with these complications so that an early diagnosis can be made and an appropriate treatment pathway initiated.

Sedation-Related Complications

One of the most frequently encountered complications of sedation related to flexible endoscopy is oversedation. The true incidence of oversedation is probably under reported in the literature, as the exact definition is not clearly established. Mild cases of oversedation may manifest as a somnolent patient with temporary hypoventilation, who responds appropriately to supplemental oxygen and verbal instructions to "take a deep breath." More significant cases may involve complete loss of airway or even cardiac arrest.

Unintended deep sedation occurs frequently. When assessing patients based on the ASA sedation criteria described above, a prospective study revealed that as many as 68 % of patients experienced at least one episode of deep sedation when the goal for endoscopy was moderate sedation [32]. Interventional procedures, specifically ERCP and EUS, were associated with increased number of patients being in a state of deep sedation. There were no patient risk factors identified as predicting in whom deep sedation might occur. Deep sedation, as an intended goal, is a safe approach to patient sedation; however, unrecognized oversedation without appropriate planning for airway management may lead to unexpected complications. Many institutions require additional training for physicians and nurses who chose to administer deep sedation.

In patients undergoing capnographic monitoring, an elevation in the expired carbon dioxide may be the first sign of sedation-induced hypoventilation. In the closely observed patient, hypercarbia and decreased respiratory rate will almost always precede hypoxemia if the etiology is oversedation. Mild cases of oversedation may respond to stimulation and noninvasive airway management, including a chin lift and supplemental oxygen. Rarely, a patient may require administration of a reversal agent, naloxone or flumazenil, as described above. This is most frequently required in the setting of recurrent hypoventilation or in patients with prolonged apnea. Temporary bag-mask ventilation or endotracheal intubation, although uncommon, may be required to maintain airway control.

Prevention is the best treatment when it comes to oversedation. Medications should be administered in a step-wise fashion, allowing time between delivery of incremental doses to obtain the desired effect. Frequent patient assessment and continuous monitoring should be performed throughout the procedure and in the recovery area. For procedures with elevated risk for oversedation, including ERCP and EUS, capnography monitoring should be considered if available. In patients with elevated risks, such as those with COPD or difficult airways, consideration should be given to an anesthesiology consult. With appropriate planning and prevention, it is rare that serious complications will occur from oversedation.

Cardiopulmonary-Related Complications

Cardiopulmonary-related complications are known potential complications of flexible endoscopy. These may be related to aspiration, cardiac arrhythmias, or medication side effects. Identification of the underlying etiology for the cardiopulmonary distress is an important first step in providing treatment.

Aspiration is a condition with which the surgical endoscopist must be familiar. There are many factors that increase the risk for aspiration during flexible endoscopy. Specifically, these include neurologic conditions, dysphagia with altered gag reflex, poor gastric emptying, obesity, and supine positioning. Emergency procedures without adequate fasting time may also increase the risk of aspiration. During an endoscopic procedure, aspiration may be large volume or may be an initially unrecognized occurrence. Patients who experience aspiration may show a broad range of clinical manifestations, ranging from mild hypoxemia without respiratory distress to complete cardiovascular collapse.

Similar to oversedation, the best treatment for aspiration is prevention. Any patient with risk factors for aspiration should be considered for general anesthesia with airway protection to prevent aspiration-related pulmonary injury. Any high-risk procedures, such as emergency cases, upper gastrointestinal bleeding cases, or gastrostomy tubes for decompression, should also prompt the endoscopist to consult his or her anesthesia colleagues.

Cardiac arrhythmias are rare as a complication of flexible endoscopy but may occur. Endoscopy often causes visceral distension, thus triggering deregulation of the autonomic nervous system of the patient. Bradycardia is more common than tacharrhythmias and often responds to decreasing the amount of abdominal visceral distension. Atropine should be available in all endoscopy suites for administration, if the patient does not promptly respond to endoscopic desufflation. Although rare, myocardial infarctions have been reported following sedation and flexible endoscopy.

Medication-Related Complications

Medication-related side effects can cover a broad range of manifestations. Hypotension is a documented side effect of many of the sedation medications described above. In patients with predisposing factors for dehydration, such as recent bowel preparation, the side effect of hypotension may be more pronounced. Often hypotension responds to fluid administration. All patients undergoing flexible endoscopy should have at least one peripheral intravenous catheter placed, with intravenous fluids readily available.

Topical anesthetics used for pharyngeal analgesia may cause methemoglobinemia with subsequent cyanosis. This may be exacerbated if these medications are administered in larger doses than recommended or in patients with altered hemoglobin, such as G6PD deficiency. Treatment for methemoglobinemia involves the intravenous administration of methylene blue.

Allergic reactions are occasionally seen following administration of sedation medications. Patients with an allergy to egg products should not receive propofol due to a documented cross reactivity. Medications to manage allergic reactions including epinephrine, steroids, and antihistamines should be readily available wherever endoscopy is performed.

Procedure-Related Complications

Complications that are procedure related in nature will be addressed in Chap. 20. It is important, however, to consider the impact that a procedural complication can have on sedation management. In situations where bleeding is encountered, it is important to have adequate intravenous access for the administration of intravenous fluids and blood products if required. In patients who have iatrogenic perforation with large volume pneumoperitoneum or in those with significant abdominal distension, special attention should be paid to the patient's pulmonary status as hypoventilation as a consequence of increased abdominal pressure may occur.

Conclusions

A thorough knowledge of the equipment required to perform an endoscopic procedure coupled with good communication among well-qualified team members, proper room setup, and meticulous monitoring of the patient while expertly providing sedation are all paramount for a safe and successful endoscopic procedure. Prompt recognition and management of complications are also critical and, with time, an inexperienced endoscopist can master all of these principles and provide expert care to his or her patients.

References

1. Riphaus A, Wehrmann T, Weber B, Arnold J, Beilenhoff U, Bitter H, et al. [S3-guidelines—sedation in gastrointestinal endoscopy]. Z Gastroenterol. 2008;46(11):1298–330.
2. East JE, Suzuki N, Arebi N, Bassett P, Saunders BP. Position changes improve visibility during colonoscope withdrawal: a randomized, blinded, crossover trial. Gastrointest Endosc. 2007;65(2):263–9.
3. East JE, Bassett P, Arebi N, Thomas-Gibson S, Guenther T, Saunders BP. Dynamic patient position changes during colonoscope withdrawal increase adenoma detection: a randomized, crossover trial. Gastrointest Endosc. 2011;73(3):456–63.
4. Standards of Practice Committee of the American Society for Gastrointestinal Endoscopy, Lichtenstein DR, Jagannath S, Baron TH, Anderson MA, Banerjee S, et al. Sedation and anesthesia in GI endoscopy. Gastrointest Endosc. 2008;68(5):815–26.
5. American Society of Anesthesiologists Task Force on Sedation and Analgesia by Non-Anesthesiologists. Practice guidelines for sedation and analgesia by non-anesthesiologists. Anesthesiology. 2002;96(4):1004–17.
6. Waring JP, Baron TH, Hirota WK, Goldstein JL, Jacobson BC, Leighton JA, et al. Guidelines for conscious sedation and monitoring during gastrointestinal endoscopy. Gastrointest Endosc. 2003;58(3):317–22.
7. Wang CY, Ling LC, Cardosa MS, Wong AK, Wong NW. Hypoxia during upper gastrointestinal endoscopy with and without sedation and the effect of pre-oxygenation on oxygen saturation. Anaesthesia. 2000;55(7):654–8.
8. Qadeer MA, Vargo JJ, Dumot JA, Lopez R, Trolli PA, Stevens T, et al. Capnographic monitoring of respiratory activity improves safety of sedation for endoscopic cholangiopancreatography and ultrasonography. Gastroenterology. 2009;136(5):1568–76. quiz 1819–20.
9. Javid G, Khan B, Wani MM, Shah A, Gulzar GM, Khan B. Role of pulse oximetry during nonsedated upper gastrointestinal endoscopic procedures. Indian J Gastroenterol. 1999;18(1):15–7.
10. Goulson DT, Fragneto RY. Anesthesia for gastrointestinal endoscopic procedures. Anesthesiol Clin. 2009;27(1):71–85.
11. Cohen LB, Wecsler JS, Gaetano JN, Benson AA, Miller KM, Durkalski V, et al. Endoscopic sedation in the United States: results from a nationwide survey. Am J Gastroenterol. 2006;101(5):967–74.
12. Petrini JL, Egan JV, Hahn WV. Unsedated colonoscopy: patient characteristics and satisfaction in a community-based endoscopy unit. Gastrointest Endosc. 2009;69(3 Pt 1):567–72.
13. Madan A, Minocha A. Who is willing to undergo endoscopy without sedation: patients, nurses, or the physicians? South Med J. 2004;97(9):800–5.
14. Chan CK, Fok KL, Poon CM. Flavored anesthetic lozenge versus Xylocaine spray used as topical pharyngeal anesthesia for unsedated esophagogastroduodenoscopy: a randomized placebo-controlled trial. Surg Endosc. 2009 [Epub ahead of print].

15. Davis DE, Jones MP, Kubik CM. Topical pharyngeal anesthesia does not improve upper gastrointestinal endoscopy in conscious sedated patients. Am J Gastroenterol. 1999;94(7):1853–6.

16. Dhir V, Swaroop VS, Vazifdar KF, Wagle SD. Topical pharyngeal anesthesia without intravenous sedation during upper gastrointestinal endoscopy. Indian J Gastroenterol. 1997;16(1):10–1.

17. Evans LT, Saberi S, Kim HM, Elta GH, Schoenfeld P. Pharyngeal anesthesia during sedated EGDs: is "the spray" beneficial? A meta-analysis and systematic review. Gastrointest Endosc. 2006;63(6):761–6.

18. Hazeldine S, Fritschi L, Forbes G. Predicting patient tolerance of endoscopy with conscious sedation. Scand J Gastroenterol. 2010;45(10):1248–54.

19. Soma Y, Saito H, Kishibe T, Takahashi T, Tanaka H, Munakata A. Evaluation of topical pharyngeal anesthesia for upper endoscopy including factors associated with patient tolerance. Gastrointest Endosc. 2001;53(1):14–8.

20. Ristikankare M, Hartikainen J, Heikkinen M, Julkunen R. Is routine sedation or topical pharyngeal anesthesia beneficial during upper endoscopy? Gastrointest Endosc. 2004;60(5):686–94.

21. Bertram G, Katzung SM, Trevor A. Basic and clinical pharmacology. 11th ed. McGraw-Hill Companies;2009.

22. Olkkola KT, Ahonen J. Midazolam and other benzodiazepines. Handb Exp Pharmacol. 2008;182:335–60.

23. Hayee B, Dunn J, Loganayagam A, Wong M, Saxena V, Rowbotham D, et al. Midazolam with meperidine or fentanyl for colonoscopy: results of a randomized trial. Gastrointest Endosc. 2009;69(3 Pt 2):681–7.

24. Peng PW, Sandler AN. A review of the use of fentanyl analgesia in the management of acute pain in adults. Anesthesiology. 1999;90(2):576–99.

25. Clark RF, Wei EM, Anderson PO. Meperidine: therapeutic use and toxicity. J Emerg Med. 1995;13(6):797–802.

26. Vanlersberghe C, Camu F. Propofol. Handb Exp Pharmacol. 2008;182:227–52.

27. Kotani Y, Shimazawa M, Yoshimura S, Iwama T, Hara H. The experimental and clinical pharmacology of propofol, an anesthetic agent with neuroprotective properties. CNS Neurosci Ther. 2008;14(2):95–106.

28. Vargo JJ, Cohen LB, Rex DK, Kwo PY. Position statement: nonanesthesiologist administration of propofol for GI endoscopy. Gastrointest Endosc. 2009;70(6):1053–9.

29. Katzung BG, Masters S, Trevor A. Basic clinical pharmacology, vol. 11. New York: McGraw-Hill Companies; 2009.

30. Weinbroum A, Rudick V, Sorkine P, Nevo Y, Halpern P, Geller E, et al. Use of flumazenil in the treatment of drug overdose: a double-blind and open clinical study in 110 patients. Crit Care Med. 1996;24(2):199–206.

31. Agostoni M, Fanti L, Gemma M, Pasculli N, Beretta L, Testoni PA. Adverse events during monitored anesthesia care for GI endoscopy: an 8-year experience. Gastrointest Endosc. 2011;74(2):266–75.

32. Patel S, Vargo JJ, Khandwala F, Lopez R, Trolli P, Dumot JA, et al. Deep sedation occurs frequently during elective endoscopy with meperidine and midazolam. Am J Gastroenterol. 2005;100(12):2689–95.

Post-procedural Considerations

6

Andrew K. Hadj and Mehrdad Nikfarjam

Introduction

Flexible endoscopy, when performed in an appropriate environment with well-defined institutional standards of care, is considered a safe and well-tolerated diagnostic and therapeutic tool. The facility must be approved to perform flexible endoscopy, carried out by qualified endoscopists. This chapter describes how patients should be managed in the post-procedure recovery unit with an emphasis on early recognition of potential complications based on the patient's risk factors (determined during preoperative evaluation—see Chap. 4), type of procedure performed and anaesthetic technique.

Standard Recovery Practices

Recovery Facility and Team

The post-procedural recovery includes the time from removal of the endoscope to discharge, varying between patient and procedure type. Patients undergoing conscious sedation may be safely transported from the procedure room to the recovery area with nursing support. Patients requiring deep sedation or general anaesthesia must have anaesthetic medical support until baseline consciousness has returned and vital observations have stabilized. Expected recovery times for standard procedures vary depending on the procedure type. Infrequently, elective patients require overnight hospital admission.

Adequate allied staffing numbers with appropriate levels of expertise are prerequisites for any office-based or institutional endoscopy service. Nursing staff should have basic life support (BLS) training and be able to undertake regular observations, which include vital signs, oxygen saturations and pain assessment. Patient service attendants and orderly staff should be available to provide assistance if required.

Post-procedural Monitoring

All vital parameters, including blood pressure, heart rate and % oxygen saturation should be recorded every 3–5 min for the first 30 min following endoscopy in patients requiring moderate to deep sedation or general anaesthesia. The level of sedation is generally repeatedly checked by frequent verbal contact. Supplemental oxygen is required in the recovery area and is administered until full consciousness is established. A vomit bowl should be available and suction accessible to allow removal fluids from the oral cavity in cases of vomiting. Patients are transferred to the ward or the day recovery centre once stable observations are noted and full consciousness is established.

Minimum standard terminology for both nursing and medical documentation post-endoscopic procedures should be utilized. This should specifically relate to procedure type, anaesthetic, surgical findings and outcomes, complications and any instituted management. Nursing documentation should include observations, patient recovery post-procedure, pain levels and specific discharge plans. Any concern or abnormal measured parameters must be documented and reported immediately to medical staff. It should be concise, accurate and legible [1]. Appropriate documentation is a medico-legal requirement.

Nursing guidelines can vary and are specific to endoscopic institutions (Table 6.1); however, a discharge score should be employed by institutions to effect safe and timely discharge [1]. The parameters should include vital signs, Glasgow Coma score, pain levels and the presence of nausea or vomiting. Any patient who has received reversal agents such as flumazenil and/or naloxone post-anaesthetic should remain in the recovery area on close observation for up to 2 h.

A.K. Hadj, M.D., B.S. • M. Nikfarjam, M.D., Ph.D., F.R.A.C.S. (✉)
Department of Surgery, University of Melbourne, Austin Health,
LTB 8, Studley Rd, Heidelberg, Melbourne, VIC 3084, Australia
e-mail: mehrdad.nikfarjam@gmail.com

J.M. Marks and B.J. Dunkin (eds.), *Principles of Flexible Endoscopy for Surgeons*,
DOI 10.1007/978-1-4614-6330-6_6, © Springer Science+Business Media New York 2013

Table 6.1 Post-procedural endoscopy protocol—management

Procedure	Immediate management	Subsequent management	Important surgical notes
Simple			
Gastroscopy	1/2 hourly observation 1 h; nil orally 1 h	Observe for aspiration risk in elderly	±Biopsy taken
Colonoscopy			
Advanced			
ERCP	1/2 hourly observation up to 2 h; nil orally 2 h	Report severe abdominal pain	±Repeated duct manipulation ±Sphincterotomy ±Failed stone extraction
Endomucosal biopsy	Endoscopic specialist guidelines	Endoscopic guidelines Report severe abdominal pain	±Significant bleeding
Stricture dilatation	1/2 hourly observation up to 2 h; nil orally 2 h	Swallow test (water) Observe for haematemesis/chest pain	±Stent in place

ERCP endoscopic retrograde cholangiopancreatography

In cases of standard upper gastrointestinal (GI) endoscopy and colonoscopy performed under moderate sedation, observations for only 30–60 min may be adequate prior to patient discharge from hospital. There are specific considerations, however, for monitoring patients after advanced endoscopic procedures. Following endoscopic retrograde cholangiopancreatography (ERCP), for instance, patients should have half-hourly observations for 2 h and nil orally. Attention should be drawn to increasing abdominal pain non-responsive to analgesia and there must be an awareness of factors during the procedure which may highlight potential post-procedural pitfalls, such as frequent pancreatic duct injection, repeated manipulation and cannulation of pancreatic duct as well as sphincterotomy.

Stricture dilatation and stenting involving the upper and lower GI tract should have management protocols similar to that of ERCP (Table 6.1). Endoscopic mucosal resection (EMR) recovery is similar to the aforementioned simple endoscopic procedures. However, there may be patient-specific recovery parameters to be followed, as directed by the endoscopist.

Discharge Information

Information given to patients at discharge should include details of post-procedural expectations, notwithstanding appropriate recovery times, adverse event symptomatology and specialist follow-up appointments. Patients should be advised to represent to the treating centre if severe symptoms develop post-discharge. Facility contact numbers should be provided to all patients discharged from endoscopic centres. A responsible individual should accompany the patient home following discharge, and the patient should be advised to not drive or operate machinery for a minimum of 24 h post-procedure.

Identification of Post-procedural Complications

Complications in the peri- and post-procedural endoscopic period are fortunately uncommon, despite the increasing frequency with which both therapeutic and diagnostic procedures are undertaken. The frequency of overall complications remains low with mortality rates during basic upper and lower endoscopy between 0.006 and 0.03 % based on large institutional reviews [2]. Overall, 90–95 % of all simple endoscopic complications are detected within 24 h post-procedure [3]. Despite the low incidence of major complications, it is critical to predict high-risk patients and recognize complications early to allow prompt intervention. In cases of delayed or missed diagnosis, such as bowel perforation during colonoscopy, mortality rates can approximate 50 % [4, 5]. This section describes general factors that should raise the awareness of the recovery room team about potential complications and specific factors related to the procedure itself, anaesthesia and infection.

Pre-procedural Risk Analysis

A pre-procedural risk evaluation should be undertaken for each patient undergoing a specific endoscopic procedure in order to minimize post-procedural complications. Details of the important elements of this evaluation are provided in Chap. 4 and include (1) significant cardiac or pulmonary disease, (2) upper respiratory disorder including sleep apnoea, (3) previous adverse reaction to sedatives or anaesthetic agents, (4) significant medication allergies including anaphylaxis, (5) alcohol or medication abuse and (6) duration since last oral intake [6]. These factors, in association with the type of procedure undertaken (standard versus advanced endoscopy), the American

Society of Anaesthesiologists (ASA) physical status of the patient and the Malampatti score (see Chap. 5) will determine the endoscopic procedure risk profile [6]. Documentation of the pre-procedural risk stratification should be recorded in all endoscopic centres and relayed by the procedure team to the recovery team. High-risk patients should always be referred to a high volume, experienced endoscopic centre [7].

Complications can occur in any patient cohort undergoing any endoscopic procedure. However it is important to recognize *high-risk procedures* and *high-risk patients* to ensure adequate preparedness of all staff involved including the recovery team.

High-Risk Procedures and Patients

High-risk procedures include any advanced endoscopy performed on any patient group and emergency procedures, including ERCP, percutaneous endoscopic gastrostomy (PEG), EMR, endoluminal dilatation and/or stenting, injection, clipping or banding for major upper gastrointestinal bleeding and complex polypectomy. High-risk patients include the elderly and any patient who has significant medical and/or surgical comorbidities (including poor cardiopulmonary reserve, end-stage renal disease, active liver failure with portal hypertension) designated by an ASA score of IV/V. Patients who are morbidly obese are also considered high risk, as many suffer from sleep apnoea or chronic respiratory failure with increased risk of respiratory depression. High-risk patients often require longer recovery times and may need intensive care support depending on the procedure type.

Upper Gastrointestinal Endoscopy

Any time-critical upper GI endoscopy for active bleeding or lodged foreign body elevates procedural risk. Profuse bleeding from oesophageal or gastric varices is often seen in portal hypertension and is considered an endoscopic emergency. Such emergency endoscopy procedures herald higher complication rates ranging from 35 to 78 % (including perforation, ulceration and aspiration) and mortality rates between 1 and 5 %. Foreign body removal, including food bolus disimpaction, has a complication rate of 5 %, most commonly from aspiration or mucosal injury [8].

Variants in upper GI anatomy, such as following gastric diversion surgery or partial/total gastrectomy, with or without Roux-en-Y reconstruction, can make upper GI endoscopy a more cumbersome and a high-risk procedure. Furthermore, patients with known anterior cervical osteophytes, Zenker's diverticulum, oesophageal strictures and malignancy are known to be at a higher risk for perforation [8].

Colonoscopy

There are several patient groups that have observably higher rates of complications following colonoscopy. Patients with any inflammatory bowel condition (Crohn's disease or ulcerative colitis), multiple diverticula or active malignancy who undergo biopsy or routine screening colonoscopy are recognized for higher rates of perforation and bleeding [9]. This is related to the friable nature of the tissue, segmental luminal stricture formation and the potential variant anatomy if previous surgical resection has been undertaken. This may be complicated by concomitant steroid use in cases of inflammatory bowel disease. Previous surgery may result in the presence of redundant bowel and abdominal wall adhesions, and wide mouth diverticula and poor colonic mobility due to previous radiation, cancer or infection have all been cited as potential high-risk factors for complications [10].

Endoscopic Retrograde Cholangiopancreatography

Risk correlation and multivariate analysis published on almost 12,000 patients undergoing ERCP at a single high volume centre demonstrated four independent determinates of patient outcome [11]. Subjects with sphincter of Oddi dysfunction or those undergoing procedures during ERCP (i.e., sphincterotomy) were at a significantly higher risk of developing complications. Patients with prior pancreatitis and those with insertion of small-calibre pancreatic stents were at significantly lower risks of complications. Perforation was statistically higher in the subgroup of patients who had undergone prior biliary diversion or foregut surgery (Billroth II gastrectomy, Roux-en-Y gastric diversion or pancreaticoduodenctomy).

Recognition of Complications

General

Recognizing a complication early in the post-procedural environment is critical to effective and safe patient management. Objective symptoms and signs together form a clinical picture to enable endoscopists to make rapid and sound clinical judgements. Pain disproportionate to that expected post-flexible endoscopy is an early warning sign. In conjunction, pain not amenable to analgesia is suggestive of a serious underlying process. Post-procedural large volume (>250 ml) haematemesis or bleeding per rectum warrants immediate resuscitation and urgent repeat endoscopy in the majority of cases if appropriate facilities are available. If the patient can be stabilized, transfer to a tertiary surgical centre may be required if bleeding cannot be controlled or intensive care support is unavailable.

Objective clinical signs are used to further evaluate and recognize complications. Shock post-endoscopy can occur from bleeding or sepsis and may manifest with hypotension, persistent tachycardia, abrupt changes in oxygen saturation, alterations in the patient's level of consciousness as measured by the Glasgow Coma Scale (GCS) and decreased urine output. Peritonitis suggests likely perforation and requires immediate investigation.

Volume depletion prior to and following colonoscopy has been recognized as a potential cause of post-procedural orthostatic hypotension related to the use of pergative agents for bowel preparation. The incidence of orthostatic hypotension is between 12 and 25 %, with the most important determinants being patient age and appropriate rehydration [12]. The use of clear fluids up to 2 h prior to anaesthesia as recommended by the ASA may reduce this complication [13]. In symptomatic patients, post-procedure intravenous hydration may be required.

Anaesthetic-Related Complications

The choice of anaesthetic will be determined by the anaesthesiologist or endoscopist, following review of the patient and procedural risk factors, as was previously discussed. True allergic reactions to sedatives employed are rare [14]. Allergic reactions can include angioedema, urticarial dermal eruptions, pruritic rash and anaphylaxis. They are usually recognized intra-operatively immediately post-administration of the culprit medication, but the reaction is sometimes not apparent until after completion of the endoscopy. Any previous known anaesthetic reactions must be documented and presented to the treating anaesthesiologist well in advance of the case. Burning sensation at injection sites and transient red wheal along the course of a vein is relatively common, is not typically indicative of an allergic reaction and does not usually require specific treatment.

Anaesthesia-related oversedation is generally recognized during the time of the procedure but may be first noted in the recovery period. This is often revealed as reduced conscious state during frequent verbal contact with patient. Respiratory depression can occur and be noted by reduced respiratory rate, reduced O_2 saturation on pulse oximetry and increased pCO_2 retention on capnography—a sensitive indicator of early respiratory depression.

Aspiration pneumonia or pneumonitis can occur in the post-procedural period. This may occur in the oversedated patient or in non-fasted patients or those with gastroparesis or gastric outlet obstruction. Aspiration must be considered in any patient who vomits during or after an endoscopic procedure, particularly if they develop a sudden decrease in oxygen saturation or become cyanotic. It may also be suspected in patients with violent coughing during or soon after an endoscopic procedure. Management includes clearance of the oral cavity of fluids, oxygen supplementation, correction of level consciousness where applicable, antibiotics and respiratory support. In serious cases, transfer to the intensive care unit is warranted.

Cardiac arrhythmias, angina and myocardial infarction can occur in the post-procedural recover period, with the risk dictated by the patient's pre-procedural medical status. Continuous supplemental oxygen is recommended in all high-risk patients, as is electrocardiogram monitoring.

Bacteremia

Bacteremia is common following some endoscopic procedures including ERCP for cholangitis or drainage of an infected pancreatic pseudocyst. It presents as a septic shower (diaphoresis, rigours and tachypnoea) and includes fevers in the post-procedural setting. It is ordinarily temporary and managed by supportive measures [15]. Antibiotics may be indicated for the underlying disease process but not usually for endocarditis prophylaxis [see Chap. 4 and guidelines from the British Society of Gastroenterology (BSG) and the American Heart Association (AHA)] [16, 17].

Procedure-Specific Complications During Recovery

Standard Endoscopy

A summary of risks associated with standard and advanced endoscopy is provided in Table 6.2. Minor post-procedural complaints after standard upper GI endoscopy and colonoscopy are common, include minor throat irritation (EGD) and abdominal discomfort from gaseous distension (EGD or Colonoscopy), and rarely require medical attention [18]. Patients can be reassured that their symptoms will be transient, particularly if they do not look unwell, have no evidence of peritonitis and have normal vital signs.

Bleeding

Early intraluminal bleeding occurs in 0.2–0.9 % for patients undergoing basic endoscopic procedures, usually with polypectomy or lesion biopsy [19, 20]. In upper GI endoscopy, bleeding is more common after gastric than oesophageal biopsy. Significant bleeding after upper GI endoscopy and colonoscopy is usually related to the inadvertent biopsy of vascular structures, such as arteriovenous (AV) malformation, haemangioma, prominent veins or variceal bleeding from portal hypertension. It presents as haematemesis or bleeding per rectum and can be delayed up to 14 days post-procedure.

Table 6.2 Summary of risks associated with standard and advanced endoscopy

Procedure	Risks	Red flags
Standard		
Gastroscopy	• Perforation • Bleeding	• Haematemesis/rectal bleeding • Disproportionate pain
Colonoscopy	• Bacteremia	• Peritonism
Advanced[a]		
ERCP	• Pancreatitis • Cholangitis • Perforation	• Severe epigastric pain • Worsening jaundice
Endomucosal Biopsy	• Bleeding • Perforation	• Haematemesis • Bleeding per rectum • Severe abdominal pain
Stricture dilatation	• Perforation • Stent migration	• Peritonism • Evidence of bowel obstruction

ERCP endoscopic retrograde cholangiopancreatography

[a]Risks for advanced endoscopy are inclusive of those for simple endoscopy with overlapping red flag considerations

Patients who have a high cardiovascular risk and on anti-coagulant therapy have a higher incidence of bleeding post-biopsy. These patients should be assessed in the peri-procedural period to determine the safest prophylactic cover, while also considering minimization of procedural and post-procedural bleeding risks (see Chap. 4 for a complete review) [21].

Early extraluminal bleeding may be occult to the surgical endoscopist but will usually present within 24 h. The likely sites in simple colonoscopy include splenic trauma at the splenic flexure, mesenteric lacerations and adhesional tears. Bleeding contained to the lesser sac or mediastinum in upper GI endoscopy is a rare event. Extraluminal bleeding is demonstrated clinically with ongoing abdominal pain, signs of peritonitis with the possibility of hemodynamic compromise and cardiovascular collapse. Management requires appropriate resuscitative measures, prompt investigation and early surgical intervention if necessary.

It is not uncommon for *delayed bleeding* to occur post-therapeutic endoscopy. Bleeding post-polypectomy usually occurs 1–14 days following the procedure, with the most frequent timeframe of between 24 and 72 h [22]. Secondary haemorrhage up to 30 days post-polypectomy has been reported [23]. Patients should be admitted to hospital with appropriate resuscitative measures undertaken and early investigation. Computed tomography (CT) angiography undertaken when site of bleeding is uncertain can aid with subsequent angiographic embolization. A comprehensive review of the management of GI bleeding is beyond the scope of this chapter, but an algorithm for the management of delayed presentation bleeding after colonoscopy is shown in Table 6.3.

Perforation

It is critical to recognize and treat suspected gastrointestinal perforation early in the post-procedural setting. Post upper GI endoscopy perforation is a rare event, with reviews suggesting an incidence of 0.03–0.06 % and mortality 0.001 % [8]. The mortality rate dramatically increases to approximate 25 % in cases of intra-thoracic perforation [24]. Post colonoscopy perforation is also rare. An overall incidence of 0.02 % is quoted in diagnostic colonoscopy and as high as 0.6 % in therapeutic colonoscopy [25]. Perforations of the sigmoid colon account for 80 % of all sites of perforation. Colonic perforation is associated with a high morbidity (40 %) and mortality (14 %) [26].

Most traumatic perforations in both upper GI endoscopy and colonoscopy are immediately obvious to the surgeon, with either excessive pain demonstrated during the procedure, visualization of the peritoneum or intra-abdominal cavity, or sudden gross distension of the abdomen [27]. If upper GI or colonic perforation is not immediately obvious upon arousal from sedation, the patient will likely demonstrate excessive abdominal pain disproportionate to that expected from the procedure later in their recovery. Clinically loss of liver dullness, abdominal distension and signs of peritonitis may be present. Cobb et al. [3] summarized the frequency of symptomatology in patients who develop colonic perforation, including abdominal pain (79 %), abdominal distension (71 %), peritoneal irritation (36 %) and tachycardia (14 %).

It is important to be aware of the possibility of extra-peritoneal perforations causing air dissection. Lumen injuries, which perforate the mesenteric side of the colon or posterior wall of the duodenum, can pass through retroperitoneum to present as crepitus in the neck, chest or scrotum. The patient may complain of ongoing chest and/or abdominal pain.

Traumatic perforations usually necessitate immediate surgical intervention and can be distinguished from pneumatic serosal tears by water-soluble contrast enema or computerized tomography (CT) [28]. In perforation secondary to barotrauma the threshold for surgery should be low.

Colonoscopic perforations are sometimes diagnosed after a delay, which can range from 1 h to several weeks post-procedure. They should be suspected in cases of increasing abdominal pain and distension especially if the pain becomes more generalized over a few hours and there is failure to pass flatus, despite clear abdominal distension [29, 30].

Perforation can be difficult to distinguish from post-polypectomy syndrome—the creation of a transmural burn on the colonic wall without perforation. It can occur after snare polypectomy or hot biopsy and causes local peritoneal irritation. The syndrome is manifest by localized tenderness, fever and tachycardia. Imaging is required to exclude free intra-abdominal air and perforation and is best done using a CT scan. Symptoms in these cases settle with supportive treatment including the administration of antibiotics.

Table 6.3 Algorithm for the management of delayed bleeding in colonoscopy

(a)	Upon presentation	Moderate blood loss (>250–500 ml)	Resuscitate
			Re-scope
			Cauterize
(b)	Secondary measures	Ongoing bleeding	Repeat colonoscopy and inject site with 1 % adrenaline 1:10,000 or clipping
(c)	Tertiary measures	Ongoing bleeding	Consider arteriogram and embolization
			Vasopressin
(d)	Surgical intervention	Ongoing bleeding	Emergency surgery

Advanced Endoscopy

The complication risks are generally greater with more advanced and therapeutic endoscopic procedures. Many of the complication types have been discussed with some more details provided.

Dilatation and Stent Placement

Dilatation and stent placement are associated with an increased risk of perforation. In cases of oesophageal dilation the perforation rate is 2–3 %, with overall with a mortality of 1 % [31]. The risks appear greatest with dilatation of caustic strictures and achalasia. Perforation rates are more varied for dilatation and stent placement in the duodenum, pylorus or colon. Migration is also a recognized complication of stent placement that is more common when utilized for treatment of non-malignant strictures. Rarely does migration of a stent in the upper GI tract results in small bowel obstruction.

Perforation of the cervical oesophagus results in neck pain, often worse with movement, and produces pharyngeal dysphagia. Subcutaneous emphysema may also be detected and management most commonly is supportive with avoidance of oral intake and coverage with antibiotics. On occasion, surgical drainage and/or repair may be required. Similar symptoms are encountered in cases of pharyngeal diverticulum rupture during standard upper GI endoscopy.

The majority of cases of upper GI perforation are recognized during the procedure. Early signs include chest pain in cases of oesophageal perforation, particularly when it occurs within the thoracic cavity. Increasing respiratory difficulty, decreased oxygen saturations, hemodynamic instability and subcutaneous emphysema may also be evident. Increasing abdominal pain and peritonitis usually develops within 24 h in cases of intra-abdominal perforation.

Signs and symptoms of upper GI or colonic perforation following dilation or stenting may also develop beyond 24 h and should prompt immediate investigation. Additional findings that should raise the suspicion of perforation is unexplained fever, signs of sepsis and general clinical deterioration.

Control of Upper Gastrointestinal Bleeding

Specific techniques utilized for treatment of upper GI bleeding have their own risks and complications. Patients with upper GI bleeding are considered high risk in particular with increased risk of aspiration. Management of non-variceal haemorrhage may involve injection of adrenaline, multipolar and bipolar coagulation and clip application. Re-bleeding risk varies with early signs including hemodynamic instability, haematemesis and melena. Perforation can occur and may present early or late depending on the site and technique used to control the bleeding.

In cases of variceal haemorrhage, endoscopic band ligation and sclerotherapy are the common treatment techniques. Band ligation is considered the safer of the two techniques. Superficial ulceration is the most common complication of this procedure. Perforation is rare, particularly when an overtube is not used. Perforation risks for sclerotherapy are significantly greater than band ligation, occurring in 2–5 % cases, and they are often delayed [32]. Minor complications such as chest pain and fever occur commonly after sclerotherapy, usually related to transmural inflammation, which resolves with conservative measures. Stricture formation leading to dysphagia can be a late complication.

Endoscopic Mucosal Resection

Endomucosal resection is commonly performed for the treatment of large polyps or early cancers, in both the upper and the lower gastrointestinal tract. Delayed bleeding is the most frequent complication and is highest in lesions exceeding 2 cm. Perforations rates vary according to the technique and location of the lesion. Late complications include luminal stenosis, particularly when near circumferential resections are undertaken.

Percutaneous Endoscopic Gastrostomy

The morbidity and mortality associated with PEG tube insertion more commonly relates to patient factors [33]. Anaesthetic-related complications such aspiration pneumonia are well described. Aspiration can also occur from reflux of PEG contents. PEG site infections and localized intra-abdominal collections are not uncommon and can be reduced by pre-operative administration of antibiotics. Minor erythema and transient localized discomfort is acceptable at the PEG site. However, a more serious infection such as necrotizing fasciitis, while rare is potentially life threatening and should be suspected if there is marked oedema or emphysema at the insertion site accompanied by fever and worsening pain.

Bleeding from the PEG site is uncommon and can be minimized by correct localization of the stomach prior to insertion. Peritonitis immediately after PEG insertion may indicate damage to small bowel or transverse colon. Peritonitis after commencement of feeding may indicate early PEG displacement, which can be confirmed by performing a contrast study through the PEG tube or abdominal CT scan. Leakage around the PEG site may be an indicative of displacement, but more commonly is caused by bumper or tube erosion (see Chap. 11).

Endoscopic Retrograde Cholangiopancreatography

Pancreatitis is the most common major complication of ERCP, with incidence ranging from 1 to 10 % [34, 35]. Post-procedural pancreatitis is strictly defined as moderate-severe abdominal pain with a consequent serum lipase elevation post-procedure requiring a minimum of two further days of hospitalization. Many institutions consider a lipase rise of between 2 and 5 times normal levels diagnostic, given the negative predictive value of 94–100 % [36]. This is a critical diagnosis and requires prompt management, as one in five cases of post-ERCP pancreatitis will be severe [35].

Haemorrhage post-ERCP occurs ordinarily in the setting of sphincterotomy. Clinically, significant haemorrhage is recognized as melena, haematemesis or a diminution of a patients' haemoglobin by >2 g/dl. It is also important to recognize that bleeding can occur up to 2 weeks post-procedure.

Perforation rates in ERCP procedures are historically quoted as 1 %, however current evidence suggests that rates are significantly lower than this. Perforation during ERCP, as with simple endoscopy, can result from trauma or pneumatic mucosal injury. The majority of perforations relate to sphincterotomy and occur in retroperitoneal location. Post-procedural back pain, fever and tachycardia raise suspicion for a retroperitoneal perforation. Abdominal CT imaging is required to confirm the diagnosis with the majority of cases managed supportively or by percutaneous drainage. Rarely, air escaping from the duodenum not only enters the right anterior pararenal space, but also communicates through the diaphragmatic hiatus and the mediastinum and into the pleural cavity. This air tracking can cause chest or abdominal wall crepitus and pneumothorax may also occur.

Cholangitis post-ERCP is seen approximately 1 % of cases [36] with the highest incidence in cases of bile duct obstruction when complete drainage is not achieved. Cholangitis may present with cardinal features of fever, right subcostal tenderness and jaundice, however it may be difficult to differentiate from pancreatitis. Adequate drainage of the obstructed biliary system is essential for proper management.

Procedural Documentation

Proper procedural documentation is an important part of the post-procedure patient management. Surgical endoscopists have a unique understanding of anatomy and relevant information required for surgery and this should be documented clearly in the procedure note with accompanying photos. Copies of the documentation should be supplied to the patient and referring physicians and information included in a database to follow conditions that will require continued surveillance at a specified interval (i.e., Barrett's oesophagus or adenomatous colonic polyps). A complete review of the important elements of procedural documentation is provided in Chap. 21.

Conclusion

Recovery from endoscopic procedures, whether in a day-surgery office or tertiary institution, should meet the minimum standards of patient care and safety requirements. Complications are fortunately rare in high-volume centres, however sound clinical judgement, identifying "red flag" indicators, and timely intervention allows for optimal patient management.

References

1. Waye JD, Rex DK, Williams CB. Colonoscopy: principles and practice. 2nd ed. New York: Wiley-Blackwell; 2003.
2. Waye JD, Kahn O, Auerbach ME. Complications of colonoscopy and flexible sigmoidoscopy. Gastrointest Endosc Clin N Am. 1996;6(2):343–77.
3. Cobb WS, Heniford BT, Sigmon LB, Hasan R, Simms C, Kercher KW, et al. Colonoscopic perforations: incidence, management, and outcomes. Am Surg. 2004;70(9):750–7. discussion 757–8.
4. Lüning TH, Keemers-Gels ME, Barendregt WB, Tan AC, Rosman C. Colonoscopic perforations: a review of 30,366 patients. Surg Endosc. 2007;21(6):994–7.
5. Roberts-Thomson IC, Teo E. Colonoscopy: art or science? J Gastroenterol Hepatol. 2009;24(2):180–4.
6. Cohen LB, Delegge MH, Aisenberg J, Brill JV, Inadomi JM, Kochman ML, et al. AGA Institute review of endoscopic sedation. Gastroenterology. 2007;133(2):675–701.
7. Salminen P, Laine S, Gullichsen R. Severe and fatal complications after ERCP: analysis of 2555 procedures in a single experienced center. Surg Endosc. 2008;22(9):1965–70.
8. Eisen GM, Baron TH, Dominitz JA, Faigel DO, Goldstein JL, Johanson JF, et al. Complications of upper GI endoscopy. Gastrointest Endosc. 2002;55(7):784–93.
9. Gedebou TM, Wong RA, Rappaport WD. Clinical presentation and management of iatrogenic colon perforations. Am J Surg. 1996;172:454–8.
10. Williams CB, Teague RH. Colonoscopy. J Gastrointest Surg. 1973;14:990–1003.
11. Cotton PB, Garrow DA, Gallagher J, Romagnuolo J. Risk factors for complications after ERCP: a multivariate analysis of 11,497 procedures over 12 years. Gastrointest Endosc. 2009;70(1):80–8.

12. Lichtenstein G. Bowel preparations for colonoscopy: a review. Am J Health Syst Pharm. 2009;66(1):27–37.
13. Standards of Practice Committee of the American Society for Gastrointestinal Endoscopy, Lichtenstein DR, Jagannath S, Baron TH, Anderson MA, Banerjee S, et al. Sedation and anesthesia in GI endoscopy. J Gastrointest Endosc. 2008;68(5):815–26.
14. Mertes PM, Maxenaire MC. Allergy and anaphylaxis in anaesthesia. Minerva Anestesiol. 2004;70(5):285–91.
15. Hirota WK, Peterson K, Baron TH. Guidelines for antibiotic prophylaxis for gastrointestinal endoscopy. Gastrointest Endosc. 2003;58:475–82.
16. Allison MC, Sandoe JA, Tighe R, Simpson IA, Hall RJ, Elliott TS, et al. Antibiotic prophylaxis in gastrointestinal endoscopy. Gut. 2009;58(6):869–80.
17. Wewalka F, Kapral C, Brownstone E, Homoncik M, Renner F, Austrian Society of Gastroenterology and Hepatology. [Antibiotic prophylaxis in gastrointestinal endoscopy–recommendations of the Austrian Society of Gastroenterology and Hepatology]. Z Gastroenterol. 2010;48(10):1225–9.
18. Zubarik R, Fleischer DE, Mastropietro C, Lopez J, Carroll J, Benjamin S, et al. Prospective analysis of complications 30 days after outpatient colonoscopy. Gastrointest Endosc. 1999;50(3):322–8.
19. Hart R, Classen M. Complications of diagnostic gastrointestinal endoscopy. Endoscopy. 1990;22(5):229–33.
20. Silvis SE, Nebel O, Rogers G, Sugawa C, Mandelstam P. Endoscopic complications. Results of the 1974 American Society for Gastrointestinal Endoscopy Survey. JAMA. 1976;235(9):928–30.
21. Constans M, Santamaria A, Mateo J, Pujol N, Souto JC, Fontcuberta J. Low-molecular-weight heparin as bridging therapy during interruption of oral anticoagulation in patients undergoing colonoscopy or gastroscopy. Int J Clin Pract. 2007;61(2):212–7.
22. Kim HS, Kim TI, Kim WH, Kim YH, Kim HJ, Yang SK, et al. Risk factors for immediate postpolypectomy bleeding of the colon: a multicenter study. Am J Gastroenterol. 2006;101(6):1333–41.
23. Ko CW, Riffle S, Michaels L, Morris C, Holub J, Shapiro JA, et al. Serious complications within 30 days of screening and surveillance colonoscopy are uncommon. Clin Gastroenterol Hepatol. 2010;8(2):166–73.
24. Pettersson G, Larsson S, Gatzinsky P, Südow G. Differentiated treatment of intrathoracic oesophageal perforations. Scand J Thorac Cardiovasc Surg. 1981;15:321.
25. Lohsiriwat V, Sujarittanakarn S, Akaraviputh T, Lertakyamanee N, Lohsiriwat D, Kachinthorn U. Colonoscopic perforation: a report from World Gastroenterology Organization endoscopy training center in Thailand. World J Gastroenterol. 2008;14(43):6722–5.
26. Garbay JR, Suc B, Rotman N, Fourtanier G, Escat J. Multicentre study of surgical complications of colonoscopy. Br J Surg. 1996;83(1):42–4.
27. Orsoni P, Berdah S, Verrier C, Caamano A, Sastre B, Boutboul R, et al. Colonic perforation due to colonoscopy: a retrospective study of 48 cases. Endoscopy. 1997;29(3):160–4.
28. Clements RH, Jordan LM, Webb WA. Critical decisions in the management of endoscopic perforations of the colon. Am Surg. 2000;66(1):91–3.
29. Panteris V, Haringsma J, Kuipers EJ. Colonoscopy perforation rate, mechanisms and outcome: from diagnostic to therapeutic colonoscopy. Endoscopy. 2009;41(11):941–51.
30. Ko CW, Dominitz JA. Complications of colonoscopy: magnitude and management. Gastrointest Endosc Clin N Am. 2010;20(4):659–71.
31. Katon RM. Complications of upper gastrointestinal endoscopy in the gastrointestinal bleeder. Dig Dis Sci. 1981;26(7 Suppl):47S–54S.
32. Tait IS, Krige JE, Terblanche J. Endoscopic band ligation of oesophageal varices. Br J Surg. 1999;86(4):437–46.
33. Schrag SP, Sharma R, Jaik NP, Seamon MJ, Lukaszczyk JJ, Martin ND, et al. Complications related to percutaneous endoscopic gastrostomy (PEG) tubes. A comprehensive clinical review. J Gastrointestin Liver Dis. 2007;16(4):407–18.
34. Elmunzer BJ, Waljee AK, Elta GH, Taylor JR, Fehmi SM, Higgins PD. A meta-analysis of rectal NSAIDs in the prevention of post-ERCP pancreatitis. Gut. 2008;57(9):1262–7.
35. Mallery JS, Baron TH, Dominitz JA, Goldstein JL, Hirota WK, Jacobson BC, et al. Complications of ERCP. Gastrointest Endosc. 2003;57(6):633–8.
36. Cartier T, Sogni P, Perruche F, Meyniard O, Claessens YE, Dhainaut JF, et al. Normal lipase serum level in acute pancreatitis: a case report. Emerg Med J. 2006;23(9):701–2.

Endoscopic Tools/Techniques for Tissue Sampling

Daniel von Renteln and Melina C. Vassiliou

Introduction

In 1932, the semiflexible endoscope was developed by Rudolph Schindler, thus permitting endoscopic inspection of the stomach [1]. A modification of the semiflexible endoscope was described in 1938, which allowed photo-documentation and introduced a working channel through which biopsies could be performed. The first fully flexible endoscope was then introduced in 1957 by Basil Hirschowitz [1]. These developments set the foundation for modern gastrointestinal endoscopy. The flexible endoscope is now an indispensable tool for the visualization and diagnosis of inflammatory, infectious, premalignant and malignant gastrointestinal diseases. Endoscopic tissue sampling is an essential part of the diagnostic process and permits histopathologic evaluation of lesions detected by endoscopy. This chapter reviews tools and techniques for endoscopic tissue sampling. Image-enhanced techniques such as virtual histology and recommended biopsy and screening protocols for the most common gastrointestinal pathologies are also discussed.

Endoscopic Instruments for Tissue Sampling

Biopsy Forceps

The standard and most commonly used biopsy forceps are single-bite cold biopsy forceps, which take a single-bite biopsy sample at one time (Fig. 7.1). Other commonly used

D. von Renteln, M.D.
Department of Interdisciplinary Endoscopy,
University Hospital, University Medical Center
Hamburg-Eppendorf, Hamburg, Germany
e-mail: renteln@gmx.net

M.C. Vassiliou, M.D., M.Ed. (✉)
Department of Surgery, Montreal General Hospital,
McGill University, Montreal, QC, Canada
e-mail: melina.vassiliou@mcgill.ca

cold biopsy forceps are equipped with an additional needle spike in the center such that two biopsies can be obtained without having to remove and reinsert the forceps. The standard and large capacity single-bite cold biopsy forceps and the available needle spike forceps go through a standard 2.8 mm endoscopic working channel (Figs. 7.2 and 7.3). There are different biopsy forceps available with round, oval, fenestrated, smooth, or serrated jaws (Fig. 7.4). There is no clear advantage or indication, however, to use a specific type of jaw over standard biopsy forceps. The so-called "jumbo biopsy forceps" can open up to 2–3 times the span of standard forceps and thus aim for larger tissue acquisition with a single bite. The specimen depth, however, is often the same compared to standard forceps [2]. Jumbo forceps usually require the use of a therapeutic endoscope with a working channel of >2.8 mm.

Biopsy forceps are the most commonly used devices for tissue sampling. They are routinely used for all endoscopic procedures and, therefore, are available in different lengths and diameters according to the endoscope and indication they are being used for. There are several biopsy forceps that also allow for the application of monopolar electrocautery. Such devices are named hot biopsy forceps (Fig. 7.5). Hot biopsy forceps allow for hemostasis during biopsy or for treatment of gastrointestinal bleeding. Hot biopsies are discouraged in general, especially if there is a plan to remove the lesion endoscopically in the future, because application of cautery can result in submucosal scarring. Cold biopsy forceps do not create submucosal scarring, and should not interfere with future endoscopic mucosal resection (EMR) in the area that was biopsied. Hot biopsies can be associated with complications including perforation and postpolypectomy syndrome, and their use should be limited to control of hemorrhage or as a tool during EMR or endoscopic submucosal dissection (ESD) [3]. Postpolypectomy electrocoagulation syndrome also referred to as post-coagulation syndrome presents as abdominal pain, fever, and leukocytosis after polypectomy (within 12 h, but can be up to 5 days)

J.M. Marks and B.J. Dunkin (eds.), *Principles of Flexible Endoscopy for Surgeons*,
DOI 10.1007/978-1-4614-6330-6_7, © Springer Science+Business Media New York 2013

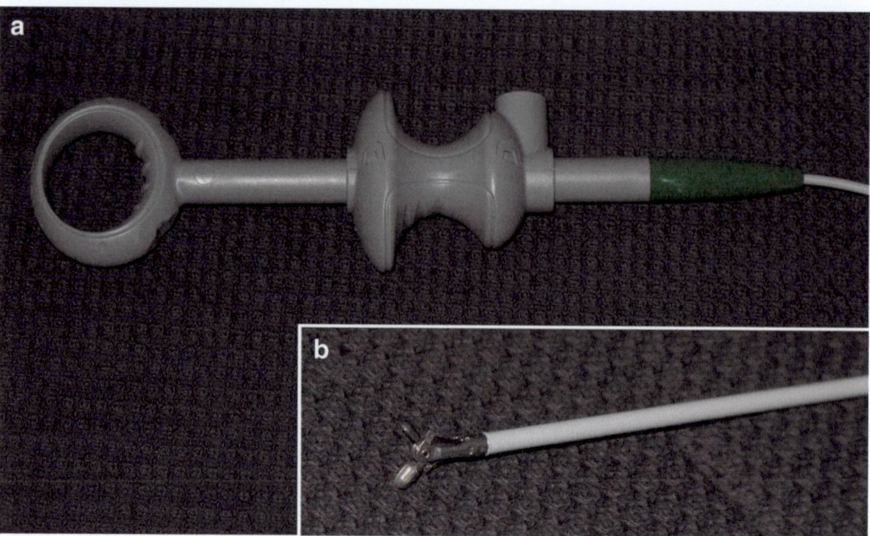

Fig. 7.1 Standard biopsy forceps. (**a**) Handle, (**b**) opened jaws

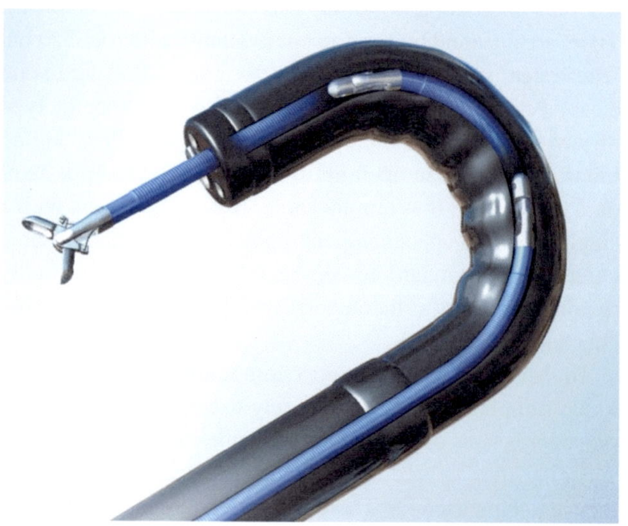

Fig. 7.2 Standard biopsy forceps used through an endoscopic working channel (Image © Olympus Medical Systems Corporation, Japan, reprint with kind permission)

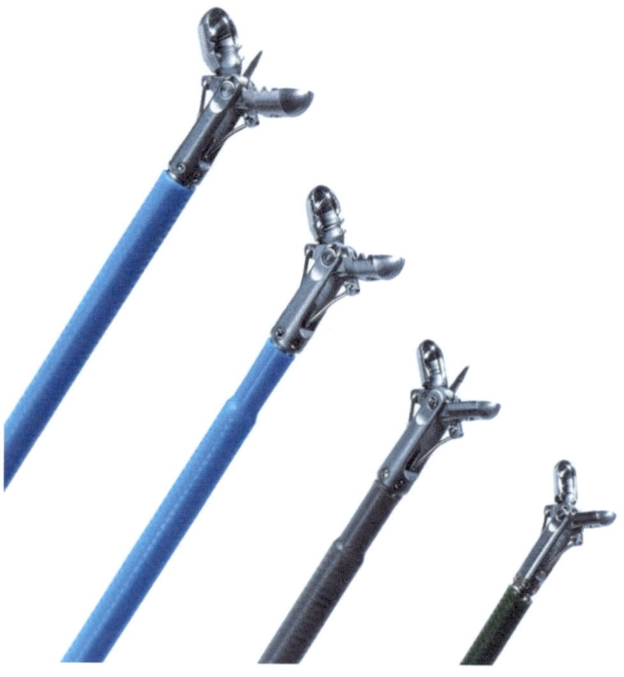

Fig. 7.3 Different size biopsy forceps with and without a central spike (Image © Olympus Medical Systems Corporation, Japan, reprint with kind permission)

without evidence of frank perforation. Treatment is usually conservative with antibiotics and bowel rest. Symptoms usually resolve without the need for surgical intervention. Delayed bleeding can occur in up to 2 % of patients after endoscopic polypectomy or biopsy [4–6]. The risk of delayed bleeding in the colon, particularly on the right side, also seems to be increased when pure coagulation current (hot forceps or snare) is used [7, 8]. This may be related to eventual sloughing of necrotic tissue from thermal injury to an area of healthy tissue that is well vascularized thus resulting in bleeding [9].

Snares

Endoscopic snares are loop-shaped metal wires that are used with or without electrocautery to resect flat or pedunculated polyps (Figs. 7.6 and 7.7). Endoscopic snares are either made of monofilament or braided wires (Fig. 7.8) and are available in various diameters (Fig. 7.9) and shapes (Fig. 7.10).

Similar to the biopsy forceps, they are used through the working channel. Snares are loaded in a plastic insulating catheter, which in general fits through a 2.8 mm endoscopic working channel. Once the insulating catheter has been introduced through the working channel, the snare wire is pushed outside of the catheter and opens into its round or oval form. Snares like biopsy forceps have handles that are in opened and closed by an assistant. Once the snare has been opened, it can be placed around the target tissue and is then carefully and gradually closed. Different electrocautery modes (cutting, coagulating, or blended electrocautery) can be used to snare resect polyps. Very small polyps cold can be removed using a cold snare technique. Snares can be used to obtain larger biopsies compared to forceps (i.e., lift and snare technique through a double channel endoscope), but are more commonly used to provide definitive endoscopic therapy for gastrointestinal polyps such as adenomas. Single-use and reusable snares are available. When using a snare resection of flat lesions submucosal infiltration with saline and a staining agent should be considered to avoid perforation (Fig. 7.11). A trap should be placed between the scope and the suction canister to allow for suction of the polyp through the channel for retrieval and subsequent histopathological analysis. If multiple pieces or larger polyps are removed that do not fit through the channel of the endoscope, a Roth net can be used for retrieval. A Roth net is similar to a snare; however, a net is secured to the rim of the snare, which allows for atraumatic retrieval of multiple mucosal lesions or larger lesions that cannot be suctioned into the scope (Figs. 7.12 and 7.13).

Snares can also be used for specialized endoscopic resection techniques (lift and cut, suck and cut, EMR) in order to remove larger specimens. Snares are made in different sizes and shapes to accommodate the targeted resection area or method (i.e., EMR with a transparent cap). For initial diagnosis of upper gastrointestinal lesions, cold biopsy forceps should be used initially. Electrocautery snare biopsy or partial removal of lesions, which may be appropriate for definitive endoscopic therapy at a later date, should not be performed given the higher risk for perforation and potential scarring of the submucosal plane.

Brush Cytology

Endoscopic cytology brushes consist of a brush tip, which is normally covered by a plastic sheath to facilitate specimen removal (Fig. 7.14). Special brush cytology catheters that can

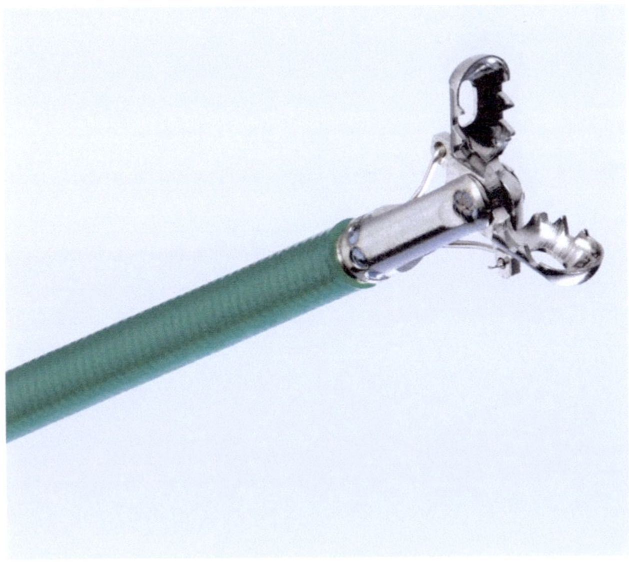

Fig. 7.4 Biopsy forceps with serrated jaw cups (Image © Olympus Medical Systems Corporation, Japan, reprint with kind permission)

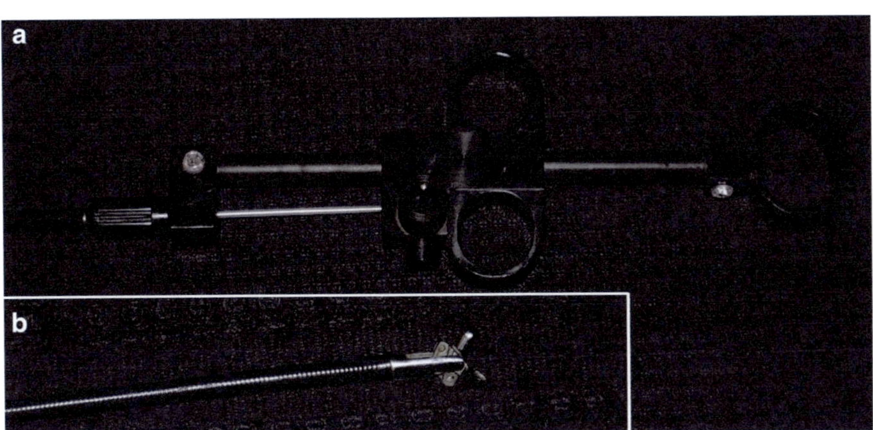

Fig. 7.5 Hot biopsy forceps. (**a**) Handle, (**b**) opened jaws

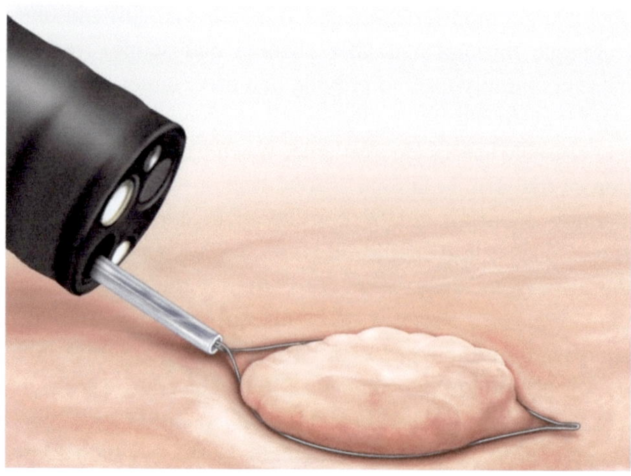

Fig. 7.6 Endoscopic snare resection of a flat polyp (Image © Olympus Medical Systems Corporation, Japan, reprint with kind permission)

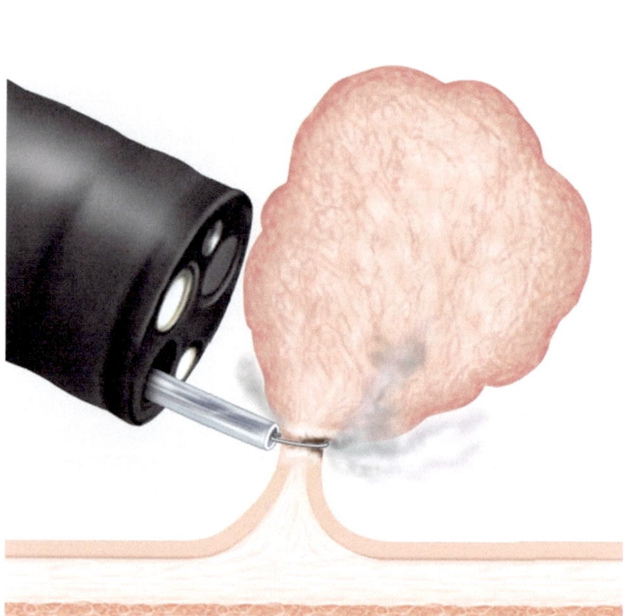

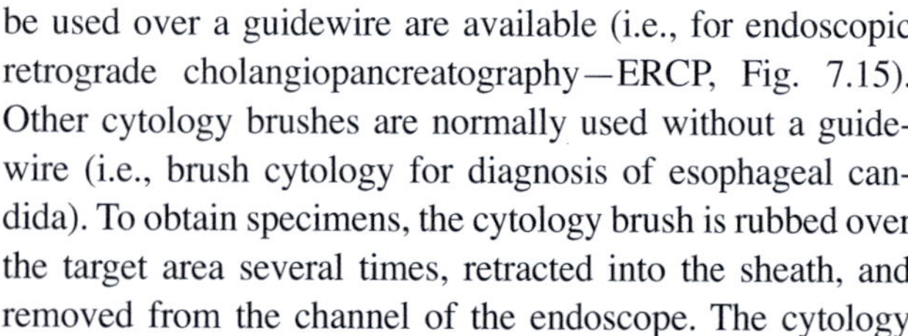

Fig. 7.7 Endoscopic snare resection of a pedunculated polyp (Image © Olympus Medical Systems Corporation, Japan, reprint with kind permission)

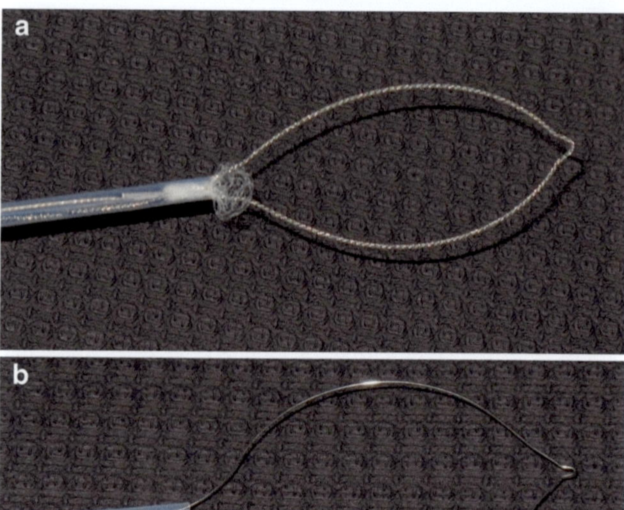

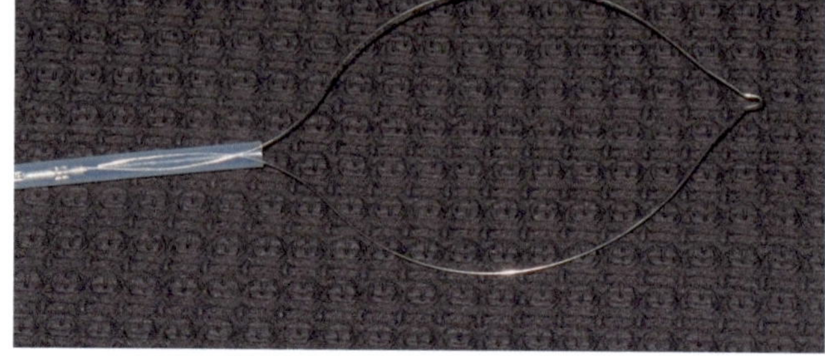

Fig. 7.8 Snares. Braided wire (**a**) and monofilament snare (**b**)

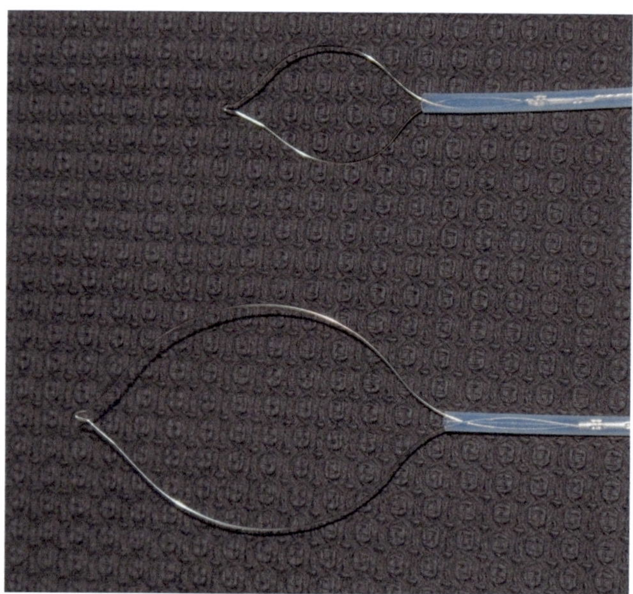

Fig. 7.9 Monofilament snares of different diameters

be used over a guidewire are available (i.e., for endoscopic retrograde cholangiopancreatography—ERCP, Fig. 7.15). Other cytology brushes are normally used without a guidewire (i.e., brush cytology for diagnosis of esophageal candida). To obtain specimens, the cytology brush is rubbed over the target area several times, retracted into the sheath, and removed from the channel of the endoscope. The cytology specimens are then wiped over glass slides or washed in an appropriate cytologic solution. Brush cytology is commonly used to obtain bile duct cytology. For bile duct and esophageal lesions, biopsy forceps are an alternative sampling tool. For the diagnosis of malignant bile duct lesions, it is recommended to obtain enough samples (i.e., 4 passes on 12 slides or combination of jaw biopsy and brush cytology) [2].

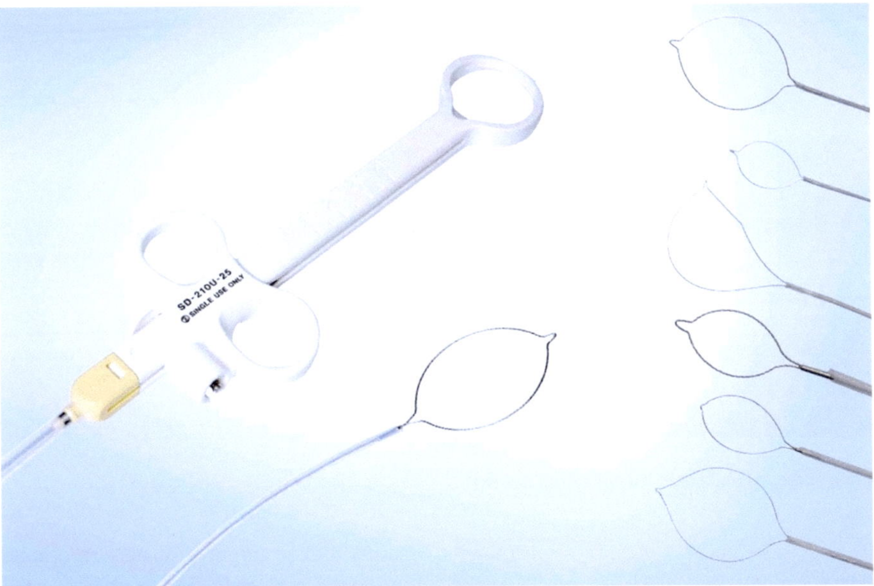

Fig. 7.10 Endoscopic snares of various shapes and diameters (Image © Olympus Medical Systems Corporation, Japan, reprint with kind permission)

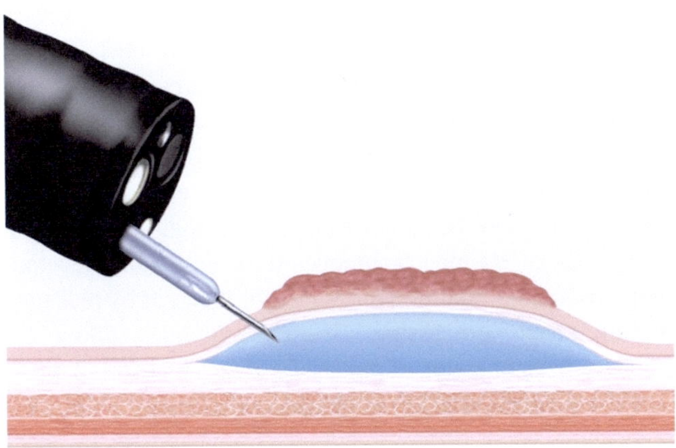

Fig. 7.11 Endoscopic submucosal injection with saline and methylene blue to lift up the lesion for safe snare removal (perforation). Epinephrine can be added to the solution to minimize the bleeding risk (Image © Olympus Medical Systems Corporation, Japan, reprint with kind permission)

Fine Needle Aspiration Cytology

For fine needle aspiration (FNA) cytology a hollow bore needle and suction is used to obtain cytology (Figs. 7.16 and 7.17). This is most commonly used in conjunction with endoscopic ultrasound (EUS) under direct visualization of the target lesion (Figs. 7.18 and 7.19, Video 7.1); however FNA specimens can also be obtained during ERCP over a guidewire (only rarely used nowadays). The standard EUS FNA devices have a hollow needle, a protective sheath, and an instrument handle for maneuvering the needle into the target tissue. Tissue acquisition is performed under EUS guidance. A vacuum syringe can be attached to apply suction in attempts

to harvest more tissue. This can sometimes lead to tissue disruption of the specimen and some EUS practitioners choose not to use suction for EUS tissue acquisition. Standard EUS needles come in sizes of 19, 22, and 25G. Routinely several passes (Fig. 7.10) of the FNA are performed to obtain enough tissue. Despite multiple passes, the samples are often only adequate for cytology in many cases. Once obtained the cytology specimens are wiped over glass slides. The slides are then fixed and can be stained for further assessment. Alternatively, the needles can be rinsed in cytoprep solution and then spun down for analysis. Newer FNA needles aim to achieve more histologically in tact specimens, similar to a core biopsy, and are flushed directly into a specimen jar as cords of tissue (Video 7.1). EUS-FNA is routinely used to obtain tissue samples from pancreaticobiliary lesions and lymph nodes or neoplasms surrounding the upper gastrointestinal tract (i.e., lymphomas or lymph node sampling to rule out metastatic disease). Large bore (19G) EUS-FNA needles can also be used to puncture and drain abscesses or infected pancreatic cysts.

Tru-Cut Endoscopic Needle Biopsy

The Tru-cut device consists of a cutting needle propelled by a spring mechanism into the target tissue. The target specimen is cut out using a removal tray inside the Tru-cut needle (Fig. 7.16). Tru-cut biopsy devices aim to collect specimens that preserve histologic architecture, but when used with flexible instruments, the biopsies are sometimes only adequate for cytology. Due to practical limitations and cost, Tru-cut devices are only used for selective indications.

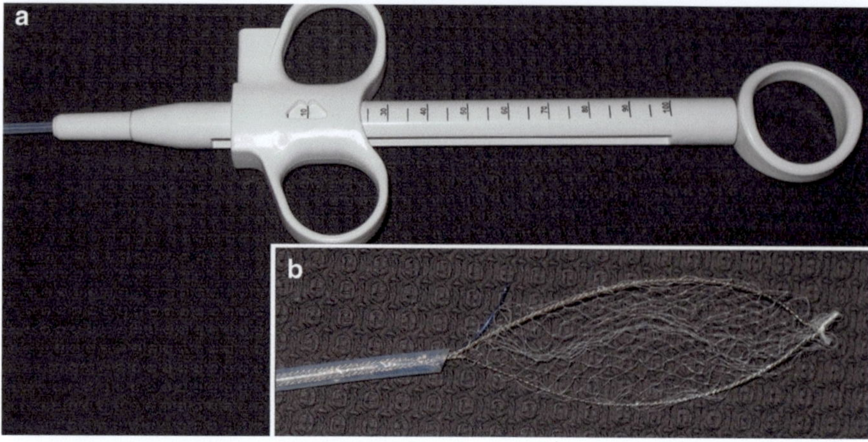

Fig. 7.12 Handle to utilize snare (**a**) and snare tip with Roth net (**b**)

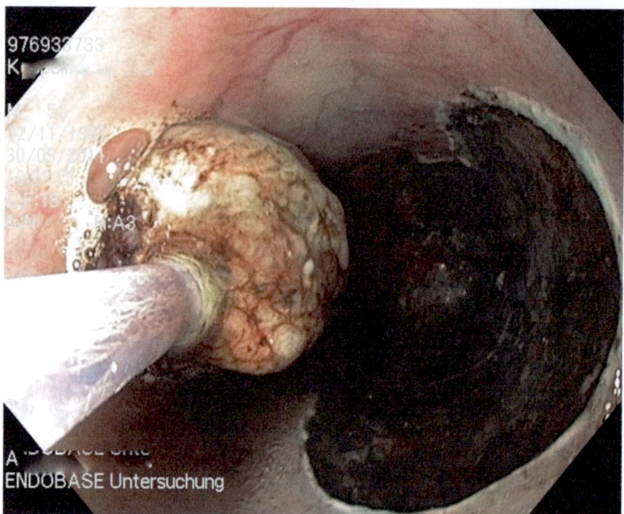

Fig. 7.13 Roth net retrieval of an EMR specimen

Enhanced Imaging and Virtual Biopsy Techniques

The clinical value of gastrointestinal endoscopy depends on detection, characterization, and confirmation of lesions. Advanced imaging techniques can help to detect lesions at an early stage and find characteristic patterns that help us to distinguish benign from malignant lesions. Modern techniques now permit the generation of real-time histologic images during endoscopy.

Chromoendoscopy and Virtual Chromoendoscopy

Topical application of stains has been used for decades to improve detection and characterization of gastrointestinal lesions and to target biopsies. Acetic acid can be used as a low-cost agent to enhance surface structures in the entire gastrointestinal tract (Fig. 7.20). The combination of acetic acid, narrow band imaging (NBI), and a transparent cap can sometimes be helpful to visualize and characterize small lesions (Figs. 7.21 and 7.22). These tissue-staining techniques (chromoendoscopy) have been shown to increase adenoma detection rates during colonoscopy [10]. Topical application of stains can help to select areas for targeted biopsy. This can improve the diagnostic yield of biopsies and reduce the number of random biopsies [10]. The use of staining techniques is not standard in most endoscopy units because they can be rather time consuming. The practical limitations of staining techniques have led to the development of "virtual" staining through light filters or by real-time digital image processing. These techniques allow for improved visualization of mucosal surfaces and vascular patterns by simply activating a light filter or an image-processing algorithm. Three different virtual chromoendoscopy techniques are available: (1) NBI (Olympus America, Center Valley, Pennsylvania, USA), (2) Fujinon Intelligent Chromoendoscopy (FICE; Fujinon Intelligent Chromo-Endoscopy, Fujinon Inc., Wayne, New Jersey, USA), and (3) the i-scan (Pentax Medical, Montvale, New Jersey, USA).

NBI narrows the wavelength of the emitted light from the light source using special filters. It eliminates the red light spectrum and increases the blue light (Fig. 7.23). The emitted light is reflected by the more superficial layers of the gastrointestinal tract. This helps to enhance surface and vascular structures. In contrast, FICE and i-scan both utilize computer algorithms to process endoscopic images and enhance surface and vascular patterns. Light filters or image processing helps to identify vascular structures, which are altered in pre-malignant and malignant lesions and to visualize surface patterns. A classification for surface patterns has been described and can be helpful in differentiating benign from malignant lesions [11]. The value of virtual chromoendoscopy has been

Fig. 7.14 Brush tip (**a**) and handle (**b**)

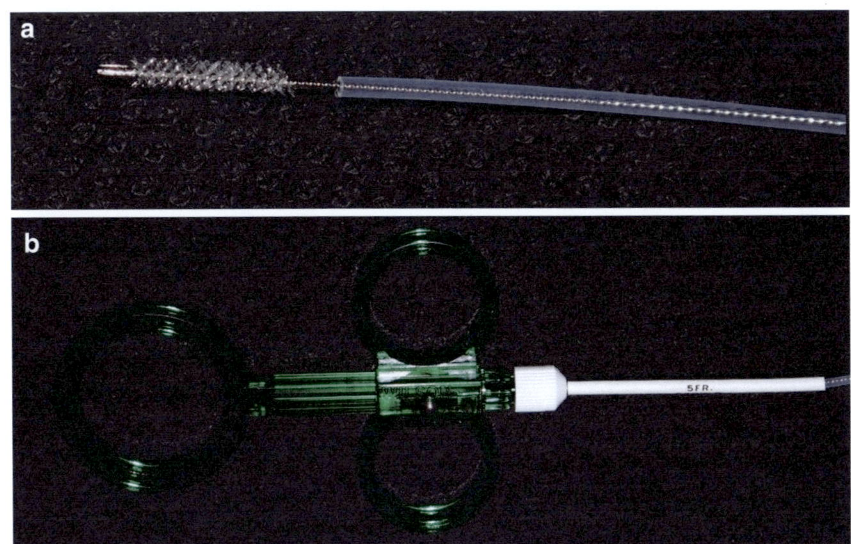

Fig. 7.15 Brush that can be used with a guidewire (Image © Olympus Medical Systems Corporation, Japan, reprint with kind permission)

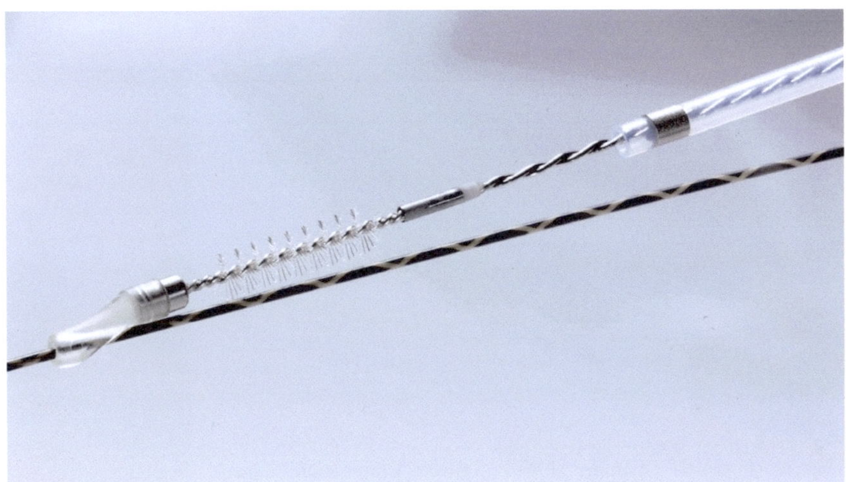

Fig. 7.16 FNA handle (**a**), Tru-cut tip (**b**), and hollow bore needle tip (**c**)

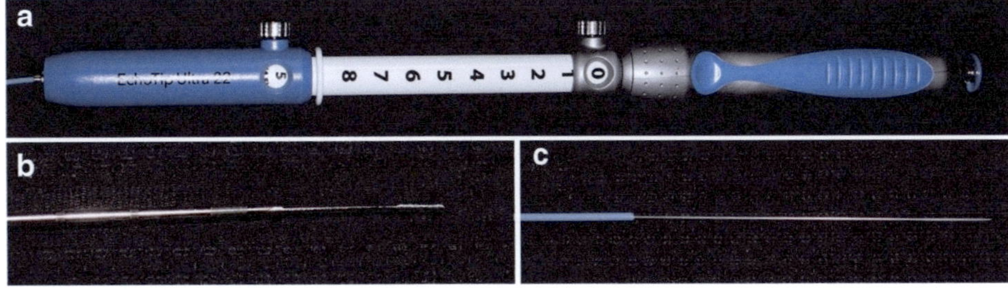

evaluated for early detection and characterization of lesions. Several studies have shown that the technique can help guide endoscopic biopsies, but the data are not conclusive [12–15]. While virtual chromoendoscopy overall does not seem to increase adenoma detection rates, it can help endoscopists to develop a more trained eye when compared to standard white light endoscopy [16, 17]. Chromoendoscopy and virtual chromoendoscopy techniques have been shown to be useful adjuncts, but are not substitutes for biopsies and histopathologic assessment.

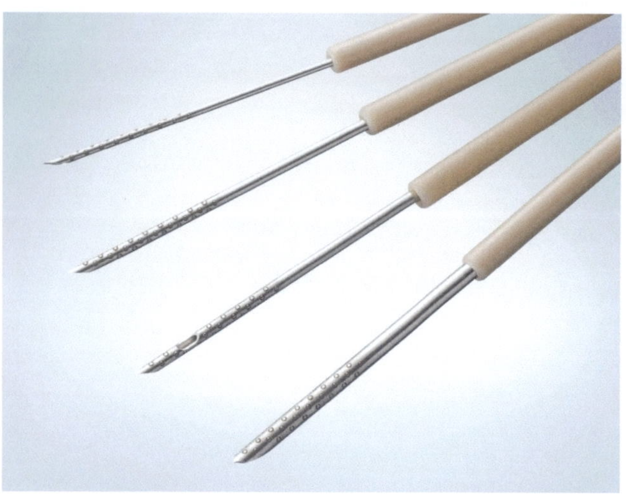

Fig. 7.17 Different sized FNA hollow bore needle tips (Image © Olympus Medical Systems Corporation, Japan, reprint with kind permission)

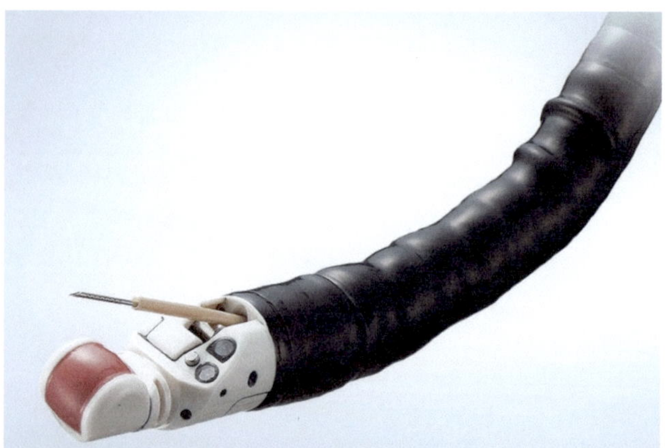

Fig. 7.18 FNA hollow used through an echo-endoscope working channel (Image © Olympus Medical Systems Corporation, Japan, reprint with kind permission)

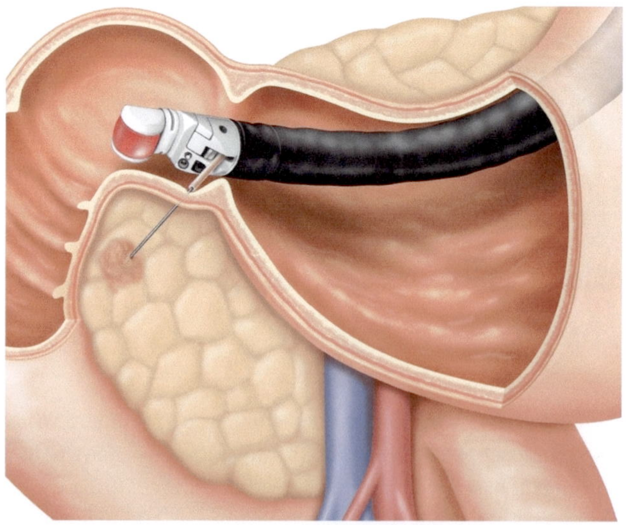

Fig. 7.19 Transduodenal EUS-FNA of a pancreatic lesion (Image © Olympus Medical Systems Corporation, Japan, reprint with kind permission)

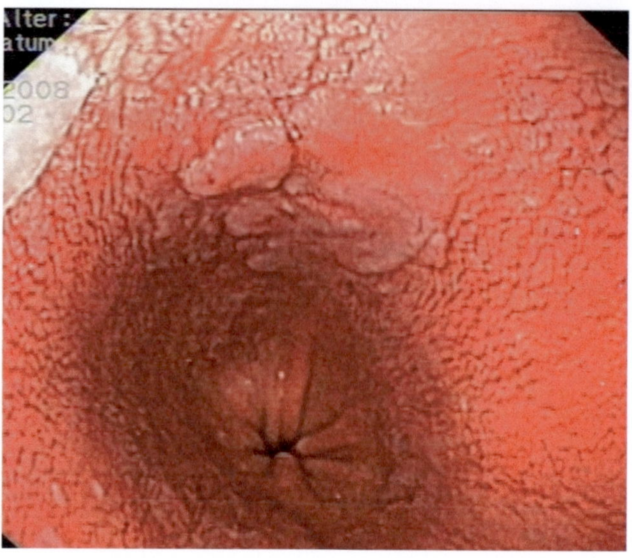

Fig. 7.20 Acetic acid stain to delineate nodular dysplastic area in a Barrett's esophagus

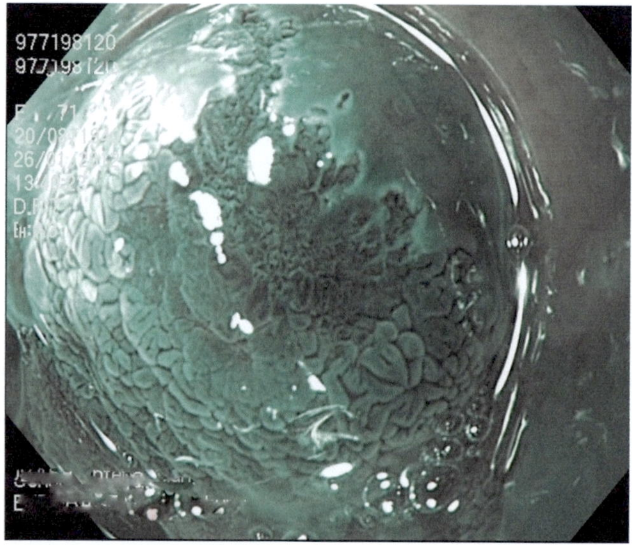

Fig. 7.21 Imaging of a small high-grade dysplastic lesion in a Barrett's esophagus by using acetic acid, NBI, and a transparent cap

Optical Coherence Tomography

Optical coherence tomography (OCT) is an imaging technique analogous to B-mode ultrasound. OCT emits light waves instead of acoustic waves to generate images. The resolution of OCT is about ten times higher compared to high-frequency ultrasound. OCT makes that it is possible to visualize microstructures [18]. OCT uses low-coherence interferometry to capture three-dimensional high-resolution images. Interferometry measures the interference produced by two light beams derived from a single source. It is a catheter-based probe system and can be used through any 2.8 mm

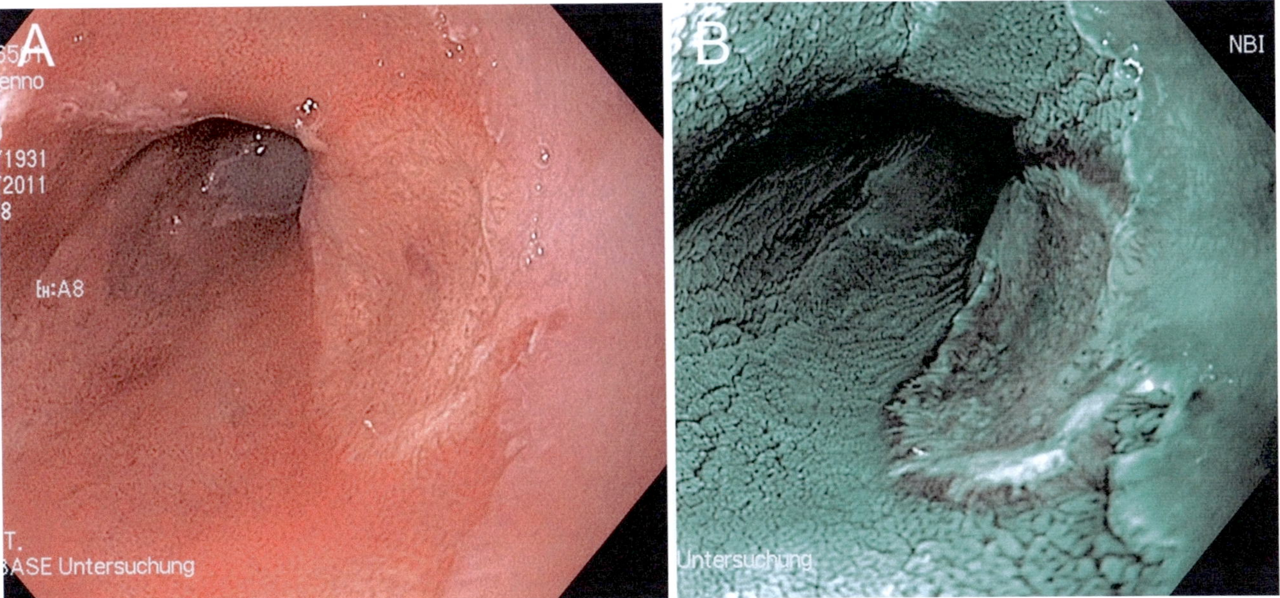

Fig. 7.22 Imaging of an adenocarcinoma within Barrett's mucosa using high-definitions white light endoscopy (**a**) and acetic acid stain combined with NBI (**b**)

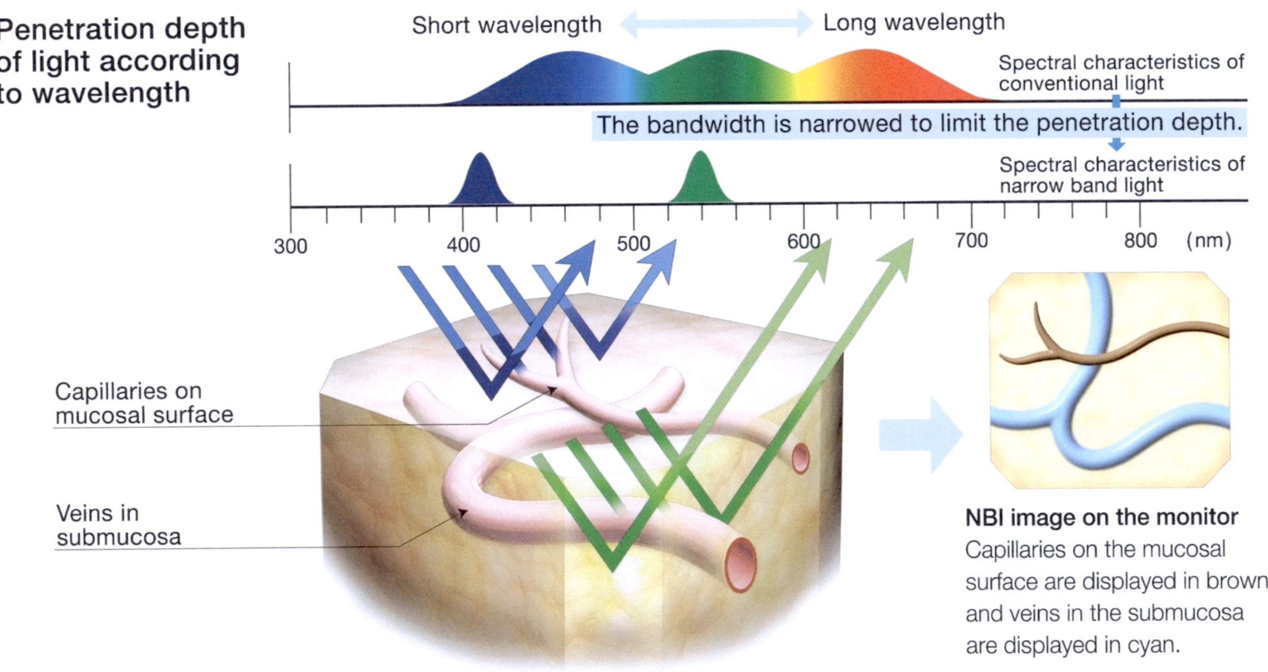

Fig. 7.23 NBI narrows the bandwidth of the emitted light in order to limit penetration depth to enhance visualization of surface and vascular structures (Image © Olympus Medical Systems Corporation, Japan, reprint with kind permission)

working channel. OCT can visualize microscopic mucosal features such as villi, crypts, and glands. Due to scattering of light by the mucosa, the sampling depth of OCT is at about 1–2 mm. OCT has been used clinically to detect buried glands in patients with Barrett's metaplasia after ablation therapy [19, 20].

Other applications currently still under investigation include the use of OCT to differentiate between mucosal and transmural inflammation in inflammatory bowel disease and to examine adenomatous versus hyperplastic polyps. The use of OCT in the biliary and pancreatic ducts has also been reported, but the role of OCT clinically is still unclear [21–23].

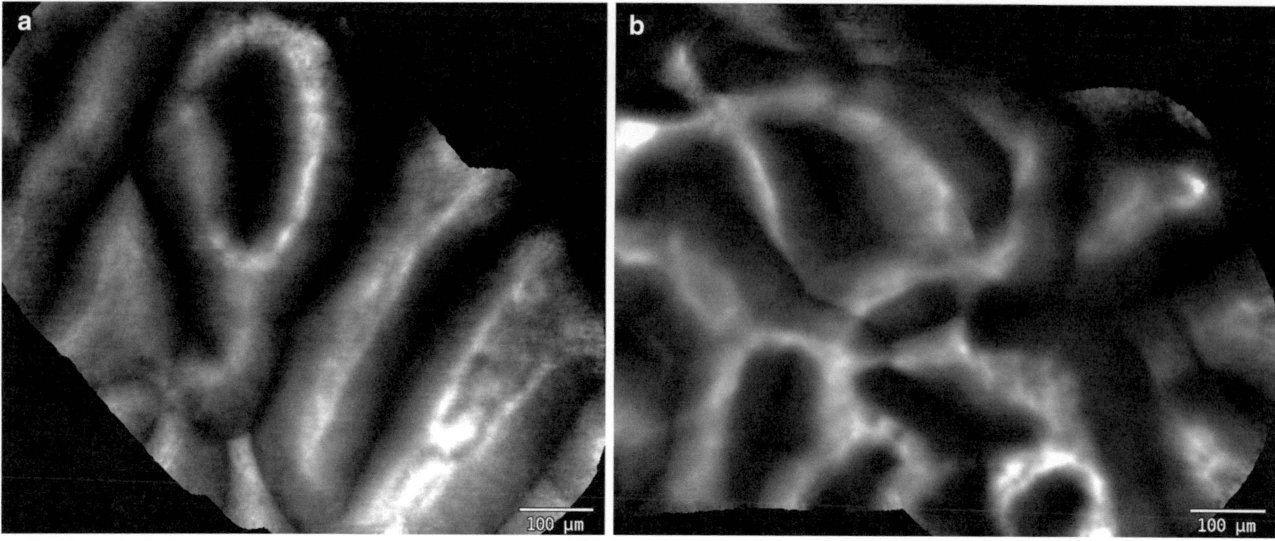

Fig. 7.24 Confocal imaging of Barrret's mucosa (**a**) and gastric cardia mucosa (**b**)

Confocal Endomicroscopy

Confocal endomicroscopy allows for in vivo real-time endoscopic assessment of cellular and subcellular mucosal structures (Fig. 7.24). Two different confocal endomicroscopy techniques are available: confocal imaging that uses tissue reflection and confocal imaging that uses tissue fluorescence. Reflectance imaging has poor resolution and, therefore, fluorescence imaging is currently the preferred method. The fluorescence confocal imaging is available as a probe-based system (Mauna Kea Technologies Inc., Newtown, PA) or an endoscope system with a confocal laser integrated into the tip of the scope (Pentax EC System). Both of these systems require the use of exogenous fluorescence agents. Available agents include fluorescein, acriflavin, and cresyl violet. Fluorescein is administered intravenously and highlights the connective tissue and capillary system during endomicroscopy. Acriflavin is applied topically and enhances the structure of mucosal cells. Endoscopic and confocal images of a target lesion can be obtained at the same time and during the same session. Confocal endomicroscopy has been used to confirm intraepithelial neoplasias for Barrett's esophagus and ulcerative colitis. Moreover, it has been used to diagnose gastric cancer, colorectal adenomas, and celiac disease. In expert hands it has demonstrated remarkable diagnostic accuracy and is helpful as a tool to target biopsies [24]. However, currently, it is not recommended for routine clinical practice or as a replacement for standard biopsy protocols.

Biopsy Protocol Recommendations for the Most Common Gastrointestinal Disorders

The biopsy recommendations outlined below are based on comparative studies, guidelines, and expert opinion.

Esophagus

Uncomplicated gastroesophageal reflux disease (GERD) can be erosive (ERD) or non-erosive (NERD). Both entities do not require routine biopsies to establish the diagnosis. For ERD, the presence of erosive lesions on endoscopy, and typical GERD symptoms are adequate. For NERD, typical symptoms with evidence of pathologic reflux on 24-h pH studies or impedance monitoring are sufficient. In patients with strictures, ulceration, or exophytic lesions, multiple biopsies should be obtained to rule out malignancy. It is recommended to obtain gastric biopsies (2× antrum, 2× body) to check for gastritis and the presence of *Helicobactor Pylori* (*H. Pylori*), in patients with GERD, although the association between *H. Pylori* infection and GERD remains elusive and unpredictable [25]. According to recommendations from the Montreal classification for GERD, Barrett's esophagus is diagnosed exclusively by histopathology [26]. Columnar-lined epithelium in the distal esophagus suspicious for Barrett's should be classified as endoscopically suspected endothelial metaplasia (ESEM) and four quadrant biopsies

Table 7.1 T stage definitions for esophageal cancer (both squamous cell and adenocarcinoma)

Primary tumor (T)[a]	
TX	Primary tumor cannot be assessed
T0	No evidence of primary tumor
Tis	High-grade dysplasia[b]
T1	Tumor invades lamina propria, muscularis mucosae, or submucosa
T1a	Tumor invades lamina propria or muscularis mucosae
T1b	Tumor invades submucosa
T2	Tumor invades muscularis propria
T3	Tumor invades adventitia
T4	Tumor invades adjacent structures
T4a	Resectable tumor invading pleura, pericardium, or diaphragm
T4b	Unresectable tumor invading other adjacent structures, such as aorta, vertebral body, trachea, etc.

From [73]

Note: cTNM is the clinical classification, pTNM is the pathologic classification

[a]At least maximal dimension of the tumor must be recorded and multiple tumors require the T(m) suffix

[b]High-grade dysplasia includes all noninvasive neoplastic epithelia that was formerly called carcinoma in situ, a diagnosis that is longer used for columnar mucosae anywhere in the gastrointestinal tract

Table 7.2 Surveillance of Barrett's esophagus [30]

No dysplasia	3 years
Low-grade dysplasia	12 months
High-grade dysplasia	Indication for definitive therapy

obtained every 1–2 cm over the complete length of the columnar lined epithelium should be obtained. The Seattle protocol, which uses samples of the esophagus in four quadrants at 1 cm intervals, is recommended in all patients with Barrett's esophagus, and specifically those with high-grade dysplasia. Up to 50 % of adenocarcinomas are missed using 2 cm biopsy intervals [27]. More recently, however, a study comparing standard, large capacity, and jumbo forceps for Barrett's biopsies found large capacity forceps using a standard scope to be superior to jumbo ones using a therapeutic endoscope [28]. A "turn and suction" technique is advocated for biopsies of the esophagus. Open forceps are kept close to the tip of the scope until the desired area is identified. The tip of the scope is then deflected towards the wall and suction is applied as the forceps are advanced and then closed [29].

Esophageal adenocarcinoma should be staged with EUS and CT scan as necessary to rule out lymph node involvement or distal metastases. If the diagnostic work up suggests a low-risk early carcinoma (T1a), endoscopic resection can be offered to selected patients, if the appropriate expertise is available. For adenocarcinoma, the risk for lymphatic spread increases with the depth of mucosal invasion (Table 7.1) [30]. After endoscopic therapy for a confirmed T1a adenocarcinoma, close surveillance is needed. Remaining or recurrent Barrett's metaplasia should be removed by EMR or ablation therapy (APC, BarrX), even if there is no dysplasia. When Barrett's with high-grade dysplasia is detected, the diagnosis should be confirmed by a second gastrointestinal pathologist [31]. If there is consensus, the patient can be referred for surgery or endoscopic therapy in selected cases. Endoscopic therapy can be accomplished using both EMR, if there are any nodules or suspicious lesions, and ablation of the remaining Barrett's mucosa. In patients with no dysplasia, surveillance can be performed every 3 years, for low-grade dysplasia every 12 months, and for high-grade dysplasia definitive treatment should be offered (Table 7.2) [30]. Although the recommendation is weak, the most recent ASGE guidelines suggest screening for Barrett's in patients with known risk factors including age older than 50 years, male sex, white race, chronic GERD, hiatal hernia, elevated body mass index, and intra-abdominal distribution of body fat [30]. For patients with symptoms of GERD that do not improve with double-dose PPI therapy, gastroscopy with biopsies of areas suspicious for metaplasia or dysplasia should be performed. If no abnormalities are seen, multiple biopsies are still recommended to rule out eosinophilic esophagitis, however, there is no data to support routine biopsies of the *z*-line without visible abnormalities [32].

For the diagnosis of eosinophilic esophagitis, separate biopsies from at least two different levels of the esophagus are recommended to confirm the diagnosis and to differentiate it from ERD. A 2-month course of proton pump inhibitor therapy is recommended prior to repeat endoscopic biopsies. The diagnosis requires at least 1 specimen with 20 or greater eosinophils per high power field. Patients with other gastrointestinal symptoms should also have gastric and duodenal biopsies to rule out eosinophilic gastroenteritis [33].

Stomach

H. Pylori infection can be diagnosed by endoscopic biopsy using a urease test (test of choice), histology (more expensive), or bacterial culture (used after eradication failure). Endoscopy is not indicated for the purpose of establishing an *H. Pylori* diagnosis. For patients suspected to be infected, it is recommended to obtain at least two biopsies from the antrum (about 3–5 cm from the pylorus) and two biopsies from the body of the stomach [34]. Urease tests on gastric biopsies have a sensitivity of 90–95 % and a specificity of 95–100 %. Sensitivity is decreased in patients with recent gastrointestinal bleeding or who use PPIs, H2 blockers, antibiotics, or bismuth-containing compounds. Obtaining tissue samples from both the antrum and the fundus is recommended for these patients and can increase the sensitivity [35].

Single antral biopsies show excellent *H. pylori* sensitivity in untreated patients. However, after effective therapy, sensitivities of biopsy tests decrease. Combined use of testing methods increases the diagnostic yield when assessing post-treatment *H. pylori* status with endoscopy, whereas the addition of multiple biopsies for each type of test is of more limited value [36]. Ideally, proton pump inhibitors, H2 blockers (2 weeks), and all antibiotics (4 weeks) should be discontinued prior to endoscopic biopsies [25]. In patients, who need to remain on PPI or who are on antibiotics multiple biopsies from the antrum and corpus in combination with a rapid urease test is recommended [37].

If a gastric ulcer is present, multiple biopsies should be obtained from both the borders and center of the lesion [38]. One biopsy of a gastric ulcer has about a 70 % sensitivity for detecting gastric cancer. Performing seven or more increases the sensitivity to 98 % [39].

In addition antral and fundic biopsies (two each) should be obtained. Gastric ulcers should be followed up after 8–12 weeks of therapy to confirm healing, and repeated biopsies to rule out carcinoma should be obtained [40]. If the ulcer does not heal after therapy and cessation of NSAIDS, surgical excision should be performed.

Focal gastric lesions, suspicious for MALT lymphoma should be extensively biopsies (>10) and gastric mapping biopsies should also be performed [41]. This includes at least four biopsies each from the antrum and corpus and two from the fundus. An additional urease test is also recommended. Testing for chronic gastritis requires a minimum of two biopsies each of the body and fundus.

Gastric polyps are rarely adenomatous or malignant; however, biopsies of several representative polyps should be obtained to confirm this. Most gastric polyps are hyperplastic with no risk of malignant transformation. Fundic gland polyps are often associated with PPI use and only require biopsies if they are large. If multiple fundic gland polyps are present, representative biopsies should be obtained. Sporadic fundic gland polyps and those occurring in patients on PPIs have essentially no risk of malignant degeneration [42–44]. Fundic gland polyps in patients with FAP, however, can harbor dysplasia in up to 40 % of cases [45]. These polyps are seen in 20–100 % of patients with FAP, are usually multiple, and occur at an earlier age [46]. Colonoscopy, therefore, should be considered in young patients with multiple fundic gland polyps who are not on PPI therapy, given the association with colonic polyps and familial adenomatous polyposis [47]. Hyperplastic polyps larger than 2 cm should be removed to rule out underlying adenomas [48]. Histology confirmed gastric adenomas should be removed endoscopically.

Subepithelial gastric lesions should be investigated by EUS. Mucosal biopsies using standard forceps are often not contributory since they do not achieve adequate depth to sample these lesions. Lesions suspicious for gastrointestinal stromal tumors (GIST) >2–3 cm, or lesions that have increased in size on repeat endoscopy after 6–12 months should be surgically removed [49]. Smaller lesions can be followed by EUS.

Duodenum

Patients with iron deficiency anemia should undergo duodenal biopsies to rule out celiac disease. Biopsies for celiac disease should include at least four duodenal biopsies—two from the bulb and two more distally. Such biopsy protocols will be sufficient to rule out or confirm suspected Giardia or Whipple's disease [50, 51].

Duodenal ulcers are normally associated with *H. Pylori* infection. Malignant duodenal ulcers are exceptionally rare. However, infiltration of the duodenum from pancreaticobiliary cancers can cause duodenal ulceration. If a very irregular appearing duodenal ulcer or other suspicious lesion is seen in the duodenum, biopsies should be performed. *H. Pylori* testing as recommended above is also essential in the presence of a duodenal ulcer.

Hepatobiliary

Tumors in this area still present a diagnostic challenge, and clinicians require clinical, radiologic, endoscopic, and histologic information to make a diagnosis. Tissue sampling through the endoscope can be performed using brush cytology, aspiration, and biopsy forceps. Often a combination of two or all three of these modalities is needed to obtain enough cells for an adequate cytologic assessment. A recent study suggests that brush cytology combined with biopsies for the diagnosis of suspected cholangiocarcinoma during ERCP may have higher yield than either technique on its own [52]. Positive results for malignancy were obtained in 41.4 % by brush cytology and in 53.4 % by forceps biopsy. Combination of both techniques resulted in an increase in diagnostic sensitivity to 60.3 % [52]. Even with combination of brush and forceps biopsy sensitivity for cholangiocarcinoma remains problematic. Alternative access routes for visualization of ductal pancreatico-hepatobiliary lesions and tissue sampling are possible by inserting a thin endoscope through the working channel of the duodenoscope into the hepatic or pancreatic duct and obtaining biopsies under direct visualization. This can be done by classical two operator mother baby endoscopy or single operator cholangioscopy (SpyGlass Direct Visualization System; Boston Scientific, Natick, MA). Some studies have indicated an advantage of cholangioscopy to increase diagnostic sensitivity [53–55]. However, not all studies show a clear benefit, image quality of mother–baby systems is limited and the two operator technique can be cumbersome and time consuming [56]. To increase image quality and endoscope handling, direct peroral cholangioscopy was recently introduced. For this technique a small diameter (>6 mm) upper endoscope is introduced over a guidewire or with a dedicated anchoring balloon system (Cook Medical, Winston-Salem, NC). Image quality is excellent compared to mother–baby systems. However, larger

Table 7.3 Surveillance recommendations after colonic polypectomy [70]

Patients with small rectal hyperplastic polyps	Considered to have normal colonoscopies, and the interval before the subsequent colonoscopy should be 10 years; an exception is patients with a hyperplastic polyposis syndrome—need to be identified for more intensive follow-up evaluation
Patients with only 1 or 2 small (<1 cm) tubular adenomas with only low-grade dysplasia	Next follow-up colonoscopy in 5–10 years; precise timing based on clinical factors (prior colonoscopy findings, family history, and preferences of the patient and judgment of the physician)
Patients with 3–10 adenomas, any adenoma >1 cm, any adenoma with villous features, or high-grade dysplasia	Next follow-up colonoscopy in 3 years if adenoma(s) are removed completely; if the follow-up colonoscopy is normal or shows only 1 or 2 small tubular adenomas with low-grade dysplasia, then the interval for the subsequent examination should be 5 years
Patients who have more than 10 adenomas at 1 examination	Should be examined at a shorter (~3 years) interval, established by clinical judgment consider the possibility of an underlying familial syndrome
Patients with sessile adenomas that are removed piecemeal	Follow-up evaluation at short intervals (2–6 months) to verify complete removal; once complete removal has been established, subsequent surveillance needs to be individualized based on the endoscopist's judgment; completeness of removal should be based on both endoscopic and pathologic assessments

clinical or comparative studies are lacking and no final conclusion on diagnostic accuracy, biopsy sensitivity, and potential risks can be made at present stage [57–61].

Inspection of the major papilla for malignant or premalignant lesions is recommended by using a side-viewing endoscope. Papillary lesions with ulcerations in patients with cholestasis and weight loss are typical for invasive carcinoma of the major papilla. Endoscopic biopsies should be obtained from all papillary lesions [62]. In the case of a bulging papilla suspicious for adenoma two biopsies are be sufficient. Larger lesions suspicious for carcinoma will require more biopsies. There is always a risk, however, for pancreatitis when biopsies of the major papilla are obtained. Therefore, unnecessary biopsies should be avoided, and care should be taken not to biopsy the area where the pancreatic duct ends into the major papilla. This is presumably in the right lower quadrant. In the case of a bulging papilla without macroscopic alterations suspicious for adenoma, an EUS can be helpful to determine intraductal adenomas. EUS has shown a higher accuracy for staging of papillary lesions and should be the next diagnostic step in the work-up of papillary lesions [63]. EMR has shown good results as definitive treatment for papillary adenomas and can be considered as treatment for early carcinoma depending on patient age and comorbidities [64, 65]. In case of a lesion that seems adequate for endoscopic resection rash ERCP and especially sphincterotomy should be avoided to enable curative and complete EMR. Biliary sphincterotomy, stenting of the biliary and pancreatic duct, should be recommended after EMR has been facilitated [64].

Colon and Rectum

Patients undergoing colonoscopy for diarrhea should have biopsies, even if the mucosa appears normal. To rule out or confirm microscopic colitis (collagenous or lymphocytic colitis which usually shows normal appearing mucosa), ulcerative colitis, or Crohn's disease, separate biopsies (two from each segment) of the terminal ileum, ascending, transverse, sigmoid colon, and rectum should be performed [66, 67]. For patients with suspected Crohn's disease, an EGD with biopsies should be added. For surveillance of ulcerative colitis, yearly colonoscopy with biopsies starting 8–10 years after the initial diagnosis is recommended for patients with pancolitis [68]. For patients with left-sided colitis, yearly colonoscopy should be performed starting 15 years after the initial diagnosis. To rule out malignancy in the setting of ulcerative colitis, biopsies should be taken in four quadrants every 10–12 cm from the cecum to the rectum [69]. Ulcerative colitis patients with high-grade dysplasia or dysplasia associated lesion or mass (DALM), independent of high- or low-grade status, should undergo proctocolectomy [69]. If the rectum is left in place, yearly endoscopic inspection should be performed. For patients with active Crohn's disease in the colon, the same surveillance protocol applies. If primary sclerosing cholangitis (PSC) is diagnosed, patients should undergo yearly colonoscopy.

All polyps in the colon should be biopsied or removed. Polyps less than or equal to 5 mm can be removed with biopsy forceps or cold snare, and larger lesions should be removed using a snare. Multiple hyperplastic polyps in the rectum can be left without obtaining biopsies [70]. All patients with adenomatous polyps need endoscopic follow-up depending on their pathology. If en bloc resection cannot be confirmed (i.e., piecemeal EMR), prompt endoscopic follow-up (in 2–6 months) with biopsies should be performed. Whenever the endoscopic removal of an adenomatous polyp is not clearly complete (en bloc, positive lateral or deep margins), repeat biopsies of the site are necessary [71]. Table 7.3 outlines the surveillance recommendations after polypectomy put forth by the US Multi-Society Task Force on Colorectal Cancer and the American Cancer Society in 2006 [70]. If there is any doubt, then early repeat colonos-

Table 7.4 Management of anticoagulation and antiplatelet agents in patients requiring endoscopy

Procedure	Condition	Management anticoagulation	Management antiplatelet
Low (diagnostic endoscopy with biopsies, ERCP+stent, EUS, etc.)	High or low	No change in anticoagulation, delay in patients with supratherapeutic INR	Clopidogrel, ticlopidine, ASA—no need to stop
High (polypectomy, EMR, sphincterotomy, dilation of stricture, EUS with FNA)	Low	Warfarin—stop 5 days prior and confirm INR ≤1.4 / Dabigatran—stop 1–2 days prior	Clopidogrel—Stop 7–10 days prior to procedure—consult cardiology and/or neurology as needed
High	High	Bridge therapy with low molecular weight heparin	Clopidogrel—Stop 7–10 days prior to procedure—consult cardiology and/or neurology
			Consider temporarily replacing with ASA
			Consider delaying procedure if possible until risk of stopping antiplatelets is more acceptable

EMR endoscopic mucosal resection, *FNA* fine need aspiration, *EUS* endoscopic ultrasound, *ERCP* endoscopic retrograde cholangiopancreatography

copy with biopsies should be considered. Early colorectal carcinomas (T1a) with low-risk characteristics such as absence of lymphovascular invasion or poor differentiation can be removed endoscopically if complete excision is feasible and can be determined [71]. If the resection is incomplete, or the lesion is high risk, surgery should be offered.

Recommendations for Tissue Sampling in Patients on Anticoagulant and Antiplatelet Agents

In determining how to manage these patients, one must always balance the risk of procedure-related bleeding (procedure risk) with the risk related to the condition (condition risk) that requires anticoagulation or antiplatelet therapy. The most common situations are outlined in Table 7.4 and based on recommendations by the American Society of Gastrointestinal Endoscopists (ASGE) [72]. Another option in patients who are at high risk for complications, if anticoagulant or antiplatelets are stopped, is to perform the diagnostic procedure, and if a more invasive intervention needs to be performed (i.e., polypectomy), patients can then be prepared and the procedure can be repeated. In most situations, patients can be restarted on therapy a few hours after the procedure. In patients with low-risk conditions, consider restarting in 3–5 days after sphincterotomy and 2 weeks after removal of a sessile polyp, when the risk of bleeding is decreased. Patients taking more than one agent such as ASA and NSAIDS or clopidogrel and ASA should be advised to stop one of the agents prior to low-risk procedures. High-risk procedures can be performed on patients taking ASA if needed.

Summary

Endoscopy is essential in the diagnosis and treatment of gastrointestinal diseases. Modern endoscopes permit detailed surface and vascular imaging. Endoscopic biopsies and tissue sampling, however, remain essential in the diagnosis and follow-up of gastrointestinal diseases. Multiple different techniques and devices have been developed to optimize diagnostic yield when used with specialized endoscopic techniques such as ERCP and EUS. Pancreatic, hepatobiliary, and submucosal neoplasms (i.e., GIST) can still be challenging, and there is room for improvement in the tissue sampling methods for these lesions. Modifications to existing techniques or the development of new technologies may help us to overcome some of the current limitations of the flexible endoscope. Certainly, the NOTES movement has spurred the creation of numerous endoscopic tools and devices. The future will tell if real-time endoscopic histopathology can replace tissue sampling. Developments in the area of endoscopic image enhancement are promising and might have the potential to change future practices. Currently, however, standard biopsy tools and recommended biopsy and surveillance protocols remain the gold standard.

References

1. Salmore R. Our heritage: a history of gastroenterology and gastroenterology nursing. Gastroenterol Nurs. 1998;21:40–3.
2. Faigel DO, Eisen GM, Baron TH, Dominitz JA, Goldstein JL, Hirota WK, et al. Tissue sampling and analysis. Gastrointest Endosc. 2003;57:811–6.
3. Gilbert DA, DiMarino AJ, Jensen DM, Katon R, Kimmey MB, Laine LA, et al. Status evaluation: hot biopsy forceps. American Society for Gastrointestinal Endoscopy. Technology Assessment Committee. Gastrointest Endosc. 1992;38:753–6.
4. Gibbs DH, Opelka FG, Beck DE, Hicks TC, Timmcke AE, Gathright Jr JB. Postpolypectomy colonic hemorrhage. Dis Colon Rectum. 1996;39:806–10.
5. Rosen L, Bub DS, Reed 3rd JF, Nastasee SA. Hemorrhage following colonoscopic polypectomy. Dis Colon Rectum. 1993;36:1126–31.
6. Waye JD, Lewis BS, Yessayan S. Colonoscopy: a prospective report of complications. J Clin Gastroenterol. 1992;15:347–51.
7. Sorbi D, Norton I, Conio M, Balm R, Zinsmeister A, Gostout CJ. Postpolypectomy lower GI bleeding: descriptive analysis. Gastrointest Endosc. 2000;51:690–6.
8. Buddingh KT, Herngreen T, Haringsma J, van der Zwet WC, Vleggaar FP, Breumelhof R, et al. Location in the right hemi-colon

is an independent risk factor for delayed post-polypectomy hemorrhage: a multi-center case-control study. Am J Gastroenterol. 2011;106:1119–24.

9. Dyer WS, Quigley EM, Noel SM, Camacho KE, Manela F, Zetterman RK. Major colonic hemorrhage following electrocoagulating (hot) biopsy of diminutive colonic polyps: relationship to colonic location and low-dose aspirin therapy. Gastrointest Endosc. 1991;37:361–4.

10. Trecca A, Gaj F, Di Lorenzo GP, Ricciardi MR, Silano M, Bella A, et al. Improved detection of colorectal neoplasms with selective use of chromoendoscopy in 2005 consecutive patients. Tech Coloproctol. 2006;10:339–44.

11. Uraoka T, Saito Y, Ikematsu H, Yamamoto K, Sano Y. Sano's capillary pattern classification for narrow-band imaging of early colorectal lesions. Dig Endosc. 2011;23 Suppl 1:112–5.

12. Cha JM, Lee JI, Joo KR, Jung SW, Shin HP. A prospective randomized study on computed virtual chromoendoscopy versus conventional colonoscopy for the detection of small colorectal adenomas. Dig Dis Sci. 2010;55:2357–64.

13. Adler A, Aschenbeck J, Yenerim T, Mayr M, Aminalai A, Drossel R, et al. Narrow-band versus white-light high definition television endoscopic imaging for screening colonoscopy: a prospective randomized trial. Gastroenterology. 2009;136:410–6.e1; quiz 715.

14. Adler A, Wegscheider K, Lieberman D, Aminalai A, Aschenbeck J, Drossel R, et al. Factors determining the quality of screening colonoscopy: a prospective study on adenoma detection rates, from 12 134 examinations (Berlin colonoscopy project 3, BECOP-3). Gut. 2013;62(2):236–41.

15. Aminalai A, Rosch T, Aschenbeck J, Mayr M, Drossel R, Schroder A, et al. Live image processing does not increase adenoma detection rate during colonoscopy: a randomized comparison between FICE and conventional imaging (Berlin Colonoscopy Project 5, BECOP-5). Am J Gastroenterol. 2010;105:2383–8.

16. Vemulapalli KC, Rex DK. Evolving techniques in colonoscopy. Curr Opin Gastroenterol. 2011;27:430–8.

17. Adler A, Pohl H, Papanikolaou IS, Abou-Rebyeh H, Schachschal G, Veltzke-Schlieker W, et al. A prospective randomised study on narrow-band imaging versus conventional colonoscopy for adenoma detection: does narrow-band imaging induce a learning effect? Gut. 2008;57:59–64.

18. Shukla R, Abidi WM, Richards-Kortum R, Anandasabapathy S. Endoscopic imaging: how far are we from real-time histology? World J Gastrointest Endosc. 2011;3:183–94.

19. Adler DC, Zhou C, Tsai TH, Lee HC, Becker L, Schmitt JM, et al. Three-dimensional optical coherence tomography of Barrett's esophagus and buried glands beneath neosquamous epithelium following radiofrequency ablation. Endoscopy. 2009;41:773–6.

20. Cobb MJ, Hwang JH, Upton MP, Chen Y, Oelschlager BK, Wood DE, et al. Imaging of subsquamous Barrett's epithelium with ultra-high-resolution optical coherence tomography: a histologic correlation study. Gastrointest Endosc. 2010;71:223–30.

21. Seitz U, Freund J, Jaeckle S, Feldchtein F, Bohnacker S, Thonke F, et al. First in vivo optical coherence tomography in the human bile duct. Endoscopy. 2001;33:1018–21.

22. Poneros JM, Tearney GJ, Shiskov M, Kelsey PB, Lauwers GY, Nishioka NS, et al. Optical coherence tomography of the biliary tree during ERCP. Gastrointest Endosc. 2002;55:84–8.

23. Arvanitakis M, Hookey L, Tessier G, Demetter P, Nagy N, Stellke A, et al. Intraductal optical coherence tomography during endoscopic retrograde cholangiopancreatography for investigation of biliary strictures. Endoscopy. 2009;41:696–701.

24. Ussui VM, Wallace MB. Confocal endomicroscopy of colorectal polyps. Gastroenterol Res Pract. 2012;2012:545679.

25. Chey WD, Wong BCY, Practice Parameters Committee of the American College of Gastroenterology. American College of Gastroenterology guideline on the management of Helicobacter pylori infection. Am J Gastroenterol. 2007;102:1808–25.

26. Vakil N, van Zanten SV, Kahrilas P, Dent J, Jones R, Global Consensus Group. The Montreal definition and classification of gastroesophageal reflux disease: a global evidence-based consensus. Am J Gastroenterol. 2006;101:1900–20; quiz 1943.

27. Reid BJ, Blount PL, Feng Z, Levine DS. Optimizing endoscopic biopsy detection of early cancers in Barrett's high-grade dysplasia. Am J Gastroenterol. 2000;95:3089–96.

28. Gonzalez S, Yu WM, Smith MS, Slack KN, Rotterdam H, Abrams JA, et al. Randomized comparison of 3 different-sized biopsy forceps for quality of sampling in Barrett's esophagus. Gastrointest Endosc. 2010;72:935–40.

29. Levine DS, Haggitt RC, Blount PL, Rabinovitch PS, Rusch VW, Reid BJ. An endoscopic biopsy protocol can differentiate high-grade dysplasia from early adenocarcinoma in Barrett's esophagus. Gastroenterology. 1993;105:40–50.

30. Spechler SJ, Sharma P, Souza RF, Inadomi JM, Shaheen NJ. American Gastroenterological Association medical position statement on the management of Barrett's esophagus. Gastroenterology. 2011;140:1084–91.

31. Hulscher JB, Haringsma J, Benraadt J, Offerhaus GJ, ten Kate FJ, Baak JP, et al. Comprehensive Cancer Centre Amsterdam Barrett Advisory Committee: first results. Neth J Med. 2001;58:3–8.

32. Kahrilas PJ, Shaheen NJ, Vaezi MF, Hiltz SW, Black E, Modlin IM, et al. American Gastroenterological Association Medical Position Statement on the management of gastroesophageal reflux disease. Gastroenterology. 2008;135:1383–91. 1391.e1–5.

33. Ammoury RF, Rosenman MB, Roettcher D, Gupta SK. Incidental gastric eosinophils in patients with eosinophilic esophagitis: do they matter? J Pediatr Gastroenterol Nutr. 2010;51:723–6.

34. van IJzendoorn MC, Laheij RJF, de Boer WA, Jansen JBMJ. The importance of corpus biopsies for the determination of Helicobacter pylori infection. Neth J Med. 2005;63:141–5.

35. Weston AP, Campbell DR, Hassanein RS, Cherian R, Dixon A, McGregor DH. Prospective, multivariate evaluation of CLOtest performance. Am J Gastroenterol. 1997;92:1310–5.

36. Laine L, Sugg J, Suchower L, Neil G. Endoscopic biopsy requirements for post-treatment diagnosis of Helicobacter pylori. Gastrointest Endosc. 2000;51:664–9.

37. Graham DY, Genta R, Evans DG, Reddy R, Clarridge JE, Olson CA, et al. Helicobacter pylori does not migrate from the antrum to the corpus in response to omeprazole. Am J Gastroenterol. 1996;91:2120–4.

38. Hatfield AR, Slavin G, Segal AW, Levi AJ. Importance of the site of endoscopic gastric biopsy in ulcerating lesions of the stomach. Gut. 1975;16:884–6.

39. Graham DY, Schwartz JT, Cain GD, Gyorkey F. Prospective evaluation of biopsy number in the diagnosis of esophageal and gastric carcinoma. Gastroenterology. 1982;82:228–31.

40. Banerjee S, Cash BD, Dominitz JA, Baron TH, Anderson MA, Ben-Menachem T, et al. The role of endoscopy in the management of patients with peptic ulcer disease. Gastrointest Endosc. 2010;71:663–8.

41. Genta RM, Graham DY. Comparison of biopsy sites for the histopathologic diagnosis of Helicobacter pylori: a topographic study of H. pylori density and distribution. Gastrointest Endosc. 1994;40:342–5.

42. Jalving M, Koornstra JJ, Wesseling J, Boezen HM, De Jong S, Kleibeuker JH. Increased risk of fundic gland polyps during long-term proton pump inhibitor therapy. Aliment Pharmacol Ther. 2006;24:1341–8.

43. el-Zimaity HM, Jackson FW, Graham DY. Fundic gland polyps developing during omeprazole therapy. Am J Gastroenterol. 1997;92:1858–60.

44. Choudhry U, Boyce Jr HW, Coppola D. Proton pump inhibitor-associated gastric polyps: a retrospective analysis of their frequency, and endoscopic, histologic, and ultrastructural characteristics. Am J Clin Pathol. 1998;110:615–21.

45. Bertoni G, Sassatelli R, Nigrisoli E, Pennazio M, Tansini P, Arrigoni A, et al. Dysplastic changes in gastric fundic gland polyps of patients with familial adenomatous polyposis. Ital J Gastroenterol Hepatol. 1999;31:192–7.

46. Domizio P, Talbot IC, Spigelman AD, Williams CB, Phillips RK. Upper gastrointestinal pathology in familial adenomatous polyposis: results from a prospective study of 102 patients. J Clin Pathol. 1990;43:738–43.

47. Lynch HT, Snyder C, Davies JM, Lanspa S, Lynch J, Gatalica Z, et al. FAP, gastric cancer, and genetic counseling featuring children and young adults: a family study and review. Fam Cancer. 2010; 9:581–8.

48. Ginsberg GG, Al-Kawas FH, Fleischer DE, Reilly HF, Benjamin SB. Gastric polyps: relationship of size and histology to cancer risk. Am J Gastroenterol. 1996;91:714–7.

49. Fletcher CD, Berman JJ, Corless C, Gorstein F, Lasota J, Longley BJ, et al. Diagnosis of gastrointestinal stromal tumors: a consensus approach. Int J Surg Pathol. 2002;10:81–9.

50. Pais WP, Duerksen DR, Pettigrew NM, Bernstein CN. How many duodenal biopsy specimens are required to make a diagnosis of celiac disease? Gastrointest Endosc. 2008;67:1082–7.

51. Green PHR, Cellier C. Celiac disease. N Engl J Med. 2007;357: 1731–43.

52. Weber A, von Weyhern C, Fend F, Schneider J, Neu B, Meining A, et al. Endoscopic transpapillary brush cytology and forceps biopsy in patients with hilar cholangiocarcinoma. World J Gastroenterol. 2008;14:1097–101.

53. Ramchandani M, Reddy DN, Gupta R, Lakhtakia S, Tandan M, Darisetty S, et al. Role of single-operator peroral cholangioscopy in the diagnosis of indeterminate biliary lesions: a single-center, prospective study. Gastrointest Endosc. 2011;74:511–9.

54. Shah RJ, Langer DA, Antillon MR, Chen YK. Cholangioscopy and cholangioscopic forceps biopsy in patients with indeterminate pancreaticobiliary pathology. Clin Gastroenterol Hepatol. 2006;4: 219–25.

55. Draganov PV, Chauhan S, Wagh MS, Gupte AR, Lin T, Hou W, et al. Diagnostic accuracy of conventional and cholangioscopy-guided sampling of indeterminate biliary lesions at the time of ERCP: a prospective, long-term follow-up study. Gastrointest Endosc. 2012;75:347–53.

56. Hartman DJ, Slivka A, Giusto DA, Krasinskas AM. Tissue yield and diagnostic efficacy of fluoroscopic and cholangioscopic techniques to assess indeterminate biliary strictures. Clin Gastroenterol Hepatol. 2012;10(9):1042–6.

57. Waxman I, Dillon T, Chmura K, Wardrip C, Chennat J, Konda V. Feasibility of a novel system for intraductal balloon-anchored direct peroral cholangioscopy and endotherapy with an ultraslim endoscope (with videos). Gastrointest Endosc. 2010;72:1052–6.

58. Moon JH, Ko BM, Choi HJ, Koo HC, Hong SJ, Cheon YK, et al. Direct peroral cholangioscopy using an ultra-slim upper endoscope for the treatment of retained bile duct stones. Am J Gastroenterol. 2009;104:2729–33.

59. Moon JH, Choi HJ, Ko BM. Therapeutic role of direct peroral cholangioscopy using an ultra-slim upper endoscope. J Hepatobiliary Pancreat Sci. 2011;18:350–6.

60. Kim HI, Moon JH, Choi HJ, Lee JC, Ahn HS, Song AR, et al. Holmium laser lithotripsy under direct peroral cholangioscopy by using an ultra-slim upper endoscope for patients with retained bile duct stones (with video). Gastrointest Endosc. 2011;74: 1127–32.

61. Choi HJ, Moon JH, Ko BM, Hong SJ, Koo HC, Cheon YK, et al. Overtube-balloon-assisted direct peroral cholangioscopy by using an ultra-slim upper endoscope (with videos). Gastrointest Endosc. 2009;69:935–40.

62. Komorowski RA, Beggs BK, Geenan JE, Venu RP. Assessment of ampulla of Vater pathology. An endoscopic approach. Am J Surg Pathol. 1991;15:1188–96.

63. Cannon ME, Carpenter SL, Elta GH, Nostrant TT, Kochman ML, Ginsberg GG, et al. EUS compared with CT, magnetic resonance imaging, and angiography and the influence of biliary stenting on staging accuracy of ampullary neoplasms. Gastrointest Endosc. 1999;50:27–33.

64. Bohnacker S, Seitz U, Nguyen D, Thonke F, Seewald S, deWeerth A, et al. Endoscopic resection of benign tumors of the duodenal papilla without and with intraductal growth. Gastrointest Endosc. 2005;62:551–60.

65. Catalano MF, Linder JD, Chak A, Sivak Jr MV, Raijman I, Geenen JE, et al. Endoscopic management of adenoma of the major duodenal papilla. Gastrointest Endosc. 2004;59:225–32.

66. Giardiello FM, Lazenby AJ, Bayless TM, Levine EJ, Bias WB, Ladenson PW, et al. Lymphocytic (microscopic) colitis. Clinicopathologic study of 18 patients and comparison to collagenous colitis. Dig Dis Sci. 1989;34:1730–8.

67. Yusoff IF, Ormonde DG, Hoffman NE. Routine colonic mucosal biopsy and ileoscopy increases diagnostic yield in patients undergoing colonoscopy for diarrhea. J Gastroenterol Hepatol. 2002; 17:276–80.

68. Itzkowitz SH, Present DH, Crohn's and Colitis Foundation of America Colon Cancer in IBD Study Group. Consensus conference: colorectal cancer screening and surveillance in inflammatory bowel disease. Inflamm Bowel Dis. 2005;11:314–21.

69. Leighton JA, Shen B, Baron TH, Adler DG, Davila R, Egan JV, et al. ASGE guideline: endoscopy in the diagnosis and treatment of inflammatory bowel disease. Gastrointest Endosc. 2006;63: 558–65.

70. Winawer SJ, Zauber AG, Fletcher RH, Stillman JS, O'Brien MJ, Levin B, et al. Guidelines for colonoscopy surveillance after polypectomy: a consensus update by the US Multi-Society Task Force on Colorectal Cancer and the American Cancer Society. Gastroenterology. 2006;130:1872–85.

71. Bond JH. Polyp guideline: diagnosis, treatment, and surveillance for patients with colorectal polyps. Practice Parameters Committee of the American College of Gastroenterology. Am J Gastroenterol. 2000;95:3053–63.

72. Anderson MA, Ben-Menachem T, Gan SI, Appalaneni V, Banerjee S, Cash BD, et al. Management of antithrombotic agents for endoscopic procedures. Gastrointest Endosc. 2009;70: 1060–70.

73. American Joint Committee on Cancer (AJCC). AJCC cancer staging manual. 7th ed. New York: Springer; 2010.

Tools and Techniques for Gastrointestinal Hemostasis

Sajida Ahad and John D. Mellinger

Introduction

Acute gastrointestinal (GI) bleeding can be amongst the most challenging GI conditions for care givers and is optimally managed in a multidisciplinary fashion. Team members can be highly variable and may include an emergency room physician, interventional radiologist or vascular surgeon, gastroenterologist, intensivist, and surgeon or surgical endoscopist. It is vital to have clear, concise and current communication among team members to optimize outcome for the patient. Each member has a critical role from initiating resuscitation promptly in the emergency room, to endoscopic diagnostic and therapeutic management, to endovascular or interventional radiologic strategies if endoscopic therapies fail, and finally to post-procedure support and monitoring of the patient. This chapter provides an in-depth look at the tools used to gain endoscopic hemostasis in the GI tract. Basic elements of the proper evaluation and preparation of a patient for endoscopic therapy of GI bleeding are also covered.

Patient Preparation

A patient with suspected GI bleeding should be carefully evaluated for hemodynamic instability and admitted to the appropriate area of the hospital for resuscitation. It is imperative to have two large bore peripheral IVs for prompt fluid resuscitation and infusion of crystalloids. Blood samples should be sent for type and cross match, complete blood count, electrolytes and coagulation studies. A nasogastric tube may be placed to confirm the diagnosis of an upper GI bleed, but is not essential if expeditious endoscopy is expected and the patient is not vomiting, and is contraindicated in variceal hemorrhage. It is important to note that a negative nasogastric aspirate for blood does not preclude an upper GI source of bleeding, particularly if the aspirate is non-bilious and therefore fails to document duodenal sampling. A urinary catheter should be placed to help monitor urinary output and guide resuscitation efforts. The patient should be given nothing per mouth. Supplemental oxygen may be necessary depending on the degree of hemorrhage and the patient's underlying cardiopulmonary status. In patients with massive upper GI bleeding and hemodynamic instability, airway protection with endotracheal intubation should be considered. Blood and blood products should be administered as dictated by the clinical course and proton pump inhibitors (PPI) should be started immediately—even before endoscopic confirmation of bleeding [1].

It is important to remember that the patient condition may dictate that the procedure be done in the intensive care unit, emergency room or operating room rather than the endoscopy suite. In such cases it is imperative to ensure that the room has at least two suction ports, supplemental oxygen outlet, emergency code cart with intubation equipment, ambu bag and a well-stocked endoscopy cart. The endoscopy nurse plays a pivotal role in such procedures as the team relies on him or her for availability of equipment and medications. The endoscopist and/or the nurse should check all endoscopic equipment prior to starting the procedure to make sure it is working properly (see Chap 3). Endoscopic and clinical scoring systems have been developed to predict the risk of re-bleeding and help triage the patient to the appropriate care environment. The Rockall Score uses age, comorbidity, presence of stigmata of recent hemorrhage and

This chapter contains a video segment that can be found by accessing the following link: http://www.springerimages.com/videos/978-1-4614-6329-0.

S. Ahad, M.D. • J.D. Mellinger, M.D., F.A.C.S. (✉)
Department of Surgery, Southern Illinois University School of Medicine, Springfield, IL, USA
e-mail: jmellinger@siumed.edu

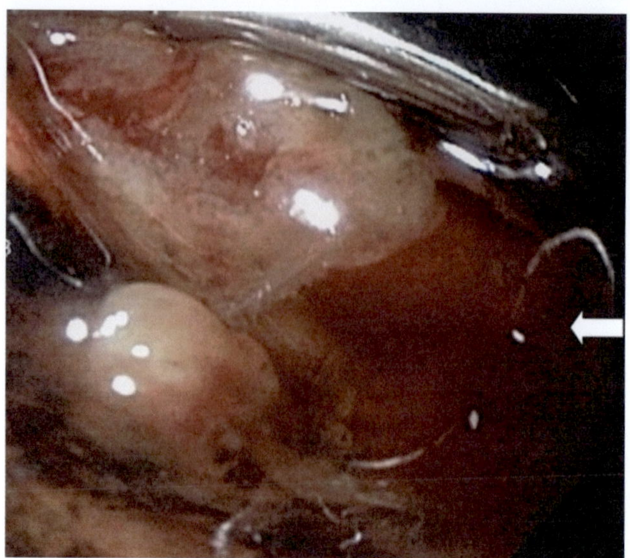

Fig. 8.1 Active bleeding from an ulcer base (*white arrow* pointing to active bleed)

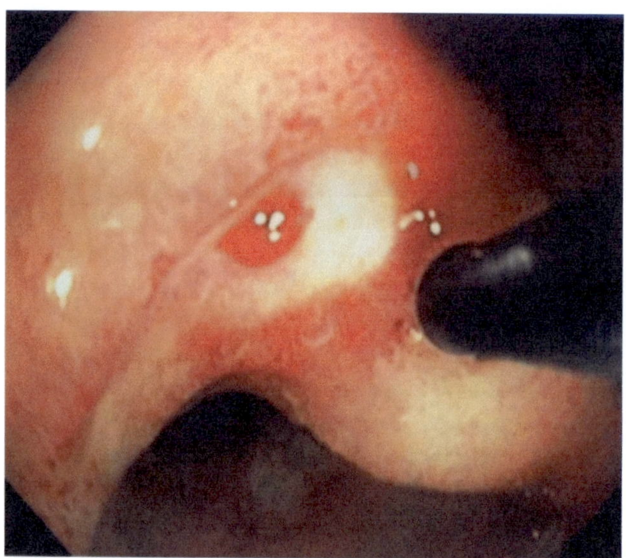

Fig. 8.2 Non bleeding visible vessel on ulcer base

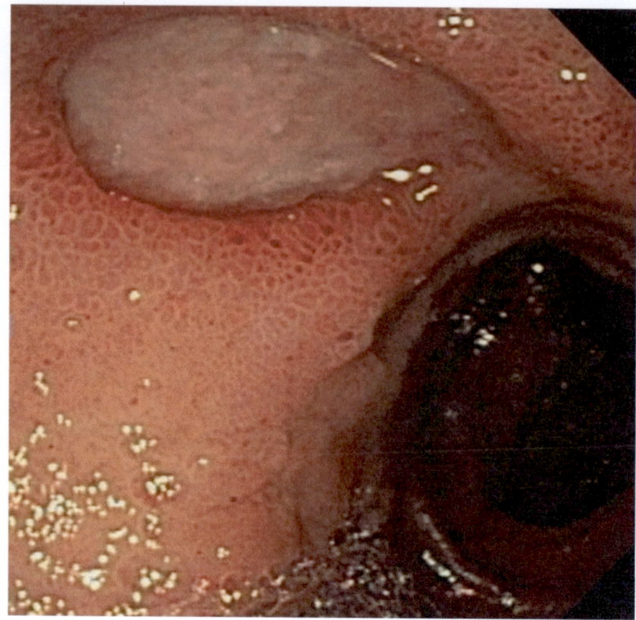

Fig. 8.3 Clean-based ulcer

Table 8.1 Endoscopic predictors of recurrent peptic ulcer hemorrhage

Endoscopic SRH	Incidence (%)	Risk of re-bleeding (%)
Major SRH		
Active bleeding	10	80–90
Non bleeding visible vessel	25	40–60
Intermediate SRH		
Adherent clot	10	25
Oozing of blood	14	10–20
Minor SRH		
Flat pigmented spot	10	13
No SRH		
Clean based ulcer	35	4–5

diagnosis to predict re-bleeding and death [2]. The Blatchford score uses laboratory and clinical variables and is calculated prior to endoscopy, making it useful for the initial triage of the patient [3]. Initial endoscopy provides valuable information not only for identification of the bleeding lesion but also to predict the risk of re-bleeding or continued hemorrhage. This risk is predicated on the appearance of the ulcer, and specifically the stigmata of recent hemorrhage. There are four such stigmata: (1) Active bleeding from an ulcer base (Fig. 8.1) which carries a 90 % risk of continued bleeding or re-bleeding without endoscopic intervention, (2) non-bleeding visible vessel (Fig. 8.2) associated with a 50 % risk of rebleed, (3) an adherent clot has a 25 % risk of re-bleeding if not removed and the underlying pathology treated, and (4) clean based ulcer (Fig. 8.3) which has minimal risk of re-bleeding (minor stigmata) (Table 8.1) [4].

Therapeutic endoscopy is usually done to stop ongoing bleeding or reduce the risk of re-bleeding. Endoscopy with endotherapy has been clearly shown to significantly decrease the need for surgical intervention. In addition endoscopy reduces the number of packed red blood cells required for transfusion and length of stay [5]. One of the greatest challenges in managing upper GI bleeding is removing intralumenal clot to visualize the bleeding source (Fig. 8.4). Traditionally, pre-endoscopic lavage was used to attempt to clear the clot, although studies have shown that this is ineffective and may

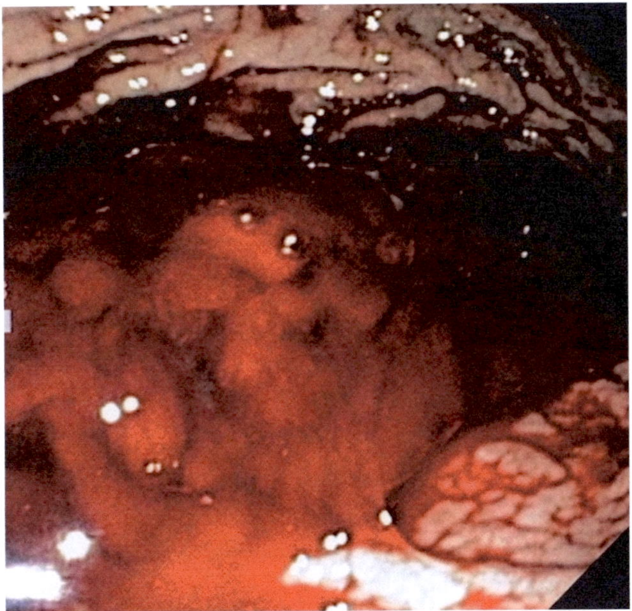

Fig. 8.4 Large amount of obscuring clot in gastric fundus and body

Table 8.2 Rockall score

Criteria	Points
Age (years)	
<60	0
60–79	1
>80	2
Shock	
Heart rate >100 beats/min	1
Systolic blood pressure <100 mmHg	2
Coexisting illness	
Coronary heart disease, congestive heart failure, etc.	2
Renal failure, hepatic failure, metastatic cancer	3
Endoscopic findings	
No lesions observed, Mallory Weiss tear	0
Peptic ulcer, erosive disease, esophagitis	1
Upper gastrointestinal cancer	2
Endoscopic stigmata of recent hemorrhage	
Clean ulcer base, flat pigmented spot	0
Blood in upper gastrointestinal tract, active bleeding, visible vessel, clot	2

Table 8.3 Glasgow-Blatchford score

Criteria	Score
Blood urea mmol/l	
6.5–<8	2
8–10	3
10–<25	4
>25	6
Hemoglobin for men	
12–<13	1
10–<12	3
<10	6
Hemoglobin for women	
10–<12	1
<10	6
Systolic blood pressure (mmHg)	
100–109	1
90–99	2
<90	3
Other parameters	
Pulse > 100	1
Presentation with melena	1
Presentation with syncope	2
Hepatic disease	2
Cardiac failure	2

delay the endoscopic intervention. Erythromycin 250 mg IV given 30 min prior to procedure has been shown to be effective as a stimulant of gastric motility through its motilin receptor agonist action, and should be utilized to facilitate clot evacuation from the stomach [6]. During the endoscopy the patient position can be changed to shift clot and liquid contents out of the way, provided that there is adequate airway protection to prevent aspiration. This maneuver will not help with adherent clots, which should be removed (with irrigation or cold snare technique) to fully evaluate the underlying lesion and direct appropriate therapy for the same. Clot removal may precipitate bleeding, thus it is recommended to inject the ulcer base surrounding the clot with epinephrine in a 1:10,000 dilution prior to clot removal.

GI hemorrhage rarely causes mortality by exsanguination, but can precipitate clinical decompensation from underlying comorbidities. A risk stratification score can be used to help direct urgency of treatment and prognosis. The two commonly used scores (Rockall and Blatchford) are used to predict the need for intervention, risk of re-bleeding and mortality (Tables 8.2 and 8.3) [2]. The Blatchford score does not require endoscopic diagnosis for risk stratification and thus can be used on initial presentation of the patient. Identification of patient at high risk for re-bleeding and mortality may help in initial triage, timing of first endoscopy and subsequent management. Endoscopy should be performed within 24 h of admission because early intervention is associated with improved patient outcomes and decreased hospital stay for both low and high-risk patients [7]. Patients who continue to bleed or re-bleed have a tenfold higher in-hospital mortality. Endoscopic therapies used to stop GI bleeding are described below.

Injection Therapy

This mode of therapy uses an injectate to infiltrate submucosally in and around the area of visible or suspected bleeding. The injectate helps halt bleeding by causing a combination of tamponade, vasospasm and/or inflammation and thrombosis. A 25-gauge sclerotherapy needle is used to inject.

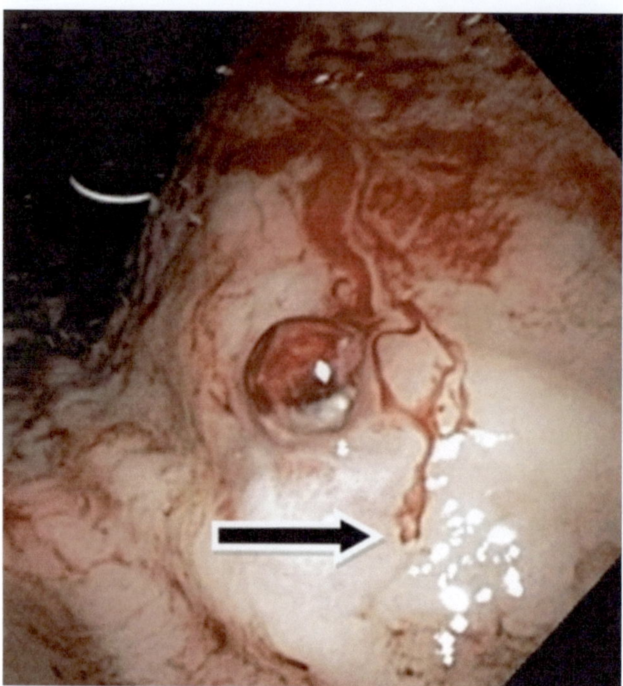

Fig. 8.5 Lesion found after clot evacuation from patient in Fig. 8.4; note blanched and raised surrounding mucosa following submucosal epinephrine injection and oozing from needle entry site (*black arrow*)

The needle is sheathed in a protective outer sleeve of plastic or metal and the endoscopist should ensure that the needle extends and retracts properly before introducing the device into the working channel of the endoscope. Once advanced beyond the tip of the endoscope, the needle should be unsheathed, or "out" only when ready to inject solution. This will minimize inadvertent injury to the surrounding tissues or the working channel of the endoscope. The intended target for injection is approached tangentially with the needle. The nurse should communicate to the surgeon the level of resistance encountered during injection, as well as injection volume as the sclerosant is administered. If the nurse feels moderate resistance during injection, then the needle is in the right place. Too little or no resistance means the needle is too superficial or too deep, possibly even in the peritoneum. With proper needle placement, a submucosal wheel will be raised as fluid is infiltrated into the tissues (Fig. 8.5). If the injected fluid leaks back towards the operating field, then the needle is too superficial. The needle should be withdrawn in such instances, and reinserted deeper into the viscous wall until the desired depth is achieved and confirmed on repeat injection. Different chemicals are used for injection therapy and include epinephrine, saline, and a variety of sclerosants such as absolute alcohol or ethanolamine.

Epinephrine

Epinephrine is the most commonly used agent for injection therapy. It causes local tamponade as well as vasospasm and promotes platelet aggregation [8]. Epinephrine is injected in a concentration of 1:10,000 in 1 ml aliquots. Up to 20 ml can be injected with some advocating the use of larger volumes of epinephrine either alone or in combination with saline. Larger volumes may be required when injecting the indurated, fibrinous base of a chronic ulcer. When injected, the resultant vasospasm of the vessel will causes blanching of the mucosa, a subtle clue that epinephrine injection is exerting its desired effect.

Epinephrine can have potential cardio-toxic effects including cardiac vasospasm, tachycardia and arrhythmias. A patient with ongoing and recent bleeding is at higher risk of suffering cardiovascular consequences due to the effects of epinephrine on the heart. Ideally the patient should be well resuscitated prior to the procedure, and ongoing efforts at replacing lost intravascular volume should continue during the course of treatment. The time to maximum cardiovascular effect of epinephrine injected submucosally is about 20 min.

Epinephrine injection is successful in the initial control of bleeding 80 % of the time [9]. Adding a second treatment modality to sclerotherapy improves outcome in high-risk bleeding ulcers [9]. Combining epinephrine injection with thermal ablation or mechanical intervention can decrease the risk of re-bleeding by 50 %. Prevention of re-bleeding decreases the need for surgery and improves survival [10]. Use of a second sclerosant in addition to epinephrine is not generally advocated because of the theoretical risk of causing transmural necrosis and perforation with such agents. Overall epinephrine is considered an excellent initial agent due to the ease of application, low cost, efficacy in initial control of hemorrhage, and availability.

Sclerosants

A sclerosing agent is used more commonly for bleeding varices. When injected into the vessel lumen it induces thrombogenesis and can trigger occlusion of a bleeding vessel. When injected into tissues surrounding the varix, it exerts its effect by inducing tamponade and subsequent inflammation and submucosal fibrosis, resulting in varix obliteration. This very same mechanism of action causes some of the side effects commonly associated with its use, including ulceration and perforation, pain, fever, infection and bleeding. It can also cause respiratory complications including pleural effusions and adult respiratory distress syndrome. There is also a 25 % risk of stricture formation long-term [11]. When used for non-variceal bleeding control, much smaller aliquots of 0.1–0.3 ml are used in contrast to 1–2 ml used for variceal hemorrhage.

In fact rarely is more than 2 ml required for non-variceal bleeding. Common sclerosants include polidocanol, ethanolamine, alcohol, and hypertonic saline or glucose. The use of sclerosants at the same site where epinephrine has been used is associated with a slightly higher risk of perforation—particularly in the gastric fundus [12, 13]. Repeat injection of sclerosants at the same site should also be avoided to minimize the risk of perforation.

Thrombin

Thrombin promotes the conversion of fibrinogen to fibrin, the end product of the coagulation cascade and main component of a primary hemostatic plug. Thrombin is available both from bovine and human sources. Thrombin use in variceal hemorrhage has yielded equivocal results in clinical trials and it is not currently considered a main line therapy for managing GI bleeding [14]. Thrombin can cause induction of antibodies causing bleeding diathesis as well as anaphylaxis in sensitized individuals.

Fibrin Glue

Fibrin glue is packaged as human fibrinogen and factor XIII in one vial and thrombin in another. A double lumen injection catheter system is used to mix the two products at the site of application because they polymerize rapidly on contact. Some fibrin glue compounds require preheating for about 20 min prior to application. Fibrin glue is resorbed from the injection site as part of a normal wound healing process and therefore does not induce intense inflammation or tissue necrosis like sclerosants [15]. In one study fibrin glue reduced re-bleeding risk when used in multiple injections compared to polidocanol, however the ultimate patient outcomes were not different between groups [16]. Due to the fact that it is technically cumbersome and relatively costly, it has not achieved wide spread use.

Cyanoacrylate

Cyanoacrylate is a synthetic resin that polymerizes rapidly when injected, thereby obliterating the lumen of the vessel. It is most commonly used for treatment of gastric varices, which account for up to 15 % of all variceal bleeds [17]. Spillage of the resin inside the endoscope or on the camera lens can cause damage to the scope. To avoid the glue from hardening prematurely it is often mixed with iodinized oil as a 5:8 mixture. Care must be taken during its use with all personnel and the patient wearing safety goggles to avoid splattering of the cornea during injection. Once injected the needle should be withdrawn quickly from the tissues to avoid cementing the needle inside the hardened resin. Cyanoacrylate resin is effective in achieving initial hemostasis in 95 % of patients in bleeding peptic ulcers [18, 19]. The glue is later expulsed from the body and replaced with fibrous tissue. Glue embolism, though uncommon (0.9 %), is a primary concern in its use. Cyanoacrylate is not Food and Drug Administration (FDA)-approved in the USA and is generally not used for non-variceal bleeds due to the availability of equally effective, more facile, and safer agents.

Mechanical Therapy

Endoclips

Since their introduction, endoclipping devices have undergone several design improvements, and several different models are now available. Clips work by grasping the mucosa, and mechanically occluding the vessel.

The endoclip device consists of two components: the deployment assembly and the clip itself. The deployment catheter delivers the clip through the endoscope to the working field. The current commercially available clip catheters fit through a 2.8 mm endoscopic biopsy channel. The deployment catheters are available either as reusable devices that require loading of clips, or disposable units with one preloaded clip on each catheter. Some types like the Resolution Clip (Boston Scientific, Natick, MA,) can be opened and closed multiple times prior to deployment allowing for more precise repositioning of the clip if necessary. Other clips have rotation capability to help achieve optimal orientation in relation to the site being addressed. The commercially available clips range in width from 8 to 12 mm when fully opened. Precise clip placement is important because a misplaced clip can make it difficult to place additional clips on the tissue. The targeted tissue is grasped in the clip prongs and manual pressure applied to approximate the prongs and assist closure (Fig. 8.6). In chronic ulcers where tough fibrinous tissue is present, clips may not work effectively and a failure rate as high as 20 % is reported in some studies (Fig. 8.7) [20]. Clips are used for control of GI bleeding in a wide variety of situations including bleeding peptic ulcer, Dieulafoy lesions, Mallory-Weis tears, and angiodysplasis as well as post-polypectomy bleeding (see Videos 8.1 and 8.2). Clips can also be used to mark the site of active bleeding to facilitate identification of the bleeding site for subsequent interventional radiologic embolization. Clips are more effectively deployed when the intended target is approached perpendicularly as tangential aim may result in poor anchoring on the viscous wall. Accordingly, endoclips may have a higher failure rate along the lesser curvature, near the cardia, and in the posterior wall of duodenum [21]. The firing mechanism of

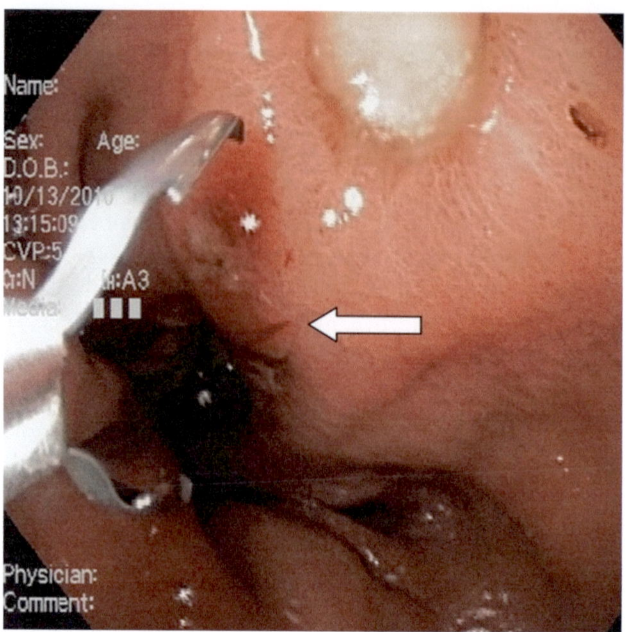

Fig. 8.6 Clip being positioned for application to bleeding area at edge of ulcer bed in patient with several adjacent ulcers (note clean bed at top of picture); *arrow* shows trail of active bleeding from bleeding point located just beyond clip jaws in field of view

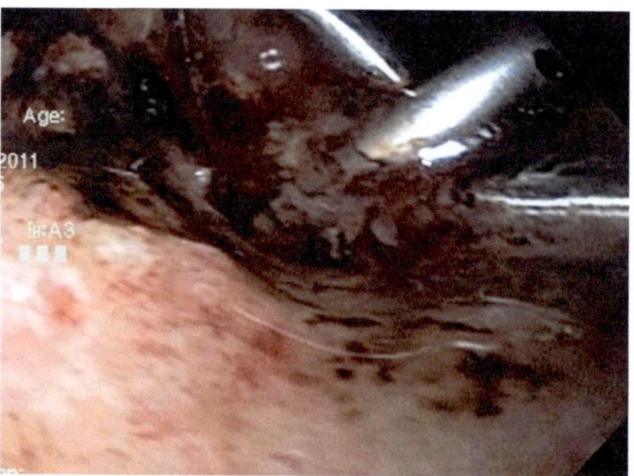

Fig. 8.7 Attempt to control bleeding from chronic, fibrous duodenal ulcer base; note multiple clips have not successfully achieved full hemostasis

the deployment assembly is weakened when the scope is retroflexed, thereby making clip application in this position more challenging. When deploying the endoclips, the jaws of the clip should extend well beyond the ulcer edge and anchor into the surrounding tissue. For very large ulcers, the visible vessel should be clipped directly. Endoclips are made of stainless steel and do not induce an inflammatory reaction in surrounding tissues. Long-term hemostasis is achieved in about 85 % percent of patients with endoclips [22]. When used as a sole means of endoscopic hemostasis, clips have lower re-bleeding rates than various injection agents [23]. In a recent meta-analysis, dual therapy was shown to decrease the risk of re-bleeding from 18.8 to 10.4 %, and risk of emergency surgery from 10.8 to 7.1 % [24]. Subanalysis showed that risk of re-bleeding decreased regardless of what type of second procedure was utilized. Other studies have shown that endoclips may be superior to heater probe devices in preventing recurrent bleeding [25].

Endoclips anchor on the mucosa and submucosa only; therefore, the risk of viscous perforation related to these is low. When using endoclips in combination with direct thermal therapy to control bleeding, caution should be exercised and use of electrocautery avoided in close proximity to endoclips. Most clips slough off within 10–14 days after application depending on type of clip used [26]. However, endoclips may remain attached to mucosa for a prolonged period of time (up to 26 months). It is important to remember that not all endoclips are magnetic resonance imaging compatible and a magnetic field can cause clip deflection [27]. Clips can also be used to help guide localization of bleeding vessels during subsequent angiography for lesions at high risk of re-bleeding [28]. Table 8.4 summarizes some of the commercially available clips.

Detachable Snares

Detachable snares are made of an outer plastic sheath with an inner metal coil that houses the hook attached to a nylon loop. The nylon loop can be tightened by adjusting the tension on the attached silicone rubber stopper. The outer

Table 8.4 Commercially available endoclips

Company	Olympus	Olympus	Boston scientific	Wilson Cook
Clip name	Rotating clip	Quick clip 2	Resolution clip	TriClip
Ready to use	No	Yes	Yes	Yes
Clip size (mm)	2.8 and 3.2	2.8	2.8	2.8 and 3.2
Max opening width (mm)	11	9.5	11	12
Rotatability	Rotatable	Rotatable	Not rotatable	Not rotatable
Reopening capability	None	None	Up to five times	none

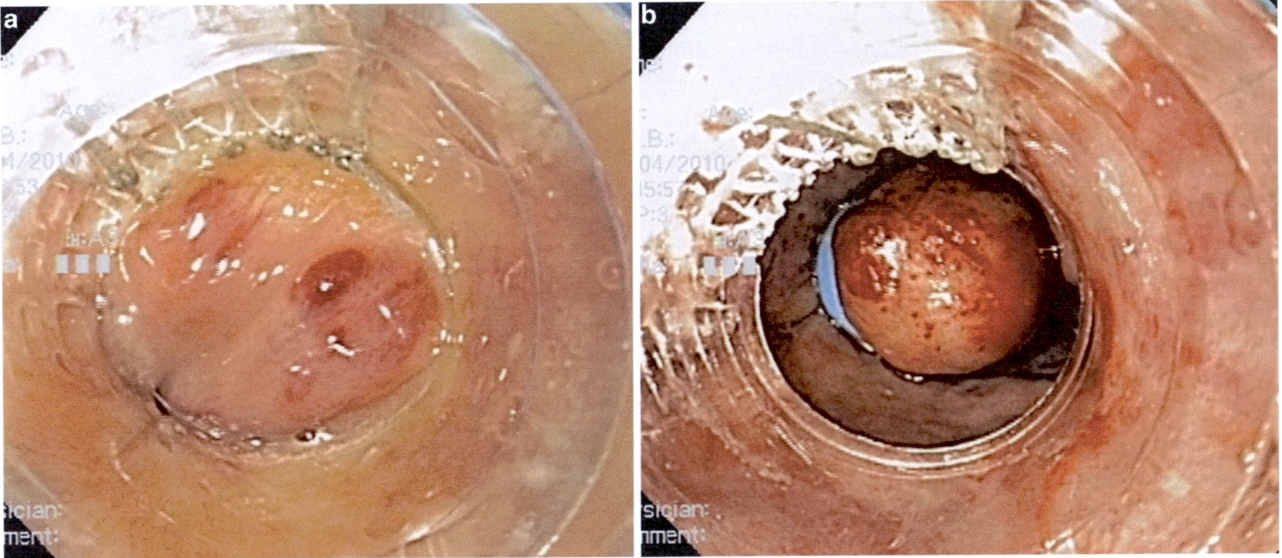

Fig. 8.8 (**a**), (**b**) Appearance of hematocystic spot on distal esophageal varix (**a**), and appearance after successful banding (**b**)

diameter of the Endoloop (Olympus Corporation, Lake Success, NY) sheath is 2.5 mm so it can be used through the working channel of a standard gastroscope or colonoscope. The nylon loop is placed around the target (often a pedunculated polyp base) and the loop tightened. The loop strangulates the blood supply to the vessel thereby halting bleeding. Care should be taken not to inadvertently transect the polyp with the loop. If used to control post-polypectomy bleeding, the polyp site should have an adequate stalk length. Endoloops may also be placed preemptively on the base of a pedunculated polyp with snare excision above the loop. Slippage of the Endoloop from a short stalked polyp may precipitate further bleeding. Endoloops have been used to ligate esophageal varices, but this can be technically challenging and risks exacerbating bleeding.

Endoscopic Band Ligation

Endoscopic band ligation (EBL) is used for both prophylaxis and treatment of esophageal varices. Banding can be used on gastric varices that are located proximally on the lesser curvature [29]. Other clinical applications include treatment of post-polypectomy bleeding, arterivenous malformations, Mallory-Weiss tears, Dieulafoy's lesions and diverticular bleeding.

A complete endoscopic examination should be performed prior to the procedure to assess for the degree and severity of varices, the presence of stigmata of recent hemorrhage, as well as presence of gastric varices. Stigmata predicting a higher risk of re-bleeding for varices include active bleeding or oozing from the varix, the "red wale sign"(red streaks on a varix), presence of adherent clot or fibin plug, and raised red spot (hematocystic spot—see Fig. 8.8) [30]. While the banding cap used for EBL will fit on the tip of a standard endoscope, it may be advisable to use a therapeutic endoscope with a 3.7 mm working channel to allow for better visualization and increased suction capability. Conversely, a smaller caliber endoscope may prove more maneuverable in the confines of the distal esophageal lumen. A transparent cap with the rubber bands preloaded is positioned on the tip of the scope. The oropharynx and upper esophageal sphincter may be difficult to negotiate with the cap in place. In this instance, flexing the patient's neck and gently advancing the endoscope while applying air insufflation and slight rotational movement helps traverse the area [31]. If the patient is intubated, temporarily deflating the balloon of the endotracheal tube may be necessary. Band ligation is performed in a distal to proximal sequence to prevent inadvertent dislodging of an already applied band by the scope. If the bleeding is from a varix present in the mid esophagus, that varix is ligated but distal non-bleeding varices are not treated during the same session. To ligate a varix, the scope is aimed towards the intended tissue and suction is applied until a "red out" is seen, indicating the mucosa and submucosa in the area of the varix have been pulled into the cap and therefore positioned suitably for band control. Firing the band prior to proper suctioning of the varix into the cap may lead to misfire and exacerbated or even torrential bleeding. Once properly deployed, the band will give the ligated varix a polyp like appearance with discoloration of overlying mucosa from strangulating the blood supply. Up to ten bands can be placed with commercially available devices in a single session without reloading [32]. Gastric varices that are small or found concurrently with esophageal varices are easily treated with

EBL. However large bleeding gastric varices may engorge and prolapsed intraluminally with blood, and the resulting submucosal tension in the varix may make it difficult to trap it in the hood of the banding device. Large varices are also more prone to ulcer formation when treated with EBL. Endoscopic obliteration by cyanoacrylate injection into the varix is more effective than EBL for gastric varix treatment [29]. EBL is safer and more effective for primary prevention of esophageal variceal bleeding when compared to beta blockade pharmacologic therapy [33]. For secondary prevention of bleeding in esophageal varices, EBL is preferred over sclerotherapy as it yields faster obliteration of varices with fewer complications [34].

Complications of EBL include post-banding ulcerations, bleeding and strictures, especially if the bands are placed in the more proximal esophagus [33]. Esophageal perforations, although rare, have been reported from overtube placement and ulcer formation. Chest pain after banding is typically temporary but rarely other interventions may be required. All patients with cirrhosis who present with variceal hemorrhage should be given prophylactic antibiotics to reduce the rate of bacterial infection, re-bleeding and improve survival (see Chap. 4) [35]. Quinolone antibiotics are most commonly used for prophylaxis in acute variceal hemorrhage in the setting of cirrhosis.

Ablative Tools

Ablative therapy refers to techniques in which intense energy is applied to targeted tissue resulting in protein coagulation, coaptation of blood vessels, and activation of the coagulation cascade resulting in thrombosis. The form of energy used varies from direct heat transfer (thermo-coagulation) to electromechanical energy (electro-coagulation). Energy is delivered via probes that fit into the working channel of the scope. The probe can then transfer this energy by direct contact with the tissue (contact method) or by hovering over the target without touching the tissue (noncontact method).

Contact Method

Contact methods include electro-coagulation and thermo-coagulation. The probe comes in direct contact with the intended target thereby maximizing energy delivery and reducing energy scatter. This principle is called coaptive coagulation, and involves the simultaneous use of pressure applied via the probe to approximate the vessel walls and limit ongoing bleeding and the resulting "heat sink" effect, along with thermal application to facilitate enduring control of bleeding (Figs. 8.9, 8.10 and 8.11). These probes can weld vessels as large as 2.5 mm in diameter.

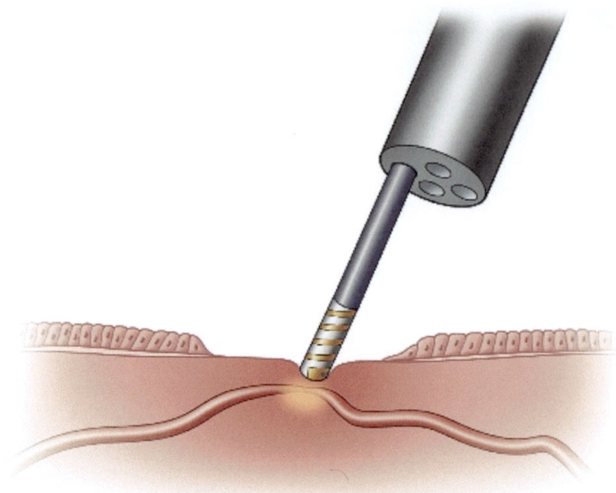

Fig. 8.9 Artist's depiction of thermal probe being applied for coaptive coagulation of vessel at ulcer base

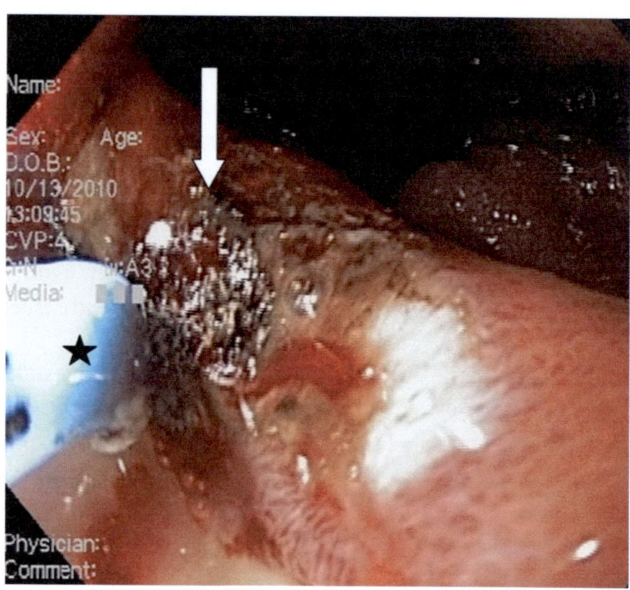

Fig. 8.10 Thermal probe application at rim of bleeding ulcer bed. Note coagulum (*white arrow*) where probe (marked with *black star*) has been in direct contact with bleeding point.

The most commonly used electro-coagulation probes apply bipolar electromechanical energy via a multipolar electrocoagulation (MPEC) device. Commercially available MPEC probes include the Gold Probe (Microinvasive, Boston Scientific Corp., Natick, MA, USA) and the Bipolar Circumactive Probe or BICAP (Circon ACMI, Stamford, CT, USA). These probes range in size from 2.3 to 3.2 mm in diameter and are therefore compatible with a 2.8 and 3.7 mm scope channels. Studies have not shown a clear benefit of the larger sized probes in outcomes in comparison the smaller probes when the technique includes epinephrine injection as well as coaptive coagulation therapy [36]. The probe is firmly applied to the tissue and the bipolar electrosurgical energy delivered

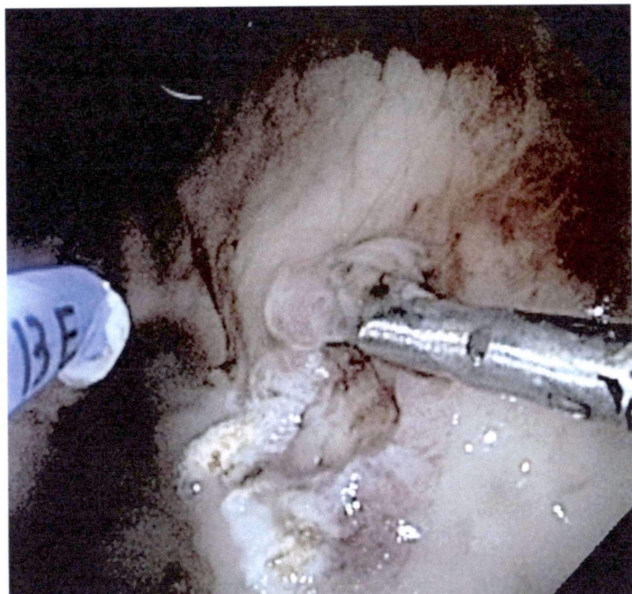

Fig. 8.11 Ulcer that required combination of epinephrine injection, multiple thermal contact probe applications, and single clip to achieve full hemostasis.

for 5–10 s using a power setting of 10–15 W. The wattage used and number of applications applied varies depending on the location in the GI tract (i.e., higher wattage and more applications in thick walled stomach versus thin walled cecum). The probes have a central channel for irrigation, and some also have a 25 gauge needle that can be used for injection if need be. The latter design can be helpful when multiple strategies for hemostasis, including injection and thermal therapy, are employed in combination. Complications of use include perforation and post-procedure ulceration with delayed bleeding.

The heater probe (Olympus, Tokyo, Japan) used thermocoagulation, or direct heat transfer, to achieve coaptive coagu-

lation. It is Teflon coated to prevent adherence to mucosa and dislodgement of the coagulum after energy application. Unlike bipolar probes, heater probes simply get hot at the tip so tissue desiccation does not limit the transfer of energy when a heater probe is used, thus potentially increasing the risk of deep tissue injury. Probes range in size from 2.3 to 3.2 mm in size and can heat up to 250 °C. The power setting is often set to 30 J and four to five bursts of energy are typically given. Effective hemostasis is indicated by whitening of the target lesion and flattening of the bleeding vessel or clot. Just like the bipolar probes, the heater probe has a central channel for irrigation that is controlled by a foot pedal [37].

Noncontact Method

Some pathologies are best treated with a noncontact method of coagulation. Argon Plasma Coagulation (APC) is monopolar electromechanical energy delivered to the target via an inert gas carrier. This allows for coagulation of the mucosa in a "painting" fashion without contact and resultant dislodgement of the coagulum. The flow of argon gas also clears the target of fluid. When the APC probe is activated, argon gas flows through the central lumen at a set rate while a high voltage spark at the tip of the probe ionizes the gas to a plasma. This plasma conducts electricity thereby transferring the energy to the tissue but with a low depth of penetration (approximately 1–2 mm) APC probes range in size from 1.5 to 3.2 mm in diameter and come in different tip configurations to allow for forward, side, or circumferential delivery. APC can be used to treat multiple lesions in a relatively short period of time. Examples of situations where this could be useful include angiodysplasias, gastric antral vascular ectasia (GAVE or watermelon stomach—see Fig. 8.12), or radiation proctitis [38]. Care should be taken to avoid

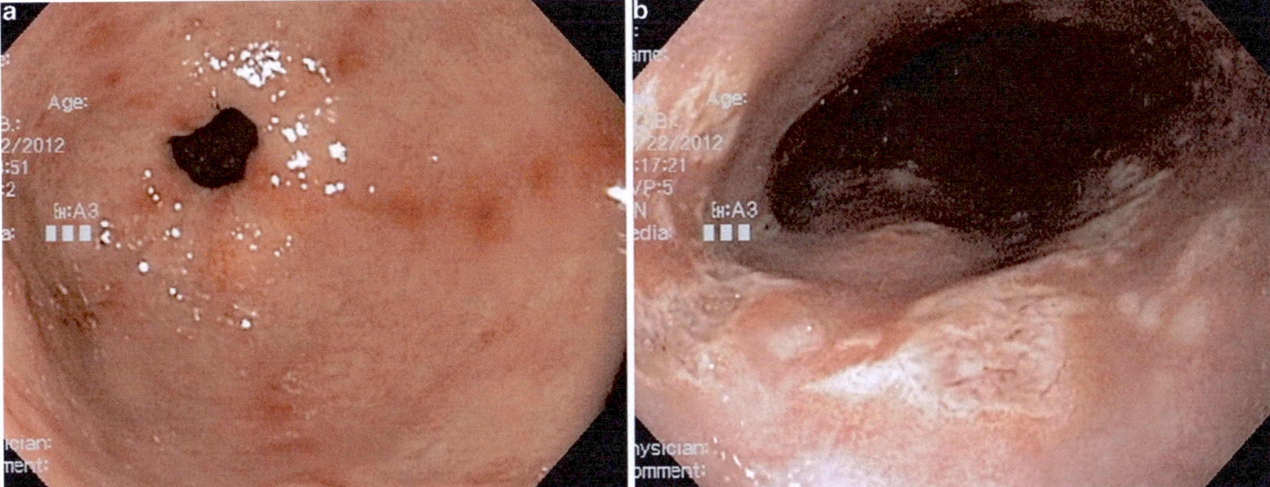

Fig. 8.12 (a), (b): GAVE in a patient with low-grade chronic gastrointestinal blood loss (a). Same area after APC treatment (b). *APC* argon plasma coagulation

Table 8.5 Modalities for endoscopic hemostasis

Anatomic site/pathology	Modalities available for hemostasis	Comments
Esophagus		
Varices	Sclerosants, EBL	
Mallory Weiss tears	*Multipolar cautery* Epinephrine injection, EBL, clips	Usually self-limited
Stomach		
Bleeding peptic ulcer	*Epinephrine + second modality* (coaptive thermal device, sclerosants, fibrin glue or clips)	Adding second modality decreases the risk of re-bleeding, surgery, and mortality
Dieulafoy's lesions	EBL, clip, electrocautery, cyanoacrylate, epinephrine, heater probe	Clip or tattoo the lesion to identify in case of recurrent bleeding
Isolated gastric varices	Sclerosant, EBL	Splenectomy if nonmalignant thrombosis of splenic vein
Watermelon stomach	APC	
Small intestine		
Angiodysplasia	APC	Use a lower power setting 20 W because of thin wall of small intestine
Ulcers	Injection, clips	
Dieulafoy's	Injection, clips, APC	Use dilute epinephrine in small bowel
Large intestine		
Diverticulosis	Injection, contact thermal devices, hemoclip, band ligation	
Hemorrhoids	EBL	Surgical consultation
Inflammatory bowel disease	Endoscopic therapy rarely useful	
Angiodysplasia	APC, injection, contact thermal devices	
Post-polypectomy bleeding	Resnaring the stalk, contact thermal, injection, clips	

EBL estimated blood loss, *APC* argon plasma coagulation

direct contact with tissue as the depth of tissue injury can increase (>4 mm). In the lumen of the GI tract, the argon must be periodically aspirated or risk perforation (0.5 % occurrence) [39]. APC treated areas ulcerate and then heal, and therefore, all foregut patients treated with this modality should be placed on PPI to facilitate healing of the attendant post-treatment ulcers.

Nd:YAG laser is another mode of noncontact energy application. Laser photocoagulation is rarely used today for hemostasis due to its relatively high cost, added safety and equipment portability issues, and risk of complications such as perforation (3 %).

The causes of GI bleeding are myriad. With so many modalities available to the modern endoscopist, the success rate if endoscopic intervention has improved. Table 8.5 summarizes some of the common causes of GI bleeding and endoscopic techniques to be considered in their management.

Recurrent Bleeding

Despite adequate initial hemostasis recurrent upper GI bleeding can happen in up to 25 % of high-risk cases. Use of PPI as well as combination endoscopic therapy can reduce recurrent bleeding rates to less than 10 % [40]. If re-bleeding occurs a second endoscopy should be done, however routine second look endoscopy is not recommended. Repeat endoscopy with control of bleeding avoids the need for surgical intervention and is effective in the majority of patients. Patients who undergo repeat thermal therapy at the same site may be at increased risk for perforation. Patients who continue to bleed after two or more sessions of endoscopic therapy should be considered for interventional angiography or surgery [41].

Evolving Technologies

As experience and expertise with Natural Orifice Transluminal Endoscopic Surgery (NOTES) has increased, more novel techniques and tools for control of GI bleeding have emerged. One such technique was initially tested for canine and porcine cardia fundoplication, and involves placement of polyester mesh tissue anchors that allows tissue to be cinched together [42]. Techniques such as this hold promise for use in GI hemostasis, and may allow the endoscopist to plicate or compress bleeding vessels in the future.

The over-the-scope-clip (OTSC) system (Ovesco Endoscopy GmbH, Tuebingen, Germany) is a newer system that allows for mechanical compression of larger areas of the GI tract. It can be used for both primary and post-interventional bleeding control. Additional uses include closure of gastrocutaneous fistula, gastrogastric fistula after bypass, iatrogenic perforations, and closure of NOTES stoma [43–46]. It is a Nitinol device that can remain in the body long-term. The OTSC cap is loaded to the tip of endoscope and the cap can be reloaded during the same procedure. It is available in two versions, traumatic and atraumatic, the former with pointed "teeth" that allows for increased anchoring capability.

Endoscopic suturing devices allow intralumenal full thickness suturing in different configurations. The Overstich Endoscopic Suturing System (Apollo Endosurgery, Austin, TX) mounts on a double channel therapeutic endoscope and allows sutures to be deployed under direct vision. It consists of three parts: the end cap, the needle driver handle, and the anchor exchange catheter. A curved arm with suture extends from the device and when the handle is closed the needle advances through the tissue. The needle is then passed over to the anchor exchange. Both absorbable and nonabsorbable sutures are available for use with the device. The system has been used in closure of marginal ulcers after gastric bypass, gastric suturing during EMR, and chronic gastrocutaneous fistula [47–49].

Summary

Therapeutic endoscopy has revolutionized the management of GI bleeding. Using modern tools and combined therapies, most GI bleeding can be stopped without the need for surgical intervention. A skilled endoscopist must have a thorough understanding of the technologies available to manage bleeding and their proper application. The method or combination of techniques chosen should depend on familiarity and expertise of the endoscopist with the tools, availability of resources within the area of practice and cost effectiveness of a given choice.

References

1. Lau JY, Leung WK, Wu JC, et al. Omeprazole before endoscopy in patients with gastrointestinal bleeding. N Engl J Med. 2007;356(16):1631–40.
2. Rockall TA, Logan RF, Devlin HB, Northfield TC. Risk assessment after acute upper gastrointestinal haemorrhage. Gut. 1996;38(3):316–21.
3. Blatchford O, Murray WR, Blatchford M. A risk score to predict need for treatment for upper-gastrointestinal haemorrhage. Lancet. 2000;356(9238):1318–21.
4. Foster DN, Miloszewski KJ, Losowsky MS. Stigmata of recent haemorrhage in diagnosis and prognosis of upper gastrointestinal bleeding. Br Med J. 1978;1(6121):1173–7.
5. Cappell MS, Friedel D. Initial management of acute upper gastrointestinal bleeding: from initial evaluation up to gastrointestinal endoscopy. Med Clin North Am. 2008;92(3):491–509. xi.
6. Coffin B, Pocard M, Panis Y, et al. Erythromycin improves the quality of EGD in patients with acute upper GI bleeding: a randomized controlled study. Gastrointest Endosc. 2002;56(2):174–9.
7. Barkun AN, Bardou M, Kuipers EJ, et al. International consensus recommendations on the management of patients with nonvariceal upper gastrointestinal bleeding. Ann Intern Med. 2010;152(2):101–13.
8. Kubba AK, Palmer KR. Role of endoscopic injection therapy in the treatment of bleeding peptic ulcer. Br J Surg. 1996;83(4):461–8.
9. Calvet X, Vergara M, Brullet E, Gisbert JP, Campo R. Addition of a second endoscopic treatment following epinephrine injection improves outcome in high-risk bleeding ulcers. Gastroenterology. 2004;126(2):441–50.
10. Brullet E, Calvet X, Campo R, Rue M, Catot L, Donoso L. Factors predicting failure of endoscopic injection therapy in bleeding duodenal ulcer. Gastrointest Endosc. 1996;43(2 Pt 1):111–6.
11. Schmitz RJ, Sharma P, Badr AS, Qamar MT, Weston AP. Incidence and management of esophageal stricture formation, ulcer bleeding, perforation, and massive hematoma formation from sclerotherapy versus band ligation. Am J Gastroenterol. 2001;96(2):437–41.
12. Dorta G, Michetti P, Burckhardt P, Gillet M. Acute ischemia followed by hemorrhagic gastric necrosis after injection sclerotherapy for ulcer. Endoscopy. 1996;28(6):532.
13. Scharnke W, Hust MH, Braun B, Schumm W. Complete gastric wall necrosis after endoscopic sclerotherapy for a gastric ulcer with visible arterial stump. Dtsch Med Wochenschr. 1997;122(19):606–9.
14. Kitano S, Hashizume M, Yamaga H, et al. Human thrombin plus 5 per cent ethanolamine oleate injected to sclerose oesophageal varices: a prospective randomized trial. Br J Surg. 1989;76(7):715–8.
15. Spotnitz WD, Prabhu R. Fibrin sealant tissue adhesive—review and update. J Long Term Eff Med Implants. 2005;15(3):245–70.
16. Rutgeerts P, Rauws E, Wara P, et al. Randomised trial of single and repeated fibrin glue compared with injection of polidocanol in treatment of bleeding peptic ulcer. Lancet. 1997;350(9079):692–6.
17. Sarin SK, Lahoti D, Saxena SP, Murthy NS, Makwana UK. Prevalence, classification and natural history of gastric varices: a long-term follow-up study in 568 portal hypertension patients. Hepatology. 1992;16(6):1343–9.
18. Cheng LF, Wang ZQ, Li CZ, et al. Treatment of gastric varices by endoscopic sclerotherapy using butyl cyanoacrylate: 10 years' experience of 635 cases. Chin Med J (Engl). 2007;120(23):2081–5.
19. Lee KJ, Kim JH, Hahm KB, Cho SW, Park YS. Randomized trial of N-butyl-2-cyanoacrylate compared with injection of hypertonic saline-epinephrine in the endoscopic treatment of bleeding peptic ulcers. Endoscopy. 2000;32(7):505–11.
20. Jensen DM, Machicado GA. Hemoclipping of chronic canine ulcers: a randomized, prospective study of initial deployment success, clip retention rates, and ulcer healing. Gastrointest Endosc. 2009;70(5):969–75.
21. Cho I, Gaslightwala I, Jensen DM, Cohen J. Endoclip therapy in the gastrointestinal tract: bleeding lesions and beyond UpToDate [online]. 2009. http://www.utdol.com/patients/content/topic.do. Accessed 27 May 2012.
22. Lin HJ, Hsieh YH, Tseng GY, Perng CL, Chang FY, Lee SD. A prospective, randomized trial of endoscopic hemoclip versus heater probe thermocoagulation for peptic ulcer bleeding. Am J Gastroenterol. 2002;97(9):2250–4.
23. Chung IK, Ham JS, Kim HS, Park SH, Lee MH, Kim SJ. Comparison of the hemostatic efficacy of the endoscopic hemoclip method with hypertonic saline-epinephrine injection and a combination of the two for the management of bleeding peptic ulcers. Gastrointest Endosc. 1999;49(1):13–8.
24. Vergara M, Calvet X, Gisbert JP. Epinephrine injection versus epinephrine injection and a second endoscopic method in high risk bleeding ulcers. Cochrane Database Syst Rev (Online). 2007(2):CD005584.
25. Cipolletta L, Bianco MA, Marmo R, et al. Endoclips versus heater probe in preventing early recurrent bleeding from peptic ulcer: a prospective and randomized trial. Gastrointest Endosc. 2001;53(2):147–51.

26. Shin EJ, Ko CW, Magno P, et al. Comparative study of endoscopic clips: duration of attachment at the site of clip application. Gastrointest Endosc. 2007;66(4):757–61.
27. Gill KR, Pooley RA, Wallace MB. Magnetic resonance imaging compatibility of endoclips. Gastrointest Endosc. 2009;70(3):532–6.
28. Eriksson LG, Sundbom M, Gustavsson S, Nyman R. Endoscopic marking with a metallic clip facilitates transcatheter arterial embolization in upper peptic ulcer bleeding. J Vasc Interv Radiol. 2006;17(6):959–64.
29. Lo GH, Lai KH, Cheng JS, Huang RL, Wang SJ, Chiang HT. Prevalence of paraesophageal varices and gastric varices in patients achieving variceal obliteration by banding ligation and by injection sclerotherapy. Gastrointest Endosc. 1999;49(4 Pt 1):428–36.
30. Merkel C, Zoli M, Siringo S, et al. Prognostic indicators of risk for first variceal bleeding in cirrhosis: a multicenter study in 711 patients to validate and improve the North Italian Endoscopic Club (NIEC) index. Am J Gastroenterol. 2000;95(10):2915–20.
31. Baron TH, Wong Kee Song LM. Endoscopic variceal band ligation. Am J Gastroenterol. 2009;104(5):1083–5.
32. Liu J, Petersen BT, Tierney WM, et al. Endoscopic banding devices. Gastrointest Endosc. 2008;68(2):217–21.
33. Sarin SK, Lamba GS, Kumar M, Misra A, Murthy NS. Comparison of endoscopic ligation and propranolol for the primary prevention of variceal bleeding. N Engl J Med. 1999;340(13):988–93.
34. Masci E, Stigliano R, Mariani A, et al. Prospective multicenter randomized trial comparing banding ligation with sclerotherapy of esophageal varices. Hepatogastroenterology. 1999;46(27):1769–73.
35. Bernard B, Grange JD, Khac EN, Amiot X, Opolon P, Poynard T. Antibiotic prophylaxis for the prevention of bacterial infections in cirrhotic patients with gastrointestinal bleeding: a meta-analysis. Hepatology. 1999;29(6):1655–61.
36. Paspatis GA, Charoniti I, Papanikolaoi N, et al. A prospective randomized comparison of 10-Fr versus 7-Fr bipolar electrocoagulation catheter in combination with adrenaline injection n the endoscopic treatment of bleeding peptic ulcers. Am J Gastroenterol. 2003;98(10):2192–7.
37. Kovacs TO, Jensen DM. Endoscopic treatment of ulcer bleeding. Curr Treat Options Gastroenterol. 2007;10(2):143–8.
38. Lecleire S, Ben-Soussan E, Antonietti M, et al. Bleeding gastric vascular ectasia treated by argon plasma coagulation: a comparison between patients with and without cirrhosis. Gastrointest Endosc. 2008;67(2):219–25.
39. Olmos JA, Marcolongo M, Pogorelsky V, Herrera L, Tobal F, Davolos JR. Long-term outcome of argon plasma ablation therapy for bleeding in 100 consecutive patients with colonic angiodysplasia. Dis Colon Rectum. 2006;49(10):1507–16.
40. Lau JY, Sung JJ, Lee KK, et al. Effect of intravenous omeprazole on recurrent bleeding after endoscopic treatment of bleeding peptic ulcers. N Engl J Med. 2000;343(5):310–6.
41. Jensen DM. Management of severe ulcer rebleeding. N Engl J Med. 1999;340(10):799–801.
42. Mellinger JD, MacFadyen BV, Kozarek RA, Soper ND, Birkett DH, Swanstrom LL. Initial experience with a novel endoscopic device allowing intragastric manipulation and plication. Surg Endosc. 2007;21(6):1002–5.
43. Heylen AM, Jacobs A, Lybeer M, Prosst RL. The OTSC(R)-clip in revisional endoscopy against weight gain after bariatric gastric bypass surgery. Obes Surg. 2011;21(10):1629–33.
44. Kouklakis G, Zezos P, Liratzopoulos N, et al. Endoscopic treatment of a gastrocutaneous fistula using the over-the-scope-clip system: a case report. Diagn Ther Endosc. 2011;2011:384143.
45. Pohl J, Borgulya M, Lorenz D, Ell C. Endoscopic closure of postoperative esophageal leaks with a novel over-the-scope clip system. Endoscopy. 2010;42(9):757–9.
46. Prosst RL, Herold A, Joos AK, et al. The 'Anal Fistula Claw': the OTSC-clip for anal fistula closure. Colorectal Dis. 2011; 14(9):1112–7.
47. Jirapinyo P, Watson RR, Thompson CC. Use of a novel endoscopic suturing device to treat recalcitrant marginal ulceration (with video). Gastrointest Endosc. 2012;76:435–9.
48. Kantsevoy SV, Thuluvath PJ. Successful closure of a chronic refractory gastrocutaneous fistula with a new endoscopic suturing device (with video). Gastrointest Endosc. 2012;75(3):688–90.
49. von Renteln D, Schmidt A, Riecken B, Caca K. Gastric full-thickness suturing during EMR and for treatment of gastric-wall defects (with video). Gastrointest Endosc. 2008;67(4):738–44.

Endoscopic Tools and Techniques for Tissue Removal and Ablation

Brian J. Dunkin

Introduction

The first snare polypectomy was performed by Wolff and Shinya in 1969 just 3 months after their report of the first successful complete colonoscopy [1]. This rapid progression from a diagnostic procedure to therapeutic intervention illustrates the driving force for the endoscopic removal of tissue from the gastrointestinal (GI) tract. Significant advances have developed since Wolff and Shinya's initial experience making colonoscopic polypectomy the most common therapeutic endoscopic procedure performed today. This chapter describes the tools and techniques used for removing tissue from the GI tract for therapeutic purposes.

Principles of Electrosurgery

Prior to undertaking endoscopic removal of tissue from the GI tract, an endoscopist must have a basic understanding of the principles of electrosurgery. Electrosurgery is the use of radiofrequency (RF) alternating current to raise intra cellular temperature in order to vaporize or coagulate tissue [2]. RF electrosurgery must be clearly distinguished from the process of cautery which is the destruction or denaturation of tissue by the passive transfer of heat from a heated instrument such as branding iron. In RF electrosurgery, energy is passed through the target tissue at a frequency in the 100 kHz to >3 MHz range. This high frequency prevents neuromuscular excitation while achieving the desired tissue effect of cutting or coagulation. An electrosurgical unit (ESU) converts the low-frequency alternating current from a household-type outlet to high frequency current in the radio wave spectrum—

i.e., radio frequency or "RF." This energy is then delivered to the instrument and target tissue in one of two pathways—monopolar or bipolar.

Monopolar energy passes from the ESU through the endoscopic device (snare, forceps, etc.) through the patient, and back to the dispersive electrode (aka "grounding pad"). There is a tissue effect at the tip of the device because there is a large concentration of current through a small area of tissue resulting in high current density at the target. The patient is not burned at the dispersive electrode, however, because the return current is "collected" over a wide surface area with low current density. Monopolar energy is used to cut, or coagulate mucosal lesions. Cutting current is delivered as a low voltage continuous waveform (Fig. 9.1) resulting in rapid heating of the tissue and vaporization of its water content. The result is a virtual explosion of the tissue with rapid division but less hemostasis. Coagulation current is delivered via a high voltage, intermittent waveform (Fig. 9.2) which results in less rapid heating of the tissue and the formation of coagulum with hemostasis. Blended currents combine features of both cutting and coagulation by changing the coagulation waveform so it is "on" through more of the energy cycle (Fig. 9.3). Blended currents can only be accessed by depressing the yellow pedal of the ESU. The most common monopolar device for resection is the polypectomy snare, but many other devices use monopolar energy as well such as biopsy forceps (aka "hot" biopsy forceps), sphincterotomes, and argon plasma coagulation (APC) catheters.

Bipolar RF energy passes from one electrical pole of the device, through the target tissue, and then into the other pole of the device. A dispersive electrode is not needed and the concentration of current between the two poles of the device prevents the spread of electrosurgical energy to surrounding tissue. In surgery, bipolar forceps are often used by neurosurgeons to desiccate delicate blood vessels in the brain without damaging surrounding tissue. In GI endoscopy, bipolar energy is most often used to ablate mucosa.

Whether using monopolar or bipolar RF energy, the endoscopist must have a firm understanding of the basis of

B.J. Dunkin, M.D., F.A.C.S. (✉)
Section of Endoscopic Surgery, MITIE℠ (the Methodist Institute for Technology, Innovation, and Education), The Methodist Hospital, Houston, TX, USA
e-mail: bjdunkin@tmhs.org

J.M. Marks and B.J. Dunkin (eds.), *Principles of Flexible Endoscopy for Surgeons*, DOI 10.1007/978-1-4614-6330-6_9, © Springer Science+Business Media New York 2013

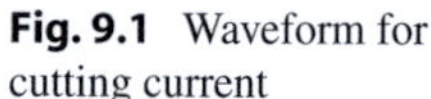

Fig. 9.1 Waveform for cutting current

Fig. 9.2 Waveform for coagulation current. Coagulation current—high voltage intermittent waveform (6 % on, 94 % off during cycle)

Fig. 9.3 Waveform for blended current. Intermittent waveform (50 % on, 50 % off in this example)

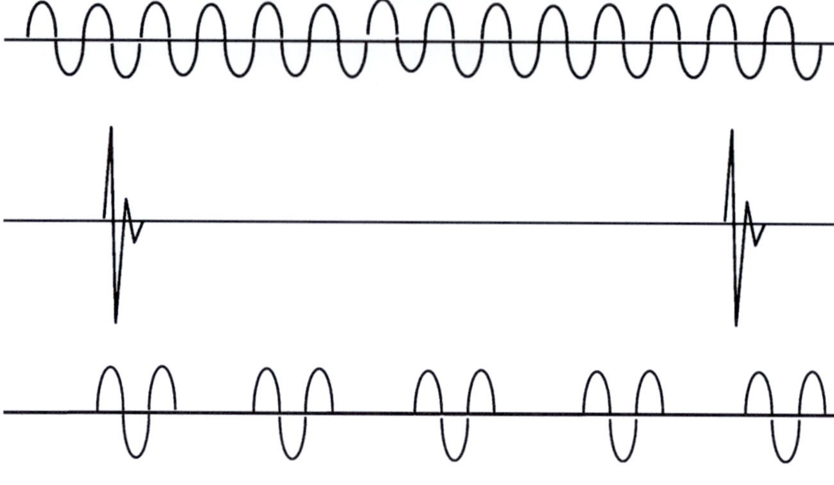

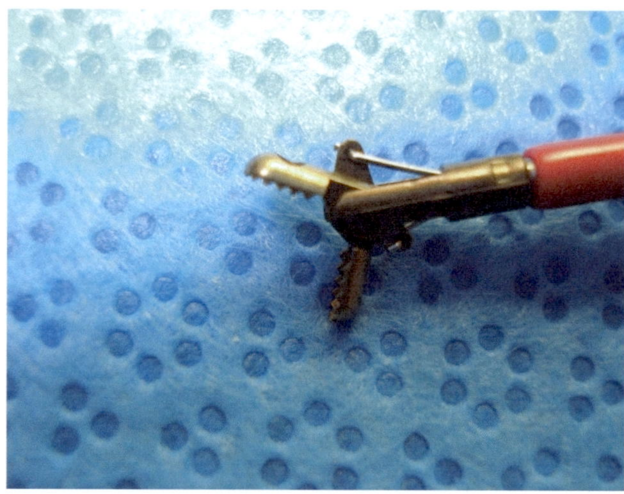

Fig. 9.4 Biopsy forceps

electrosurgery, be very familiar with the ESU he or she is using, and know the proper settings of that unit to achieve the desired tissue effect without injuring the patient. A more complete discussion of electrosurgical energy and its specific application to the GI tract can be found in the SAGES Manual on the Fundamental Use of Surgical Energy (FUSE) [3].

Tissue Removal

During GI endoscopy, mucosal lesions are frequently encountered that require removal. These lesions can range in size from a few millimeters to many centimeters. This section reviews methods for removing tissue beginning from the smallest lesions and progressing to much larger ones.

Biopsy Forceps

Endoscopic biopsy forceps are frequently used to sample or remove tissue in the GI tract (Fig. 9.4). They range in size and

configuration and the endoscopist must be familiar with what is available in his or her unit. Traditionally, standard biopsy forceps fit down the 2.8 mm working channel of a diagnostic gastroscope and had a cup length of 2.0–2.3 mm. In contrast, "jumbo" forceps required a 3.2 mm working channel but had cup lengths up to 4 mm. Modern biopsy forceps have a cup length of 3 mm allowing acquisition of tissue samples almost as large as that of a jumbo forceps without requiring a therapeutic working channel. The cup of the forceps can have a serrated or cutting edge, and often a needle is placed in the "crotch" of the forceps to aid fixation on the target tissue and to hold the first specimen if a second "bite" is going to be taken. Multiple studies have compared standard biopsy forceps and "jumbo" forceps with different tip configurations. In general, the jumbo forceps retrieve larger surface area samples, but not deeper, and there is no clear advantage to the needle. A serrated edge appears to be best [4–6].

The simplest method to manage small polyps is biopsy forceps removal. "Diminutive" polyps 1–3 mm in size and can be removed completely with "cold" biopsy. The forceps is passed through the working channel of the endoscope into the lumen of the GI tract. The scope and forceps are then rotated to align the polyp with the working channel, and the tissue grasped. A gentle pull on the forceps then tears the polyp off the surrounding mucosa with very little bleeding. The area should be reexamined to see if additional "bites" are necessary. The most significant advantage of cold forceps polypectomy is that it avoids the application of RF energy which illuminates the risk of complications such as perforation or post-polypectomy syndrome (see Tips and Tricks section) [7].

An alternative to cold forceps polypectomy for diminutive polyps is "hot biopsy." A "hot" biopsy forceps delivers monopolar electrosurgical energy to the jaws to enable tissue destruction. During "hot" biopsy, the lesion is grasped with the forceps and lifted away from the underlying submucosa. Brief applications of RF energy are then applied until a white zone of coagulum is visible at the base of the polyp. In theory, this technique allows sampling of the lesion to determine its pathology while destroying any remaining tissue to minimize recurrence or continued growth. Although still practiced, there is controversy about the efficacy of the hot biopsy technique. A report by Gilbert et al. showed that the hot biopsy technique failed to reduce the incidence of colorectal cancer and was not associated with complete obliteration of the lesion [8]. Further the procedure risks deep tissue injury with the consequent complications of bleeding, perforation, and post-polypectomy syndrome. In a study by Mönkemüller et al. pathologists blinded to the fashion in which the specimen was acquired (hot vs. cold biopsy) found a significant rate of architectural distortion and tissue fragmentation in samples acquired by hot biopsy [9]. In addition, Tappero et al. described using the cold biopsy technique as an alternative to hot biopsy in 210 consecutive patients where 288 polyps less than 5 mm were excised without diathermy [10]. They reported this alternative to be safe and comparable to the conventional hot biopsy technique in adequacy of tissue acquisition for histopathology. Given these results, many endoscopists have abandoned the hot biopsy technique.

Snare Excision

When removing lesions in the GI tract larger than a few millimeters, the monopolar snare is most commonly used. Like biopsy forceps, snares come in a variety of sizes and configurations. Typically they are constructed of braided wire in the shape of an oval, crescent, or hexagon and connected to a control handle with an insulted plastic sheath (Fig. 9.5). Sizes range for 1.1–4 cm and special features are sometimes incorporated such as rotation to aid positioning, and the addition of an injection needle so that submucosal injections can be administered at the same time as snare excision without having to exchange devices.

To snare excise a lesion, the endoscope is positioned so that the lesion is in-line with the working channel and the snare is passed through the scope, opened, and placed over the polyp. It is most effective to place the plastic insulation sheath at the "crotch" of the snare against the base of the polyp and then close the snare so that the wire is drawn back to the polyp against the insulation (Fig. 9.6a), otherwise closure of the snare might result in the wire pulling off the polyp (Fig. 9.6b). Once the target tissue is captured in the snare, it can then be excised with or without RF energy.

Polyps 3–5 mm in size may be cold snare excised. After the snare has been tightened around the tissue it is closed completely to result in a cold guillotine resection. A small amount of inconsequential bleeding is common. The advantage of this technique is minimal risk of post-polypectomy bleeding or perforation with rapid acquisition of tissue without thermal artifact [11].

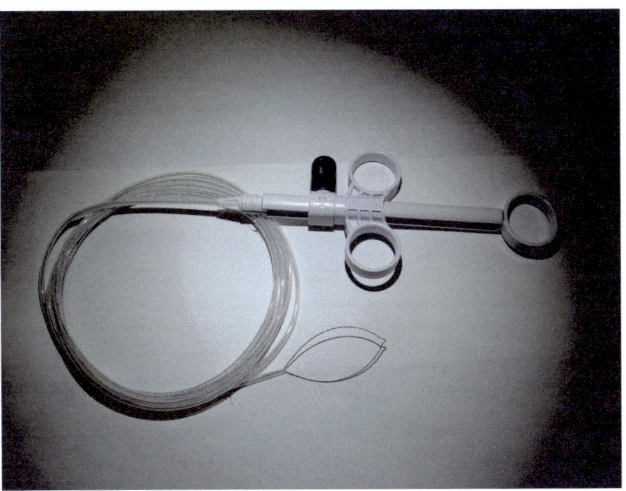

Fig. 9.5 Polypectomy snare

Polyps larger than 5 mm are usually snare excised using RF energy. The snare is positioned as described above, and when "snug" around the base of the polyp, slowly closed as RF energy is applied. The smallest snare and lowest energy setting to achieve the desired effect should be used. Exact energy settings vary according to location in the GI tract, patient body habitus, and the amount of tissue to be divided. Blended or pure coagulation current should be used. Pure cutting current results in the highest post-polypectomy bleeding rates [12]. Blended and pure coagulation currents seem to be equally effective, although blended current may have a higher risk of immediate post-polypectomy bleeding compared to pure coagulation which more often bleeds 2–8 days later. Pedunculated polyps should be snared along the stalk of the polyp at a safe distance away from the surround bowel wall as the stalk represents an extension of normal mucosa and does not need to be excised completely. Sessile polyps ≤2 cm may be snare excised in one piece similar to pedunculated polyps. The snare is simply placed flush to the mucosa and the lesion drawn into the snare. Removal of sessile polyps is associated with an increased risk of perforation from inadvertent snare excision of the underlying muscularis propria and care must be taken to elevate the tissue away from the bowel wall prior to applying RF energy.

Adjuncts to Polypectomy

An important adjunct to the safe removal of sessile polyps is the saline lift technique. Prior to snare excision, saline is injected into the submucosal layer beneath the lesion creating a cushion between the mucosa and the underlying muscularis propria (Fig. 9.7). The elevated tissue is then snare excised. Some endoscopists choose to add epinephrine (1:10,000 dilution) to improve hemostasis and/or methylene

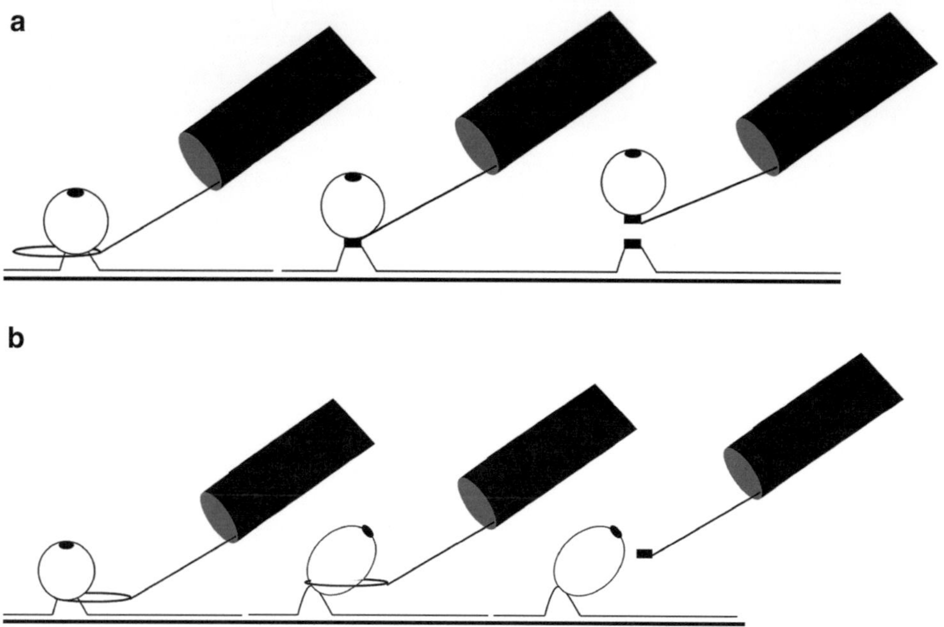

Fig. 9.6 (**a**) Proper technique for snare polypectomy. (**b**) Improper technique for snare polypectomy

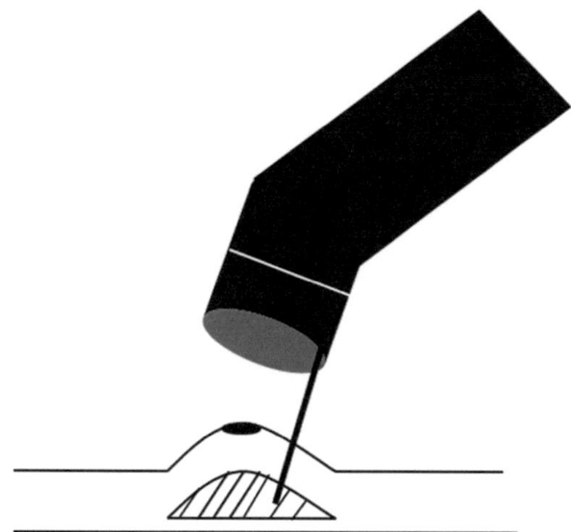

Fig. 9.7 Submucosal injection

blue to more clearly stain the submucosa for better assessment of the completeness of resection or evidence of perforation. Sessile polyps larger than 2 cm should be excised piecemeal, usually in combination with a saline lift (Fig. 9.8). APC may be used to destroy any residual tissue around the periphery of the resection margin after piecemeal excision. APC is a form of monopolar electrosurgery where argon gas is used to conduct the RF energy rather than a metallic device. When argon gas is excited by RF energy, it becomes a plasma which conducts electricity. The advantage of APC is that it is a noncontact method of RF energy delivery that enables rapid painting of surfaces without coagulum sticking to the device. When using APC in the lumen of the GI tract the endoscopist must be careful to continually aspirate the gas or risk bowel overdistention and/or perforation.

Removing pedunculated polyps with thick stalks may be associated with less post-procedure bleeding if the stalk is first injected with epinephrine [13]. Some have also advocated "preconditioning" the stalk by applying short bursts of pure coagulation current until the tissue blanches, followed by blended current to complete the excision. Another option for prevention of post-polypectomy bleed is to place an endoloop [14]. The endoloop is a detachable oval-shaped nylon snare. It is deployed in the same way as a standard snare but when tightened it can be separated from the delivery device and left behind to strangle the polypectomy stalk. The endoloop is placed around the stalk or base of the polyp prior to polypectomy and the snare excision is then performed "above" the endoloop, leaving it behind to slough off over time. Endoscopic clips can be used in an identical fashion. Kouklakis et al. randomized 64 patients with polyps greater than 2 cm in size to receive either epinephrine injection or a combination of endoloop and endoclip placement. The combination of endoloop and clip was superior to epinephrine alone with a 3 % post-polypectomy bleed rate compared to 12 % [15].

Tips and Tricks

Performing procedures within the closed lumen of the GI tract and working through the instrument channel of an endoscope present unique opportunities for complications during flexible GI endoscopy. This section provides guidance on avoidance of these complications, recognition of their occurrence, and management.

Fig. 9.8 Piecemeal snare
polypectomy

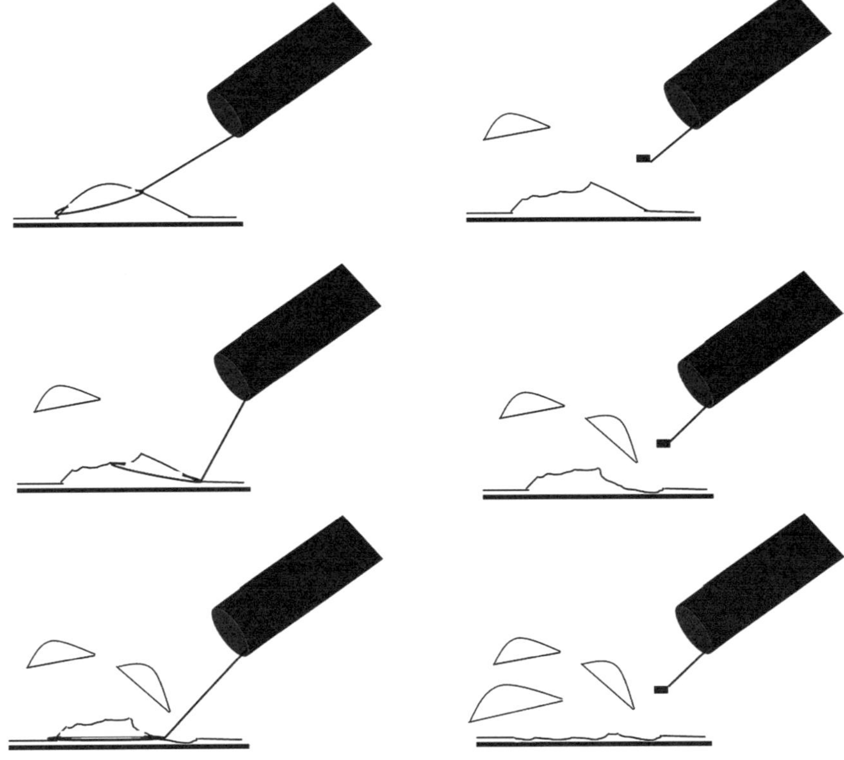

Post-polypectomy Syndrome

This complication is the result of full thickness thermal injury to the colonic wall following polypectomy. Patients usually initially feel well and are discharged from the endoscopy suite after their procedure only to return later that day or the next with abdominal pain and fever. On examination they have localized tenderness suggesting possible colonic perforation. However, on computer tomography (CT) imaging there is no evidence of perforation. The full thickness thermal injury has resulted in localized inflammation and peritoneal irritation without perforation. These patients are managed with supportive therapy (i.e., intravenous fluids, antibiotics, and bowel rest) and monitored closely with serial examinations. Most resolve their symptoms without operative intervention. The correct application of electrosurgical energy coupled with safety adjuncts like tenting of the mucosa during resection and saline lift will help to avoid this complication.

Unintentional Coupling

Unintentional direct coupling is the inadvertent application of energy to tissue that is in contact with either the device or target tissue. A unique opportunity for unintentional direct coupling occurs during removal of large pedunculated polyps. As energy is applied to the snare, the tip of the polyp may rest against the opposite wall of the colon (Fig. 9.9) resulting in the unintentional delivery of energy to that site and risking thermal damage or perforation. To avoid this problem, the polyp should be rapidly moved back and forth

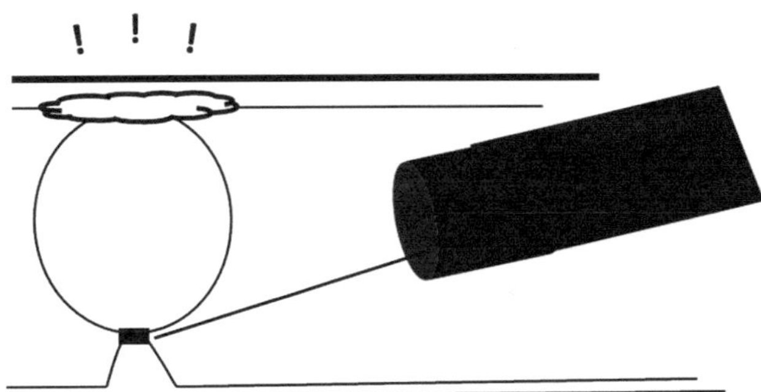

Fig. 9.9 Unintentional direct coupling to the wall opposite a large pedunculated polyp

during application of energy by "jiggling" the snare. In this way, even if there is direct coupling, it will occur for only a very brief period of time over multiple areas of the opposite wall and thus minimizes significant energy delivery or thermal damage.

Incorrect Management of the Polypectomy Snare

A unique aspect of GI endoscopy is that the devices are often "operated" by the assistant while the endoscopist targets the tissue. During snare polypectomy it is important that the assistant not tighten the snare too quickly while the energy is being applied. This can either result in a cold guillotine of the lesion with resultant bleeding, or embedding of the snare wire into the polyp tissue which increases the surface area in contact with the snare and decreases current density. In this "buried snare" scenario, increased levels of energy must be applied to cut through the polyp which risks full thickness thermal damage. When dealing with a buried snare, switching to pure cutting current may help complete the polypectomy while avoiding collateral thermal damage.

Endoscopic clips are frequently used to control bleeding or serve as a radiopaque marker. If clips have been applied near the base of a polyp, it is important to avoid placing a snare over these clips. Direct coupling between the snare and clips can result in the unintentional delivery of thermal energy to another part of the GI mucosa and possible deep thermal damage or perforation.

Difficult Access

At times, polyps are difficult to visualize because they are behind a mucosal fold or around the bend of a colonic flexure. There are three strategies for managing these difficult situations. The first is to simply change the patient's position. Placing a patient in right lateral decubitus position straightens the splenic flexure. Supine position can gain access to the right colon or change the orientation of a polyp to make it easier to access. The second method is to use the saline lift technique to "deliver" the polyp into view. Injection of saline just proximal to a sessile polyp partially hidden behind a fold will rotate the polyp into the lumen and distally and aid in visualization. The third technique is to retroflex the endoscope within the lumen of the GI tract. The method requires the endoscopist to be experienced in how much force can be applied through the deflection wheels of the endoscope and in the technique of retroflexion, but can be accomplished quite readily in most areas of the GI tract. A pediatric colonoscope may aid in retroflexion in the right colon and cecum, and a gastroscope can be used to retroflex in the left colon. Retroflexion is routinely performed in the distal rectum with a standard adult colonoscope.

Tissue Retrieval

After snare excision of a polyp the tissue must be retrieved for pathological evaluation. If the lesion is less than 1 cm in size, it may be aspirated through the working channel of the colonoscope and captured in a suction trap connected to the umbilicus of the scope. Larger lesions require use of the colonoscope and various tools for complete retrieval. If there is no need to visualize the remaining lumen of the colon, or if the lesion is in the left colon and it is not difficult to reintroduce the scope after polyp removal, the polyp may be simply suctioned up against the tip of the colonoscope and then both the scope and polyp are removed together under direct vision. If the suction method is unsuccessful, the polyp may be grasped with either a forceps or snare. If a piecemeal excision is being

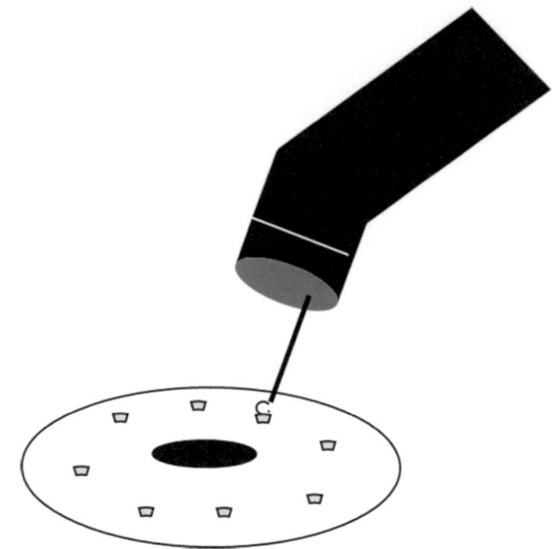

Fig. 9.10 Marking the periphery of a lesion prior to EMR

done, or the polyp cannot be grasped with snare or forceps, a retrieval net (Roth Net®, US Endoscopy, Mentor, Ohio) is available that can be passed through the working channel of the colonoscope, opened in the GI lumen, and used to "scoop" the specimens into the net which is closed around them. An advantage of the retrieval net is not only secure capture of the lesion, but maintenance of visualization during continued withdrawal. By positioning the net away from the lens of the endoscope, the remainder of the GI lumen can be inspected. Finally, if repeated introductions of the endoscope are required to retrieve all the excised tissue, it may be advantageous to use an overtube. The overtube is mounted on the colonoscope prior to introduction into the colon. When the scope has been passed to the desired depth, the overtube is advanced over the colonoscope and into the colon. With the overtube in place, the colonoscope can be reintroduced into the colon easily and repeatedly.

Endoscopic Mucosal Resection

At times, it is desirable to remove a GI lesion en bloc for more accurate pathologic evaluation. In the colon, this may simply require snare excision with or without saline lift. In the esophagus it is difficult to perform a saline lift snare excision, and more advanced techniques may be required. One technique available is endoscopic mucosal resection (EMR). Using EMR, 2 cm full thickness mucosal resection down to the muscularis mucosa can be achieved. There are two main methods of performing EMR: non-suction ("lift-and-cut") and suction ("suck-and-cut") techniques. Both techniques begin by marking the planned resection margins with brief bursts of cautery using an endoscopic snare with the wire minimally deployed (Fig. 9.10).

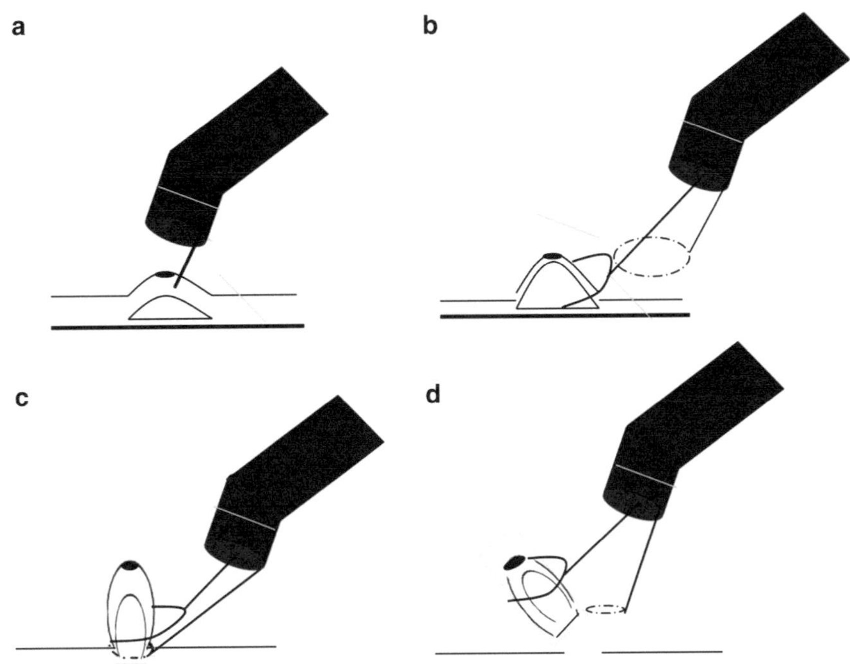

Fig. 9.11 The lift and cut technique for EMR. (**a**) Submucosal injection; (**b**) passage of a grasping forceps through the open polypectomy snare; (**c**) tightening of the snare at the base of the lesion; (**d**) completion of the snare excision

"Lift-and-Cut" Technique

The original strip-off biopsy technique described by Tada et al. in 1984 utilized a double channel endoscope and the lift-and-cut technique similar to a saline lift polypectomy (Fig. 9.11) [16]. The injection was originally done with saline, but other solutions have been used to gain better maintenance of the bleb including hypertonic saline (3.75 % NaCl), 20 % dextrose, or sodium hyaluronate [17]. Indigo carmine (0.004 %) is often added to the injectate to stain the submucosa and provide a better evaluation of the depth of resection. Submucosal injection can also be used to determine if a lesion is appropriate for endoscopic resection. Lack of elevation of a lesion with submucosal injection indicates deep submucosal involvement and is a relative contraindication to proceeding with EMR. After creating the submucosal elevation, the lesion is grasped with a rat-tooth forceps that has been passed through an open polypectomy snare. The forceps lifts the lesion and the snare is pushed down around its base and resection ensues.

"Suck-and-Cut" Technique

In this method, the lesion is aspirated into a cap attached to the tip of the endoscope and then resected. The most common methods utilize either a cap (EMR-C) or a band ligating device (EMR-L). For EMR-C (Fig. 9.12), a specialized cap is fitted to the end of the endoscope providing a chamber for aspiration of mucosa. The lesion is elevated with a submucosal injection and a crescent shaped snare is mounted into the distal inner rim of the cap. The lesion is then aspirated into the cap and the snare tightened around its base. The snared "pseudopolyp" is then excised with monopolar energy. The special EMR caps come in various sizes and shapes, the largest of which is 18 mm in diameter.

When performing EMR-L (Fig. 9.13), submucosal injection may not be required. This technique utilizes a variceal band ligator to ligate the mucosal lesion and create a pseudopolyp. The banded tissue is then simply snare excised either above or below the band.

Both EMR-C and EMR-L are limited in their capacity to accomplish en bloc resection. The maximum diameter amenable to one-piece excision is approximately 20 mm. If multiple resections are required, they should be accomplished at the initial setting if possible as submucosal lift may not be attainable once scar tissue has formed.

Endoscopic Submucosal Dissection

Endoscopic submucosal dissection (ESD) allows for larger en bloc resections and begins similar to EMR by marking the periphery of the lesion with small cautery burns. A margin of at least 5 mm is planned and marks are placed approximately every 2 mm (Fig. 9.14a). A submucosal injection is then accomplished around the periphery of the lesion utilizing a solution such as sodium hyaluronate with indigo carmine so that the elevation will persist throughout the procedure (Fig. 9.14b). A circumferential incision is then made to isolate the lesion using an ESD electrosurgical knife (Fig. 9.14 c, d). There are a number of ESD knifes to choose from (Fig. 9.15):

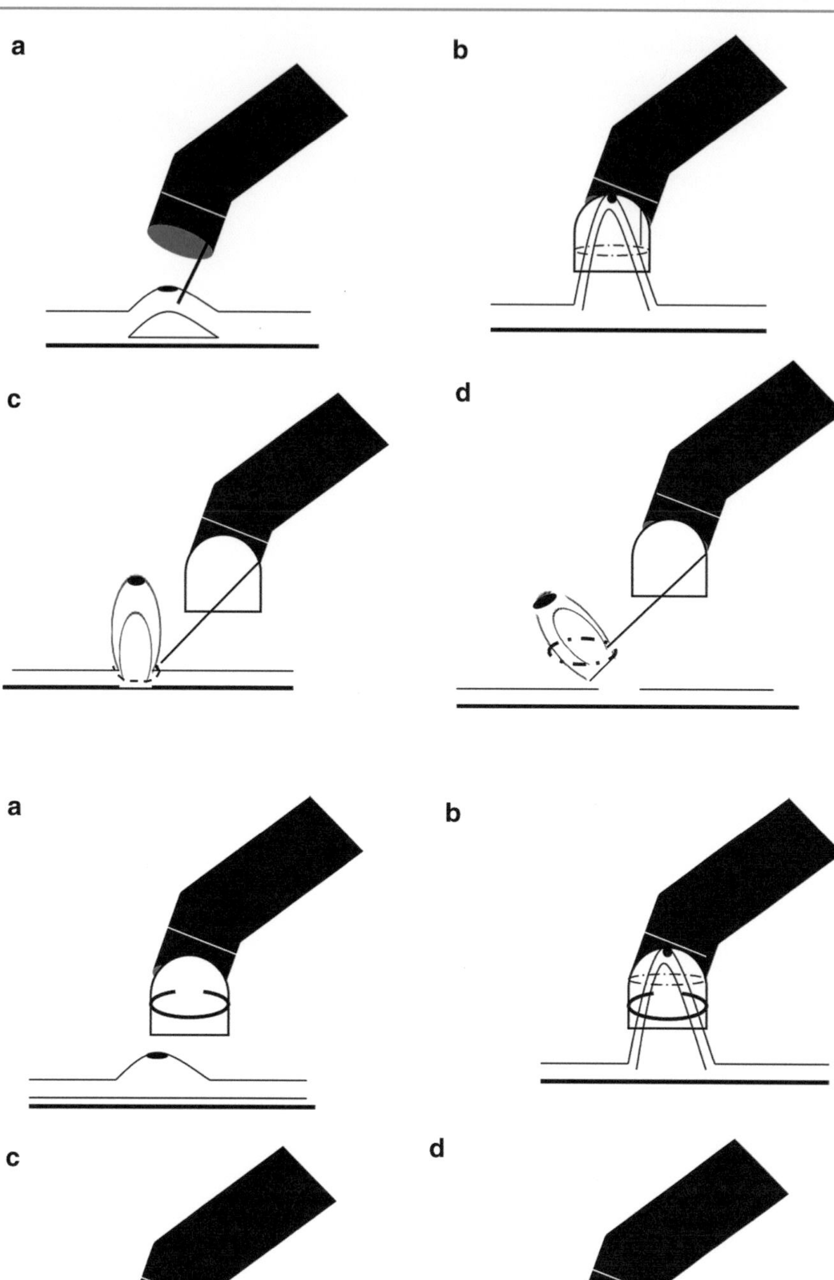

Fig. 9.12 EMR using a cap and snare technique. (**a**) Submucosal injection; (**b**) aspiration of target tissue into the cap with a pre-mounted snare; (**c**) tightening of the snare around the base of the lesion; (**d**) completion of the snare excision

Fig. 9.13 EMR with a band ligator. (**a**) Placement of the cap of the band ligator over the target tissue; (**b**) aspiration of the target tissue into the cap; (**c**) placement of a ligation band around the base of the target tissue; (**d**) snare excision of the lesion beneath the ligating band

Needle Knife

This knife has a fine tip and small contact area, which allows sharp incision. Because of its sharp nature, it can easily cause perforation if not controlled carefully. Mucosal incisions are usually begun with a needle knife, but then a switch is made to a protected tip knife to minimize the risk of perforation.

IT Knife

The insulated tip knife is a needle knife with the tip covered by a ceramic ball. This blunt, nonthermal tip reduces the risk of perforation. A second generation IT knife has a conducting surface on the bottom of the ball tip to allow for better tissue division when drawing back on the knife.

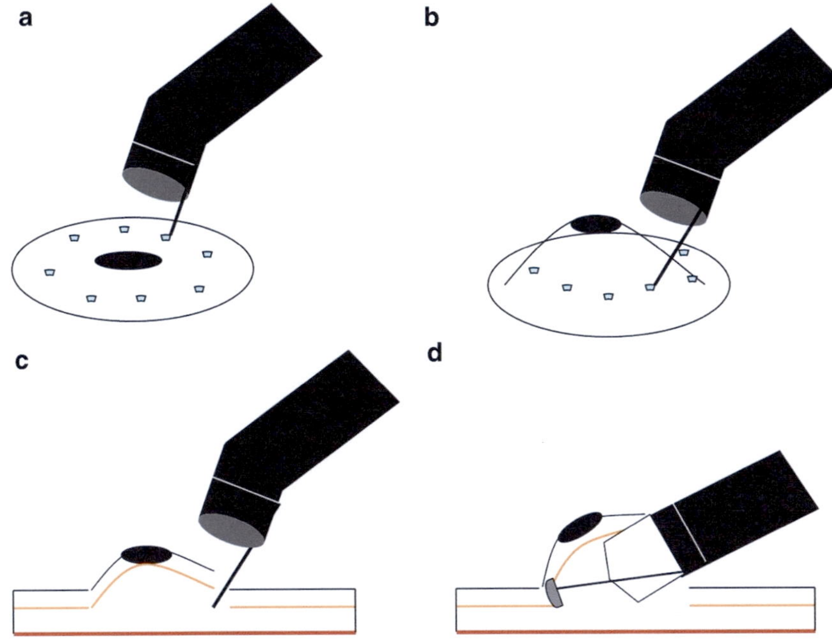

Fig. 9.14 Technique of ESD. (**a**) Marking of the planned resection margin; (**b**) submucosal injection; (**c**) incision into the submucosa with an ESD knife; (**d**) elevation of the lesion off the muscularis mucosa with dissection into the submucosal plane using an endoscopic cap

Hook Knife

This is a needle knife with the distal 1 mm of the tip bent at a right angle. The knife also rotates for optimal positioning.

Flex Knife

This knife has a rounded tip made of a twisted wire like a snare. Its length can be adjusted as needed. The shaft of the catheter is flexible with a thickened tip that acts as a tissue stop to minimize the chance of perforation.

Triangle Tip Knife

The TT knife has a triangular conductive tip that facilitates cutting mucosa. This knife was designed to be used for all parts of the ESD procedure.

Once the circumferential incision is complete, additional solution is injected into the submucosa in the center to obtain a more complete lift. One of the ESD knives is then used to excise the lesion in the submucosal plane. Meticulous hemostasis is critical in order to facilitate visualization, and the lesion is often positioned opposite the ground to utilize gravity to clear the field. A transparent hood is often mounted on the end of the endoscope to facilitate visualization and dissection into the submucosal plane.

Mucosal Ablation

This technique refers to a method of destroying the mucosa of the GI tract while preserving the underlying structures in an effort to treat mucosal-based diseases. After ablation, the treated area heals with non-diseased mucosa. The technique has most commonly been applied to Barrett's esophagus (BE) and intramucosal esophageal adenocarcinoma. Barrett's esophagus is a change in the type of cells lining the esophagus, transitioning from normal squamous epithelium to a columnar epithelium similar to that seen in the intestine. It is a known risk factor for the development of esophageal adenocarcinoma. The risk of progressing from BE to esophageal cancer is further defined by the degree of dysplasia (low or high) and length of the Barrett's segment. Some studies have shown that a patient with BE has a 30-fold increased risk of developing esophageal cancer when compared to a patient without Barrett's. This risk has led practitioners to pursue ablation of Barrett's prior to progression to adenocarcinoma.

The ideal ablative endoscopic therapy would remove metaplastic or dysplastic tissue down to, but not through, the muscularis mucosa. This would avoid stricture formation or transmural injury. The current modalities for ablating BE fall into two categories: thermal and cryogenic.

Thermal

The majority of the endoscopic therapies for treating BE with dysplasia fall into this category. They include multipolar electrocoagulation (MPEC), APC, photodynamic therapy (PDT), and bipolar radiofrequency ablation (RFA).

Multipolar Electrocoagulation

This is a bipolar electrosurgical probe 7 or 10F in diameter passed through the working channel of the endoscope. It is essentially bipolar energy conducted between adjacent wire wraps on the tip of the catheter. The gold color of the wires results in the catheter commonly being referred to as a

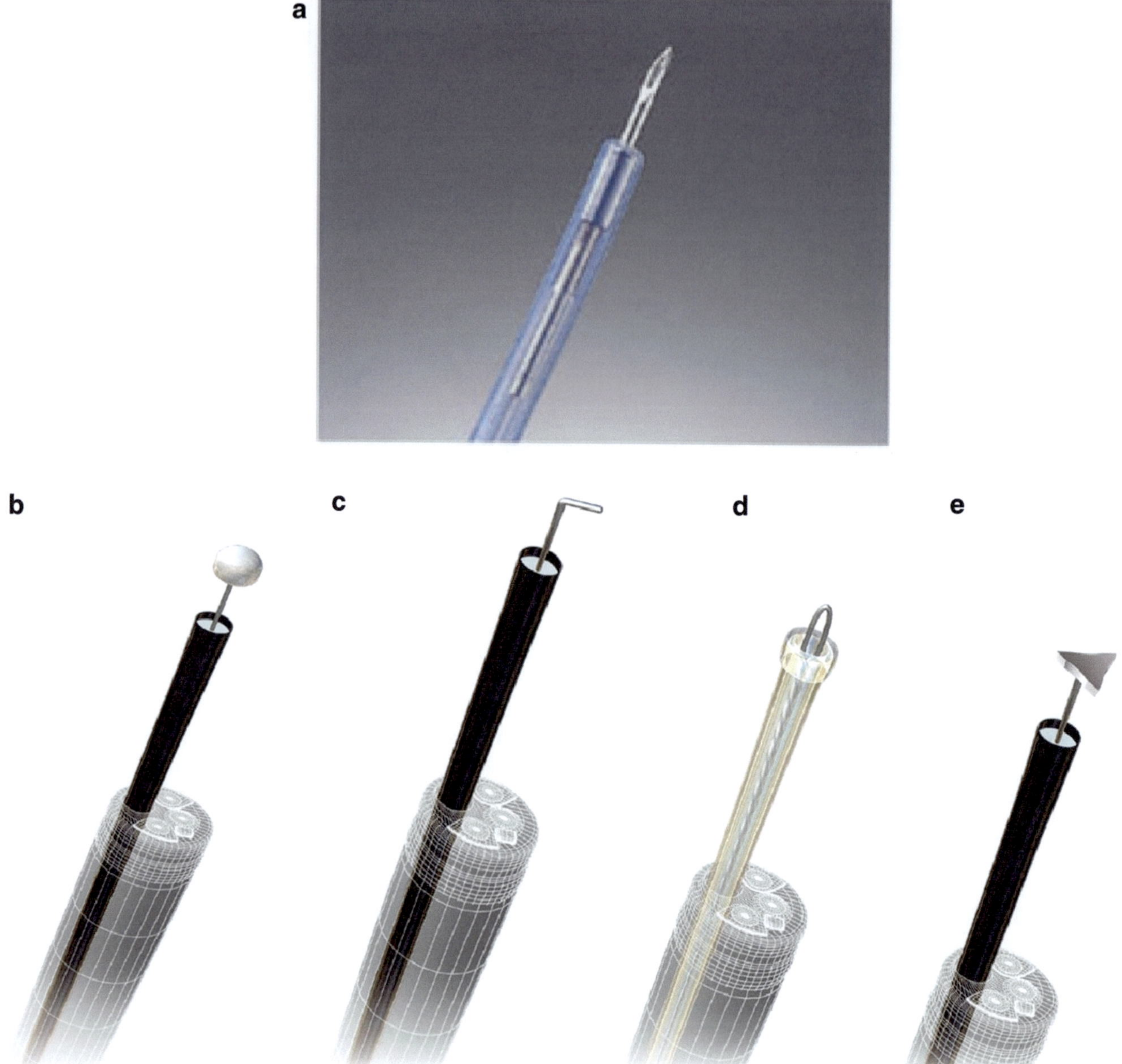

Fig. 9.15 (**a**) Needle knife; (**b**) insulated tip (IT) knife; (**c**) hook knife; (**d**) flex knife; (**e**) triangular tip (TT) knife

"gold probe" (see Fig. 9.10). Some MPEC catheters have injection needles and irrigation ports integrated into them. One advantage of using MPEC for mucosal ablation is that it uses a readily available energy source that is familiar to endoscopists. Typical energy settings range between 15 and 20 W.

In a review of published MPEC data done by Sampliner 292 patients with non-dysplastic Barrett's esophagus (BE) and 4 with low grade dysplasia were treated [18]. On average, 92 % of patients had resolution of their BE with a range of 72–100 %. Two strictures developed in this group and complications were mostly minor but included transient fever, chest pain, and odynophagia. Application of this technique is somewhat tedious because of its "point-and-shoot"

nature. MPEC is usually used in combination with another modality such as PDT which has the ability to rapidly treat larger areas of BE, leaving the MPEC for "clean-up" of residual areas on follow-up endoscopy.

Argon Plasma Coagulation

APC is simply high frequency monopolar electromechanical energy delivered to the target tissue using argon gas as a conductor. The advantage of using APC is that the probe can deliver the energy without touching the tissue, thus avoiding fouling with coagulum. The gas also allows the operator to "paint" larger surfaces quickly and the depth of thermal energy is fairly well controlled at 1–3 mm. The APC probe is a

7-French or 10-French catheter that has a forward-firing, side-firing, or radially firing tip. It is passed down the working channel of the endoscope and applied under direct endoscopic vision. Typical energy settings for the generator are 30–90 W and an argon gas flow rate of 1–2 l/min. Lower energy settings cause less penetration of the thermal energy into the tissues. The flow of argon gas can over insufflate the stomach or bowel and must be aspirated during the procedure.

A comprehensive report of using APC to treat BE by Franchimont et al. reviews nine studies examining ablation of non-dysplastic BE in 333 patients [19]. One to eight treatment sessions were required resulting in 55–100 % of patients obtaining eradication of their BE. This variability reflects varying treatment regimens (different power settings and number of treatment sessions), acid suppression regimens, and length of follow-up. There were five perforations and eight strictures reported in this review with up to 68 % of patients in one series relapsing back to BE at 12 month follow-up. In summary, APC does not seem to be an effective de novo treatment for BE because of a relatively high serious complication rate and the frequent finding of recurrent disease on follow-up. This "point-and-shoot" technology, like MPEC, is mainly used as an adjunct to another treatment modality for "clean-up."

Photodynamic Therapy

PDT uses a combination of laser light and a photosensitizing agent to effect tissue destruction. Two photosensitizing drugs are most commonly used—Sodium porfimer (Photofrin II, Axcan Pharma, Montreal, Quebec, Canada) and 5-amino levulinic acid (5-ALA). The photosensitizing drug is given to the patients 48–72 h before their endoscopy. Sodium porfirmer results in photosensitivity for 30–90 days so these patients must avoid exposure to sunlight for a significant period of time. The photosensitizer is taken-up preferentially in abnormal tissue with a higher metabolic activity level resulting in a degree of selectivity of tissue destruction to the abnormal epithelium.

Forty eight to seventy two hours after the patient receives the photosensitizing agent, endoscopy is performed to deliver light to the treatment area. Laser light is the only source of photoradiation strong enough to elicit the tissue destruction desired in the GI tract. Two lasers were commercially available—the Laserscope Model 630XP Dye Module (San Jose, California, USA) and the Diomed 630 PDT Laser (Cambridge, UK). Currently, neither is available in the USA. The Laserscope is a tunable dye KTP:YAG laser delivering 7 W at 630 nm wavelength. The Diomed laser delivers 2 W at 630 nm. The laser fiber can be positioned manually within the lumen of the esophagus, or centered with a positioning balloon. PDT therapy has only been approved by the FDA for treatment of BE with high grade dysplasia (HGD). 200 J/cm are delivered for flat HGD while 300 J/cm is used for nodular disease.

Overholt et al. reported on 103 patients followed for 51 months. Forty three percent had complete clearance of their BE and 94 % cleared their HGD. However, 30 % developed strictures which can be refractory to dilation [20]. The PHO-BAR trial is an international, multicenter trial enrolling 200 patients treated at 30 centers. Patients with BE and HGD were randomized to receiving PDT plus omeprazole, or omeprazole alone [21]. At 12 months follow-up, 41 % of the PDT treated patients had no residual BE and 72 % had no more HGD. This was statistically better than the omeprazole only group that had only 38.6 % resolution of the HGD. The PDT also resulted in a threefold decrease in the development of esophageal adenocarcinoma in these patients.

In summary, PDT is an effective therapy for clearing BE with HGD but is associated with a significant stricture rate, frequently causes odynophagia, fever, and chest pain, and requires patients to deal with photosensitivity for a significant period of time. Because of the severe mucosal damage caused by PDT, its use should be reserved for only treating BE with HGD.

Bipolar Radiofrequency Ablation

The only commercially available RFA device for treating BE is the HALO^{360} System (Covidien, Delaware, USA) approved by the FDA in 2001 (Fig. 9.16). The System includes the HALO^{360+} circumferential ablation catheter (Fig. 9.17) and the HALO^{90+} and HALO^{60+} focal ablation catheters (Figs. 9.18a, b). The HALO^{360+} catheter is a balloon-based bipolar electrode array used for treating circumferential segments of BE. The HALO^{90+} (13×20 mm treatment area) and HALO^{60+} (60% of the treatment area of the HALO^{90+}) ablation catheters provide primary or secondary "spot" treatments for smaller areas such as islands and tongues. Barrett's epithelium is approximately 500 μm thick so the HALO^{FLEX} energy generator and the HALO ablation catheter electrode arrays are designed to apply a uniform, superficial depth of ablation between ~500 and 1,000 μm. This achieves an ideal ablation depth down to, but not through, the muscularis mucosa which decreases the risk of post-procedure stricture.

Circumferential Ablation Steps: Using standard endoscopic techniques under moderate sedation, the HALO^{360+} ablation catheter facilitates rapid ablation of long and short circumferential segments of BE. The procedure begins by sizing the internal diameter of the esophagus to guide the correct choice of circumferential ablation catheter. The endoscope is introduced into the esophagus to identify anatomic landmarks and the length of Barrett's epithelium. A guidewire is inserted and the endoscope exchanged off the wire. The HALO^{360+} sizing balloon is introduced over the guidewire and the inner diameter of the esophagus measured. The sizing balloon is then removed, leaving the guidewire in place. Based on the smallest sizing measurement, the appropriate ablation catheter is selected.

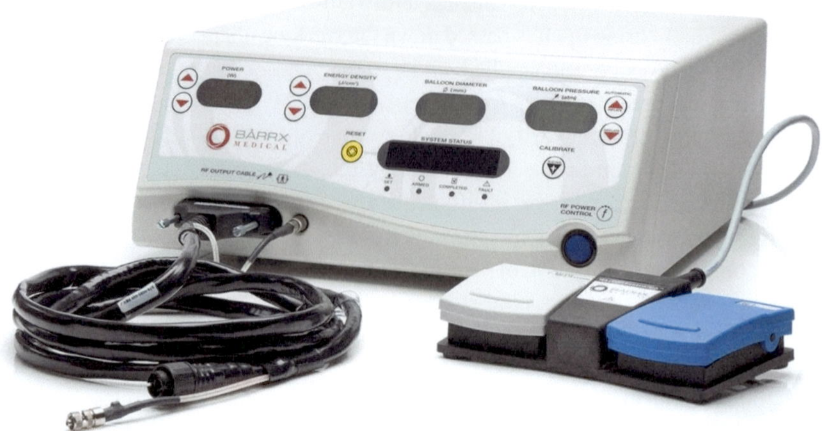

Fig. 9.16 HALO^FLEX generator

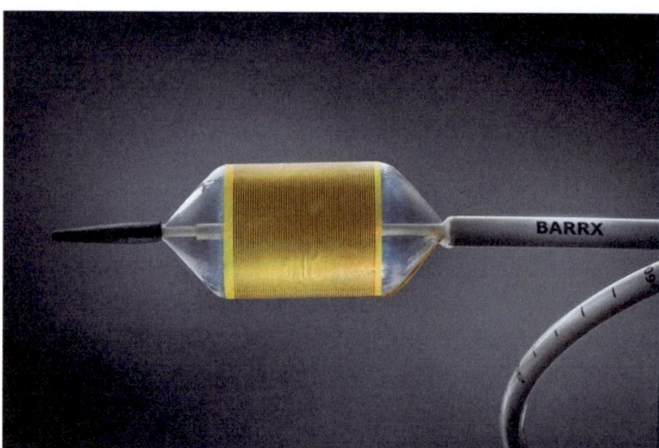

Fig. 9.17 HALO^{360+} circumferential RFA ablation catheter

After sizing the esophagus, the appropriate HALO^{360+} ablation catheter is introduced over the guidewire and into the esophagus with the endoscope reinserted alongside. The balloon electrode is positioned under direct visualization so that the proximal edge is slightly above the top of the intestinal metaplasia (Fig. 9.19). The balloon is automatically inflated and energy applied at 300 W and 10 or 12 J/cm^2 (10 J/cm^2 for non-dysplastic BE; 12 J/cm^2 for low grade dysplasia, HGD, or intramucosal esophageal adenocarcinoma). The electrode is then moved distally by 3 cm, aligning the proximal edge with the distal edge of the ablation zone and inflation and ablation repeated (Fig. 9.20). This process continues until the top of the gastric folds is reached.

The coagulum is then removed from the ablation zone using the HALO EMR—type cap mounted on the tip of the gastroscope. The surface of the ablation catheter is cleaned with water outside of the body and reintroduced over the guidewire. The endoscope is reinserted alongside the ablation catheter and the ablation steps repeated for a total of two treatment applications to the entire area of BE.

Focal Ablation Steps: The HALO^{90+} and HALO^{60+} catheters enable physicians to provide primary treatment for short segments of BE including focal areas such as islands and small tongues. The HALO^{90+} or HALO^{60+} ablation catheter are mounted to the end of the endoscope and introduced into the esophagus under direct vision. The anatomic landmarks are identified and measured. The endoscope is then deflected to bring the electrode into contact with the targeted tissue and ablation energy delivered at 12 J/cm^2. This step is repeated immediately for a total of two treatments to each targeted area. After this initial treatment, the coagulum is removed from the ablation zones using the edge of the HALO^{90+} or HALO^{60+} catheter. The endoscope and ablation catheter are removed and cleaned outside the body with water and then reintroduced and the ablation steps repeated for a total of four treatment applications to each targeted area.

The use of endoscopic RFA therapy in patients with dysplasia is supported by the results of several randomized, controlled trials. In a U.S. multicenter, randomized, sham-controlled trial of RFA involving 127 patients with dysplasia in BE (64 LGD, 63 HGD patients), subjects were randomized to receive either RFA or a sham procedure (control group). At 1 year, intention-to-treat analyses revealed complete eradication of dysplasia in 90.5 % of patients with LGD in the RFA group, compared to 22.7 % of those in the control group ($p < 0.001$). Similarly, complete eradication was found in 81.0 % patients with HGD in the RFA group compared to 19.0 % in the control group ($p < 0.001$). Complete eradication of the *all* Barrett's metaplasia was 77.4 % in the RFA group versus 2.3 % in the control group ($p < 0.001$). Post-RFA complications occurred in 6 (7 %) of the 84 patients who received RFA, including one self-limited upper GI bleed and five mild esophageal strictures [22]. There were no perforations or deaths. Other studies from Europe and USA show quite similar results [23–26].

While questions remain about the long-term efficacy of RFA for BE, this technology has already revolutionized the management of BE patient's with dysplasia and the current clinical results suggest that it is a step closer to

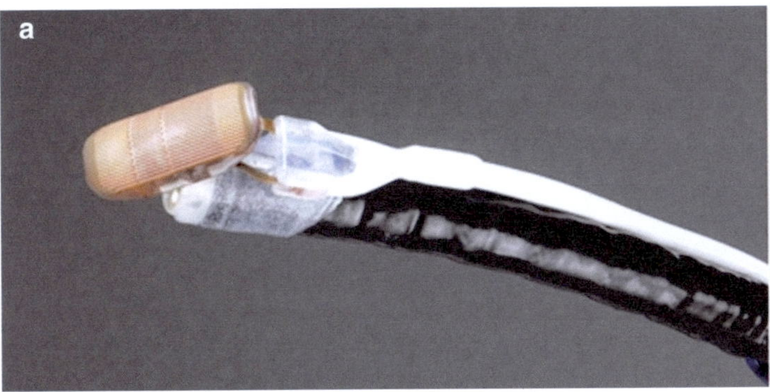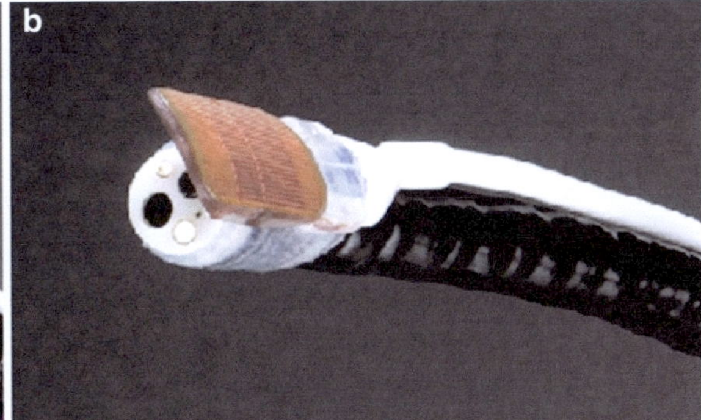

Fig. 9.18 (**a**, **b**) HALO[90+] focal RFA ablation catheter

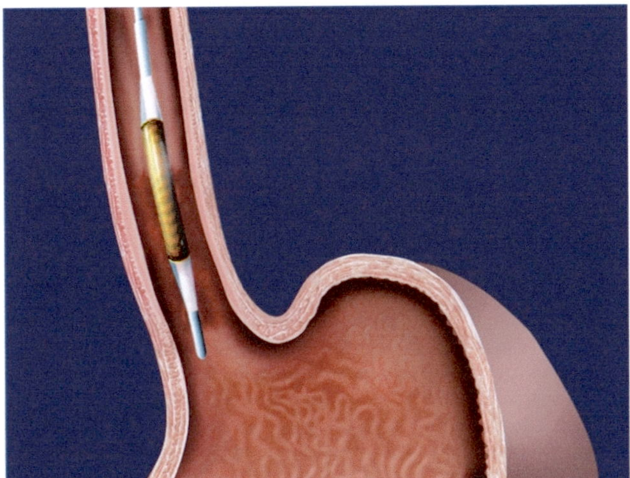

Fig. 9.19 Positioning the HALO[360+] RF ablation catheter at proximal end of the targeted treatment area

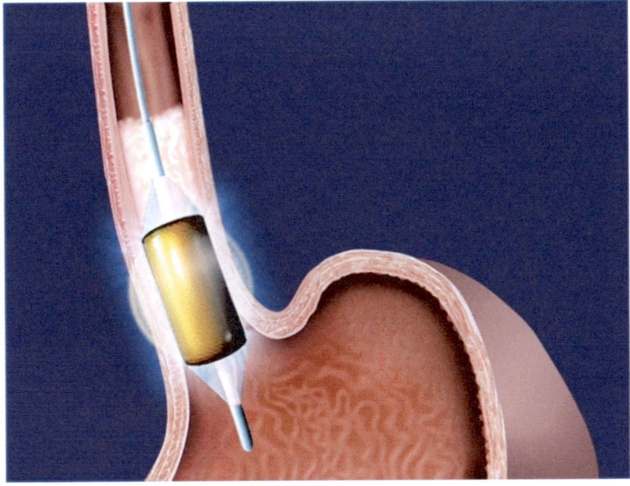

Fig. 9.20 Repositioning the HALO[360+] RF ablation catheter to treat more distal disease

achieving the ideal ablative therapy which resolves the Barrett's esophagus completely and removes the patient from the surveillance cycle. One limitation of RFA is the inability to effectively ablate nodular disease. As a result, it is often combined with EMR where mucosal resection is used to remove nodular disease and to determine if there is evidence of invasive carcinoma, and the remaining "flat" BE is ablated with RFA. Some groups have reported 100 % success in eradicating intramucosal carcinoma using this technique [27].

Cryotherapy

High pressure nitrous oxide or low pressure liquid nitrogen can be used as a cryogen to ablate esophageal mucosa. This is sprayed onto the mucosa using a 7-French or 9-French probe. The probe is connected to a delivery device which has a console for monitoring the cryogen release and a dual control foot pedal to control delivery and warm the catheter. It is a "point-and-shoot" technology that requires the endoscopist to spray the area of treatment.

The mechanism of injury to the mucosa is distinct from thermal. Cryoablation of the mucosa causes apoptosis and cryonecrosis resulting in transient ischemia and stimulation of the immune system. This distinct ablation mechanism may allow cryotherapy to work on segments of Barrett's esophagus that have not responded to other modalities. The ability of the cryogen to work with blood in the field and to treat nodular disease also differentiates it from thermal therapy. There is, however, limited published clinical data on cryotherapy and its role in ablation of GI mucosa continues to evolve.

Summary

Removal and ablation of mucosal tissue of the GI tract has revolutionized the management of digestive diseases. Performing these procedures with safety and efficacy requires a thorough knowledge of the devices, techniques, and principles of electrosurgical energy. With a solid foundation in excising mucosal-based diseases, advanced therapeutic endoscopists may be well positioned to progress to full thickness intralumenal resection in the future.

References

1. Wolff WI. Colonoscopy: history and development. Am J Gastroenterol. 1989;84(9):1017–25.
2. Munro MG. Principles of radiofrequency energy for surgery. In: Feldman L, Fuchshuber P, Jones DB, editors. The SAGES manual on the fundamental use of surgical energy (FUSE). New York: Springer; 2012. p. 15–60.
3. Dunkin BJ, Lyons CD. Electrosurgical energy in gastrointestinal endoscopy. In: Feldman L, Fuchshuber P, Jones DB, editors. The SAGES manual on the fundamental use of surgical energy (FUSE). New York: Springer; 2012. p. 107–22.
4. Berstein DE, Barkin J, Reiner DK, et al. Standard biopsy forceps versus large-capacity forceps with and without needle. Gastrointest Endosc. 1995;41(6):573–6.
5. Woods KL, Anand BS, DPhil RA, et al. Influence of endoscopic biopsy forceps characteristics on tissue specimens: results of a prospective randomized study. Gastrointest Endosc. 1999;49(2):177–83.
6. Abudayyeh S, Hoffman J, El-Zimaity HT, Graham DY. Prospective, randomized, pathologist-blinded study of disposable alligator jaw biopsy forceps for gastric mucosal biopsy. Dig Liver Dis. 2009;41:340–4.
7. Rex DK. Preventing colorectal cancer and cancer mortality with colonoscopy: what do we know and what do we want to know? Endoscopy. 2010;42:320–3.
8. Gilbert DA, DiMarino AJ, et al. Status evaluation: hot biopsy forceps. American Society for Gastrointestinal Endoscopy. Technology Assessment Committee. Gastrointest Endosc. 1992;38(6):753–6.
9. Mönkemüller KE, Fry LC, et al. Histological quality of polyps resected using the cold versus hot biopsy technique. Endoscopy. 2004;36(5):432–6.
10. Tappero G, Gaia E, et al. Cold snare excision of small colorectal polyps. Gastrointest Endosc. 1992;38(3):310–3.
11. Way JD. New methods of polypectomy. Gastrointest Endosc Clin N Am. 1997;7:413.
12. Rey JF, Bellenhoff U, Neumann CS, Dumonceau JM. European society of gastrointestinal endoscopy (ESGE) guideline: the use of electrosurgical units. Endoscopy. 2010;42:764–71.
13. Dobrowolski S, Dobosz M, Babicki A, et al. Prophylactic submucosal saline-adrenaline injection in colonoscopic polypectomy: prospective randomized study. Surg Endosc. 2004;18:990–3.
14. Iishi H, Tatsuta M, Narahara H, et al. Endoscopic resection of large pedunculated colorectal polyps using a detachable snare. Gastrointest Endosc. 1996;44:594–7.
15. Kouklakis G, Mpoumponaris A, Gatopoulou A, et al. Endoscopic resection of large pedunculated colonic polyps and risk of postpolypectomy bleeding with adrenaline injection versus endoloop and hemoclip: a prospective, randomized study. Surg Endosc. 2009;23(12):2732–7.
16. Tada M, Shimada M, Murakami F, et al. Development of strip-off biopsy (in Japanese with English abstract). Gastroenterol Endosc. 1984;26:833–9.
17. Fujishiro M, Yahagi N, Kashimura K, et al. Comparison of various submucosal injection solutions for maintaining mucosal elevation during endoscopic mucosal resection. Endoscopy. 2004;36:579–83.
18. Sampliner RE. Barrett's esophagus: electrocoagulation. Gastrointest Endosc. 1999;49(3):S17–S9.
19. Franchimont D, Van Laethem J, Deviere J. Argon plasma coagulation in Barrett's esophagus. Gastrointest Endosc Clin N Am. 2003;13(3):457–66.
20. Overholt BF, Panjehpour M, Halberg DL. Photodynamic therapy for Barrett's esophagus with dysplasia and/or early stage carcinoma: long term results. Gastrointest Endosc. 2003;58(2):183–8.
21. Overholt BF, Lightdale CJ, Wang KK, et al. Photodynamic therapy with porfimer sodium for ablation of high-grade dysplasia in Barrett's esophagus: international, partially blinded, randomized phase III trial. Gastrointest Endosc. 2005;62:488–98.
22. Shaheen NJ, Sharma P, Overholt BF, et al. Radiofrequency ablation in Barrett's esophagus with dysplasia. N Engl J Med. 2009;360:2277–88.
23. May A, Gossner L, Pech O, et al. Local endoscopic therapy for intraepithelial high-grade neoplasia and early adenocarcinoma in Barrett's oesophagus: acute-phase and intermediate results of a new treatment approach. Eur J Gastroenterol Hepatol. 2002; 14:1085–91.
24. Sharma VK, Wang KK, Overholt BF, et al. Balloon-based, circumferential, endoscopic radiofrequency ablation of Barrett's esophagus: 1-year follow-up of 100 patients. Gastrointest Endosc. 2007;65:185–95.
25. Gondrie JJ, Peters FP, Curvers WL, et al. Radiofrequency ablation of Barrett's esophagus containing high-grade dysplasia. Gastrointest Endosc. 2007;65:137–9.
26. Ganz RA, Overholt BF, Sharma VK, et al. Circumferential ablation of Barrett's esophagus that contains high-grade dysplasia: a US multicenter registry. Gastrointest Endosc. 2008;68:35–40.
27. Gondrie JJ, Pouw RE, Sondermeijer CM, et al. Stepwise circumferential and focal ablation of Barrett's esophagus with high-grade dysplasia: results of the first prospective series of 11 patients. Endoscopy. 2008;40:359–69.

Eric M. Pauli and Jeffrey M. Marks

Introduction

Clinically significant luminal narrowing—whether the result of a benign, malignant, or postsurgical processes—represents a group of conditions commonly encountered by the surgeon performing endoscopy. While the introduction of proton pump inhibitors (PPIs) has reduced the incidence of benign peptic strictures of the esophagus requiring endoscopic dilation, the bariatric surgical revolution of the late 1990s has resulted in a large population of patients in need of similar endoscopic therapies. This chapter reviews currently available methodology for the management of strictures and stenoses found during the course of endoscopic evaluation of the gastrointestinal (GI) tract.

Overview of the Techniques for Stricture Management

Despite the disparate origins of strictures of the GI tract, the two main methods of endoscopic management, dilation and stenting, can be applied to a multitude of circumstances. Pharmacological therapy, such as triamcinolone acetate injection represent adjuncts to these measures and are briefly discussed in this chapter. The methods described below have

This chapter contains a video segment that can be found by accessing the following link: http://www.springerimages.com/videos/978-1-4614-6329-0.

E.M. Pauli, M.D.
Department of Surgery, Penn State Hershey Medical Center, Hershey, PA, USA
e-mail: epauli@hmc.psu.edu

J.M. Marks, M.D., F.A.C.S., F.A.S.G.E. (✉)
University Hospitals Case Medical Center, Cleveland, OH, USA
e-mail: Jeffrey.marks@uhhospitals.org

applications specific to diseases of both the upper and lower GI tract. The individual therapy selected will be determined by the nature of the disease process, the anticipated treatment outcome, and the experience and preference of the surgical endoscopist.

Dilation

Overview

Currently available dilators come in three classes: Weighted Bougie Dilators, Wire-Guided Bougie Dilators, and Balloon (Hydrostatic/Pneumatic) Dilators. Weighted bougie dilators have the longest history of use and are available with a tapered tip (Maloney Style) and a rounded tip (Hurst Style) (Fig. 10.1). Tungsten has largely replaced mercury filled versions due to concerns of leakage and reclamation of mercury. While still popular in foregut surgical procedures (such as sizing for Nissen fundoplication), weighted bougies have been supplanted by wire-guided polyvinyl-chloride dilators (Savary-Gilliard Style or Amplatz Style) (Fig. 10.1) for stricture management due to their ease of use and the security of performing the dilation over a wire that guides the device through the stricture [1–5]. Hydrostatic and pneumatic dilators come in two types; over-the wire (OTW) balloons (including achalasia balloons) that function akin to wire-guided bougienade and through-the-scope (TTS) balloons that pass through the working channel of the endoscope either with or without a guidewire.

The surgeons overall experience with a particular method plays a large role in the success of dilation, and indeed, direct comparisons between mechanical dilation and balloon dilation have yielded conflicting results [5–9]. Some authors favor the results provided by mechanical dilators, which taper gradually over many centimeters and apply force in both the axial and radial vector during their forward motion [10]. This is in contrast to controlled radial expansion (CRE) balloon

J.M. Marks and B.J. Dunkin (eds.), *Principles of Flexible Endoscopy for Surgeons*,
DOI 10.1007/978-1-4614-6330-6_10, © Springer Science+Business Media New York 2013

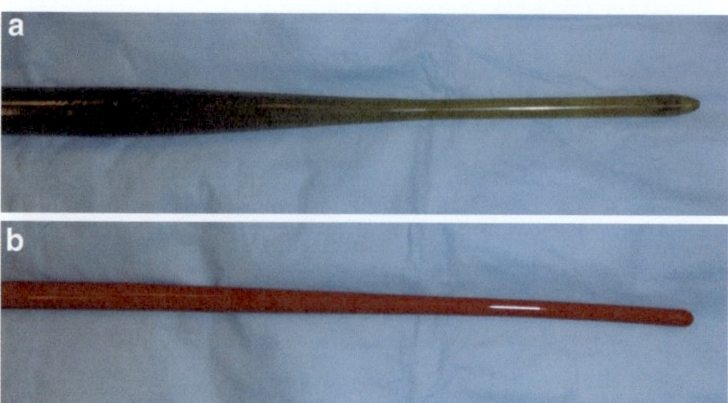

Fig. 10.1 Savory-Gilliard wire-guided (**a**) and rounded tip weighted (Hurst) (**b**) dilators

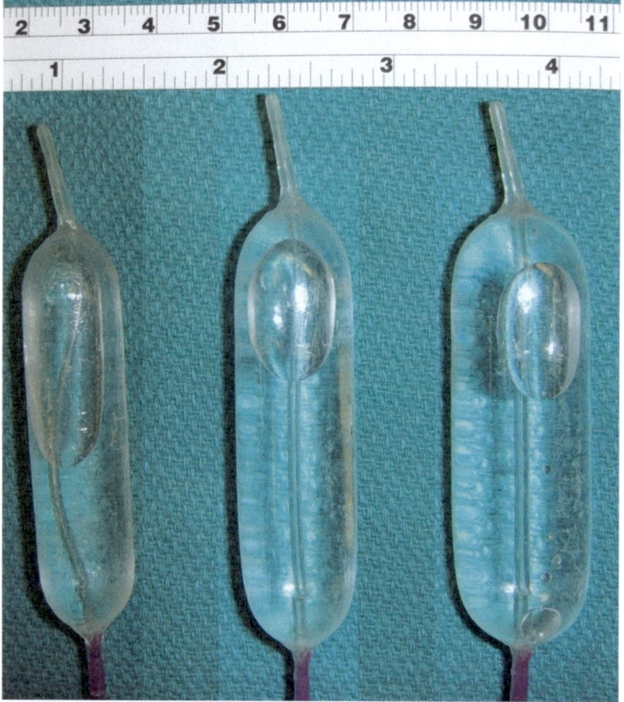

Fig. 10.2 A single controlled radial expansion (CRE) balloon inflated to its three distinct, pressure-controlled diameters

dilators, which dilate in three 1.0–1.5 mm intervals and which provide a much larger radial dilating force over the entire 5.5–8 cm balloon length simultaneously (Fig. 10.2) [10–13].

Regardless of the dilation method to be employed, the diameter of the dilator selected is critical to reducing the risk of perforation during the procedure [14, 15]. Pre-procedural imaging or estimates based on endoscopic visualization are commonly employed methods to determine initial dilator size, which should be approximately the same diameter as the strictured lumen. Commercially available endoscopic measuring devices or the open jaw of an endoscopic biopsy forceps are also useful for determining luminal diameter.

Fluoroscopy is frequently employed during the course of mechanical and balloon dilatation procedures, both during wire passage and during dilation itself. Wire advancement under fluoroscopy helps to confirm passage into the lumen distal to the stricture. This is of particular benefit in circumstances where the stricture cannot first be traversed by the endoscope to confirm normal lumen beyond [4]. During esophageal mechanical dilation, for example, fluoroscopy may be of particular benefit in patients with hiatal hernias [16]. Fluoroscopic visualization of balloon dilation is accomplished by using dilute (typically 1/2–1/3 strength) water soluble radiopaque contrast. This permits appropriate balloon positioning relative to the stricture location and allows visualization of the dilation itself; the "waist" the stricture creates in the balloon should disappear if the procedure is successful (Fig. 10.3) [10]. Interestingly, the literature is split on whether fluoroscopy is beneficial, with some authors reporting therapeutic benefit and decreased morbidity from reduced perforation risk, while others noting that it is unnecessary and exposes the patient and staff to ionizing radiation [6, 16–21].

Patient Selection and Preparation

Successful dilation depends on the etiology, the complexity, and the length of the stricture (see disease specific sections below). Coagulopathy, if present, should be reversed (International Normalizing Ratio less than 1.3) and anticoagulants should be withheld before the procedure. Although bacteremia occurs during the course of dilation [21, 22] current consensus recommendations do not support the use of prophylactic antibiotics even in high-risk populations [24–26]. See Chap. 4 for more detailed recommendations on the peri-procedural management of anticoagulation and antibiotic prophylaxis. Patients can be positioned in a left lateral decubitus position or supine and are generally fasted overnight.

Technique of Weighted Mechanical Dilation

Following upper endoscopy to document the location and diameter of the stricture, an appropriate sized Maloney dilator is selected and passed into the esophagus blindly. It is advanced to and beyond the stricture. The surgeon assesses for resistance with passage and inspects the withdrawn bougie for blood, both of which suggest successful dilatation. Increasingly larger bougies are passed generally following the "rule of threes," that is, not exceeding three dilator sizes above where significant resistance is first felt [27] and not dilating the stenotic segment by more than six French beyond the first bougie used [28]. Repeat endoscopy is then performed to assess for successful dilation and to assess for bleeding or other complications.

Technique of Wire-Guided Mechanical Dilation

Following upper endoscopy to document the location and diameter of the stricture, a Savary-Gillard or other guidewire

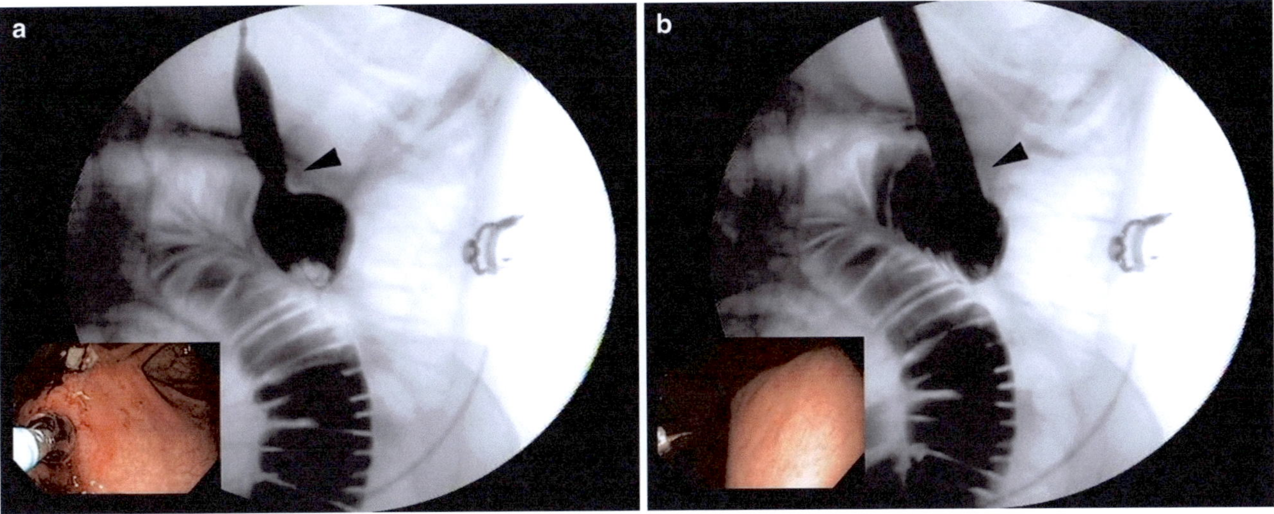

Fig. 10.3 Fluoroscopic images of a through the scope dilating balloon demonstrating the "waist" which represents the area of stricture (**a**) and ablation of the "waist" as the balloon completes dilation

is passed through the instrument channel of the endoscope. Endoscope traversal of the stricture before wire passage is preferable, but not always possible. Use of a pediatric or slim adult endoscope may be useful to accomplish this. Fluoroscopy can be used to confirm wire position and stability as the endoscope is withdrawn over the wire. Dilators are then passed down the wire utilizing similar technique to the Maloney dilation method described above with repeat endoscopic and possibly fluoroscopic evaluation at the conclusion of the procedure.

Technique of Over-the-Wire Balloon Dilation

OTW balloon dilation (such as that commonly used for the management of achalasia), proceeds in a manner identical to wire-guided mechanical dilation. The balloon catheter is advanced over the wire under fluoroscopic guidance. Radiopaque markers within the catheter allow appropriate positioning and permit conformation of balloon location during inflation.

Technique of Through-the-Scope Balloon Dilation

After identification of the stricture, an appropriately sized TTS balloon (available sizes range from 6 to 20 mm [18–54 French]) is passed through the endoscope channel. The balloon can be passed over a 0.035″ (0.89 mm) guidewire if the stricture is located adjacent to a bend that the balloon sheath may have difficulty navigating. An attempt should be made to situate the stricture in the mid portion of the balloon and the endoscope should be positioned just above the stricture. The sheath of the balloon is held tightly against the control section of the endoscope with one hand and the endoscope held tightly against the bite block with the other while the balloon is inflated. These maneuvers minimize

prograde and retrograde migration of the balloon during inflation. Balloons are inflated to nominal diameter as determined by atmospheres of pressure on the package insert. CRE balloons are unique in that they inflate to three distinct, pressure-controlled diameters. Rather than exchange to a different, larger diameter balloon, the atmospheres of pressure are increased to achieve a larger diameter (Fig. 10.2). This permits dilation to three different sizes with one balloon, minimizing the number of balloons necessary to complete the procedure and the time spent with instrument exchanges. If contrast agent is used to inflate the balloon, rather than water, fluoroscopy can be employed to document full balloon inflation by observing waist ablation. See Video 10.1 for an overview of TTS balloon dilation.

Complications

Regardless of the location or etiology of the stricture, bleeding and perforation are the most serious complications of dilation. These complications occur in 0.5% of esophageal dilations and in around 0–10% of dilations done for all other locations in the GI tract [28–36].

The most feared complication of dilation is perforation, which can result in localized or diffuse spillage of luminal contents. Perforation risk varies greatly depending on the location of the stricture within the GI tract and on the etiology of the stricture. Colon stricture dilation typically has rates higher than esophageal dilation. Malignancy, severe inflammation (eosinophilic esophagitis, inflammatory bowel disease), prior radiation exposure, prior perforation, high inflation pressures, endoscopist inexperience and the blind passage of dilators are all identified as risk factors for procedural perforation [21, 32, 35–40].

Table 10.1 Classification of esophageal perforations after dilation procedure

Type of perforation	Characteristics	Management strategy
Type I	Intramural perforation	Antibiotics, NPO
Type II	Transmural perforation	Antibiotics, NPO, TPN, possible stent placement
Type III	Transmural perforation with mediastinal leakage	Antibiotics, NPO, TPN, possible stent placement, surgical exploration, repair, and drainage

NPO nil per os, *TPN* total parenteral nutrition

Benign esophageal strictures carry a 0.1–0.3% risk of perforation in the largest series although much of this data is based on weighted mechanical dilation methods infrequently used in current endoscopy units [2, 4, 41]. Table 10.1 provides an overview of the classification of esophageal perforations after dilation procedures. Perforation rates can be as high as 13–48% for balloon dilation procedures for radiation and corrosive strictures, although the vast majority of these are type 1 (intramural) or type 2 (transmural without mediastinal spillage) ruptures [39, 42]. Malignant esophageal lesions can also be safely dilated, with a perforation rate of 0–1.3% [43–45].

Perforation rates for dilation of pyloric and gastric outlet obstructions (including surgical anastomotic strictures) are generally low, and the risk of perforation appears to relate primarily to the maximum diameter of dilation [33, 46–51].

Perforation rates for colorectal strictures are generally higher than those for foregut strictures, although most studies on this topic are small, retrospective case series. Rates range from 1.6 to 8%, and are similar for strictures related to inflammatory bowel disease or benign anastomotic strictures [31, 32, 36–38, 52, 53].

Clinically significant bleeding after all types of stricture dilation is uncommon, but may occasionally require immediate or delayed endoscopic therapy; most commonly thermal cautery or endoclip application. Bacteremia occurs transiently in as many as 45% of dilation procedures, but clinically significant complications of this bacteremia are only noted in the occasional case report [22, 23, 54, 55].

Stenting

Overview

Self-expanding-metal stents (SEMS) were first introduced in 1989 for the relief of malignant obstruction of the biliary tree [56]. It was quickly recognized that the use of an expandable tubularized metal stent had potential benefit for other malignant and recalcitrant strictures of the GI tract. Over the last

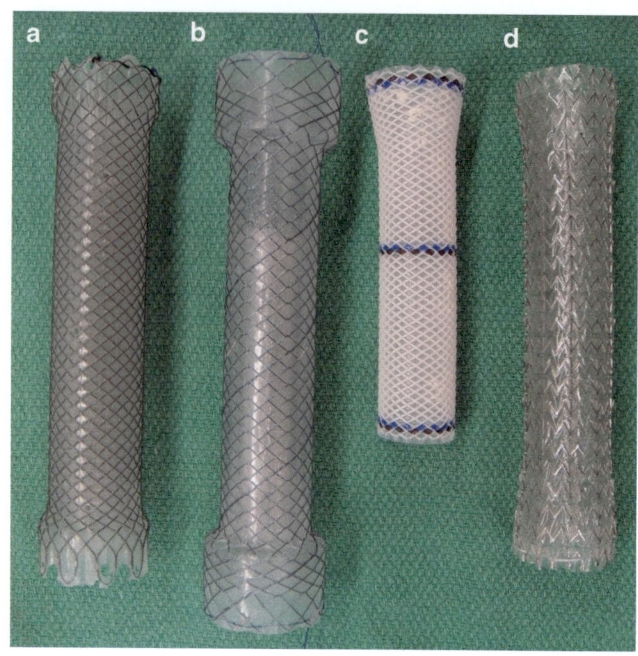

Fig. 10.4 Various self-expanding metal (**a**, **b**, **d**) and plastic (**c**) fully covered enteral stents

two decades, SEMS and, more recently, self-expanding plastic stents (SEPS) have gained popularity and shown tremendous therapeutic potential for stricture/obstructions of the esophagus, gastric outlet and colon. Stents currently have an evolving role in the management of enteric fistulae, perforations and anastomotic leaks, although many of these uses are not in line with the Food and Drug Administration (FDA)-approved indication for the devices. A more detailed discussion of the use of stents for this purpose can be found in Chap. 12.

Self-expanding enteral stents were designed as a replacement for rigid polyvinyl or rubber endo-prosthesis tubes (pulsion tubes), which required a large diameter to place, had a narrow inner diameter and unacceptably high rates of pain, perforation, and death [57]. In comparison, expandable stents can be placed across more narrow strictures, achieve a larger inner diameter and have lower rates of peri-procedural morbidity and mortality [58–63]. Rigid endoprostheses are of historical significance in developed nations, but are still commonly used in Central Asia and Africa where esophageal cancer rates are high and SEMS are cost prohibitive [64–66].

Stent Morphology

SEMS consist of woven, knit or laser-cut tubular metal mesh alloys of varying shapes and diameters (depending on manufacturer) held tightly within a constraining system in a delivery catheter (either OTW or TTS) (Fig. 10.4). The base metal is stainless steel, Nitinol (nickel and titanium alloy), or

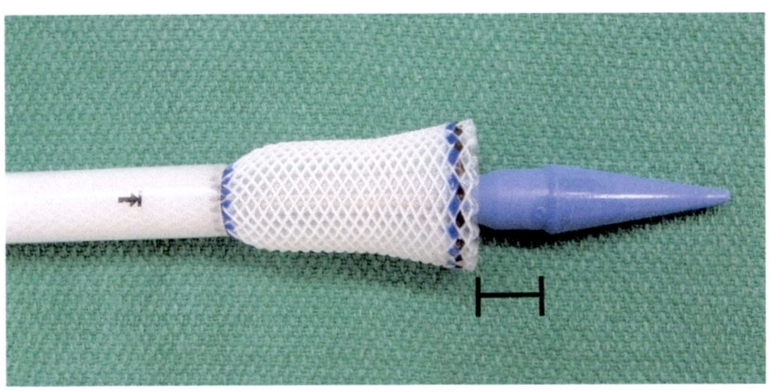

Fig. 10.5 Self-expanding plastic stent being released from its constraining system. Note that as the stent is expanding, it has shortened, as evidenced by the distance between the collared end of the delivery system and the top of the stent

Elgiloy (chromium, cobalt, and nickel alloy). After positioning with endoscopic and/or fluoroscopic guidance, the constraining system is removed, which causes a simultaneous increase in stent diameter and decrease in stent length (Fig. 10.5) [67]. The degree of stent expansion and shortening varies from stents of different manufacturers with newer generation non-braided designs exhibiting virtually no shortening when deployed [68, 69]. Familiarity with the degree of shortening of the stent to be deployed is critical to successful placement.

First generation SEMS were bare metal, which embedded themselves in the tumor and surrounding tissue with pressure necrosis. With time, the struts of these stents migrate through the mucosa and into the submucosa where a fibrous reaction embeds the stent in collagen [70, 71]. Rapid ingrowth of tumor and granulation tissue through the open mesh construct ensues [57]. While this results in lower rates of stent migration after 3 weeks, increased rates of tumor ingrowth and recurrent dysphagia (as high as 30% in some series) are observed [72–74]. Such ingrowth may not be of clinical concern in patients with limited life expectancy or in whom stent placement will be followed shortly by surgical resection of the involved segment of the GI tract. Uncovered stents are still commonly used for treatment of extra-luminal compression, where tumor ingrowth is not a concern [75]. Unfortunately, in these circumstances, granulation tissue overgrowth commonly results in stent occlusion.

Current generation stents cover the metal weave with polyester or silicone (so called covered SEMS) to resist tumor and granulation tissue ingrowth [76]. While efficacious in this regard, fully covered stents are more difficult to deploy (larger delivery systems, less flexible stent) and have a higher rate of migration, particularly at the gastroesophageal junction [77]. To counteract this migration risk, manufacturers offer fully covered stents with widely flared ends or partially covered stents with bare metal ends that permit some degree of luminal anchorage [75–78]. Covered SEMS also have a

role in the management of luminal perforations, postsurgical anastomotic leaks, and benign or malignant fistulae. A more detailed discussion of this topic can be found in Chap. 12.

In 2001, a self-expanding polyester braid stent with a full silicone covering was introduced to the market (Polyflex®, Boston Scientific, Natick, MA). This stent allows minimal ingrowth of tissue, which permits easier repositioning and removal, making it an attractive alternative to SEMS for benign disease requiring only temporary stenting [79]. Unfortunately, SEPS appear to have a higher migration rate (50–82% in the largest series) despite the fact that the plastic exerts more radial force than their SEMS counterparts [57, 80–88].

Stent Delivery Systems

Similar to endoscopic balloons, enteral stents come in a TTS delivery system and a non-TTS delivery system. Both delivery systems function as over the wire method, with endoscopic evaluation and wire placement occurring before stent deployment. Due to channel diameter constraints and stent deployment system size, TTS stents are only available in uncovered (bare metal) variety in the USA. Non-TTS stents are available in fully covered, partially covered and fully uncovered varieties, but their delivery system rigidity makes them deployable only in the very proximal and very distal GI tract. SEMS and SEPS have similar functioning delivery systems; however, the diameter of the SEPS is larger than that of SEMS, which can make passage of the device through a tight stricture or past an obstructing mass more difficult.

Patient Selection and Preparation

Enteral stents are indicated in malignant stricture-obstruction of the esophagus, gastric outlet, and colon and for upper GI strictures that are recalcitrant to repeated balloon or mechanical dilatation [61, 75, 89]. They also have a role in relief of distal obstructions that are exacerbating a more proximal anastomotic insufficiency or fistula. It should be noted that colon, pancreatic, gastric, and esophageal cancers are frequently detected in patients over 65 years of age who frequently have multiple underlying comorbid conditions [90]. Coagulopathy related to malnutrition or malignancy should be corrected. Stenting can be accomplished under conscious sedation in a left lateral decubitus position, but many surgeons perform the procedure in supine position under general anesthesia with an endotrachial tube to minimize the risk of aspiration in patients with obstruction of the GI tract [78]. Patients receiving upper GI tract stents should be kept NPO. Patients receiving colonic stents for subtotal obstruction, enemas permit distal colon evacuation and improve visualization. Current guidelines do not specifically address the need for prophylactic antibiotics during stent placement [24–26]. Some authors have suggested that prophylactic antibiotics should be considered in patients with complete obstruction and a markedly dilated colon because introduction of air during the procedure may promote microperforation and bacteremia [91].

Technique

Endoscopy is undertaken to identify the location of the lesion to be stented. Pre-procedural cross sectional imaging provides an invaluable roadmap for stent placement procedures as it can identify the location and the length of the lesion to be stented. Contrast fluoroscopy (either prograde or retrograde) also provides anatomical data about the location of the stricture and can also provide information about the degree of obstruction and the diameter of patent lumen (if any). As with dilatation procedures, endoscopic visualization of the GI tract beyond the lesion is preferable to facilitate wire passage, although it is not mandatory. This may require the use of a slim endoscope. In all cases, fluoroscopy is beneficial during the procedure. Blind passage of a guide wire should not be attempted [72].

The proximal and distal margins of the stenosis can be marked with mucosal clips, external skin markers or with submucosal injection of contrast material to permit fluoroscopic identification of the area to be covered with the stent. Luminal injection of contrast can help define stricture length, identify the distal lumen and aid in correct passage of catheters and guidewires [69]. Pre-stenting dilation of upper GI lesions (esophagus, gastric, small bowel) has been advocated previously, but current data suggest that this is not advisable due to an increased risk of perforation [92–96]. Pre-stenting dilation may also increase the risk of early stent migration and is rarely necessary [96, 97]. The exception to this rule is lesions with a diameter less than 9–10 mm that will not permit passage of the stent delivery system. Even in tight strictures, the stent will assume nominal expansion diameter in a matter of days without pre-dilation. For malignant colonic strictures, use of a 15 mm TTS balloon to dilate the lesion has been reported to increase stent deployment rates without increasing perforations [98–100].

If the endoscope is capable of traversing the lesion, a stiff guidewire with a floppy tip (such as a 0.038″ Savory or Amplatz type wire) is passed 15–20 cm beyond the lesion under direct endoscopic and/or fluoroscopic guidance. If the stricture cannot be traversed with the endoscope, a standard hydrophilic biliary guidewire preloaded in a biliary catheter can be used to navigate the lesion. The catheter is advanced over the biliary guidewire into the distal bowel. Contrast injection through the catheter can then be used confirm distal luminal position. The biliary guidewire can then be exchanged for a stiffer 0.038″ Savory type wire that will support stent insertion. Alternatively, the biliary guide wire can be used to support stent insertion.

Pre and intra-procedural imaging as well as endoscopic visualization of the lesion are used to determine the length of lumen to be stented. A minimum of 1–2 cm of stent coverage proximal and distal to the lesion is desirable and helps guide the length of the stent used (a minimum of 2–4 cm longer than the lesion).

For non-TTS stent insertion, the endoscope is withdrawn over the wire. Fluoroscopy confirms that the guidewire has not migrated during this process. The stent is loaded on the wire and advanced into position. Wetting the guidewire, adequately lubricating the stent delivery device and liberally using fluoroscopy all make advancement progress easier. The delivery system is stiff at its tip and therefore has poor support and poor mechanical advantage for forward advancement in curved areas of the GI tract (body of the stomach, duodenum, sigmoid colon) and may require manual external compression. Endoscopic pull assistance with a grasping forceps or a snare can be utilized in circumstances where forward advancement by push is not successful [101, 102]. The stent is deployed using the manufacturer specific system under fluoroscopic guidance to ensure appropriate position and to minimize migration during deployment. Some surgeons pass an endoscope parallel to the delivery system and observe the deployment under direct endoscopic visualization. Most stent delivery systems permit recapture and reposition of the device if it has not been fully deployed if the surgeon is not satisfied with position during deployment.

For TTS stent insertion, the endoscope remains in position after the guidewire is passed. A therapeutic endoscope with a 3.7 mm working channel is necessary to accommodate the 10Fr stent delivery system, and an endoscope exchange over the wire may be necessary if a non-therapeutic endoscope was used initially. The stent is passed over the wire, through the endoscopic channel and deployed using the method described above for TTS balloon inflation to prevent migration. Due to the shortening of the stent as it is deployed, constant readjustment of the stent delivery system and endoscope is necessary to ensure appropriate positioning of the device as deployment progresses.

The deployed stent is evaluated with fluoroscopy to document location and to assess for complete deployment. Contrast injection demonstrates stent patency and can assess for inadvertent perforation (Fig. 10.6; Videos 10.1 and 10.2).

Anti-migratory Measures

The major force limiting early stent migration is the radial tension exerted on the luminal wall. In an attempt to further reduce the risk of migration, authors have proposed a number of endoscopic methods to protect against stent migration or to reduce the risk of recurrent migration in the setting of a second procedure being performed for a migrated stent. Perhaps the most common method employed is the placement of an endoscopic clip to mechanically couple the proximal portion of the stent and the mucosa. Such clip application has been demonstrated to reduce the early risk of stent migra-

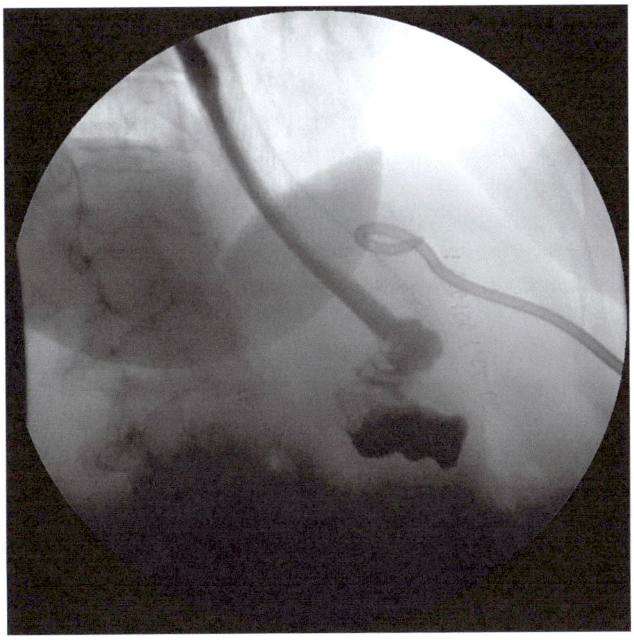

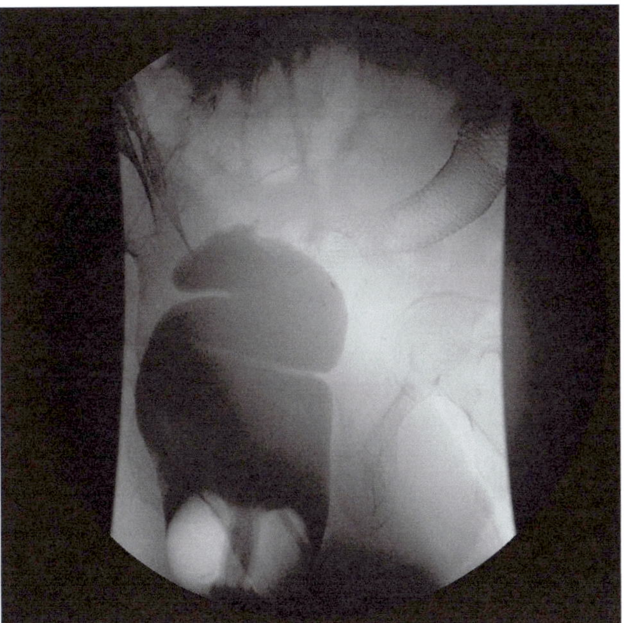

Fig. 10.6 Fluoroscopic examination of a newly deployed SEMS demonstrates good position across the gastroesophageal junction lesion with prompt passage of contrast through the stent

Fig. 10.8 Barium enema examination demonstrates occlusion of a recto-sigmoid stent in patient with recurrent obstructive symptoms

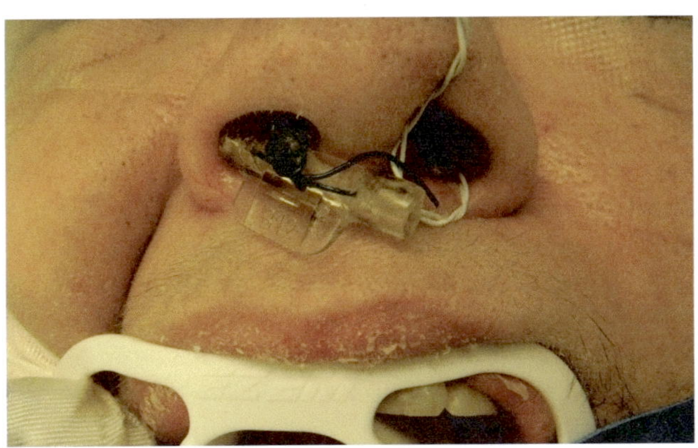

Fig. 10.7 Nasal bridal composed of monofilament suture endoscopically looped through the interstices of the stent, then retrieved through each nostril and secured through nasal cannula tubing to prevent skin damage to the nasal septum

tion, providing time for tissue ingrowth to further prevent migration [103–107]. Clip application is this manner is quick and familiar to most endoscopists.

Other authors have advocated the use of suture or umbilical tape passed through the interstices of the stent and subsequently secured to the nasal septum or earlobe (Fig. 10.7) [108, 109]. More recently, Blackmon and colleagues described a novel method of trans-cervical esophageal pexy that utilizes an ultrasound probe to guide the deployment of a suture-passing needle lateral to the trachea, medial to the carotid artery through the stent and into the esophagus [110].

In our practice, we have also employed current generation endoscopic suturing devices, such as the Overstitch (Apollo Endosurgery, Austin, TX), to secure enteral stents.

Complication

Due to the underlying disease processes, complications remain common in patients receiving enteral stents. Fortunately, stent deployment malfunction and misplacement rates are below 1% [64]. Peri-procedural complications including aspiration, pain and bleeding occur in as many as 10–20% of patients undergoing upper GI stent placement [111, 112]. Upper and lower GI bleeding resulting from tumor friability and mucosal tearing occur in 3–8% and 0–5% of cases respectively and is generally self-limited [111, 113]. Perforation rates range from <1% during esophageal and gastroduodenal stenting to 4.5–7% with colon stent placement [64, 93, 113–116].

Re-intervention due to stent fracture, migration and obstruction (from tumor ingrowth, granulation tissue formation or food bolus obstruction) is necessary in 10–50% of stented patients depending upon the type of stent utilized [116–120]. Partial stent migration is managed by repositioning or by insertion of an overlapping stent. Complete migration is usually managed with removal and replacement of a new stent. Migration results from undersizing of the initial stent, from tumor shrinkage in the face of neo-adjuvant or palliative chemo-radiation and from pre-stent placement dilation [98–100, 117, 121, 122]. Several studies have reported a higher risk of stent migration with fully covered stents in comparison to uncovered stents. The plastic coating prevents tissue ingrowth (granulation or tumor), which creates a longer-term patency rate but affords a significantly higher risk of migration [71, 113, 123, 124].

Stent obstruction (Fig. 10.8) from stool or food bolus impaction can be managed with endoscopic intervention. Risk of stent obstruction from food may be minimized by maintaining a low-residue diet, although there is no prospective data to support this practice. Tumor or granulation tissue obstruction is treated with placement of an additional stent within the first stent (typically a fully covered stent within an occluded uncovered stent) [125]. The radial tension of the new stent causes tissue necrosis over time and reestablishes luminal patency. This maneuver may also permit removal of the previously occluded stent, if necessary.

Enteral stent have a well-documented history of erosion. Such erosions can result in full thickness perforation of the GI tract and in the formation of fistulae (such as broncho-esophageal and aorto-esophageal fistula) [126–129]. Such perforations and fistulae represent life threatening situations with a high mortality.

Management of Specific Disease Processes

Benign Esophageal Strictures

Chronic gastroesophageal reflux disease remains the primary etiology of the majority (60–70%) of benign esophageal strictures although the incidence is decreasing as a result of proton pump therapy [130–134]. The remaining 30–40% is made up of strictures due to caustic ingestions, radiation therapy, and eosinophilic esophagitis.

Both balloon and mechanical dilation techniques are effective in treating benign strictures and head to head comparisons between the two methods have not demonstrated the superiority of either technique [5, 7–9]. Most patients with simple esophageal strictures require 1–3 dilations to relieve their symptoms, although 25–35% of patients require serial dilations beyond these three [134]. Simple strictures are more likely to respond to a single dilation session, whereas more complex strictures are more likely to require multiple sessions with higher recurrence and complication rates [3, 135]. While generally successful, benign strictures occasionally fail to respond to repeated dilation. In these cases, some authors have attempted adjunct therapy with intra-lesional steroid injection and placement of SEPS [136].

Steroid injection works through an incompletely understood mechanism [137]. Triamcinolone acetonide (Kenalog, Bristol-Myers Squibb, Princeton, NJ) in 10–40 mg/ml concentrations is injected into 4–6 locations within the stricture with a 23-gauge sclerotherapy needle. Aliquot size ranges from 0.25 to 1 ml depending on the concentration of steroid used. Dilation then proceeds with balloon or mechanical devices. Studies have shown reduced stricture recurrence rates and a decreased need for additional dilation sessions [138, 139].

SEPS have been advocated for the management of refractory benign esophageal strictures. A recent review of the use of SEPS in 130 patients with esophageal strictures demonstrated that only 52% were symptom free at 1-year post-stenting [140]. Stent migration and a need for endoscopic re-intervention were seen in as many as 20% of patients. Although not approved for benign disease, fully covered SEMS have an evolving role in the management of refractory strictures. They have a lower migration rate compared to SEPS, have a smaller diameter deployment system and are easily removable due to poor tissue ingrowth. Uncovered metal stents have no role in the management of benign esophageal disease due to prohibitively high rates of major complications (migration, erosion, fistula formation and recurrent stricture) [141–144].

Endoscopic electrosurgical incision of refractory esophageal strictures using a papillatome catheter or needle–knife has been advocated by some authors, but has not been thoroughly evaluated for safety or for long term success [145–150].

Malignant Esophageal Stricture/Obstructions

Per-oral dilation of esophageal malignancy can temporarily restore lumen patency to a diameter adequate to permit adequate swallowing in more than 90% of patients, although it should be noted that this data is from series using weighted mechanical dilators (and not hydrostatic balloons) [43, 44]. Such dilation is possible in the vast majority of patients and has a low perforation rate (1.3%). The largest series of hydrostatic dilation of esophageal cancers was conducted to permit endoscopic ultrasound (EUS) staging of the lesions. This series had a similar perforation rate as weighted mechanical dilation (1.4%), but there was no evaluation of the short-term success rate [151]. Unfortunately, repeat dilation procedures are needed every few weeks to maintain luminal patency [44, 45, 152].

Enteral stents offer advantages over per-oral dilation; they have a similar complication profile, but offer durable esophageal patency in as high as 95% of patients after one therapeutic endoscopic session [153–155]. For patients who are surgical candidates, stents can alleviate obstructive symptoms, permitting disease staging and preoperative chemoradiation in surgical candidates. In such patients, the stent is resected with the surgical specimen at the time of operation.

Stents are not advocated for high lesions (within 2 cm of the upper esophageal sphincter), however, due to an intense foreign body sensation and pain [89, 156]. Most sources recommend the use of a fully covered enteral stent for esophageal cancer, to minimize the risk of tumor or granulation tissue overgrowth, which would necessitate repeat endoscopic evaluations. No single fully covered SEMS has demonstrated efficacy over another in terms of complication profile or efficacy [157].

Foregut Anastomotic Strictures

Endoscopic dilation is the treatment of choice for foregut anastomotic strictures. The majority of such strictures occur as the result of esophagectomy (with anastomosis in the neck or chest) or after Roux-en-Y gastric bypass procedure for morbid obesity. Both weighted mechanical dilators and hydrostatic balloons have been used with similar success rates in terms of symptom relief and with similar complication profiles. Most endoscopists prefer the use of TTS balloon dilation, as it permits dilation under direct visualization.

One to three dilation sessions are required to successfully dilate foregut anastomotic strictures, although this number rises dramatically for specific types of anastomotic structures (such as cervical anastomotic strictures after esophagectomy) [47, 158–162]. Dilation was successful in relieving symptoms of dysphagia in 83–93% of patients with a perforation rate of between 1 and 3% [62, 158, 161].

Gastroduodenal Outlet Obstructions

Stent placement for relief of gastroduodenal outlet obstructions (GDOO), which occur as the result of unresectable pancreatic, gastric or biliary cancer, have been advocated by many authors [121, 163–165]. Stents confer a similar rate of early symptom relief (upwards of 90% in some series), early resumption of diet, and lower peri-procedural morbidity and mortality than formal surgical bypass procedures [123, 165–168]. Unfortunately, major complications and need for repeat interventions are more common (as high as 40%) in patients treated with stents [166, 168, 169], suggesting that stents may be better for patients with short life expectancy or in who surgical bypass in contraindicated.

For GDOO management, uncovered SEMS are utilized as they provide good luminal anchorage (to minimize the risk of migration) and do not cover the duodenal papilla (to avoid biliary obstruction) [69]. Moreover, the delivery system of fully covered SEMS (which are not available in a TTS system) cannot be readily placed in patients with otherwise fully intact anatomy. The presence of a SEMS in the duodenum makes access to the biliary tree difficult, however, and patients with risk of biliary tract obstruction should have a metal biliary stent placed prior to the placement of a duodenal stent. However, if necessary, biliary stents can be placed by a trans-hepatic route at a later time.

In patients with GDOO deemed not surgical candidates and in whom enteral stent placement is not feasible (or has failed), the placement of a decompressive PEG tube has been show to be relieve symptoms and to improve quality of life [170–173].

Malignant Colorectal Obstructions

Seven to twenty-nine percent of patients with colorectal cancer present with high-grade or complete bowel obstructions, and it is well established that such obstructions negatively affect outcomes in patients undergoing definitive surgery for their disease [174, 175]. Moreover, these high-grade obstructions are commonly found in patients with unresectable disease. Colon obstructions from extrinsic masses are also seen in patients with cervical, ovarian and prostate cancer. Enteral stents serve a critical role in all of these patients; converting an emergent surgical procedure into an elective one in the former group, and providing palliation of advanced disease in the latter.

Stent placement for preoperative decompression has numerous advantages over emergency surgery: medical stabilization of the patient including correction of fluid and electrolyte abnormalities, reestablishment of enteral nutrition to counteract malnutrition from bowel obstruction, avoidance of a two stage surgical procedure with a high morbidity and mortality, avoidance of stoma formation, administration of a bowel preparation, administration of preoperative chemotherapy and radiation (for rectal lesions) and colonoscopic examination of the remaining colon to evaluate for synchronous colon lesions or polyps. When stents are placed in this setting, they are resected en bloc with the surgical specimen.

As with GDOO, placement of colon stents for malignancy is associated with fewer early complications and more late complications when compared to surgical palliation [96, 116]. However, many late complications (such as stent occlusion and migration) are manageable endoscopically, making colonic stent placement an acceptable alternative to palliative surgery for colonic obstructions [176].

Benign Colorectal Obstructions

While malignant obstructions of the colon are the most common indication for stent placement, there is a growing body of literature to support their use in patients with benign stricture-obstructions of the colon and rectum. Ischemic, diverticular, Crohns', radiation-induced and anastomotic strictures have all been successfully managed with enteral stent placement [177–182]. While most case series in the literature describe small number of patients, technical success rates are high (76–100%) [177–179, 181, 182]. As with any stent placement, technical complications, including perforation, fistula formation, and migration can occur [2, 77, 179–181].

References

1. Kozarek RA. Esophageal dilation. Mayo Clin Proc. 1992;67:299–300.
2. Piotet E, Escher A, Monnier P. Esophageal and pharyngeal strictures: report on 1,862 endoscopic dilatations using the Savary-Gilliard technique. Eur Arch Otorhinolaryngol. 2008;265:357–64.
3. Siersema PD. Treatment options for esophageal strictures. Nat Clin Pract Gastroenterol Hepatol. 2008;5:142–52.
4. Pereira-Lima JC, Ramires RP, Zamin Jr I, et al. Endoscopic dilation of benign esophageal strictures: report on 1043 procedures. Am J Gastroenterol. 1999;94:1497–501.

5. Scolapio JS, Pasha TM, Gostout CJ, et al. A randomized prospective study comparing rigid to balloon dilators for benign esophageal strictures and rings. Gastrointest Endosc. 1999;50:13–7.

6. Ho SB, Cass O, Katsman RJ, et al. Fluoroscopy is not necessary for Maloney dilation of chronic esophageal strictures. Gastrointest Endosc. 1995;41:11–4.

7. Shemesh E, Czerniak A. Comparison between Savary-Gilliard and balloon dilatation of benign esophageal strictures. World J Surg. 1990;14:518.

8. Cox JG, Winter RK, Maslin SC, et al. Balloon or bougie for dilatation of benign esophageal stricture? Dig Dis Sci. 1994;39:776.

9. Saeed ZA, Winchester CB, Ferro PS, et al. Prospective randomized comparison of polyvinyl bougies and through-the-scope balloons for dilation of peptic strictures of the esophagus. Gastrointest Endosc. 1995;41:189.

10. Kozarek RA. To stretch or to shear: a perspective on balloon dilators. Gastrointest Endosc. 1987;33:459–61.

11. Adele JE. The physics of esophageal dilatation. Hepatogastroenterology. 1992;39(6):486–9.

12. Lindahl H, Rintala R. Shear stress in the performance of esophageal dilation: comparison of balloon dilation and bougienage. Radiology. 1989;172:983–6.

13. Goldstein JA, Barkin JS. Comparison of the diameter consistency and dilating force of the controlled radial expansion balloon catheter to the conventional balloon dilators. Am J Gastroenterol. 2000;95(12):3423–7.

14. Saeed ZA. Balloon dilatation of benign esophageal stenoses. Hepatogastroenterology. 1992;39(6):490–3.

15. Riley SA, Attwood SAE. Guidelines on the use of oesophageal dilatation in clinical practice. Gut. 2004;53:i1–6.

16. McClave SA, Brady PG, Wright RA, et al. Does fluoroscopic guidance for Maloney esophageal dilation impact on the clinical endpoint of therapy: relief of dysphagia and achievement of luminal patency. Gastrointest Endosc. 1996;43(2 Pt 1):93–7.

17. Kozarek RA, Patterson DJ, Ball TJ, et al. Esophageal dilation can be done safely using selective fluoroscopy and single dilating sessions. J Clin Gastroenterol. 1995;20:184–8.

18. Tucker LE. The importance of fluoroscopic guidance for Maloney dilation. Am J Gastroenterol. 1992;87(12):1709–11.

19. Wang YG, Tio TL, Soehendra N. Endoscopic dilation of esophageal stricture without fluoroscopy is safe and effective. World J Gastroenterol. 2002;8(4):766–8.

20. Raymondi R, Pereira-Lima JC, Valves A, et al. Endoscopic dilation of benign esophageal strictures without fluoroscopy: experience of 2750 procedures. Hepatogastroenterology. 2008;55(85): 1342–8.

21. Hernandez LJ, Jacobson JW, Harris MS. Comparison among the perforation rates of Maloney, balloon, and Savary dilation of esophageal strictures. Gastrointest Endosc. 2000;51(4): 460–2.

22. Bautista-Casasnovas A, Varela-Cives R, Estévez Martínez E, et al. What is the infection risk of oesophageal dilatations? Eur J Pediatr. 1998;157:901–3.

23. Nelson DB, Sanderson SJ, Azar MM. Bacteremia with esophageal dilation. Gastrointest Endosc. 1998;48:563–7.

24. ASGE Standards of Practice Committee, Banerjee S, Shen B, Baron TH, et al. Antibiotic prophylaxis for GI endoscopy. Gastrointest Endosc. 2008;67(6):791–8.

25. Wilson W, Taubert KA, Gewitz M, et al. Prevention of infective endocarditis: guidelines from the American Heart Association. Circulation. 2007;116(15):1736–54.

26. Nishimura RA, Carabello BA, Faxon DP, et al. ACC/AHA 2008 guideline update on valvular heart disease: focused update on infective endocarditis. Circulation. 2008;118:887–96.

27. Langdon DF. The rule of three in esophageal dilation. Gastrointest Endosc. 1997;45(1):111.

28. Tulman AB, Boyce HW. Complications of esophageal dilation and guidelines for their prevention. Gastrointest Endosc. 1981;27(4):229–34.

29. Lemberg B, Vargo JJ. Balloon dilation of colonic strictures. Am J Gastroenterol. 2007;102:2123–5.

30. Silvis SE, Nebel O, Rogers G, et al. Endoscopic complications: results of the 1974 American Society for Gastrointestinal Endoscopy Survey. JAMA. 1976;235:928–30.

31. Kozarek RA. Hydrostatic balloon dilation of gastrointestinal stenoses: a national survey. Gastrointest Endosc. 1986;32(1):15–9.

32. Couckuyt H, Gevers AM, Coremans G, et al. Efficacy and safety of hydrostatic balloon dilatation of ileocolonic Crohn's strictures: a prospective longterm analysis. Gut. 1995;36(4):577–80.

33. Lau JYW, Chung SCS, Sung JJY, et al. Through-the-scope balloon dilation for pyloric stenosis: long-term results. Gastrointest Endosc. 1996;43(2):98–101.

34. Ahmad J, Martin J, Ikramuddin S, et al. Endoscopic balloon dilation of gastroenteric anastomotic stricture after laparoscopic gastric bypass. Endoscopy. 2003;35(9):725–8.

35. Singh VV, Draganov P, Valentine J. Efficacy and safety of endoscopic balloon dilation of symptomatic upper and lower gastrointestinal Crohn's disease strictures. J Clin Gastroenterol. 2005; 39(4):284–90.

36. Breysem Y, Janssens JF, Coremans G, Vantrappen G, et al. Endoscopic balloon dilation of colonic and ileo-colonic Crohn's strictures: longterm results. Gastrointest Endosc. 1992;38(2):142–7.

37. Blomberg B, Rolny P, Jarnerot G. Endoscopic treatment of anastomotic strictures in Crohns disease. Endoscopy. 1991;23: 195–8.

38. Sabate JM, Villarejo J, Bouhnik Y, et al. Hydrostatic balloon dilatation of Crohn's strictures. Aliment Pharmacol Ther. 2003; 18:315–8.

39. Swaroop VS, Desai DC, Mohandas KM, et al. Dilation of esophageal strictures induced by radiation therapy for cancer of the esophagus. Gastrointest Endosc. 1994;40:311–5.

40. Marshall JB, Afridi SA, King PD, et al. Esophageal dilation with polyvinal (American) dilators over a marked guidewire; practice and safety at one center over a 5-yr period. Am J Gastroenterol. 1996;91(8):1503–6.

41. Mandelstam P, Sugawa C, Silvis SE, et al. Complications associated with esophagogastroduodenoscopy and with esophageal dilation. Gastrointest Endosc. 1976;23(1):16–9.

42. Choi GB, Shin JH, Song HY, et al. Fluoroscopically guided balloon dilation for patients with esophageal stricture after radiation treatment. J Vasc Interv Radiol. 2005;16:1705–10.

43. Heit HA, Johnson LF, Siegel SR, et al. Palliative dilation for dysphagia in esophageal carcinoma. Ann Intern Med. 1978;89: 629–31.

44. Cassidy DE, Nord HJ, Boyce HW. Management of malignant esophageal strictures: role of esophageal dilation and peroral prosthesis. Gastroenterology. 1981;75:173.

45. Boyce Jr HW. Palliation of advanced esophageal cancer. Semin Oncol. 1984;11:186–95.

46. Kim JH, Shin JH, Bae JI, et al. Gastric outlet obstruction caused by benign anastomotic stricture: treatment by fluoroscopically guided balloon dilation. J Vasc Interv Radiol. 2005;16:699–704.

47. de Lange EE, Shaffer Jr HA. Anastomotic strictures of the upper gastrointestinal tract: results of balloon dilation. Radiology. 1988;167:45–50.

48. DiSario JA, Fennerty MB, Tietze CC, et al. Endoscopic balloon dilation for ulcer-induced gastric outlet obstruction. Am J Gastroenterol. 1994;89:868–71.

49. McMahon MJ, Greenall MJ, Johnston D, Goligher JC. Highly selective vagotomy plus dilatation of the stenosis compared with truncal vagotomy and drainage in the treatment of pyloric stenosis secondary to duodenal ulceration. Gut. 1976;17:471–6.

50. Johnston D, Lyndon PJ, Smith RB, Humphrey CS. Highly selective vagotomy without a drainage procedure in the treatment of haemorrhage, perforation, and pyloric stenosis due to peptic ulcer. Br J Surg. 1973;60:790–7.

51. Delaney P. Preoperative grading of pyloric stenosis: a long term clinical and radiological follow-up of patients with severe pyloric stenosis treated by highly selective vagotomy and dilatation of the stricture. Br J Surg. 1978;65:157–60.

52. Dinneen MD, Motson RW. Treatment of colonic anastomotic strictures with 'through the scope' balloon dilators. J R Soc Med. 1991;84(5):264–6.

53. Shreden K, Wug SN, Myrvold HE. Balloon dilation of rectal strictures. Acta Chri Scand. 1987;153:615–7.

54. Botoman VA, Surawicz CM. Bacteremia with gastrointestinal endoscopic procedures. Gastrointest Endosc. 1986;32(5):342–6.

55. Niv Y, Bat L, Motro M. Bacterial endocarditis after Hurst bougienage in a patient with a benign esophageal stricture and mitral valve prolapse. Gastrointest Endosc. 1985;31(4):265–7.

56. Huibregtse K, Cheng J, Coene PP, et al. Endoscopic placement of expandable metal stents for biliary strictures—a preliminary report on experience with 33 patients. Endoscopy. 1989;21(6):280–2.

57. Schembre DB. Recent advances in the use of stents for esophageal disease. Gastrointest Endosc Clin N Am. 2010;20(1):103–21.

58. Knyrim K, Wagner H-J, Bethge N, et al. A controlled trial of an expansile metal stent for palliation of esophageal obstruction due to inoperable cancer. N Engl J Med. 1993;329:1302–7.

59. De Palma GD, di Matteo E, Romano G, et al. Plastic prosthesis versus expandable metal stents for palliation of inoperable esophageal thoracic carcinoma: a controlled prospective study. Gastrointest Endosc. 1996;43(5):478–82.

60. Roseveare CD, Patel P, Simmonds N, et al. Metal stents improve dysphagia, nutrition and survival in malignant oesophageal stenosis: a randomized controlled trial comparing modified Gianturco Z-stents with plastic Atkinson tubes. Eur J Gastroenterol Hepatol. 1998;10(8):653–7.

61. Siersema PD, Hop WC, Dees J, et al. Coated self-expanding metal stents versus latex prostheses for esophagogastric cancer with special reference to prior radiation and chemotherapy: a controlled, prospective study. Gastrointest Endosc. 1998;47(2):113–20.

62. Sanyika C, Corr P, Haffejee A. Palliative treatment of oesophageal carcinoma—efficacy of plastic versus self-expandable stents. S Afr Med J. 1999;89(6):640–3.

63. Yakoub D, Fahmy R, Athanasiou T, et al. Evidence-based choice of esophageal stent for the palliative management of malignant dysphagia. World J Surg. 2008;32(9):1996–2009.

64. Ramirez FC, Dennert B, Zierer ST, Sanowski RA. Esophageal self-expandable metallic stents—indications, practice, techniques, and complications: results of a national survey. Gastrointest Endosc. 1997;45:360–4.

65. Bolzan HE, Spatola J, Luna R, et al. Endoesophageal prosthesis as palliative treatment for malignant esophageal stenosis: cooperative study of the Northwest of the Buenos Aires Province. Acta Gastroenterol Latinoam. 1999;29(1):21–4.

66. Heniford BT. Personal communication, August 19, 2011.

67. Baron TH. Expandable metal stents for the treatment of cancerous obstruction of the gastrointestinal tract. N Engl J Med. 2001; 344(22):1681–7.

68. Chan AC, Shin FG, Lam YH, et al. A comparison study on physical properties of self-expandable esophageal metal stents. Gastrointest Endosc. 1999;49:462–5.

69. Katsanos K, Sabharwal T, Adam A. Stenting of the upper gastrointestinal tract: current status. Cardiovasc Intervent Radiol. 2010;33(4):690–705.

70. Bethge N, Sommer A, Gross U, et al. Human tissue responses to metal stents implanted in vivo for the palliation of malignant stenoses. Gastrointest Endosc. 1996;43:596–602.

71. Simmons DT, Barron TH. Technology insight: enteral stenting and new technology. Nat Clin Pract Gastroenterol Hepatol. 2005;2:365–74.

72. Baerlocher MO, Asch MR, Dixon P, et al. Interdisciplinary Canadian guidelines on the use of metal stents in the gastrointestinal tract for oncological indications. Can Assoc Radiol J. 2008;59:107–22.

73. Song HY, Jung HY, Park SI, et al. Covered retrievable expandable nitinol stents in patients with benign esophageal strictures: initial experience. Radiology. 2000;217:551–7.

74. Vakil N, Gross U, Bethge N. Human tissue responses to metal stents. Gastrointest Endosc Clin N Am. 1999;9:359–65.

75. Sabharwal T, Morales JP, Salter R, et al. Esophageal cancer: self-expanding metallic stents. Abdom Imaging. 2005;30:456–64.

76. Kim ES, Jeon SW, Park SY, et al. Comparison of double-layered and covered Niti-S stents for palliation of malignant dysphagia. J Gastroenterol Hepatol. 2009;24:114–9.

77. Sabharwal T, Hamady MS, Chui S, et al. A randomized prospective comparison of the Flamingo Wallstent and Ultraflex stent for palliation of dysphagia associated with lower third oesophageal carcinoma. Gut. 2003;52:922–6.

78. Morgan R, Adam A. The radiologist's view of expandable metallic stents for malignant esophageal obstruction. Gastrointest Endosc Clin N Am. 1999;9:431–5.

79. Dai YY, Gretschel S, Dudeck O, et al. Treatment of oesophageal anastomotic leaks by temporary stenting with self-expanding plastic stents. Br J Surg. 2009;96(8):887–91.

80. Verschuur EM, Repici A, Kuipers EJ, et al. New design esophageal stents for the palliation of dysphagia from esophageal or gastric cardia cancer: a randomized trial. Am J Gastroenterol. 2008;103:304–12.

81. Broto J, Asensio M, Vernet JM. Results of a new technique in the treatment of severe esophageal stenosis in children: poliflex stents. J Pediatr Gastroenterol Nutr. 2003;37:203–6.

82. Repici A, Conio M, De Angelis C, et al. Temporary placement of an expandable polyester silicone-covered stent for treatment of refractory benign esophageal strictures. Gastrointest Endosc. 2004;60:513–9.

83. Evrard S, Le Moine O, Lazaraki G, et al. Self-expanding plastic stents for benign esophageal lesions. Gastrointest Endosc. 2004;60:894–900.

84. Karbowski M, Schembre D, Kozarek R, et al. Polyflex self-expanding, removable plastic stents: assessment of treatment efficacy and safety in a variety of benign and malignant conditions of the esophagus. Surg Endosc. 2008;22:1326–33.

85. Garíca-Cano J. Dilation of benign strictures in the esophagus and colon with the Polyflex stent: a case series study. Dig Dis Sci. 2008;53:341–6.

86. Barthel JS, Kelley ST, Klapman JB. Management of persistent gastroesophageal anastomotic strictures with removable self-expandable polyester silicon-covered (Polyflex) stents: an alternative to serial dilation. Gastrointest Endosc. 2008;67: 546–52.

87. Pennathur A, Chang AC, McGrath KM, et al. Polyflex expandable stents in the treatment of esophageal disease: initial experience. Ann Thorac Surg. 2008;85:1968–72.

88. Dua KS, Vleggaar FP, Santharam R, et al. Removable self-expanding plastic esophageal stent as a continuous, non-permanent dilator in treating refractory benign esophageal strictures: a prospective two-center study. Am J Gastroenterol. 2008;103:2988–94.

89. Sabharwal T, Morales JP, Irani FG, et al. Quality improvement guidelines for placement of esophageal stents. Cardiovasc Intervent Radiol. 2005;28:284–8.

90. Burstein HJ, Mayer RJ. Gastrointestinal cancer. In: Hunter CP, Johnson KA, Muss HB, editors. Cancer in the elderly. New York: Marcel Dekker; 2000. p. 325–8.

91. Baron TH, Dean PA, Yates MR, et al. Expandable metal stents for the treatment of colonic obstruction: techniques and outcomes. Gastrointest Endosc. 1998;47:277–86.

92. Zollikofer CL, Jost R, Schoch E, Decurtins M. Gastrointestinal stenting. Eur Radiol. 2000;10:329–41.

93. Morgan R, Adam A. Use of metallic stents and balloons in the esophagus and gastrointestinal tract. J Vasc Interv Radiol. 2001;12:283–97.

94. Lopera JE, Brazzini A, Gonzales A, Castaneda-Zuniga WR. Gastroduodenal stent placement: current status. Radiographics. 2004;24:1561–73.

95. Sabharwal T, Irani FG, Adam A. Quality assurance guidelines for placement of gastroduodenal stents. Cardiovasc Intervent Radiol. 2007;30:1–5.

96. Small AJ, Coelho-Prabhu N, Baron TH. Endoscopic placement of self-expandable metal stents for malignant colonic obstruction: long-term outcomes and complication factors. Gastrointest Endosc. 2010;71(3):560–72.

97. Sebastian S, Johnston S, Geoghegan T. Pooled analysis of the efficacy and safety of self-expanding metal stenting in malignant colorectal obstruction. Am J Gastroenterol. 2004;99:2051–7.

98. Rey JF, Romanczyk T, Greff M. Metal stents for palliation of rectal carcinoma: a preliminary report on 12 patients. Endoscopy. 1995;27(7):501–4.

99. Spinelli P, Mancini A. Use of self-expanding metal stents for palliation of rectosigmoid cancer. Gastrointest Endosc. 2001;53(2):203–6.

100. Baron TH, Rey JF, Spinelli P. Expandable metal stent placement for malignant colorectal obstruction. Endoscopy. 2002;34(10):823–30.

101. Maetani I, Tada T, Shimura J, et al. Technical modifications and strategies for stenting gastric outlet strictures using esophageal endoprostheses. Endoscopy. 2002;34:402–6.

102. Hyodo T, Yoshida Y, Imawari M. A new endoscopic metallic stenting method for duodenal stenosis: a preliminary report. J Gastroenterol. 1999;34:577–81.

103. Shim CS, Cho YD, Moon JH, et al. Fixation of a modified covered esophageal stent: its clinical usefulness for preventing stent migration. Endoscopy. 2001;33(10):843–8.

104. Park SY, Park CH, Cho SB, et al. The usefulness of clip application in preventing migration of self-expandable metal stent in patients with malignant gastrointestinal obstruction. Korean J Gastroenterol. 2007;49(1):4–9.

105. Kato H, Fukuchi M, Miyazaki T, et al. Endoscopic clips prevent self-expandable metallic stent migration. Hepatogastroenterology. 2007;54(77):1388–90.

106. Kim ID, Kang DH, Choi CW, et al. Prevention of covered enteral stent migration in patients with malignant gastric outlet obstruction: a pilot study of anchoring with endoscopic clips. Scand J Gastroenterol. 2010;45(1):100–5.

107. Vanbiervliet G, Filippi J, Karimdjee BS, et al. The role of clips in preventing migration of fully covered metallic esophageal stents: a pilot comparative study. Surg Endosc. 2012;26(1):53–9.

108. Kim JH, Yoo BM, Lee KJ, et al. Self-expanding coil stent with a long delivery system for palliation of unresectable malignant gastric outlet obstruction: a prospective study. Endoscopy. 2001;33(10):843–8.

109. Yimcharoen P, Heneghan HM, Tariq T, et al. Endoscopic stent management of leaks and anastomotic strictures after foregut surgery. Surg Obes Relat Dis. 2011;7(5):628–36.

110. Blackmon SH, Santora R, Schwarz P, et al. Utility of removable esophageal covered self-expanding metal stents for leak and fistula management. Ann Thorac Surg. 2010;89:931–7.

111. Lee SH. The role of oesophageal stenting in the nonsurgical management of oesophageal strictures. Br J Radiol. 2001;74(886):891–900.

112. Katsanos K, Sabharwal T, Koletsis E, et al. Direct erosion and prolapse of esophageal stents into the tracheobronchial tree leading to life-threatening airway compromise. J Vasc Interv Radiol. 2009;20:1491–5.

113. Khot UP, Lang AW, Murali K, et al. Systematic review of the efficacy and safety of colorectal stents. Br J Surg. 2002;89(9):1096–102.

114. Dormann A, Meisner S, Verin N, et al. Self-expanding metal stents for gastroduodenal malignancies: systematic review of their clinical effectiveness. Endoscopy. 2004;36(6):543–50.

115. Baron TH. Expandable gastrointestinal stents. Gastroenterology. 2007;133:1407–11.

116. Watt AM, Faragher IG, Griffin TT, et al. Self-expanding metallic stents for relieving malignant colorectal obstruction: a systematic review. Ann Surg. 2007;246(1):24–30.

117. Lo SK. Metallic stenting for colorectal obstruction. Gastrointest Endosc Clin N Am. 1999;9(3):459–77.

118. Rozanes I, Poyanli A, Acuna B. Palliative treatment of inoperable malignant esophageal strictures with metal stents: one center's experience with four different stents. Eur J Radiol. 2002;43(3):196.

119. Morgan RA, Ellul JP, Denton ER, et al. Malignant esophageal fistulas and perforations: management with plastic-covered metallic endoprostheses. Radiology. 1997;204(2):527.

120. May A, Hahn EG, Ell C. Self-expanding metal stents for palliation of malignant obstruction in the upper gastrointestinal tract. Comparative assessment of three stent types implemented in 96 implantations. J Clin Gastroenterol. 1996;22(4):261.

121. Mauro MA, Koehler RE, Baron TH. Advances in gastrointestinal intervention: the treatment of gastroduodenal and colorectal obstructions with metallic stents. Radiology. 2000;215(3):659–69.

122. Ludwig D, Dehne A, Burmester E, Wiedemann GJ, Stange EF. Treatment of unresectable carcinoma of the esophagus or the gastroesophageal junction by mesh stents with or without radiochemotherapy. Int J Oncol. 1998;13:583–8.

123. Yim HB, Jacobson BC, Saltzman JR, et al. Clinical outcome of the use of enteral stents for palliation of patients with malignant upper GI obstruction. Gastrointest Endosc. 2001;53:329–32.

124. Vakil N, Morris AI, Marcon N, et al. A prospective, randomized, controlled trial of covered expandable metal stents in the palliation of malignant esophageal obstruction at the gastroesophageal junction. Am J Gastroenterol. 2001;96:1791–6.

125. Yoon JY, Jung YS, Hong SP, et al. Outcomes of secondary stent-in-stent self-expandable metal stent insertion for malignant colorectal obstruction. Gastrointest Endosc. 2011;74(3):625–33.

126. Grundy A, Glees JP. Aorto-oesophageal fistula: a complication of oesophageal stenting. Br J Radiol. 1997;70:846–9.

127. Hendra KP, Saukkonen JJ. Erosion of the right mainstem bronchus by an esophageal stent. Chest. 1996;110:857–8.

128. Schweigert M, Dubecz A, Stadlhuber RJ, et al. Risk of stent-related aortic erosion after endoscopic stent insertion for intrathoracic anastomotic leaks after esophagectomy. Ann Thorac Surg. 2011;92(2):513–8.

129. Van Hooft JE, Fockens P, Marrinelli AW, et al. Premature closure of the Dutch Stent-in I study. Lancet. 2006;368(9547):1573–4.

130. Marks RD, Richter JE. Peptic strictures of the esophagus. Am J Gastroenterol. 1993;88(8):1160.

131. Spechler SJ. AGA technical review on treatment of patients with dysphagia caused by benign disorders of the distal esophagus. Gastroenterology. 1999;117:233–54.

132. Marks RD, Richter JE, Rizzo J, et al. Omeprazole versus H2-receptor antagonists in treating patients with peptic stricture and esophagitis. Gastroenterology. 1994;106(4):907–15.

133. Barbezat GO, Schlup M, Lubcke R. Omeprazole therapy decreases the need for dilatation of peptic oesophageal strictures. Ailment Pharmacol Ther. 1999;13(8):1041–5.

134. Jha S, Levine MS, Rubesin SE, et al. Detection of strictures on upper gastrointestinal tract radiographic examinations after laparoscopic Roux-en-Y gastric bypass surgery: importance of projection. AJR Am J Roentgenol. 2006;186:1090–3.

135. Kim JH, Song HY, Kim H, et al. Corrosive esophageal strictures: long-term effectiveness of balloon dilation in 117 patients. J Vasc Interv Radiol. 2008;19:736–41.

136. Zein NN, Greseth JM, Perrault J. Endoscopic intralesional steroid injections in the management of refractory esophageal strictures. Gastrointest Endosc. 1995;41(6):596–8.

137. Russell SB, Trupin JS, Myers JC, et al. Differential glucocorticoid regulation of collagen mRNAs in human dermal fibroblasts. Keloid-derived and fetal fibroblasts are refractory to down-regulation. J Biol Chem. 1989;264(23):13730–5.

138. Kochhar R, Makharia GK. Usefulness of intralesional triamcinolone in treatment of benign esophageal strictures. Gastrointest Endosc. 2002;56(6):829.

139. Ramage Jr JI, Rumalla A, Baron TH, et al. A prospective, randomized, double-blind, placebo-controlled trial of endoscopic steroid injection therapy for recalcitrant esophageal peptic strictures. Am J Gastroenterol. 2005;100(11):2419–25.

140. Repici A, Hassan C, Sharma P, et al. Systematic review: the role of self-expanding plastic stents for benign oesophageal strictures. Ailment Pharmacol Ther. 2010;31(12):1268–75.

141. Ackroyd R, Watson DI, Devitt PG, et al. Expandable metallic stents should not be used in the treatment of benign esophageal strictures. J Gastroenterol Hepatol. 2001;16:484–7.

142. Fiorini A, Fleischer D, Valero J, et al. Self-expandable metal coil stents in the treatment of benign esophageal strictures refractory to conventional therapy: a case series. Gastrointest Endosc. 2000;52:259–62.

143. Sandha GS, Marcon NE. Expandable metal stents for benign esophageal obstruction. Gastrointest Endosc Clin N Am. 1999;9:437–46.

144. Wadhwa RP, Kozarek RA, France RE, et al. Use of self-expandable metallic stents in benign GI diseases. Gastrointest Endosc. 2003;58:207–12.

145. Burdick JS, Venu RP, Hogan WJ. Cutting the defiant lower esophageal ring. Gastrointest Endosc. 1993;39(5):616–9.

146. Krevsky B, Pusateri Jr JP. Laser lysis of an esophageal web. Gastrointest Endosc. 1989;35(5):451–3.

147. Ibrahim A, Cole RA, Qureshi WA, et al. Schatzki's ring: to cut or break an unresolved problem. Dig Dis Sci. 2004;49(3):379–83.

148. Hordijk ML, Siersema PD, Tilanus HW, Kuipers EJ. Electrocautery therapy for refractory anastomotic strictures of the esophagus. Gastrointest Endosc. 2006;63:157–63.

149. Schubert D, Kuhn R, Lippert H, Pross M. Endoscopic treatment of benign gastrointestinal anastomotic strictures using argon plasma coagulation in combination with diathermy. Surg Endosc. 2003;17:1579–82.

150. Beilstein MC, Kochman ML. Endoscopic incision of a refractory esophageal stricture: novel management with an endoscopic scissors. Gastrointest Endosc. 2005;61:623–5.

151. Jacobson BJ, Shami VM, Faigel DO, et al. Through-the-scope balloon dilation for EUS staging of stenosing esophageal cancer. Dig Dis Sci. 2007;52(3):817–22.

152. Lundell L, Leth R, Lind T, et al. Palliative endoscopic dilation of carcinoma of the esophagus and esophagogastric junction. Acta Chir Scand. 1989;155(3):179–84.

153. Acuna B, Rozanes I, Akpinar S, et al. Palliation of malignant esophageal strictures with self-expanding nitinol stents: drawbacks and complications. Radiology. 1996;199(3):648–52.

154. Saxon RR, Morrison KE, Lakin PC, et al. Malignant esophageal obstruction and esophagorespiratory fistula: palliation with a polyethylene-covered Z-stent. Radiology. 1997;202(2): 349–54.

155. Ell C, May A, Hahn EG. Gianturco-Z stents in the palliative treatment of malignant esophageal obstruction and esophagotracheal fistulas. Endoscopy. 1995;27(7):495–500.

156. Choi EK, Song HY, Kim JW, et al. Covered metallic stent placement in the management of cervical esophageal strictures. J Vasc Interv Radiol. 2007;18:888–95.

157. Sreedharan A, Harris K, Crellin A, et al. Interventions for dysphagia in oesophageal cancer. Cochrane Database Syst Rev. 2009;(4):CD005048.

158. Ikeya T, Ohwada S, Ogawa T. Endoscopic balloon dilation for benign esophageal anastomotic stricture: factors influencing its effectiveness. Hepatogastroenterology. 1999;46(26):959–66.

159. Ahamad J, Martin J, Ikramuddin S, et al. Endoscopic balloon dilation of gastroenteric anastomotic stricture after laparoscopic gastric bypass. Endoscopy. 2003;35(9):725–8.

160. Peifer KJ, Shiels AJ, Azar R, et al. Successful endoscopic management of gastrojejunal anastomotic strictures after Roux-en-Y gastric bypass. Gastrointest Endosc. 2007;66(2):248–52.

161. Ukleja A, Afonso BB, Pimentel R, et al. Outcome of endoscopic balloon dilation of strictures after laparoscopic gastric bypass. Surg Endosc. 2008;22(8):1746–50.

162. Go MR, Muscarella P, Needleman BJ, et al. Endoscopic management of stomal stenosis after Roux-en-Y gastric bypass. Surg Endosc. 2004;18(1):56–9.

163. Adler DG, Baron TH. Endoscopic palliation of malignant gastric outlet obstruction using self-expanding metal stents; experience in 36 patients. Am J Gastroenterol. 2002;97(1):72–8.

164. Binkert CA, Jost R, Steiner A, et al. Benign and malignant stenosis of the stomach and duodenum; treatment with self-expanding metallic endoprostheses. Radiology. 1996;199(2):335–8.

165. Shaw JM, Bornman PC, Krige JE, et al. Self-expanding metal stents as an alternative to surgical bypass for malignant gastric outlet obstruction. Br J Surg. 2010;97(6):872–6.

166. Jeurnink SM, van Eijck CH, Steyerberg EW, et al. Stent versus gastrojejunostomy for the palliation of gastric outlet obstruction: a systematic review. BMC Gastroenterol. 2007;7:18.

167. Cho YK, Kim SW, Hur WH, et al. Clinical outcomes of self-expandable metal stent and prognostic factors for stent patency in gastric outlet obstruction caused by gastric cancer. Dig Dis Sci. 2010;55(3):668–74.

168. Jeurnink SM, Steyerberg EW, van Hooft JE, et al. Surgical gastrojejunostomy or endoscopic stent placement for the palliation of malignant gastric outlet obstruction (SUSTENT study): a multicenter randomized trial. Gastrointest Endosc. 2010;71(3): 490–9.

169. Jeurnink SM, Steyerberg EW, Hof G, et al. Gastrojejunostomy versus stent placement in patients with malignant gastric outlet obstruction: a comparison in 95 patients. J Surg Oncol. 2007;96:389.

170. Cannizzaro R, Bortoluzzi F, Valentini M. Percutaneous endoscopic gastrostomy as a decompressive technique in bowel obstruction due to abdominal carcinomatosis. Endoscopy. 1995;27(4):317–20.

171. Shike M, Wallach C, Bloch A, Brennan MF. Combined gastric drainage and jejunal feeding through a percutaneous endoscopic stoma. Gastrointest Endosc. 1990;36:290–2.

172. Laval G, Arvieux C, Stefani L, et al. Protocol for the treatment of malignant inoperable bowel obstruction: a prospective study of 80 cases at Grenoble University Hospital Center. J Pain Symptom Manage. 2006;31:502–12.

173. Pothuri B, Montemarano M, Gerardi M, et al. Percutaneous endoscopic gastrostomy tube placement in patients with malignant bowel obstruction due to ovarian carcinoma. Gynecol Oncol. 2005;96:330–4.

174. Deans GT, Krukowski ZH, Irwin ST. Malignant obstructions of the left colon. Br J Surg. 1994;81:1270–6.

175. Fielding LP, Phillis RKS, Fry JS, et al. Prediction of outcome after emergency curative resection for large bowel cancer. Lancet. 1986;18:904–7.
176. Lee HJ, Hong SP, Cheon JH, et al. Long-term outcome of palliative therapy for malignant colorectal obstruction in patients with unresectable metastatic colorectal cancers: endoscopic stenting versus surgery. Gastrointest Endosc. 2011;73(3):535–42.
177. Suzuki N, Saunders BP, Thomas-Gibson S, et al. Colorectal stenting for malignant and benign disease: outcomes in colorectal stenting. Dis Colon Rectum. 2004;47(7):1201–7.
178. Forshaw MJ, Sankararajah D, Stewart M, Parker MC. Self-expanding metallic stents in the treatment of benign colorectal disease: indications and outcomes. Colorectal Dis. 2006;8(2):102–11.
179. Small AJ, Young-Fadok TM, Baron TH. Expandable metal stent placement for benign colorectal obstruction: outcomes for 23 cases. Surg Endosc. 2008;22(2):454–62.
180. Modarai B, Forshaw M, Parker MC, Stewart T. Self-expanding metallic stents in the treatment of benign colorectal anastomotic strictures: a word of caution. Tech Coloproctol. 2008;12(2):127–9.
181. Keränen I, Lepistö A, Udd M, et al. Outcome of patients after endoluminal stent placement for benign colorectal obstruction. Scand J Gastroenterol. 2010;45(6):725–31.
182. Saida Y, Enomoto T, Takabayashi K, et al. Outcome of 141 cases of self-expandable metallic stent placements for malignant and benign colorectal strictures in a single center. Surg Endosc. 2011;25:1748–52.

Endoscopic Techniques for Enteral Access

11

Samuel Ibrahim, Kevin El-Hayek, and Bipan Chand

Introduction

Tools and techniques for enteral access have changed dramatically in large part due to advancements in the fields of endoscopy, laparoscopy, and radiology. Percutaneous endoscopic gastrostomy (PEG) tube placement is now the standard of gastric feeding access since its development by Gauderer and Ponsky in 1980 [1]. The percutaneous endoscopic technique allows for safe and feasible access without the need for general anesthesia or laparotomy in the majority of patients. Using the principles of this initial innovation, minimally invasive methods to access the gastrointestinal tract have expanded tremendously. In this chapter, we outline the evolution of minimally invasive tools and techniques for enteral access.

This chapter contains a video segment that can be found by accessing the following link: http://www.springerimages.com/videos/978-1-4614-6329-0.

S. Ibrahim, M.D.
Department of General Surgery, Cleveland Clinic Foundation, Cleveland, OH, USA

K. El-Hayek, M.D.
Surgical Endoscopy, Department of Bariatric and Metabolic Institute, Cleveland Clinic Hospital, Cleveland, OH, USA

B. Chand, M.D., F.A.C.S. (✉)
Associate Professor of Surgery, Minimally Invasive Surgery, Loyola University, Maywood, IL, USA
e-mail: bchand@lumc.edu

Percutaneous Endoscopic Gastrostomy

Indications

For over 30 years, PEG tubes have been widely used to provide enteral feeding for patients with functionally normal gastrointestinal tract with inadequate oral intake. More recently, enteral tubes have also been placed to provide decompression in various conditions leading to gastrointestinal obstructions. These two indications make up the vast majority of all PEG placements. The conditions for which patients are commonly referred for insertion of a PEG tube are outlined in Table 11.1.

Contraindications

There are very few relative and even fewer absolute contraindications to PEG tube placement. A list of each is highlighted in Table 11.2. A caveat to these contraindications is that PEG placement should be performed only in patients with some hope of recovery. While there is no defined time limit, a patient with an expected survival on the order of days should not be offered PEG placement unless by palliative measures it will aid in discharge from a hospital setting. Over the past several decades, many former absolute contraindications have shifted to the relative category. Likewise, many relative contraindications have been overcome by medical and surgical advancements. For example, patients with coagulopathy can be rapidly corrected prior to PEG placement with only a mild increased risk. Likewise, patients with severe ascites can have a paracentesis prior to PEG placement with the addition of T-fasteners to secure the gastrostomy site to the anterior abdominal wall. Many of these advancements are described below. Specific to stomach access, while the concept of transillumination is

Table 11.1 Indications and conditions for which patients are commonly referred for insertion of a PEG tube

Long-term feeding	Gastric decompression
• Neurologic disorders	• Chronic small bowel obstruction
• Oropharyngeal and upper gastrointestinal malignancy	• Gastric outlet obstruction
	• Severe delayed gastric emptying

Table 11.2 Contraindications for PEG insertion

Absolute	Relative
• Diffuse peritonitis	• Coagulopathy
• Esophageal or pharyngeal obstruction	• Acute severe illness
	• Anorexia
	• Previous gastric surgery
	• Localized peritonitis
	• Ascites
	• Gastric outlet obstruction

preferable, failure of transillumination is not an absolute contraindication to PEG tube insertion [2]. Old age should also not be a contraindication for PEG insertion as in a recent study there was no difference in mortality in patients older or younger than 80 years, except in patients with dementia [3]. Sanders et al. conducted a retrospective cohort analysis of 361 consecutive adult patients over a 5-year period. Patients were categorized into the following four groups: group 1: oropharyngeal malignancy; group 2: acute monohemispheric stroke; group 3: dementia; and group 4: miscellaneous (head injury, motor neuron disease, multiple sclerosis, Parkinsonism, cerebral palsy, and HIV). The overall mortality for the entire cohort was 28 % at 1 month and 63 % at 1 year. These high mortality rates are most often secondary to the underlying disease and not typically related to the procedure.

Pull-Type PEG

Three principal methods of PEG insertion have been described. The first description of PEG placement was the pull technique, described by Gauderer and Ponsky in 1980 [1].

Setup and Equipment

It is preferable to perform all endoscopic enteral access procedures with two individuals in either an endoscopy suite or at the patient's bedside in an ICU. One individual performs the endoscopy while the second individual works at the abdominal side for PEG insertion. The key equipment necessary to perform a pull-type PEG include a scalpel, syringe with small-gauge needle, local anesthetic, large-gauge needle with or without catheter, looped wire, polypectomy snare, and gastrostomy tube. The endoscopist, with the assistance of the nurse, will handle the polypectomy snare and gastrostomy tube, while the bedside assistant will manage the syringe and needle, local anesthetic, scalpel, needle with catheter, and looped wire.

Technique

The patient is maintained in the supine position with both arms secured with soft restraints. Intravenous antibiotics should be given and completed within 1 h of the procedure start time. Proper monitoring should be performed including pulse oximetry, cycling blood pressures, and cardiac rhythm. Intravenous antibiotics should be administered prior to the start of the procedure [4]. If the patient is wearing a gown, this should be taped to the upper chest and exposure should be obtained from the xiphoid process to the level just below the umbilicus. The bedside assistant prepares the skin with an aseptic solution and drapes the upper abdomen while the endoscopist performs a standard diagnostic endoscopy after appropriate sedation. Following completion of the diagnostic endoscopy, the stomach should be fully insufflated and the light directed toward the anterior gastric wall. Ideal access in any percutaneous endoscopic method involves three components. These components are highlighted in Fig. 11.1 and include transillumination, finger indentation, and the "safe-tract" technique [5]. If the assistant is having a difficult time identifying the endoscope light, it is helpful to turn off the room lights and use the "X-illumination" function of the videoendoscope. Transillumination indicates that the inflated stomach is closely apposed to the anterior abdominal wall without intervening tissue or viscera (e.g., the colon). With one finger, the assistant gently depresses the abdominal wall to locate an appropriate site for access. Recommended placement is on the anterior aspect of the stomach, proximal to the incisura and midway between the greater and lesser curvature of the stomach. This site is most often chosen to decrease the potential of injuring the major gastric vasculature. At this point, the endoscopist should easily see a discrete point of luminal depression. Finally, the "safe-tract" technique is employed. Here, the assistant engages the small-gauge needle with a half filled syringe of local anesthetic at the selected site. The assistant slowly advances the needle maintaining negative pressure while monitoring the syringe for aspiration of air. Once the assistant aspirates air, he or she should clearly verbalize "Air." At this point, the endoscopist should see the needle and clearly verbalize "Needle." If the assistant aspirates air and the endoscopist cannot see the needle tip, the needle is presumed to be within another bowel lumen (likely colon) and a different position is selected. Once confirmation of safe access to the stomach is obtained, the bedside assistant infiltrates the skin level and makes an incision roughly 1.5 times the diameter of the selected PEG tube. Making a larger incision appears to decrease the incidence of infection around the tube site, as the tube will be pulled through mouth, esophagus, and

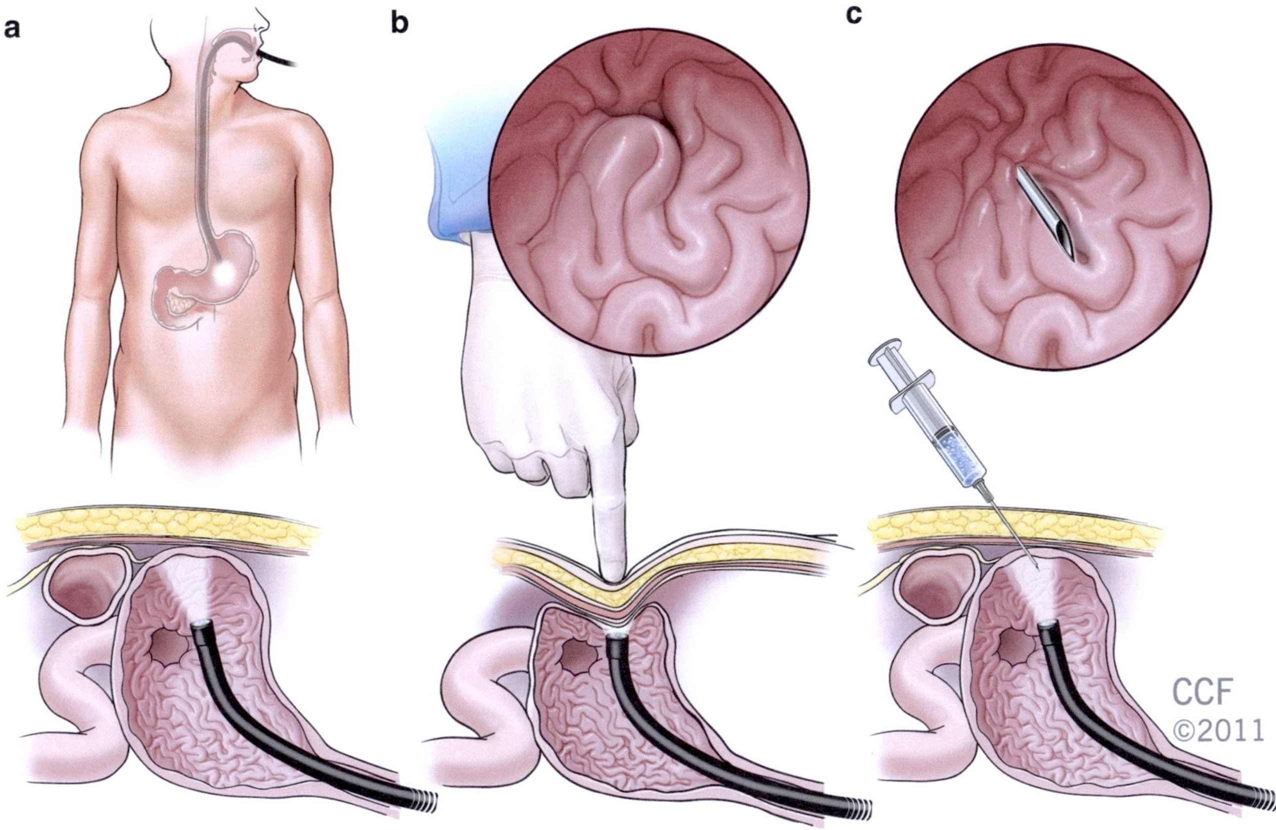

Fig. 11.1 Safe percutaneous endoscopic enteral access. (**a**) Transillumination. (**b**) Finger indentation. (**c**) "Safe-tract" technique. *With permission © Cleveland Clinic Foundation*

stomach before exiting the skin. Next, the endoscopist positions an open polypectomy snare against the anterior stomach wall at the expected entry site. The assistant advances the larger needle with or without a catheter through the skin incision and into the stomach through the open snare. If the snare does not encircle the needle at this point, the endoscopist should reposition the snare. If the needle carries a sheath, the endoscopist confirms that the sheath has entered the stomach prior to withdrawal of the needle. The assistant then inserts the looped wire through the needle or sheath and into the stomach. Next, the assistant withdraws the needle or sheath while the endoscopist lassos the looped wire. The endoscopist should tighten the snare and withdraw the endoscope, snare, and looped wire through the patient's mouth. The assistant should maintain control of the wire at the skin level so that it is not pulled completely into the stomach, thus losing access. The PEG catheter has a tapered end that terminates in a suture loop. The endoscopist passes one loop through the other in such a fashion that the PEG catheter is securely fastened to the wire. Reinsertion of the endoscope is not mandatory at this stage; however, this maneuver allows for investigation of the gastrostomy site for immediate signs of bleeding [6, 7]. In order to facilitate this step, the endoscopist uses the snare to hold the flange of

the PEG against the tip of the endoscope and allows the assistant to safely "pull" the PEG and endoscope into the gastrointestinal tract. The steps to this portion of the procedure involve pulling the wire/PEG/endoscope tip complex into the mid esophagus, at which point the assistant stops and the snare is opened to release the flange. The PEG is then further pulled into the stomach to release it from the snare. The endoscopist then removes the snare and continues to follow the PEG into the stomach. This technique allows the endoscope to gain reentry into the esophagus with minimal difficulty. After the tapered portion has exited the anterior abdominal wall, the rubber tube of the catheter will be seen. Some catheters have marks to identify the length of the tube within the subcutaneous tract. The assistant should continue to pull until resistance indicates that the bumper of the PEG tube is engaged on the stomach wall. The endoscopist, having followed the PEG into the stomach, observes the entry site and confirms hemostasis. Visual confirmation of adequate position of the bumper, which should be snug but not tight against the gastric wall, is the final maneuver prior to securing the catheter with the selected external bumper, clamp, and access port. When external markings are present, the endoscopist should document at which level the tube has been secured.

Push-Type PEG

The push-type PEG was introduced by Sacks-Vine et al. and proved to be as safe and feasible as the pull-type PEG [8].

Setup and Equipment

Again, the patient is placed in a supine position and receives pre-procedural intravenous antibiotics. The anterior abdominal wall from the rib cage up to the pelvic brim is prepped and draped in the usual fashion. The key equipment necessary to perform a push-type PEG include a scalpel, syringe with small-gauge needle, local anesthetic, large-gauge needle with or without catheter, stiff guidewire, polypectomy snare, and gastrostomy tube.

Technique

Following standard endoscopy an appropriate location on the anterior gastric wall is chosen. Following the same steps as in pull-type PEG, the stomach is accessed and the stiff guidewire pulled through the mouth. At this point, the gastrostomy tube is advanced or "pushed" over the guidewire through the mouth and into appropriate position. The gastrostomy tube tip has a firm dilating portion which serves to dilate the anterior gastric wall, subcutaneous tissue, and skin in an antegrade fashion. Reinsertion of the endoscope is preferable to confirm adequate positioning of the gastrostomy tube. Securing the tube is performed in a fashion analogous to pull-type PEG.

Introducer-Type PEG

The introducer-type PEG technique was first described by Russell et al. in 1984 [9]. This method utilizes the Seldinger technique to place a balloon gastrostomy into the stomach under endoscopic guidance. The gastrostomy balloon must remain inflated to maintain tube position. Dislodgment of the tube may result if the balloon is inadvertently deflated. The principal advantage of this method is that the tube is not pulled or pushed through the mouth and therefore decreases the risk of infection and tumor seeding in instances of head and neck malignancy. Ease of tube dislodgment is a major disadvantage, and the authors prefer the pull-type technique for this reason.

Setup and Equipment

The patient is prepared in a similar fashion to the pull-type technique. Necessary equipment for this procedure include needle, scalpel, stiff guidewire, dilator, sheath, and balloon gastrostomy tube. Prior to commencing procedure, the endoscopist should confirm that the gastrostomy tube passes easily through the sheath and that the balloon functions well.

Technique

A diagnostic endoscopy is once again performed, and the stomach insufflated for apposition to the abdominal wall. Appropriate tube placement is again chosen based on transillumination, finger indentation, and the "safe-tract" technique. Following infiltration of local anesthetic, an incision large enough for easy passage of the catheter is then made. Under endoscopic vision, the assistant advances the needle through the anterior abdominal wall and into the stomach. The stiff guidewire is passed through the needle and the needle is withdrawn. Next, using the Seldinger technique, the assistant first passes the dilator and then the sheath over the guidewire. Firm but gentle pressure and a twisting motion facilitate their passage. The endoscopic view confirms passage of needle, wire, dilator, and finally sheath into the stomach. Occasionally the dilator or the sheath will tent up the mucosa of the stomach rather than directly entering the lumen. The endoscopist can apply counterpressure with the closed tip of a biopsy forceps, or increase the insufflation of the stomach. The sheath must fully enter the stomach to successfully complete the procedure. The balloon gastrostomy tube is lubricated and advanced into the stomach through the sheath. Next, the sheath is peeled away from the tube. The balloon is inflated and the tube gently pulled back so that the stomach is barely indented by pressure of the balloon. Finally, the gastrostomy is secured in place. Too much tension on the catheter may lead to pressure necrosis of the gastric wall; too little may allow leakage around the tube.

Outcomes of Different PEG Techniques

Evolution of various PEG techniques came out of theories that the push and introducer methods might improve upon the pull method. The introducer method is believed to carry less risk of peristomal infection because it avoids passage of the tube through the oropharynx as is necessary in the pull and push methods [10]. Development of the introducer technique was also believed to improve tract maturation following PEG placement, although a recent study found no difference in stoma tract maturation between the pull-type method and a novel introducer kit with T-fasteners in a porcine model. Van Dyck et al. analyzed the outcome and short-term complications of pull and introducer methods in oncology patients with esophageal or head and neck cancer [11]. There were actually more complications using the introducer versus the pull method in this study. This group suggested using the conventional pull-type PEG in this subset of patients whenever possible.

Table 11.3 Complications of insertion of a percutaneous endoscopic gastrostomy (PEG) tube

Early	Late
• Hemorrhage	• Peristomal leakage or infection
• Tube dislodgement (immature tract)	• Tube malfunction
	• Tube dislodgement (mature tract)
• Wound infection	• Tube degradation
• Injury to intraabdominal viscera (liver, bowel, spleen)	• Peritonitis
	• Skin or gastric ulceration
• Sedation related (aspiration, cardiopulmonary compromise)	• Granulation around PEG
	• Gastric fistula after removal of PEG
	• Gastric outlet obstruction
	• Buried bumper syndrome
	• Gastrocolonic fistula

Complications

A prospective study during a 6-year period from Germany identified a 13.5 % complication rate for PEG insertion, with infection being the most common complication (11.1 %) [12]. The rate of infection was higher in cancer patients (20.5 %) than patients with nonmalignant diseases (5.5 %). The risk factors for infection were cancer, radiation exposure, and cirrhosis. Most centers recommend preoperative antibiotics for all patients within 1 h of procedure to decrease infection rates, as the procedure is considered "clean-contaminated" [4]. Peristomal bleeding (0.5 %) occurred after a mean of 8 ± 4.5 days. There was no statistically significant difference between patients with or without anticoagulants, or in those with an increased INR. Peritonitis requiring surgery was observed in 1.3 % of patients and there were no procedure-related deaths. Srinivasan et al. identified the complications in the pediatric population [13]. Erythema at the PEG site is the most common (15.4 %). Other complications include abscess formation, bumper migration to subcutaneous tissue, and inadvertent removal of the tube. A more complete list of complications following PEG insertion is given in Table 11.3.

Management of Complications

Most PEG complications can be treated non-operatively or with repeat endoscopy. Peristomal bleeding is usually at the skin level. This can be controlled by placing a U-shaped stitch around the tube or cauterization with silver nitrate. Occasionally repeat endoscopy is required to control mucosal bleeding at the intra-luminal gastrostomy site. Two methods of hemorrhage control should be employed intra-luminally (i.e., endoscopic clips, cautery, sclerotherapy, argon beam coagulation). Patients who bleed on therapeutic anticoagulation must have the risks and benefits of continued anticoagulation carefully weighed, as bleeding may continue without

coagulopathy correction. Cellulitis around the tube site is typically alleviated with a short course of intravenous or oral antibiotics. If an abdominal wall abscess forms, incision and drainage should be performed.

The most significant major complication is early tube dislodgement, which can lead to spillage of the gastric contents and enteral feeds within the abdominal cavity. The traditional and most conservative management of this complication has been emergent laparotomy. Advancements in minimally invasive surgery allow for appropriately trained surgeons to offer a laparoscopic approach when indicated. T-fasteners have recently been used as an adjunct to the standard pull technique for PEG placement in patients deemed to be at high risk for early tube dislodgement. T-fasteners serve by approximating the stomach to the anterior abdominal wall, thus minimizing the need for emergent laparotomy in cases of early tube dislodgement. Patients who experience early tube dislodgement have significantly higher morbidity and mortality than those who do not have this complication [14–17]. Figure 11.2 shows a decision tree following PEG dislodgement [17].

PEG with Jejunal Extension

Indications

Indications for PEG with jejunal extension (PEG-JET) placement include patients with aspiration risk, delayed gastric emptying, or who require jejunal feedings secondary to underlying medical conditions (e.g., pancreatitis). Patients with altered gastric anatomy may also be candidates for a PEG with jejunal limb extension when indicated.

Contraindications

Contraindications of PEG-JET are similar to those described above and highlighted in Table 11.2. Essentially, a patient must be an appropriate candidate for a PEG procedure to be a candidate for a PEG-JET, as the primary access remains within the stomach.

Setup and Equipment

As in PEG placement, the patient is placed in a supine position with arms secured. A surgical endoscopist will sometimes be called upon to place a primary PEG-JET or to replace an existing PEG with an "all-in-one" PEG-JET tube through an old gastrostomy tract.

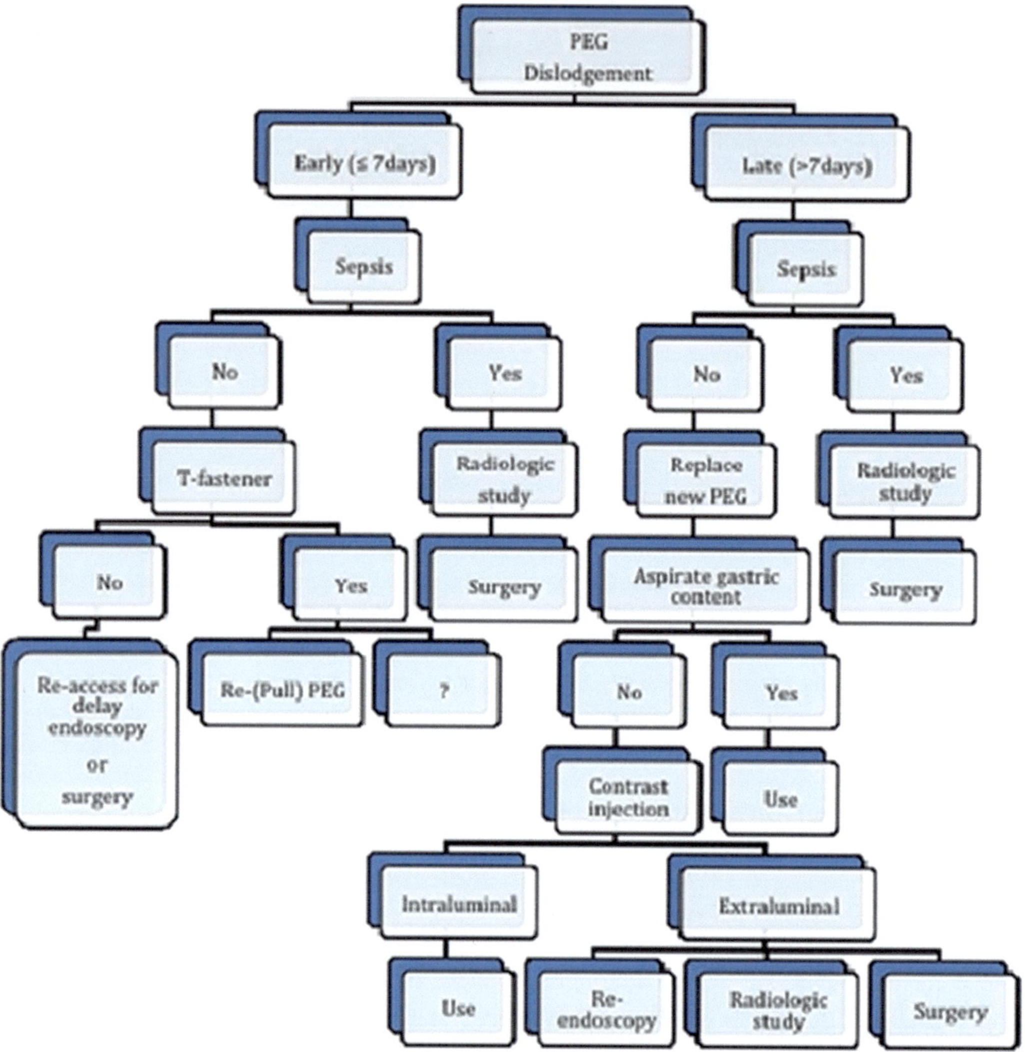

Fig. 11.2 Decision tree following PEG dislodgement

Technique

When a patient does not have a prior existing PEG placed, gastric access is first obtained via one of the above-described methods of PEG placement. Once PEG access is achieved, a jejunal extension tube is advanced through the PEG and into the jejunum. There are multiple techniques for guiding the tube within the jejunum. One technique involves first placing a guidewire into the stomach and advancing this guidewire endoscopically into the jejunum. Often, it is helpful to use a pediatric colonoscope for maximal advancement into the jejunum. Next, the jejunal extension tube can be advanced over the guidewire. Fluoroscopy is a helpful adjunct when the tube does not advance easily over the guidewire. When a patient presents with a long-standing PEG and a well-formed tract, an "all-in-one" PEG-JET tube can be used. The principal advantage with this type of tube is access to both the stomach and jejunum ports. To place this variation, a guidewire can once again be placed through the PEG and into the jejunum. The entire tube can then be exchanged over the wire as in the jejunal extension method. Alternatively, a suture loop can be placed around the tip of the jejunal portion of the tube, and this can be directly advanced endoscopically to confirm jejunal placement. The loop can then be secured to the jejunal mucosa with an endoscopic clip. There are many commercially available endoscopic clips; however, the most useful are those that can be opened and closed prior to engagement with the tissue. This feature will allow the endoscopist several attempts at grasping and pulling the tube into the jejunum. A key point is to withdraw the endoscope carefully once the tube is secured so as not to drag the tube back within the gastric lumen. Because of the frequency of such an occurrence, the authors prefer fluoroscopic advancement of the jejunal port over a guidewire. A final variation on this technique involves the advancement of a small-caliber endoscope (i.e., XP) through the existing PEG site and into the jejunum. In this case, a guidewire is placed directly through the working channel and the scope is exchanged over the guidewire. The tube can then be advanced over the guidewire.

Troubleshooting Tips

When advancing the PEG-JET tube or jejunal extension through the PEG tube, some difficulty may arise in securing the tube within the jejunum. When placing the tube under direct endoscopic vision, the tube can become adherent to the endoscope shaft and can therefore withdraw with the endoscope. One technique to avoid this pitfall is to slowly withdraw with small clockwise and counterclockwise torque maneuvers to "shake off" the jejunal tube. In the guidewire technique, sometimes advancing of the tube causes the guidewire to loop within gastric lumen. In this case, it is helpful to ensure that the guidewire is placed as far as possible within the jejunum, and that there is a slight amount of tension on the guidewire while advancing the tube. This will prevent bending of the guidewire and the ultimate loss of jejunal access. Despite adherence to these troubleshooting tips, up to a third of all cases result in retrograde dislodgement, and mean functional duration is roughly 2 months [14, 15]. This can be a frustrating occurrence for the patient who is left with a long tube in the stomach, defeating the purpose of the procedure. Reasons for this occurrence include the multiple fixed angles (at the skin entry site, stomach entry site, pylorus, and ligament of Treitz) the tube must take to traverse the stomach and duodenum, which create fulcrums on which the tube can dislodge into the stomach. If many attempts at placing this tube are unsuccessful, alternative options for jejunal access are recommended.

Direct Percutaneous Endoscopic Jejunostomy

Indications and Contraindications

Indications for a direct percutaneous endoscopic jejunostomy (DPEJ) tube are similar to those listed above. Other indications include patients with altered GI anatomy and a need for long-term enteral access. An example of this includes patients with Roux-en-Y anatomy with either mechanical or functional oral feeding limitations. A DPEJ in this case can offer a more durable feeding option while

the primary issue is being addressed. Relative and absolute contraindications for DPEJ are similar to PEG as listed in Table 11.2. There are also unique contraindications to DPEJ. The author's preference is to perform a DPEJ only when direct jejunal apposition to the abdominal wall can be obtained with endoscopic assistance. This is often the case when an ante-colic, ante-gastric Roux-limb or efferent limb has been fashioned surgically. While the authors have experience with DPEJ on patients with normal gastrointestinal anatomy, risk of inadvertent bowel injury is higher in these cases. Likewise, when a jejunal limb is fashioned in either a retro-colic or a retro-gastric position, higher risk of inadvertent bowel injury is assumed. Whenever possible, reviewing prior operative reports and imaging is recommended in such cases.

Technique

A pediatric colonoscope is preferable to a standard upper endoscopy so that maximal advancement into the jejunum can be achieved. Next, using the standard transillumination, finger indentation, and "safe-tract" techniques as described above, a position on the abdominal wall is chosen for DPEJ placement. In patients without prior intestinal surgery, the preferable position for placement of a DPEJ is just distal to the ligament of Treitz. This will ensure that placement occurs at a reasonable distance from the transverse colon and allows for future endoscopic access if needed. A standard gastrostomy tube can be placed in any of the above-mentioned methods. The bumper should be secured loosely at the skin level. If there is a concern for tube dislodgement post procedure, endoscopic T-fasteners can be used to pexy the jejunal limb to the anterior abdominal wall. Several points directly around the gastrostomy tube are chosen. Following placement, instillation of contrast and fluoroscopy can further assist in ensuring luminal placement without any tube leakage (see Video 11.1).

Laparoscopic Assisted Enteral Access

Endoscopic enteral access cannot be safely obtained for a number of reasons. Some of these reasons include the relative contraindications as listed in Table 11.2. When this is the case, laparoscopic assistance can aid in safe placement of enteral tubes. First, laparoscopic access is achieved and the abdomen insufflated. In cases of severe ascites, fluid can be aspirated from the abdomen to help promote adhesion formation and visceral apposition, as well as decrease the risk of bacterial contamination of the ascites. When a suitable position on the stomach or the jejunum is chosen, the site can then be pexied to the abdominal wall with transfascial suture fixation. Once the sutures are pulled up to the abdominal wall, a gastrostomy or jejunostomy tube can be placed using any of the above-described methods, depending on the ease of endoscopic visualization. Final position can be verified laparoscopically prior to completion of the case (see Video 11.2).

Radiologic Assisted Enteral Access

Radiologic assisted endoscopic access can be attempted either primarily or following unsuccessful endoscopic attempts. One indication of radiologic assisted gastric access is in the setting of acute bowel obstruction with severe remnant gastric distension in patients with a history of Roux-en-Y gastric bypass. Likewise, if an endoscope cannot be passed into the stomach due to an obstructive process, gastric access can often be obtained via radiologic assistance. Another indication for radiologic assisted enteral access is in the setting of patients with a history of gastrostomy or jejunostomy who no longer have access. Following removal of an enteral tube, the tract can close within several hours. However, even if the tract cannot be safely recannulated, bowel serosa often remains apposed to the abdominal wall secondary to adhesions. Therefore, access can be gained with fluoroscopy and contrast guidance for replacement of the tube. Typical modalities for radiologic assisted enteral access include fluoroscopy, ultrasound, and computed tomography (CT). The advantages of fluoroscopy and ultrasound include "real-time" identification of the enteral lumen as well as verification of needle access. Disadvantages include user variability and limited imaging with regard to surrounding structures. Principal advantages of CT include excellent special recognition and image quality. Disadvantages include use of static images to direct placement, cost, and increased radiation exposure. Regardless of the modality used, the principal techniques are often the same. The organ of interest is identified, needle and wire access is obtained, serial dilation is performed to accommodate tube placement, and finally tube is placed using Seldinger technique. Frequently, a smaller bore double-pigtail catheter (8–12 French) is used initially, though this can be dilated over several sessions.

Recent Advancements in Enteral Access Techniques

Placement of DPEJ via Proximal Enterocutaneous Fistula

In challenging situations such as proximal small bowel enterocutaneous fistulae, often the only option for nutrition is via TPN. The same principles of DPEJ can be used to achieve feeding access distal to a proximal enterocutaneous fistula. In this technique, a small endoscope is advanced through the fistula. In order to ensure distal placement, the duodenum and stomach should be identified if possible. Once the afferent limb is identified, the endoscopist can advance through the efferent limb and place a distal feeding tube.

T-Fasteners

One adjunct to PEG placement involves the use of endoscopically placed T-fasteners for stomach wall apposition. Placement of T-fasteners is highlighted in Fig. 11.3. T-fasteners can be used in a variety of clinical situations including concern for early tube dislodgement, ascites, and DPEJ. By placing T-fasteners, the bowel surrounding the tube is more securely apposed to the anterior abdominal wall. In cases when a tube is inadvertently dislodged, one is not obligated to emergently repair the enterotomy and replace the tube. Instead, access can be regained in a more controlled setting [16]. Likewise, in cases with massive ascites, T-fasteners can help to promote adhesion formation prior to re-accumulation of fluid within the abdomen.

SliC Technique

The SliC technique, as a variation to the introducer technique, was described by Sabnis et al. in 2006 [17]. Examples of patients who qualify for a SliC procedure include those who have near-obstructing head and neck malignancies whereby passing a standard endoscope is not possible or where there is concern for tumor seeding through the PEG tract. In this procedure, a small-bore endoscope (i.e., pediatric endoscope or XP endoscope) is placed within the stomach. Using T-fasteners, the stomach wall is apposed to the anterior abdominal wall. Next, using a 7–8 mm dilating laparoscopic trocar set, the stomach is entered under endoscopic visualization. Following this, an 18 French malecot tube is advanced through the trocar and the trocar is subsequently removed. The malecot catheter is then secured to the skin.

Percutaneous Transhepatic Access

Another method for access to the gastrointestinal tract is via a percutaneous transhepatic route. Indications for this type of access include altered anatomy with a difficult-to-access gastric or biliopancreatic limb. In this procedure, the right or left intrahepatic bile ducts are accessed percutaneously and a guidewire is advanced through the ampulla and into the duodenum. Once this access is achieved, a

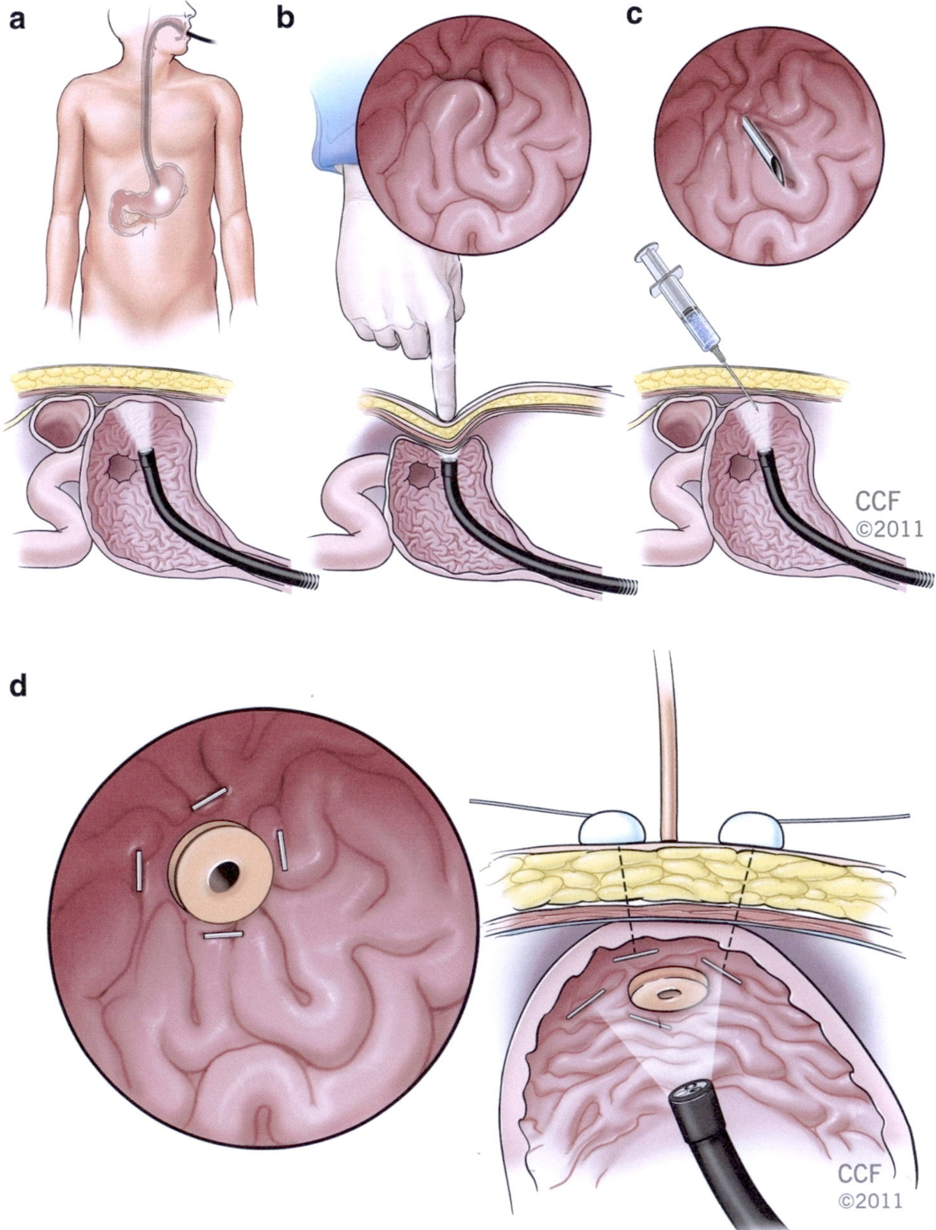

Fig. 11.3 Placement of endoscopic T-fasteners. (**a**) Enteral access with T-fastener needle. (**b**) T-fastener deployment. (**c**) Final securing of T-fastener. (**d**) Final image with enteral tube and T-fasteners. *With permission © Cleveland Clinic Foundation*

pigtail catheter can be placed directly into the duodenum. While this procedure is typically performed for biliary obstruction, if a tube with sideholes only at the tip is chosen, it can also be used for enteral feeds or biliary limb decompression.

Conclusion

Since the advent of PEG tube placement, there has been a tremendous evolution of tools and techniques for access to the gastrointestinal tract. This evolution has ultimately expanded options for clinicians and patients alike as we move from a "one-size-fits-all" mentality to one of individualized medicine. As technology and equipment continue to improve, so to will the options for enteral access.

References

1. Gauderer MW, Ponsky JL, Izant Jr RJ. Gastrostomy without laparotomy: a percutaneous endoscopic technique. J Pediatr Surg. 1980;15(6):872–5.
2. Stewart JA, Hagan P. Failure to transilluminate the stomach is not an absolute contraindication to PEG insertion. Endoscopy. 1998; 30(7):621–2.
3. Malmgren A, Hede GW, Karlstrom B, et al. Indications for percutaneous endoscopic gastrostomy and survival in old adults. Food Nutr Res. 2011;55.
4. Banerjee S, Shen B, Baron TH, et al. Antibiotic prophylaxis for GI endoscopy. Gastrointest Endosc. 2008;67(6):791–8.
5. Foutch PG, Talbert GA, Waring JP, Sanowski RA. Percutaneous endoscopic gastrostomy in patients with prior abdominal surgery: virtues of the safe tract. Am J Gastroenterol. 1988;83(2):147–50.
6. Odelowo OO, Dasaree L, Hamilton Y, et al. Is repeat endoscopy necessary after percutaneous endoscopic gastrostomy? J Assoc Acad Minor Phys. 2002;13(2):57–8.
7. Sartori S, Trevisani L, Nielsen I, Tassinari D, Abbasciano V. Percutaneous endoscopic gastrostomy placement using the pull-through or push-through techniques: is the second pass of the gastroscope necessary? Endoscopy. 1996;28(8):686–8.
8. Foutch PG, Woods CA, Talbert GA, Sanowski RA. A critical analysis of the Sacks-Vine gastrostomy tube: a review of 120 consecutive procedures. Am J Gastroenterol. 1988;83(8):812–5.
9. Russell TR, Brotman M, Norris F. Percutaneous gastrostomy. A new simplified and cost-effective technique. Am J Surg. 1984; 148(1):132–7.
10. Horiuchi A, Nakayama Y, Kajiyama M, Fujii H, Tanaka N. Nasopharyngeal decolonization of methicillin-resistant Staphylococcus aureus can reduce PEG peristomal wound infection. Am J Gastroenterol. 2006;101(2):274–7.
11. Van Dyck E, Macken EJ, Roth B, Pelckmans PA, Moreels TG. Safety of pull-type and introducer percutaneous endoscopic gastrostomy tubes in oncology patients: a retrospective analysis. BMC Gastroenterol. 2011;11:23.
12. Richter-Schrag HJ, Richter S, Ruthmann O, Olschewski M, Hopt UT, Fischer A. Risk factors and complications following percutaneous endoscopic gastrostomy: a case series of 1041 patients. Can J Gastroenterol. 2011;25(4):201–6.
13. Srinivasan R, Irvine T, Dalzell M. Indications for percutaneous endoscopic gastrostomy and procedure-related outcome. J Pediatr Gastroenterol Nutr. 2009;49(5):584–8.
14. Udorah MO, Fleischman MW, Bala V, Cai Q. Endoscopic clips prevent displacement of intestinal feeding tubes: a long-term follow-up study. Dig Dis Sci. 2010;55(2):371–4.
15. Zopf Y, Rabe C, Bruckmoser T, Maiss J, Hahn EG, Schwab D. Percutaneous endoscopic jejunostomy and jejunal extension tube through percutaneous endoscopic gastrostomy: a retrospective analysis of success, complications and outcome. Digestion. 2009; 79(2):92–7.
16. Timratana P, El-Hayek K, Shimizu H, Kroh M, Chand B. Percutaneous endoscopic gastrostomy (PEG) with T-fasteners obviates the need for emergent replacement following early tube dislodgement. Surg Endosc. In press.
17. Sabnis A, Liu R, Chand B, Ponsky J. SLiC technique. A novel approach to percutaneous gastrostomy. Surg Endosc. 2006;20(2): 256–62.

Ahmed Sharata and Lee L. Swanstrom

Background

Since the first attempts at intestinal anastomoses, leaks and fistulas have been a constant problem. In particular, the rising prevalence of morbid obesity and corresponding increase in the volume of bariatric surgery have led to a mounting experience with associated gastrointestinal (GI) anastomotic complications. Anastomotic or staple-line leaks after GI surgery are relatively uncommon complications, but quite morbid and potentially lethal.

Although it is a relatively uncommon surgery, esophagectomy has a substantial risk of anastomotic leak or fistulization due to its lack of serosa and relative ischemia of its reconstruction options. There is between a 3 and 21 % rate of esophageal anastomotic leaks and they can become fistulas to mediastinal structures including vascular (usually fatal) or pulmonary (highly morbid). There is also a small but real incidence of spontaneous (Boerhaave's) and iatrogenic upper GI tract perforations [1, 2].

Leaks following colonic resection occur between 1 and 11 % of the time, depending on its location, status of neoadjuvant cancer treatments, and other patient-specific risk factors. Iatrogenic perforation from endoscopy is a rare

complication. Risks of colonoscopic perforation (0.12 %) and mortality (0.01 %) are found in the literature. Common sites of perforation include the sigmoid colon (53 %), followed by the cecum (24 %). The mechanisms of perforation include blunt or torque injury (55 %), followed by polypectomy (27 %) and thermal injuries (18 %).

After Roux-En-Y gastric bypass (RYGB), leaks occur in 2–5 % of cases while after laparoscopic sleeve gastrectomy (LSG), leaks from the staple-line occur in 2.7 % of cases [3, 4]. The risk of some complications can be minimized by concentrating surgeries at Centers of Excellence having high-volume, fellowship-trained surgeons but even with this, leaks are an inescapable fact of GI surgery. Postoperative leaks traditionally carry an overall morbidity of 53 % and mortality of 0.5–10 % [5, 6]. This is somewhat deceptive however, since as many as 50 % of patients may be asymptomatic with leaks detected only on radiographic studies [5]. When either acute or chronic events occur, surgeons, radiologists, and gastroenterologists have a variety of management options, including endoscopic therapies.

The majority of existing data on GI leaks and their management centers on the most common procedures, traditional or laparoscopic esophageal and colorectal surgery or bariatric procedures. Endoscopic treatment strategies may attempt to bypass a leak (stenting) or to occlude the orifice (clips, plugs, glues, or suture). In addition there are some novel new therapies being described such as catheter-based negative pressure therapy. These complications require a thoughtful, often multispecialty, and frequently long-term approach to management.

This chapter contains a video segment that can be found by accessing the following link: http://www.springerimages.com/videos/978-1-4614-6329-0.

A. Sharata, M.D.
Department of General and Minimally Invasive Surgery,
Oregon Clinic, Portland, OR, USA

L.L. Swanstrom, M.D. (⊠)
Division of Gastrointestinal and Minimally Invasive Surgery,
The Oregon Clinic, Oregon Health and Sciences University,
Portland, OR, USA
e-mail: lswanstrom@orclinic.com

Etiology and Classification

Both the etiology and a management pathway may be suggested by the time at which a leak appears. The literature suggests a classification of leaks by their time to diagnosis: (1) early leaks: evident <3 days after surgery; (2) intermediate

J.M. Marks and B.J. Dunkin (eds.), *Principles of Flexible Endoscopy for Surgeons*,
DOI 10.1007/978-1-4614-6330-6_12, © Springer Science+Business Media New York 2013

leaks: occurring or detected between 4 and 7 days after surgery; and (3) late leaks/fistulas: apparent 8 or more days after surgery. In early leaks, the local inflammatory and the systemic responses to peritoneal contamination can be dramatic but are also sometimes limited. At a later stage, inflammatory responses are likely at their height; with friable tissue and substantial contamination, traditional surgical remedies frequently fail [7]. For late leaks, local inflammation may have subsided but chronic healing as a fistulous tract may hamper spontaneous closure. Fistulas resulting from such leaks are often associated with strictures as well making treatment a complex process requiring synchronous application of multiple techniques. Fistulas may present in a dramatic fashion—such as high-output enteric fistulas or enteropulmonary fistulas leading to cough and pneumonias. They can also be very subtle in presentation, involving elusive fevers, recurrent abscesses, or as a loss of the benefits of the weight loss surgery from gastro-gastric fistula (GGF) after RYGB often presenting. They can also form to other hollow viscous with variable effects or to the skin along a drain tract.

While both technical and host factors contribute, early postoperative leaks are most commonly attributed to a technical flaw. A leak presenting four or more days after surgery may be due to ischemia at the staple line or anastomosis, poor nutrition, or other host factors. Colorectal leaks can occur at the site of any anastomosis but are more often seen with low pelvic anastomosis, secondary to tension and/or ischemia. Enteric leaks can also be associated with trauma to the bowel wall through rough manipulations or stray energy burns. Esophageal anastomoses leak often enough that it is the major justification for performing the anastomoses in the neck—where leaks are less morbid. With gastrectomy or gastric bypass, most leaks occur at the gastrojejunostomy [5, 6, 8]. After a sleeve gastrectomy, most leaks occur at the former angle of His, where the staple line meets the esophagogastric junction (EGJ) [9, 10]. After ligation of the short gastric arteries, this area may be particularly susceptible to ischemia-related perforation. Also a functional pylorus creating pressure in the narrow, tubular stomach has been implicated in the etiology of these leaks [7]. Despite sound surgical principles, ischemia or technical failure may occur unpredictably. The time at which a leak occurs and the associated etiology offer valuable treatment information.

Diagnosis

An early postoperative leak after GI surgery can be challenging to diagnose. The abdominal exam is often not reflective of the severity of internal soiling. The most sensitive indicator of leak in most cases is isolated tachycardia. While normally laparoscopic patients feel well and ambulate on the night of and day after surgery, patients who complain of

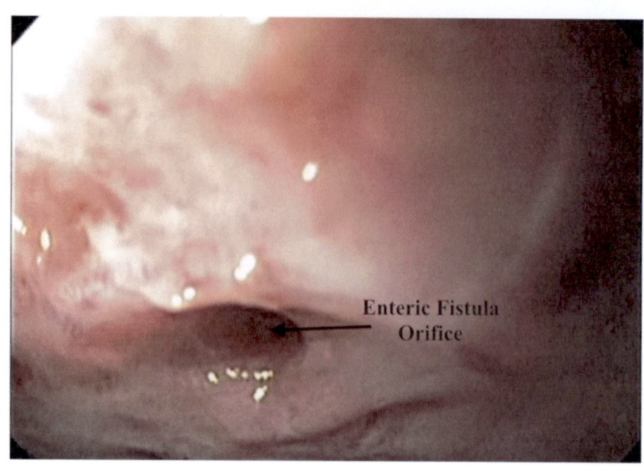

Fig. 12.1 Endoscopic view of enteric fistula

severe pain, are not ambulating, or otherwise deviate from the standard postoperative course should prompt suspicion of a leak. Computed tomography performed with oral, water-soluble contrast provides the most information and has a near-100 % sensitivity [11]. Contrast esophagograms or upper GI series to evaluate the foregut have often been employed but are not very sensitive [12]. For the lower GI tract, contrast enemas are more accurate. If not diagnosed early, these patients will rapidly develop florid sepsis with rapid respiratory failure.

Acute, self-limited leaks or small, intermediate leaks may present late as chronic fistulas. These can present insidiously, months to years after surgery, with nonspecific abdominal complaints such as pain or malaise. Additionally, fistulas between the gastric pouch and gastric remnant can occur after bypass surgery and may present with weight regain. With appropriate clinical suspicion, upper endoscopy or contrast upper or lower GI radiographs will usually make the diagnosis. Endoscopic examination will often demonstrate a granulated fistula tract, often too small to permit passage of the endoscope (Fig. 12.1). Contrast radiographs should be reviewed directly by the clinician; radiologists seeing contrast pass from one part of the GI tract to another through the fistula may misinterpret the study as normal. Cross-sectional imaging may exclude other diagnoses or reveal occult abscesses but is unlikely to show a fistula directly. Without specific symptoms or gross findings on clinical exam, these diagnoses rely on the astute clinician.

Management

Traditional care for anastomotic complications after gastrointestinal surgery has been to obtain source control surgically, treat the systemic sepsis medically, and allow the leak to heal naturally. Iatrogenic or spontaneous perforations have traditionally been considered an acute surgical emergency.

Table 12.1 Results of operative and nonoperative therapy

Author (Ref)	Year	# of patients	Success rate (%)	Days to healing
Sypropoulos et al. [8]	2011	30	63	33.2
De Aretxabala et al. [10]	2011	5	80	30
Csendes et al. [13]	2010	16	100	45
Casella et al. [9]	2009	5	40	38
Ballesta et al. [5]	2008	36	97	–
Thodiyil et al. [14]	2008	33	100	17
Gonzalez et al. [6]	2007	36	88	–

Patients with severe sepsis, or who are hemodynamically unstable, should be aggressively resuscitated prior to interventions for source control. Nonoperative and endoscopic therapies should be attempted only in a hemodynamically stable patient. If source control is established or the patient is minimally symptomatic, radiological or endoscopic drainage of any peritoneal fluid collections is reasonable and increasingly used as a primary therapy. Broad-spectrum antimicrobials and close monitoring are essential adjuncts.

Early/Intermediate

Early diagnosis of acute leaks yields the best prognosis for the patient. The greatest number of therapeutic possibilities exists in this setting. Though there is little comparative data, a variety of effective solutions are available and endoscopic treatments are becoming increasingly used. In the appropriate setting, a regimen of drainage, antimicrobials, nil per os, and nutritional support (parenteral or jejunal) results in closure within 5 weeks in 90 % of patients (Table 12.1) [5, 6, 8–10, 13, 14]. Surgical exploration and repair with drainage show similar efficacy in early but not intermediate leaks. Primary surgical repair performed after 2–3 days or in the face of significant peritoneal contamination is unlikely to succeed, but may be treatable endoluminally [7]. In both early and intermediate leaks, endoscopic therapies offer important alternatives to classical therapy.

Therapies using endoscopic clips, glue, plugs, or suturing are increasingly used for acute perforations. Most iatrogenic or acute perforations can be controlled using endoscopic clips or suturing devices and optimally should be addressed at the time of the injurious endoscopy. Postoperative anastomotic leaks occurring within 3 days of surgery can sometimes be successfully treated with drainage, antimicrobials, and nutritional support alone. Operative intervention and suture repair have merit for early but not intermediate leaks. Primary stenting offers early oral intake but may not speed healing and is associated with migration or other stent complications. Failure of initial operative or nonoperative management can result in a complex leak or even GI fistulas requiring a multipronged approach.

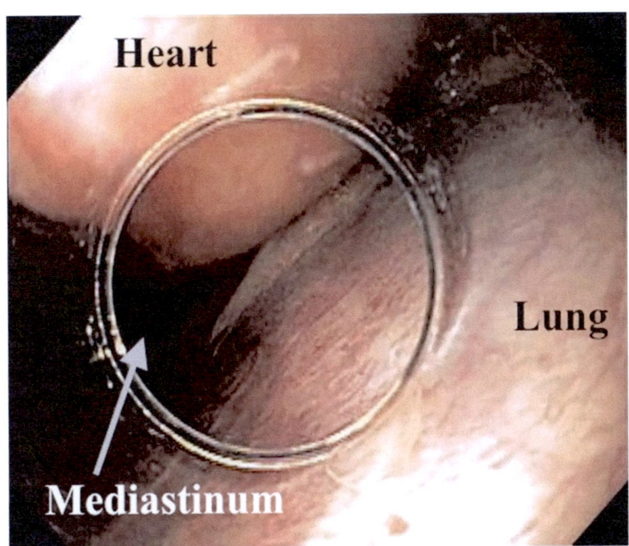

Fig. 12.2 Endoscope passed through the enterotomy and into the mediastinum to perform lavage and debridement

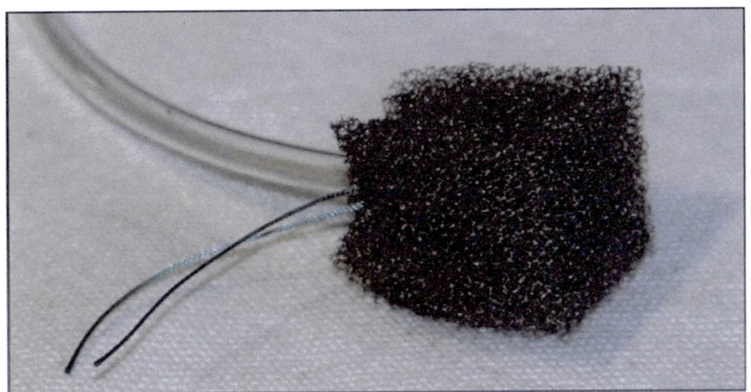

Fig. 12.3 Endoscopic vacuum-assisted closure sponge fixed to a nasoduodenal tube. Negative pressure wound therapy has recently been described as a method to speed healing of late enteric perforations with associated abscess cavities

For intermediate or older leaks transluminal endoscopy has been employed for abdominal drainage. Entering the soiled peritoneal, mediastinal, or retroperitoneal cavity through the leak, endoscopic debridement, necrosectomy, and irrigation have all been described (Fig. 12.2). Transnasal drainage catheters can traverse the leak and be left in the peritoneum to drain the abscess [15]. After allowing for systemic and local contamination to decrease, the trans-nasal peritoneal drain may be removed and the leak will seal if continuing contamination is avoided. Recently reports that draw on the cutaneous wound healing success using negative pressure sponge treatments have applied this technology to anastomotic leaks with extraluminal abscess cavities (Fig. 12.3). These anecdotal reports have shown great promise. Though endoscopic abdominal drainage can address localized peri-enteric collections, significant widespread peritoneal contamination likely still requires operative lavage and drainage.

Table 12.2 Results of endoscopic stenting: early and late leaks

Study/year	# of patients	Indication	Time to start (weeks)	Success (%)	Migration (%)	Complications[a]	Time to healing
Iqbal/2011 [16]	17	All	<1	41	37	4 migrations, erosions, or perforations	49 days
De Aretxabala/2011 [10]	4	Failed, non-op	<1	75	50		6 weeks
Jurowich/2011 [41]	3	1 primary, 2 failed non-op	<1	100	0		
Tan/2010 [18]	8	Failed non-op	<1	50	50	1 GI bleed	6 weeks
Blackmon/2010 [17]	5	Failed non-op	<1	100	40	1 bleeding, 1 erosion	30 days
Eubanks/2008 [20]	11	Failed non-op	<1	91	58	3 migrations	35 days
Edwards/2008 [42]	5	Failed non-op	<1	100	50		44 days
Fukumoto/2007 [43]	4	Failed non-op	<1	75	50		6 weeks
Bege/2011 [15]	22	Failed non-op	>4	41	59		86 days
Spyropoulos/2011 [8]	8	Failed non-op	>1	100	0	1 GI bleed	43.2 days
Blackmon/2010 [17]	5	Failed non-op	>1	100	40	1 bleeding, 1 erosion	30 days
Casella/2009 [9]	3	Failed non-op	>1	100	33		55 days
Toussaint/2009 [27]	3	"Large" leak	>2	33	0		
Eubanks/2008 [20]	2	Failed non-op	>1	50	58		35 days
Serra/2007 [21]	5	Failed non-op	>1	80	20		12 weeks
Salinas/2006 [19]	17	Failed non-op	>1	94	6	2 mucosal tears	12 weeks

[a]Requiring surgery

Endoscopic stenting using covered stents diverts enteric contents past the leak while maintaining GI continuity. In studies employing routine stenting for early leaks, healing was complete for >75 % of patients at the predetermined time of initial stent removal: usually 3–6 weeks. Despite comparable success, it must be remembered that they are not without drawbacks. Stent morbidity includes a >40 % likelihood of stent migration, frequently requiring repeat endoscopy or potentially surgical removal in ~25 % of cases (Table 12.2). Less commonly, stents have resulted in clinically significant bleeding and gastrointestinal erosion requiring surgery [16–18]. Stenting does allow for oral intake if successful but there is no evidence to suggest faster or more complete healing.

Late

When presenting or diagnosed late, leaks can be associated with significant and persistent soiling. Similarly, leaks that have failed previous management may have fibrotic inflammation or friable granulation tissue complicating treatment. In series with late leaks, nonoperative strategies had between 40 and 80 % rates of success (Table 12.1) [8, 10, 17]. Failure requiring alternative treatments was higher in these patients compared to those with earlier therapy within the same series. However, in most of these series, failures of nonoperative and operative therapies have responded to stenting.

Fully covered esophageal stents can improve healing by minimizing soiling and inflammation of the wound. Stents are traditionally employed as second-line therapy after failure of operative intervention or nonoperative management after 4 weeks (Table 12.2). Casella reported three stents placed for failed nonoperative management of leaks after sleeve gastrectomy. All fistulas sealed within 62 days of stent placement [9]. In 2006 Salinas reported similar success with stenting after 1–3 weeks [19]. These stents were left in situ for 2–4 months, demonstrating complete healing on contrast esophagogram when removed. As part of a larger series, Blackmon presented 10 leaks and Spyropoulos presented 12 leaks after bariatric surgery, which were all successfully treated with endoscopic stenting [8, 17]. Some series of stenting have less success. Eubanks and Serra have 50–80 % success with closure of delayed fistulas with stents alone [20, 21]. Despite the failure of initial therapy, stents alone were successful in a median of 97 % of patient in these studies. When late failure becomes more complicated, other therapies are available.

Glue, fistula plugs, and endoscopic suturing are only a few of the other modalities attempted for closure of fistulas (Videos 12.1–12.3). Though most series are small, early results are promising. Injection of fibrin glue, biologic and degradable, into the leak orifice was uniformly successful in 4 series of 11 patients in total [9, 22–25]. Half of the patients required a median of three endoscopic injections, administered every other day. Concerns that fibrin would be rapidly degraded have been only theoretical. No adverse events have been described.

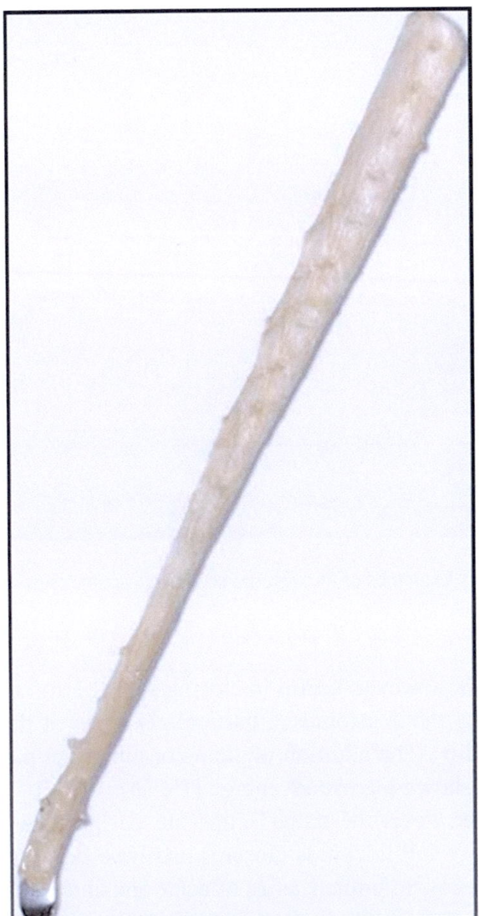

Fig. 12.4 An example of a biologic matrix fistula plug

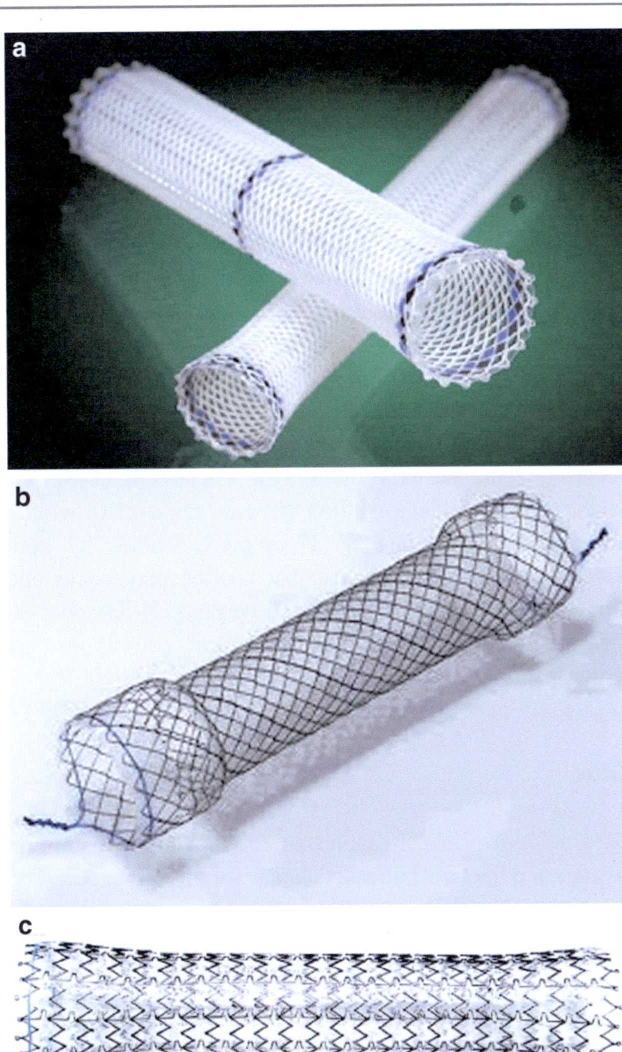

Fig. 12.5 Covered enteric stents (**a**) plastic, (**b**) partially covered, (**c**) fully covered

In theory, fibrin glue not only seals the leak but also provides a matrix and co-stimulatory molecules to enhance wound healing. Similarly, biologic scaffolding fistula plugs can provide a matrix for tissue ingrowth for healing a chronic fistula (Fig. 12.4). Even with large fistulas (~1.5 cm or wider), plug insertion appears successful in over 80 % of events [26–28]. Endoscopic suturing of leaks creates plications of adjacent mucosa, which are then closed over the defect [29]. Abrading or denuding the defect of granulation or epithelium promotes healing at the site and may facilitate adhesion of flanking plications [30, 31]. Increasingly complex fistulas may require several technologies simultaneously.

A few series have examined outcomes of multimodality therapy for complex fistulas after GI procedures. Employing a combination of transluminal debridement, endoclips, injectable glue, and stenting, Bege et al. achieved 100 % success with endoscopic management of a series of bariatric surgery patients [15]. In this series of 22 patients, 25 of 27 patients had fistulas larger than 10 mm and 59 % had multiple or complex fistulas, including 3 esophago-bronchial and 1 gastric-colonic. Notably, patients required a median of 4.4 endoscopies (range 2–16) before resolution at a mean of 86 days.

Though many treatment modalities exist for late presenting GI leaks, the variable presentation and response to standard treatment present a challenge. Surgical rectification should be avoided unless absolutely necessary.

Technologies

Stents

Stents are an endoscopic means to divert the stream of GI contents past a leak. As such, stents must be covered, fully or partially (Fig. 12.5). While partially covered stents migrate less, fully covered stents prevent tissue ingrowth and are easier to remove with less trauma to the underlying mucosa [32]. Migration is the most common complication with esophageal and gastric stent placement. In a series of 70 migrated stents, only 3 stents required operative removal for complications [33]. Among covered stents, there appears no difference in migration rates between self-expanding plastic and metal stents [20]. Anchoring the proximal edge of the stent to prevent distal migration has been attempted with clips and endoscopic suturing. The results are promising but variable [15, 34]. Anatomic constrictions such as the pylorus and gastro-esophageal junction can help to hold stents in place. The combination of overlapping stents, and bridging across natural junctions, may provide the best means of securing stents placed in the foregut. There is no consensus on the timing of stent migration and early removal, providing adequate time for healing, is optimal. Studies by both Eisendrath and Song suggest that healing may occur and stents may be removed in under 6 weeks [35]. Esophageal stenting provides a valuable adjunct for perforations and leaks despite fairly high rates of migration.

Glue

Bioglues are primarily indicated for treatment of chronic fistulae and the only published data is for this indication. The endoscopic injection of glue into the site of anastomotic leakage has been anecdotally reported and it can occlude the orifice and prevent continued soiling at least in some cases. Some studies have used fibrin glue injection as primary therapy but it frequently required multiple applications [9, 22–25]. More commonly, this modality is an adjunct to endoscopic stenting or other closure techniques [8, 15, 30]. Both fibrin and cyanoacrylate-based products have been tried and while both may be used without risk of damage to the endoscope, there are no comparative studies to suggest superiority of a particular product. In theory, cyanoacrylate products will withstand the digestive environment; however, fibrin glues permit tissue growth through a potentially stimulatory matrix. While glue injection may be adequate as sole therapy for small leaks or fistulas, the best role for this modality may be in conjunction with stenting.

Clips

Endoscopic clips come in a variety of sizes and configurations but classically are a through-the-scope bi-legged unit specially designed to approximate mucosa (Fig. 12.6). There is little data to recommend the use of standard endoscopic clips in the closure of anastomotic leaks after GI or bariatric surgery due to the typically fibrotic and thickened nature of most anastomotic leaks.

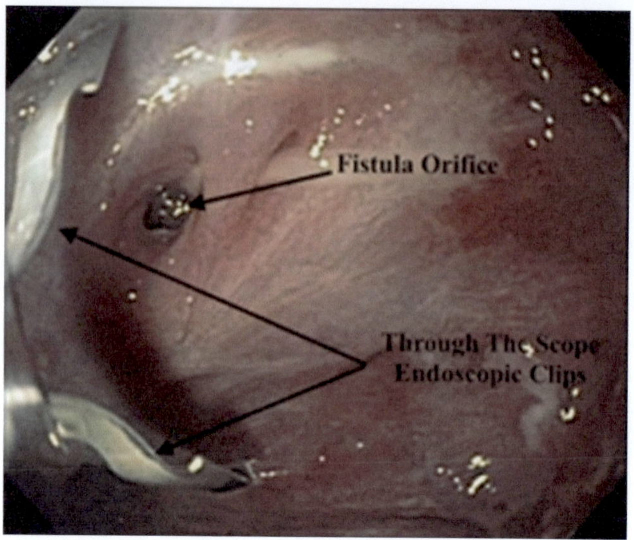

Fig. 12.6 Examples of through-the-scope endoscopic clips

Clips are, however, useful in closing acute perforations not involving the anastomosis, particularly some of the newer larger clips. The addition of stents or glue to clip closures has not shown a great advantage [15, 36].

Larger, "over-the-scope" clips are designed to achieve aggressive full-thickness closures and have been used with good success in limited series of acute and chronic closures; however the data is limited to a small number of patients (Fig. 12.7) [37, 38]. Denuding of epithelialized tissue at the site of a leak or a fistula may enhance the success of closure with a clip. This may be done either mechanically, using a cytology brush, or with energy sources such as argon plasma coagulation [39, 40]. The NOTES experience has indicated that clips are a safe and effective closure technology for many acute and elective enterotomies. The new generation of over-the-scope clips may even be able to repair anastomotic leaks.

Suturing

Endoscopic suturing for early leaks has only been described anecdotally to date. In the United States, currently endoscopic tissue apposition devices include the OverStitch (Apollo, Austin, Texas), the G-Prox (USGI Medical, San CApistrano, CA), and the TAS (Ethicon, Blue Ash, OH) (Fig. 12.8). In a canine model, endoscopic tissue apposition after mucosal ablation was more successful than suturing alone [31]. Case reports of endoscopic suturing have involved late fistulas with good success by incorporating healthy, less inflamed tissue adjacent to the site of leak [29, 30]. As endoscopic suturing technology improves, this procedure may find greater application.

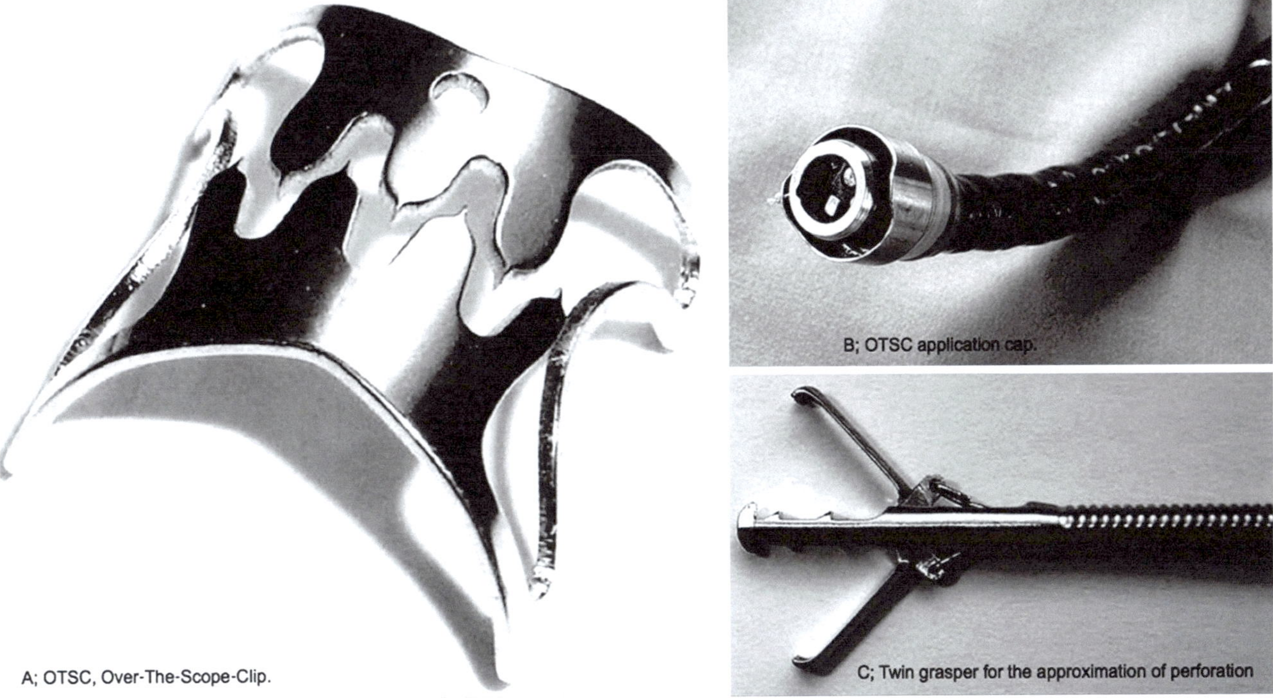

Fig. 12.7 An over-the-scope full-thickness endoscopic closure clip

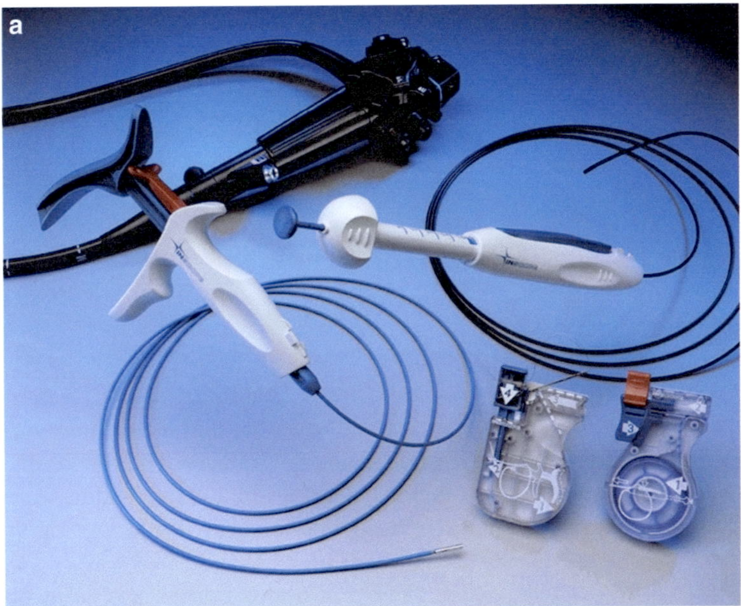

Fig. 12.8 A variety of endoscopic suturing devices are currently on the market: (**a**) TAS (Ethicon), (**b**) G-Prox (USGI), (**c**) OverStitch (Apollo Medical)

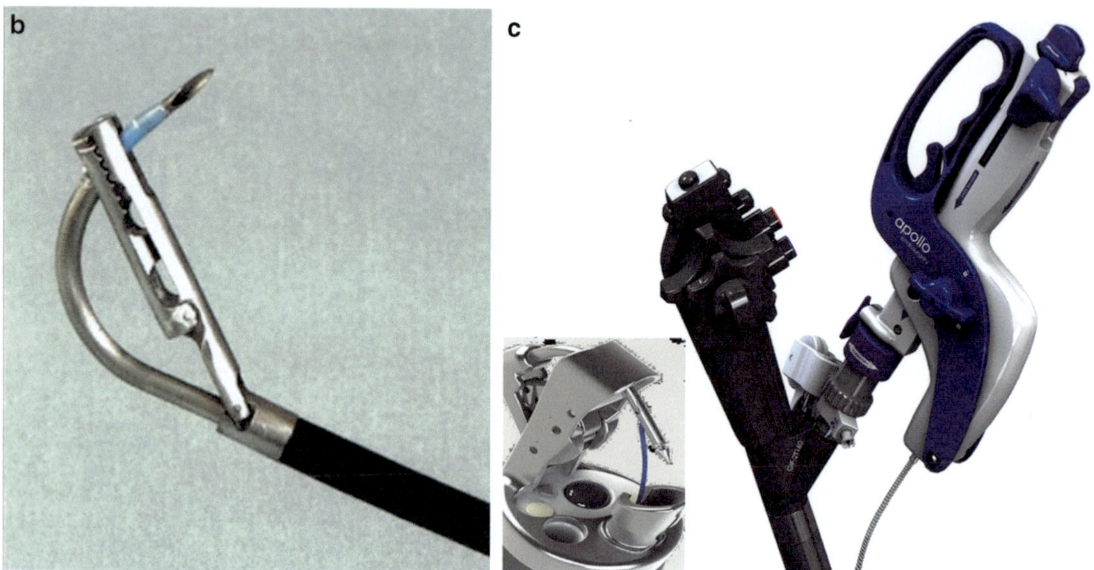

Fig. 12.8 (continued)

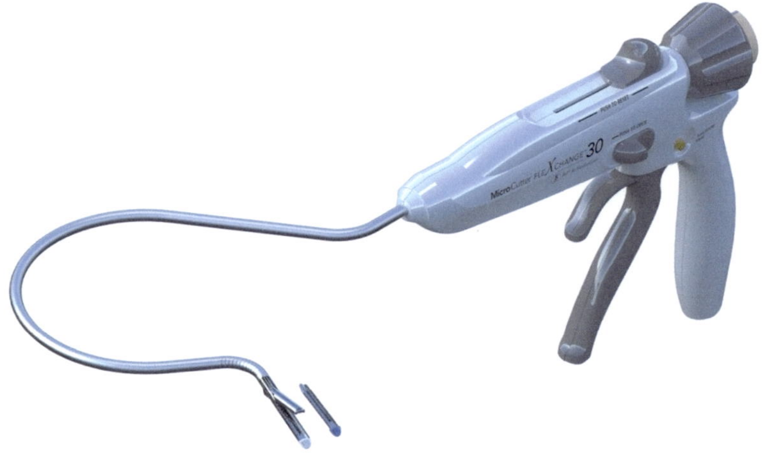

Fig. 12.9 While as of yet only existing in prototype form, in the future endoscopic stapling devices will truly broaden the applications and success of endoscopic damage control options. *With permission from Cardica*

Staplers

Linear staplers have become the gold standard for enteric closures for laparoscopic and open GI surgeries. New developments have made the possibility of a flexible endoscopic stapler a true possibility—although none are available on the market today (Fig. 12.9).

Conclusions

Though uncommon, staple-line or anastomotic leaks after GI surgery are highly morbid events and challenging to treat. Traditional operative drainage, systemic antibiotics, nil per os, and nutritional supplementation remain the standard of care. The role of endoscopic therapy in drainage, enteric bypass, and treatment of the actual leak is in evolution but is increasingly the first-line treatment (Fig. 12.10).

Covered enteric stents, endoscopic clips, biologic glues, and, increasingly, endoscopic suturing technologies have become the tools of choice for the endoscopic surgeon. These tools are steadily converting enteric leaks and fistulas from open surgical emergencies to low-morbidity endoscopic procedures. The winners in this scenario are our patients and the surgeons with the skills and foresight to master these new technologies.

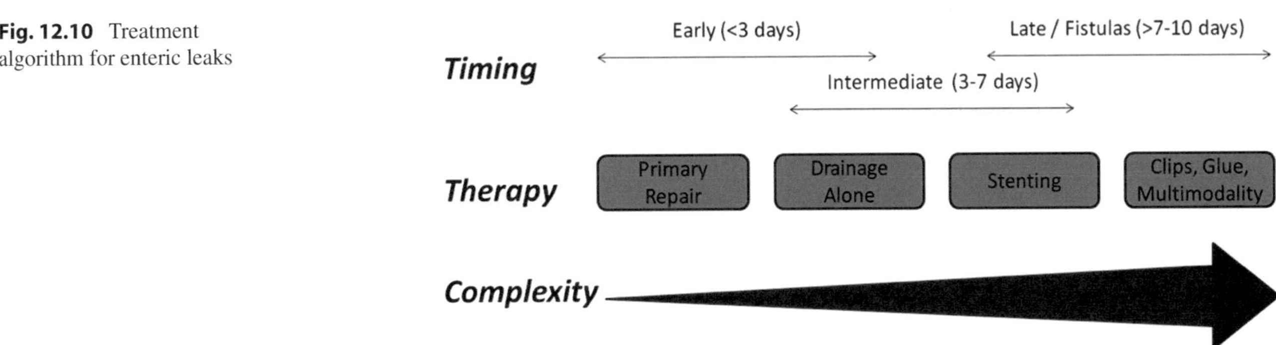

Fig. 12.10 Treatment algorithm for enteric leaks

References

1. Ohri SK, Liakakos TA, Pathi V, Townsend ER, Fountain SW. Primary repair of iatrogenic thoracic esophageal perforation and Boerhaave's syndrome. Ann Thorac Surg. 1993;55:603–6.
2. Pasricha PJ, Fleischer DE, Kalloo AN. Endoscopic perforation of the upper digestive tract: a review of their pathogenesis, prevention and management. Gastroenterology. 1994;106:787–802.
3. Anon. ASMBS guideline on the prevention and detection of gastrointestinal leak after gastric bypass including the role of imaging and surgical exploration. Surg Obes Relat Dis. 2009;5(3): 293–6.
4. Anon. Updated position statement on sleeve gastrectomy as a bariatric procedure. Surg Obes Relat Dis. 2010;6(1):1–5.
5. Ballesta C, Berindoague R, Cabrera M, Palau M, Gonzales M. Management of anastomotic leaks after laparoscopic Roux-en-Y gastric bypass. Obes Surg. 2008;18(6):623–30.
6. Gonzalez R, Sarr MG, Smith CD, et al. Diagnosis and contemporary management of anastomotic leaks after gastric bypass for obesity. J Am Coll Surg. 2007;204(1):47–55.
7. Deitel M, Gagner M, Erickson AL, Crosby RD. Third International Summit: current status of sleeve gastrectomy. Surg Obes Relat Dis. 2011;7(6):749–59.
8. Spyropoulos C, Argentou M-I, Petsas T, et al. Management of gastrointestinal leaks after surgery for clinically severe obesity. Surg Obes Relat Dis Off J Am Soc Bariatric Surg. 2011. http://www.ncbi.nlm.nih.gov/pubmed/21616725. Accessed 23 Oct 2011.
9. Casella G, Soricelli E, Rizzello M, et al. Nonsurgical treatment of staple line leaks after laparoscopic sleeve gastrectomy. Obes Surg. 2009;19(7):821–6.
10. de Aretxabala X, Leon J, Wiedmaier G, et al. Gastric leak after sleeve gastrectomy: analysis of its management. Obes Surg. 2011;21(8):1232–7.
11. Lyass S, Khalili TM, Cunneen S, et al. Radiological studies after laparoscopic Roux-en-Y gastric bypass: routine or selective? Am Surg. 2004;70(10):918–21.
12. Doraiswamy A, Rasmussen JJ, Pierce J, Fuller W, Ali MR. The utility of routine postoperative upper GI series following laparoscopic gastric bypass. Surg Endosc. 2007;21(12):2159–62.
13. Csendes A, Braghetto I, León P, Burgos AM. Management of leaks after laparoscopic sleeve gastrectomy in patients with obesity. J Gastrointest Surg. 2010;14(9):1343–8.
14. Thodiyil PA, Yenumula P, Rogula T, et al. Selective nonoperative management of leaks after gastric bypass: lessons learned from 2675 consecutive patients. Ann Surg. 2008;248(5):782–92.
15. Bège T, Emungania O, Vitton V, et al. An endoscopic strategy for management of anastomotic complications from bariatric surgery: a prospective study. Gastrointest Endosc. 2011;73(2):238–44.
16. Iqbal A, Miedema B, Ramaswamy A, et al. Long-term outcome after endoscopic stent therapy for complications after bariatric surgery. Surg Endosc. 2011;25(2):515–20.
17. Blackmon SH, Santora R, Schwarz P, Barroso A, Dunkin BJ. Utility of removable esophageal covered self-expanding metal stents for leak and fistula management. Ann Thorac Surg. 2010;89(3):931–6. Discussion 936–7.
18. Tan JT, Kariyawasam S, Wijeratne T, Chandraratna HS. Diagnosis and management of gastric leaks after laparoscopic sleeve gastrectomy for morbid obesity. Obes Surg. 2010;20(4):403–9.
19. Salinas A, Baptista A, Santiago E, Antor M, Salinas H. Self-expandable metal stents to treat gastric leaks. Surg Obes Relat Dis. 2006;2(5):570–2.
20. Eubanks S, Edwards CA, Fearing NM, et al. Use of endoscopic stents to treat anastomotic complications after bariatric surgery. J Am Coll Surg. 2008;206(5):935–8. Discussion 938–9.
21. Serra C, Baltasar A, Andreo L, et al. Treatment of gastric leaks with coated self-expanding stents after sleeve gastrectomy. Obes Surg. 2007;17(7):866–72.
22. Kowalski C, Kastuar S, Mehta V, Brolin RE. Endoscopic injection of fibrin sealant in repair of gastrojejunostomy leak after laparoscopic Roux-en-Y gastric bypass. Surg Obes Relat Dis. 2007;3(4): 438–42.
23. Papavramidis ST, Eleftheriadis EE, Apostolidis DN, Kotzampassi KE. Endoscopic fibrin sealing of high-output non-healing gastrocutaneous fistulas after vertical gastroplasty in morbidly obese patients. Obes Surg. 2001;11(6):766–9.
24. Papavramidis ST, Eleftheriadis EE, Papavramidis TS, Kotzampassi KE, Gamvros OG. Endoscopic management of gastrocutaneous fistula after bariatric surgery by using a fibrin sealant. Gastrointest Endosc. 2004;59(2):296–300.
25. Papavramidis TS, Kotzampassi K, Kotidis E, Eleftheriadis EE, Papavramidis ST. Endoscopic fibrin sealing of gastrocutaneous fistulas after sleeve gastrectomy and biliopancreatic diversion with duodenal switch. J Gastroenterol Hepatol. 2008;23(12):1802–5.
26. Maluf-Filho F, Hondo F, Halwan B, et al. Endoscopic treatment of Roux-en-Y gastric bypass-related gastrocutaneous fistulas using a novel biomaterial. Surg Endosc. 2009;23(7):1541–5.
27. Toussaint E, Eisendrath P, Kwan V, et al. Endoscopic treatment of postoperative enterocutaneous fistulas after bariatric surgery with the use of a fistula plug: report of five cases. Endoscopy. 2009; 41(6):560–3.
28. Kim Z, Kim YJ, Kim YJ, Goo DE, Cho JY. Successful management of staple line leak after laparoscopic sleeve gastrectomy with vascular plug and covered stent. Surg Laparosc Endosc Percutan Tech. 2011;21(4):e206–8.
29. Overcash WT. Natural orifice surgery (NOS) using StomaphyX for repair of gastric leaks after bariatric revisions. Obes Surg. 2008;18(7):882–5.

30. Schweitzer M, Steele K, Mitchell M, Okolo P. Transoral endoscopic closure of gastric fistula. Surg Obes Relat Dis. 2009;5(2):283–4.

31. Felsher J, Farres H, Chand B, Farver C, Ponsky J. Mucosal apposition in endoscopic suturing. Gastrointest Endosc. 2003;58(6):867–70.

32. van Boeckel PGA, Sijbring A, Vleggaar FP, Siersema PD. Systematic review: temporary stent placement for benign rupture or anastomotic leak of the oesophagus. Aliment Pharmacol Ther. 2011;33(12):1292–301.

33. Ko H-K, Song H-Y, Shin JH, et al. Fate of migrated esophageal and gastroduodenal stents: experience in 70 patients. J Vasc Interv Radiol. 2007;18(6):725–32.

34. Vanbiervliet G, Filippi J, Karimdjee BS, et al. The role of clips in preventing migration of fully covered metallic esophageal stents: a pilot comparative study. Surg Endosc. 2011. http://www.ncbi.nlm.nih.gov/pubmed/21792721. Accessed 12 Dec 2011.

35. Eisendrath P, Cremer M, Himpens J, et al. Endotherapy including temporary stenting of fistulas of the upper gastrointestinal tract after laparoscopic bariatric surgery. Endoscopy. 2007;39(7):625–30.

36. Merrifield BF, Lautz D, Thompson CC. Endoscopic repair of gastric leaks after Roux-en-Y gastric bypass: a less invasive approach. Gastrointest Endosc. 2006;63(4):710–4.

37. Seebach L, Bauerfeind P, Gubler C. "Sparing the surgeon": clinical experience with over-the-scope clips for gastrointestinal perforation. Endoscopy. 2010;42(12):1108–11.

38. Conio M, Blanchi S, Repici A, Bastardini R, Marinari GM. Use of an over-the-scope clip for endoscopic sealing of a gastric fistula after sleeve gastrectomy. Endoscopy. 2010;42 Suppl 2:E71–2.

39. Bhardwaj A, Cooney RN, Wehrman A, Rogers AM, Mathew A. Endoscopic repair of small symptomatic gastrogastric fistulas after gastric bypass surgery: a single center experience. Obes Surg. 2010;20(8):1090–5.

40. Spaun GO, Martinec DV, Kennedy TJ, Swanström LL. Endoscopic closure of gastrogastric fistulas by using a tissue apposition system (with videos). Gastrointest Endosc. 2010;71(3):606–11.

41. Jurowich C, Thalheimer A, Seyfried F, Fein M, Bender G, Germer CT, et al. Gastric leakage after sleeve gastrectomy-clinical presentation and therapeutic options. Langenbecks Arch Surg. 2011;396(7):981–7. Epub 2011 May 10.

42. Edwards CA, Bui TP, Astudillo JA, de la Torre RA, Miedema BW, Ramaswamy A, et al. Management of anastomotic leaks after Roux-en-Y bypass using self-expanding polyester stents. Surg Obes Relat Dis. 2008;4(5):594–9. Discussion 599-600. Epub 22 Aug 2008.

43. Fukumoto R, Orlina J, McGinty J, Teixeira J. Use of Polyflex stents in treatment of acute esophageal and gastric leaks after bariatric surgery. Surg Obes Relat Dis. 2007;3(1):68–71. Discussion 71–2. Epub 27 Dec 2006.

Endoscopic Considerations in Morbid Obesity

Vimal K. Narula, Dean J. Mikami, and Jeffrey W. Hazey

Introduction

Obesity is a serious public health crisis associated with increased morbidity and mortality and decreased quality of life. According to the World Health Organization (WHO), in 2005 there were approximately 1.6 billion overweight adults and at least 400 million obese adults worldwide [1]. The prevalence of obesity has increased so rapidly over the last few decades that it is now considered a global epidemic.

In the USA, the National Health and Nutrition Examination Surveys (NHANES), conducted by the Center for Disease Control (CDC), study the prevalence of obesity by using directly measured heights and weights. Studies have shown that currently there are 72 million obese adults (i.e., BMI ≥ 30 kg/m^2). Interestingly, while the prevalence has more than doubled over the last four decades (from 13.4 % in 1960–1962 to 35.1 % in 2005–2006 for adults aged 20–74 years) [2], it seems to have reached a plateau over the last 3 years [3–5]. However, when Ogden et al. compared the distribution of BMI between 1976–1980 and 2005–2006 they observed that, among adults, the distribution of BMI has shifted to the right, reflecting the change in prevalence of superobesity (i.e., BMI ≥ 50 kg/m^2), which increased from 0.9 % in 1960–1962 to 6.2 % in 2005–2006 among adults [4].

Surgical treatments have become the most successful therapy for morbid obesity in the USA. The number of operations performed has increased significantly in the last decade, and weight loss with gastric bypass approaches 60–80 % of excess body weight in large series. While morbidity from surgical treatments has improved over the same time period, the most common operation performed, laparoscopic Roux-en-Y gastric bypass, still carries anastomotic leak rates of 0.5–3 %. Surgical mortality rates are low (<1 %), but the incidence of significant morbidity still approaches 20–30 % [5, 6].

Bariatric surgical procedures are divided into restrictive (i.e., adjustable gastric banding, vertical banded gastroplasty, sleeve gastrectomy), malabsorptive (biliopancreatic diversion with/out duodenal switch), or a combination of both (Roux-en-Y gastric bypass). Of the various procedures, Roux-en-Y gastric bypass and adjustable gastric banding are the most commonly performed procedures. While bariatric surgery has been shown to be extremely effective for long-term weight loss, the mortality rate, albeit low, is not zero [i.e., 0.28 % (95 % confidence interval (CI), 0.22–0.34) and 0.35 % (95 % CI, 0.12–0.58)] at ≤ 30 days and >30 days, respectively [7]. Additionally, there are procedure-specific risks [8, 9], and shared complications including, incisional hernias, wound infections, fistula, or leaks [10].

Interventional gastrointestinal endoscopy has also seen significant improvements over the last decade, and overall interest in endoluminal therapies for morbid obesity has increased accordingly. Endoscopic treatments for GI bleeding, biliary pathology, and premalignant tumors of the GI tract have decreased the morbidity of intervention compared to surgical treatments. In the obese population, endoscopic procedures that produce weight loss equivalent to surgical treatments may help further reduce the risk of morbidity and mortality.

This chapter contains a video segment that can be found by accessing the following link: http://www.springerimages.com/videos/978-1-4614-6329-0.

V.K. Narula, M.D., F.A.C.S. • J.W. Hazey, M.D., F.A.C.S. (⊠)
Division of General and Gastrointestinal Surgery, Department of Surgery, The Ohio State University, Columbus, OH, USA
e-mail: Jeffrey.Hazey@osumc.edu

D.J. Mikami, M.D., F.A.C.S.
Department of Gastrointestinal Surgery, Wexner Medical Center at the Ohio State University, Columbus, OH, USA

J.M. Marks and B.J. Dunkin (eds.), *Principles of Flexible Endoscopy for Surgeons*,
DOI 10.1007/978-1-4614-6330-6_13, © Springer Science+Business Media New York 2013

More recently, there has been emerging interest in transoral techniques for preoperative, stand-alone, or revisional bariatric procedures [11]. Considering that transoral surgery is performed exclusively through the gastrointestinal tract via a flexible endoscope, the value of this approach lies in the possibility of an ambulatory weight loss procedure that may be safer and more cost effective compared with laparoscopic approaches. By extension, this may allow bariatric procedures to be performed on individuals who are currently precluded due to multiple comorbidities, older age, super-obesity (BMI $\geq$ 50 kg/m^2), mild obesity (BMI 25–30 kg/m^2), atypical anatomy (i.e., adhesions secondary to any abdominal surgery, a history of gastric resection, or bowel resection) or disease states that affect the bowel (i.e., Crohn's disease).

Primary Endoluminal Bariatric Procedures

Primary procedures are divided into malabsorptive or restrictive. Malabsorptive procedures, designed to bypass the absorptive surface of the intestine (i.e., biliopancreatic diversion with/out a duodenal switch), is achieved with use of a duodenal–jejunal bypass sleeve/stent (DJBS) or the ValenTx sleeve secured at the GE junction. Restrictive devices include intragastric balloons, endoluminal suturing, endoluminal stapling, and the transoral restrictive implant system. These are designed to mimic restrictive laparoscopic procedures (i.e., adjustable gastric banding, vertical banded gastroplasty, sleeve gastrectomy).

Endoluminal Malabsorptive Procedures

Intraluminal Stents

Duodenal–Jejunal Bypass Sleeve

The duodenal–jejunal bypass sleeve (DJBS; The EndoBarrier, GI Dynamics Inc., Lexington, MA, USA) is an endoluminal malabsorptive procedure that effectively bypasses the proximal small intestine using a 60 cm long fluoropolymer sleeve anchored in the duodenum (Fig. 13.1). Under general anesthesia, the device is delivered using both fluoroscopy and endoscopy. The implant is delivered using an over-the-wire catheter system and is contained within a capsule at the distal end of the catheter Fig. 13.2. Once the capsule is placed in the duodenum, an inner catheter is pushed and the bowel negotiated with the aid of an atraumatic ball attached to the distal end of the catheter. The sleeve is attached to the catheter, which pulls the sleeve out of the capsule. Once the sleeve is fully deployed, the anchor is deployed from the capsule to sit within the duodenal bulb. The anchor is self-expanding, and the barbs engage the duodenal tissue to

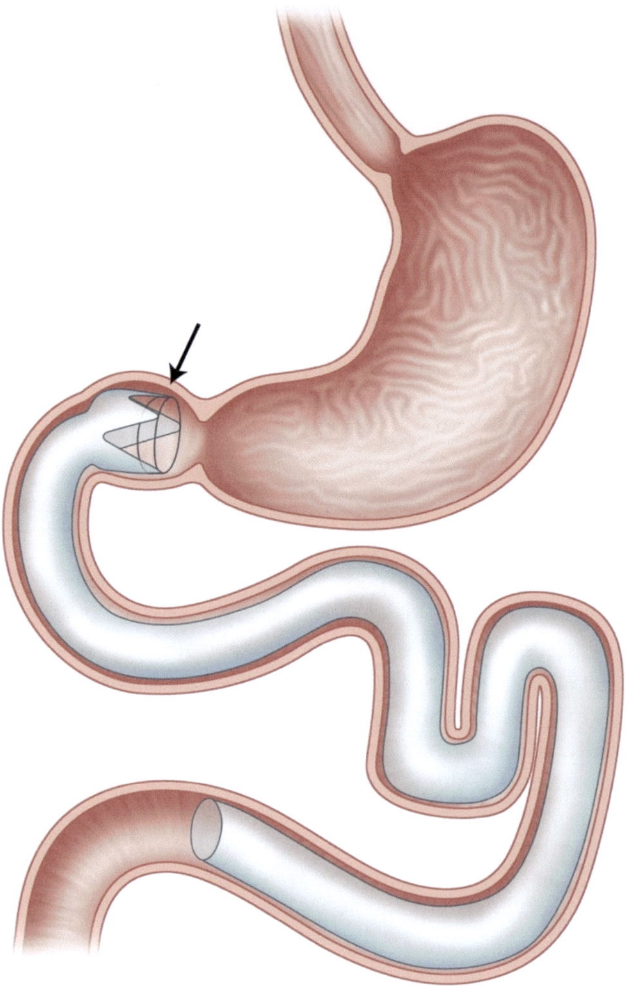

Fig. 13.1 Schematic of the Endobarrier sleeve anchored in the duodenum just beyond the pylorus

prevent movement Fig. 13.3. Contrast is flushed to ensure patency of the sleeve, and the sleeve and ball are detached from the catheter, which is removed from the bowel, leaving the implant in place [12].

Rodriguez-Grunert et al. [12] reported on the first human experience, delivering and retrieving the DJBS in 12 patients. Primary outcome measures examined the incidence and severity of adverse events, with secondary measures focused on %EWL and changes in comorbid status. The mean implant and explant times were 26.6 and 43.3 min, respectively. The device remained in place for 12 weeks in 10 of 12 patients, with early retrieval (i.e., 9 days) in 2 patients due to intractable abdominal pain. Most adverse events related to implantation occurred within the first 2 weeks and included abdominal pain, nausea and vomiting. During explantation, there was one partial pharyngeal tear, and one esophageal tear. All patients had implant site inflammation. In terms of weight loss, at 12 weeks the average %EWL in 10 of 12 patients was 23.6 %, with all patients achieving at least a

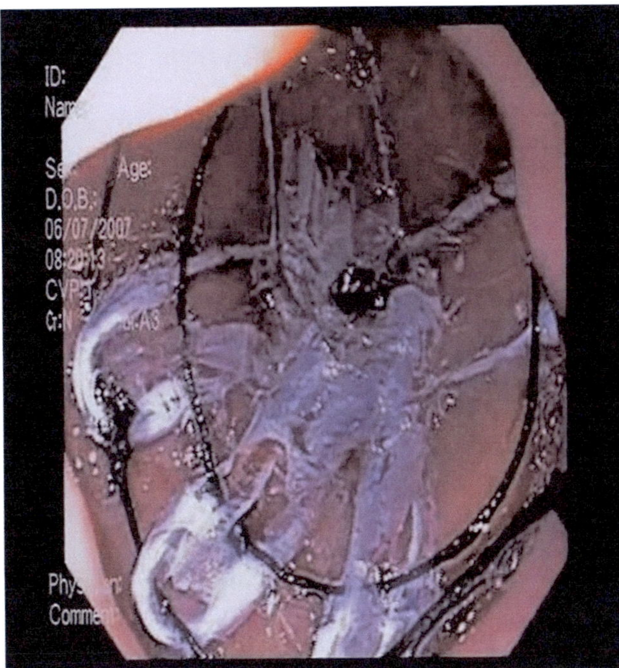

Fig. 13.2 An endoscopic view of the Endobarrier sleeve inlet within the wall of the duodenum

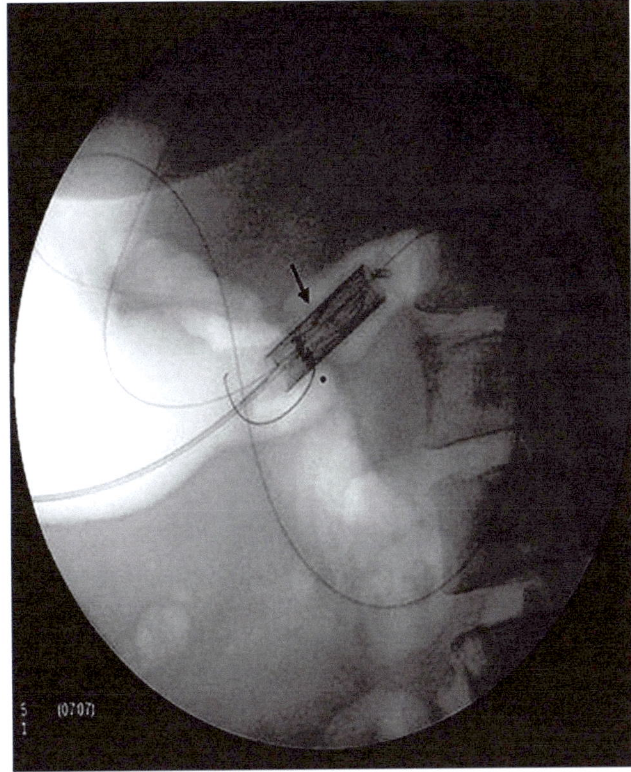

Fig. 13.3 Fluoroscopic view of the Endobarrier sleeve during deployment

10 % EWL. Finally, of the four diabetic patients, all had normal fasting plasma glucose levels for the entire 12 weeks without the need for oral hypoglycemics, and three of four patients had decreased HA1c of $\geq$0.5 % by week 12.

Tarnof et al. [13] conducted an open-label, multicenter, prospective randomized control trial comparing the effect of the DJBS with a low fat diet, to a low fat diet alone for 12 weeks. The device was implanted in 25 patients, and 14 patients comprised the control arm. Both groups received counseling at baseline, consisting of a low calorie diet, with advice on exercise/behavior modification. The study demonstrated that 20 of 25 device subjects maintained the sleeve for 12 weeks. Five of twenty-five device subjects had to have the device explanted early due to upper GI (UGI) bleeding ($n=3$), anchor migration ($n=1$) and sleeve obstruction ($n=1$). At 12 weeks the average %EWL was 22.1 % and 5.3 % for the device and control group respectively. In terms of improvement (reduction of diabetic medications) or resolution of (cessation of diabetic medications) diabetes, four patients had type 2 diabetes; one in the control group and three in the device group. Within 1 week, all four patients had improved HbA1c levels, and one diabetic in the device arm had complete resolution of diabetes at 12 weeks.

Adverse events from DJBS include nausea, pain, pseudopolyp, and inflammation at implant site, device dislocation or rotation, GI bleed, and constipation [12–15]. In larger series, most patients experienced at least one of these complications, though the majority of them were minor. No complications of distal migration or obstruction have been reported.

ValenTx Endoluminal Sleeve

The ValenTx (ValenTx, Inc. Carpinteria CA, USA) endoluminal bypass therapy accomplishes the restrictive and malabsorptive components of the Roux-en-Y gastric bypass procedure, by placement of an implantable device that does not require surgery, gastric stapling, or permanent changes to the patient's anatomy. An implantable sleeve is placed at the GE junction endoscopically (Fig. 13.4). This sleeve extends into the proximal jejunum hence, bypassing the stomach (Fig. 13.5).

In a collaborative study led by physicians from the University of California San Diego Medical Center and the Imperial College of London, and conducted at the Hospital San Jose de Monterrey in Monterrey, Mexico, 12 patients underwent the implantation of the ValenTx bypass sleeve during a 12-week trial. Patients completing the study achieved an average excess weight loss of 39.5 % [16]. The ValenTx endoluminal sleeve is not approved in the USA by the Food and Drug Administration (FDA) and is still undergoing further clinical trials.

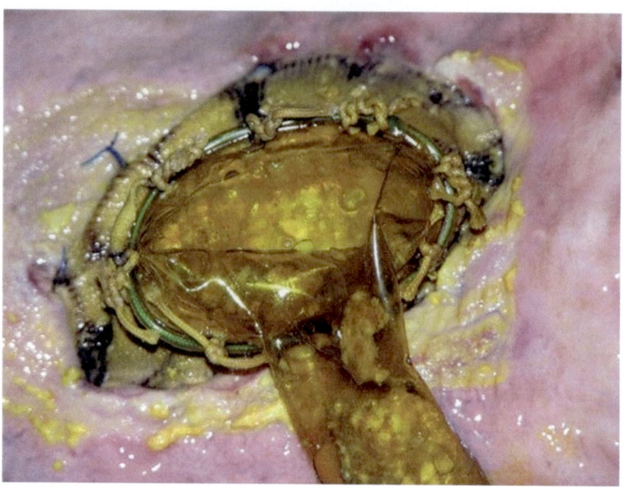

Fig. 13.4 Schematic of the ValenTx sleeve anchored at the GE junction

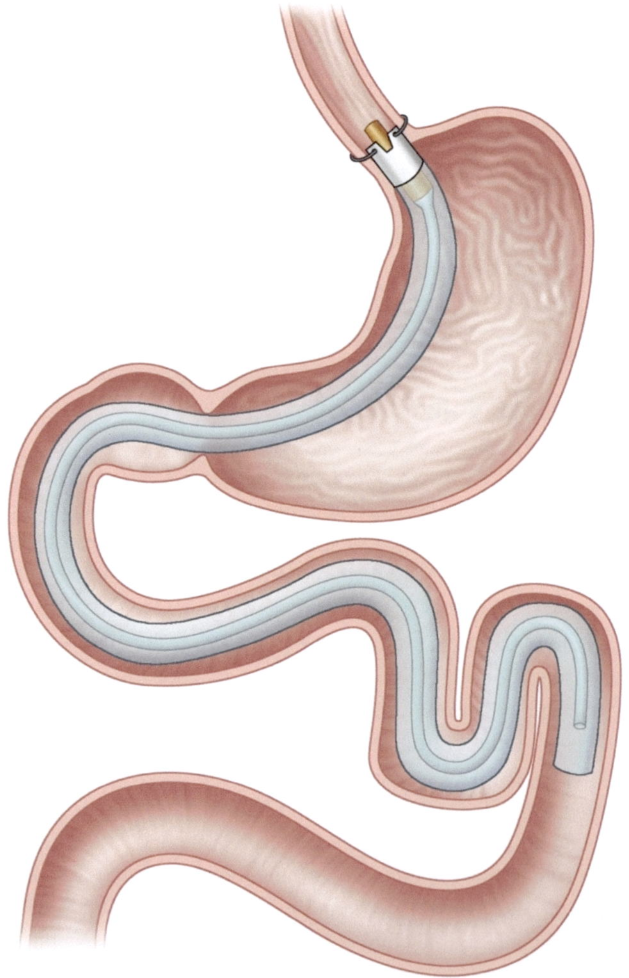

Fig. 13.5 Explant view from the gastric side of the ValenTx sleeve anchored at the GE junction

Endoluminal Restrictive Procedures

Transoral Endoscopic Restrictive Implant System

The transoral endoscopic restrictive implant system [BaroSense Trans-oral Endoscopic Restrictive Implant System (TERIS); BaroSense, Redwood City, CA] endoscopically implants a prosthetic device at the level of the cardia, creating a small gastric reservoir. The procedure requires formation of five gastric plications with insertion of five silicone anchors, followed by attachment of the gastric restrictor (Fig. 13.6) [17].

Specifically, the plications are created at the level of the cardia, 3 cm distal to the GE junction. The first plication is created just above the lesser curve of the stomach using an articulating endoscopic circular stapler, which, through suction, can acquire a full-thickness gastric plication, compress the tissues and create two concentric rings of 3.5-mm staples reinforced by a plastic ring. The stapler also excises the tissues within the ring to create a plication hole. Then utilizing a double lumen cannulation guide, the endoscope along with the silicone anchors and an articulated guide with an anchor grasper are inserted. The proximal end of the silicone anchor is pulled, under direct visualization, through the plication hole and then released. Once all five anchors are placed, they are each attached to locking anchor graspers using a multiple-lumen guide and a 5-mm endoscope. The five proximal handles of the anchor graspers are passed through the five apertures in the gastric restrictor and are used to guide the gastric restrictor down to the level of the anchors. Under direct visualization, the proximal ends of the silicone anchors are brought inside the gastric restrictor, to lock it in place.

The initial feasibility and safety of this technique in 20 human subjects is being examined by Biertho et al. in a randomized, uncontrolled, open label, single group Phase I human trial. A published report on their first case demonstrated that there were no intraoperative or postoperative complications and the patient was discharged home on postoperative day 2 tolerating a soft diet. At 3 and 6 months, the percent excess weight loss was 21 % and 26 % respectively [17].

Considering the novelty of the TERIS system, further investigation into the safety and efficacy of the device in the short and long-term, and comparison to a control group in a randomized fashion is warranted.

Endo Cinch Suturing System

The Endo Cinch Suturing System (Bard, Murray Hill, NJ) has been used in animate models and human trials [18, 19]. The device is mounted on an operating upper endoscope and

Fig. 13.6 Schematic of the BaroSense restrictive mechanism placed in the proximal stomach

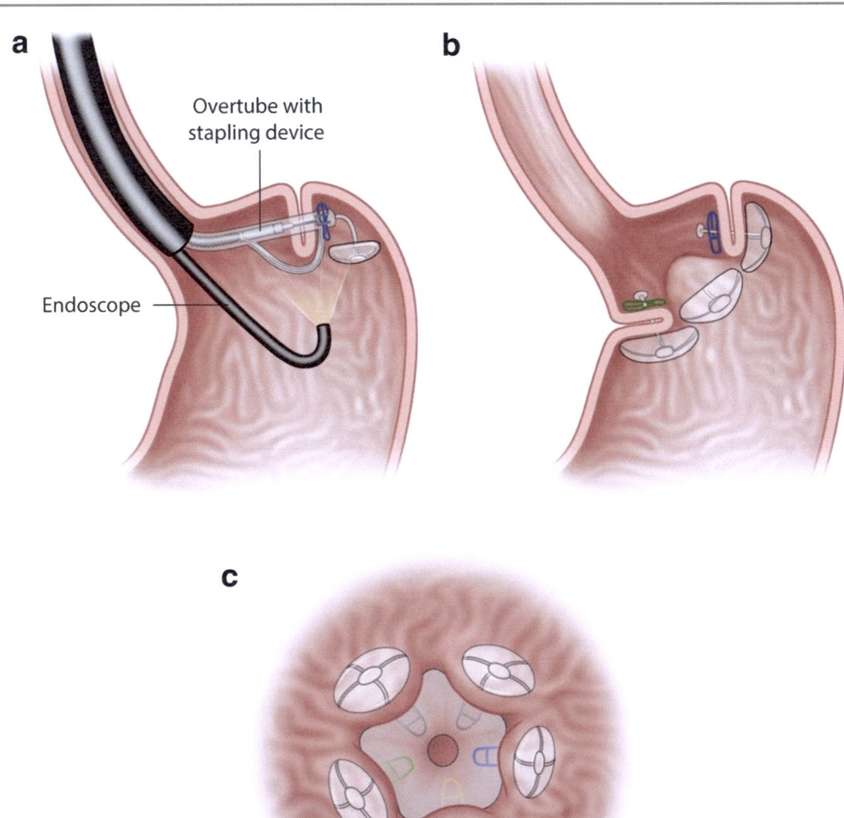

placed within the stomach. Using several running polypropylene sutures, a vertical gastroplasty is created by approximating the anterior and posterior surfaces of the stomach and excluding the greater curvature side of the body and antrum (Fig. 13.7). Fogel et al. reported 64 patients treated with endoscopic gastroplasty followed for 1 year. Morbidly obese patients in this study had a mean EWL of 58 % [19]. Although the Bard Endocinch system has been trialed extensively in the treatment of GERD, few trials looking at its utility treating morbidly obese patients have been published.

TOGa System

The TOGa system (Transoral gastroplasty system; Satiety, Palo Alto, CA) is an endoscopic stapling device that is used to create a gastric sleeve from the angle of His to the mid portion of the stomach. Performed along the lesser curvature, it is similar to a laparoscopic sleeve gastrectomy, only without resection. A multicenter phase I trial conducted outside the USA by Deviere et al. included 21 patients [17 female, age 43.7 (22–57) years, BMI 43.3 (35–53) kg/m^2]. There were no serious adverse events reported and the most commonly reported procedure or device-related adverse events

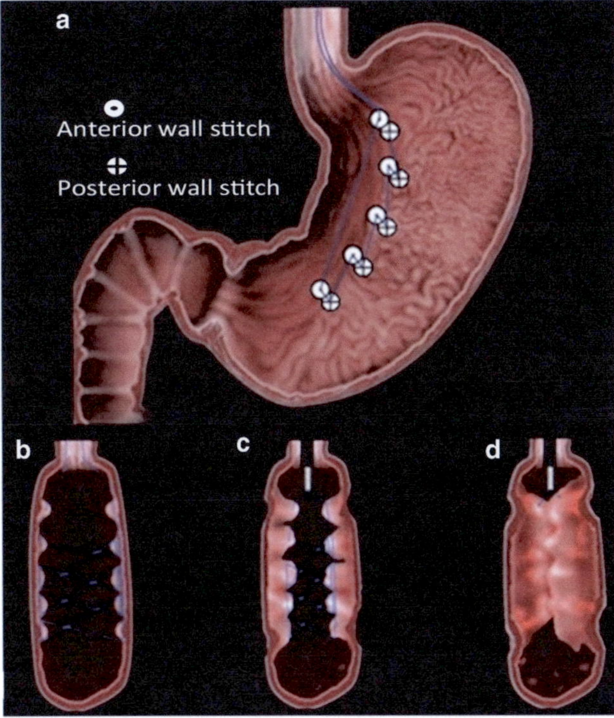

Fig. 13.7 Illustration of the gastroplasty created by the Endocinch suturing system

were vomiting, pain, nausea, and transient dysphagia. At 6-month endoscopy, all patients had persistent full or partial stapled sleeves. Patients lost an average 17.6 pounds at 1 month, 24.5 pounds at 3 months, and 26.5 pounds at 6 months post-treatment (excess weight loss of 16.2 %, 22.6 %, and 24.4 %, respectively) [20].

Subsequently, the European Trial published at the end of 2011 reviewed 53 of 67 patients at 12 month follow-up and found an excess BMI loss of 33.9, 42.6, and 44.8 % at 3, 6, and 12 months, respectively [21].

Transoral Gastric Volume Reduction Procedure

Transoral gastric volume reduction (TRIM procedure) performed using the Restore Suturing System (Bard-Davol, Warwick, RI) utilizes a multistitch endoscopic suturing system placed through the wall of the stomach. It uses interrupted polypropylene sutures to achieve gastric mucosal apposition, starting 10 cm distal to the gastroesophageal junction. Several plications are then created moving proximally along the greater curvature. Initial experience with use of this device has shown no major complications in the periprocedural period, and long-term follow-up is ongoing [22].

Space-Occupying Procedures

Intragastric Balloon Placement

Since the 1980s, many attempts at developing an endoscopically placed intragastric balloon device have been made. These devices occupy a significant volume of the stomach and accomplish two goals. First, they produce satiety by filling the stomach; second, they may slow gastric emptying and decrease transit time. At this time, no intragastric balloon devices are approved for use in the USA by the FDA; however, several are available in Europe and South America.

The most widely used device is the BioEnterics Intragastric Balloon (BIB) (Allergan, Irvine CA). The balloon is a spherical device made of silicone. It is placed endoscopically into the gastric fundus under either general anesthesia or conscious sedation, and then it is filled with 400–700 mL of saline mixed with methylene blue. The dye alerts the patient to balloon rupture that may occur during the treatment period. The balloon is radiopaque, which allows balloon position and migration to be evaluated by either plain films or fluoroscopy. Patients are placed on a liquid diet and antiemetics post procedure. The most common complications are nausea and vomiting, which in some series are seen in the majority of patients. The balloon is left in place for 6 months,

at which time it is removed. The risk of balloon migration or deflation increases beyond this time interval, and removal is therefore recommended [23]. Balloon removal is performed by endoscopically deflating the device and then removing it through the mouth. Its use has been described as a primary treatment for morbid obesity and as a bridge to surgical therapy in super obese patients [24].

Weight loss results with BIB therapy have been promising in the short term. Genco et al. conducted a double blind crossover study comparing BIB to sham endoscopy in 32 patients with a mean body mass index (BMI) of 43.7 kg/m^2. The treatment groups were then crossed at 3 months. The group treated with BIB had significantly better mean excess weight loss (EWL) at 3 months. Interestingly, the initial treatment group continued to lose weight after crossing over to blinded balloon removal, which may be related to improvement in eating habits and ongoing satiety even after balloon removal [25]. Lopez-Nava and colleagues followed 714 patients treated at a single center with mean EWL of 41 % at 6 months. A subset of patients underwent repeat balloon placement after 6 months and continued to lose weight [26]. Evans and Scott reported a series of 69 balloon placements in patients with a mean BMI of 46.3 kg/m^2. At 7-month follow-up, the mean EWL was 18 %. Notably within this series, 18 balloon displacements were identified, 3 requiring laparotomy for removal. Vomiting was the most common complication, occurring in 31 patients [23].

Long-term outcomes, however, have been mixed. Few series document protocol-driven follow-up beyond 6 months. Lopez-Nava followed 148 patients who did not undergo further bariatric procedures after initial 6 months of balloon therapy. Over half of these patients gained at least 50 % of the weight lost with balloon therapy at 2-years follow-up [26]. Dastis et al. followed 100 patients with mean BMI of 35 kg/m^2 for 30 months. Only 63 % had successful weight loss at 6 months; at 30 months, only 24 % were successful. Mean weight loss for the study population at 30 months was only 5.8 kg [27]. These studies suggest that the BIB as a primary endoscopic therapy for weight loss is not likely to achieve long-term efficacy equivalent to surgical treatments at this time.

It has been suggested that patients with BMI > 50 have an increased risk of morbidity and mortality with Roux-en-Y gastric bypass, though the data has not been definitive [28, 29]. In these patients, consideration of staged surgical procedures has been suggested and performed with good results [30]. To that end, the BIB has been applied in a staged fashion. Spyropoulos et al. reported 26 patients with mean BMI of 65 kg/m^2 who underwent BIB placement that achieved a mean EWL of 22 %. Improvement was seen in sleep apnea, diabetes, and hypertension in several of the patients. Nearly all patients subsequently underwent biliopancreatic diversion with good outcomes [31]. Gottig and colleagues reported similar findings in 75 with mean BMI of 68.2 kg/m^2 patients treated with balloon placement. Subsequently, 69 patients underwent gastric bypass after EWL of 20 % with balloon [32].

Few studies comparing balloon therapy to surgical therapy have been completed and none in a randomized fashion. Two studies examining BIB versus sleeve gastrectomy demonstrated conflicting results. Milone et al. compared weight loss at 6 months in 20 super obese patients undergoing laparoscopic sleeve gastrectomy to the results of two nonrandomized trials of BIB at other centers. Mean weight loss in the surgical cohort was 45 kg, compared to 18 kg and 26 kg for the balloon cohorts [33]. A case control study by Genco and colleagues showed no difference in excess weight loss at 6 and 12 months between groups of patients undergoing sleeve gastrectomy and balloon therapy [34].

Heliosphere Bag

The Heliosphere Bag (Heliosphere Medical Implants, UK) is an air-filled bag placed within the fundus after diagnostic endoscopy. After its approval for use in the UK, two series of its use were reported. Patients were treated for 6 months. Weight loss outcomes appeared similar to other endoscopic therapies [35, 36], but frequent complications of migration and obstruction have led to its withdrawal from the market [37].

Stationary Antral Balloon

Lopasso reported on the use of a stationary balloon placed within the gastric antrum in 26 patients. Inclusion criteria included a BMI of greater than 25 kg/m^2. The distal tip of a conical-shaped balloon sits within the proximal duodenum. It is filled with 180 mL of saline mixed with green dye. Its shape creates an intermittent gastric outlet obstruction. It is hypothesized that the duodenal anchor also stimulates inhibitory signals that augment the feeling of satiety. Results of 6-month treatment were somewhat disappointing, as only nine patients were able to complete the study; the others required early removal of the balloon due to either malfunction or side effects. Weight loss was reported as a mean of 11 kg in patients completing the treatment [38].

Silimed Gastric Balloon

The Silimed Gastric Balloon (Silimed, Rio de Janeiro, Brazil) is a silicone based intragastric prosthesis that is mounted on a sheath for delivery. The sheath is attached to the tip of the endoscope, and the balloon is placed in the fundus. It is then filled with both radiopaque contrast material and methylene blue to alert rupture or migration. The initial series of 16 patients treated with the device demonstrated a reduction in mean BMI from 27.5 to 24.5 kg/m^2 [39].

Complications of Endoscopic Balloons

Gastric balloon therapy carries a risk of several complications and side effects as documented in the studies referenced above, including nausea, vomiting, deflation, gastritis, and intolerance. Nausea and vomiting are common in the first week occurring in up to 90 % of patients but this tends to improve with time. In approximately 18 % of patients the nausea and vomiting persist after 3 weeks. Abdominal pain can be seen in up to 46 % of patients and reflux esophagitis can be seen in up to 11 %. Deflation or rupture of the balloon is seen in 19–27 % of patients that may contribute to migration or small bowel obstruction in up to 4 %. In rare cases (<0.2 %) gastric necrosis or perforation can occur necessitating emergent operation [40]. Rossi et al. reported an increase in the incidence and severity of erosive esophagitis in patients treated with balloons [41]. Severe complications including obstruction, perforation, and even death have been reported [40–44].

Adjustable Totally Implantable Intragastric Prosthesis

The adjustable totally implantable intragastric prosthesis (ATIIP-Endogast) (Districlass Medical S.A., France) is unique device that incorporates techniques used in both percutaneous endoscopic gastrostomy (PEG) tube placement as well as adjustable gastric band placement. It is placed under endoscopic guidance using a technique similar to a PEG tube placed using the introducer technique. The device is connected to silicone tubing that attaches to port that can be accessed percutaneously to adjust the volume of the balloon. The prosthesis is filled with 300 mL of air after insertion. A multicenter series of 57 patients demonstrated mean EWL of 40 % at 1 year. Seven wound infections at the port sites were seen in this series [45].

Given the lack of level 1 evidence for primary endoscopic treatment of obesity, it is difficult to recommend these procedures as a definitive treatment at this time. They may have a role as bridge therapy for the super and super-super obese that ultimately will require surgery. Refinements in device design and materials may allow their use for longer periods of time with greater efficacy. Randomized trials of devices compared to sham procedures need to be completed to further examine their role in the spectrum of treatments for obesity.

Neural Alteration Procedures

Gastric Electrical Stimulation in Obesity

Morbid obesity results from alterations in food intake and reduced activity in most individuals. It has been postulated that morbid obesity results from dysregulation of peripheral and central neurohumoral pathways that control the food intake. Thus the interest in gastric electrical stimulation (GES) methods to reduce the food intake and to promote weight loss via action on gastric motor and afferent function and on extragastric neurohumoral activities

Several gastric stimulation protocols have demonstrated weight reduction in morbidly obese patients and in animal models of obesity as well. The methods of stimulus for obesity are different that the ones for gastroparesis. The first method involves the laparoscopic implantation of the Transcend Gastric Stimulator (Medtronic, Minneapolis, MN, USA). The concept is to increase the feeling of satiety thus reducing the food intake. It employs an implantable, pacemaker like device that delivers low level electrical stimulation to the stomach. The stimulation electrodes are sutured to the outer lining of the stomach along the lesser curvature and connected to a device that is implanted underneath the skin on the abdomen similar to as laparoscopic gastric band port. An external remote programmer is used to control the device. The procedure is done laparoscopically with 4–6 ports and requires about 1 h to complete. It is proposed as a less aggressive and invasive procedure than gastric bypass [46]. Although this method may inhibit gastric motor function, it is believed to decrease food intake by primarily acting on vagal afferent pathways [47].

The second method is the Tantalus system (MetaCure, Orangeburg, NY, USA) and it involves the surgical placement of three electrode pairs. One pair is in the fundus and detects food intake, and the two other pairs are in the antrum and they detect intrinsic slow waves and deliver stimuli in synchrony with these slow waves [48]. Gastric stimulation begins when food enters the stomach and is only delivered postprandially [49]. The device augments antral contractions and this phasic activity enhances satiety that is elicited by postprandial gastric distension [50].

The first gastric stimulator for the treatment of morbid obesity was implanted by Cigaina in 1995 and two individuals from this group that were followed for longer than 5 years lost 38 % and 67 % of their excess body weight [51]. Four subsequent trials have been done using this method. A European trial consisting of 65 obese patients showed similar weight reduction [52]. Another multicenter European Laparoscopic Obesity Stimulation Survey trial had 69 patients with a mean BMI of 41 kg/m². They had a mean weight loss of 21 lbs in excess of their body weight [53]. In

the USA a sham controlled trial in 103 patients showed no greater weight loss at 7 months in those with the device activated vs. the sham group. However, in an open label Dual Lead Implantable Gastric Electrical Stimulation Trial (DIGEST), 30 patients reported a 23 % reduction in the excess body weight loss at 16 months [54]. This was associated with reduction in appetite and enhancement of satiety.

Other studies of 12–24 obese patients reported an excess body weight loss of 24–30 % at 9–36 months after implantation of the Medtronic device [51, 55]. An added bonus as with any weight loss procedure is that patients reported that their symptoms of GERD and glucose intolerance improved. Complications of the implantable gastric stimulator include intragastric lead perforations after surgery and lead dislodgements in 20–25 % of patients [55]. Other side effects along with induction of satiety have been bloating, abdominal pain and nausea. However, in 2005 Medtronic issued a press release stating that in a double blind study with 200 patients, the Transcend device did not meet its study endpoint. Currently this device is being used in Canada and Europe, but is not FDA approved in the USA [47].

Of note is that most of the studies have been done with the Medtronic stimulator. However one study has reported benefits of the Tantalus gastric modulation device [48]. In 12 patients body weight decreased from 129±5 to 120±6 kg after 20 weeks. Furthermore, in nine patients that are followed up for 52 weeks weight decreased to 112±4 kg. Weight reduction had a direct correlation with improved hypertension. Like its counterpart the Tantalus device is available in Europe but not FDA approved in the USA.

In summary, GES may have a therapeutic potential for obesity but it has failed to produce consistent and positive weight loss in morbidly obese patients in double blinded placebo controlled studies. The results in the open label use were more promising. New wireless gastric electronic stimulators are in development eliminating the need for laparoscopic placement. The new generation of stimulators have been placed endoscopically and tested in animals [51].

Secondary Bariatric Procedures

Endoscopic Treatment of Weight Gain After Bariatric Surgery

Transoral procedures are also being investigated in the context of revisional bariatric surgery. Specifically, while Roux-en-Y Gastric bypass remains the gold-standard surgery for weight loss (i.e., %EWL at 2 years of 61.6 % [56]; early and late mortality of 0.16 % and 0.09 % respectively [7], inadequate loss and/or weight regain is reported as high as 25–30 % after gastric bypass or other bariatric procedures [57, 58]. The etiology of weight regain is multifactorial [59], and includes inadequate long-term management of psychological, dietary, or medical issues, as well as anatomical aberrancies.

Focusing on the anatomy, initial investigations must include an esophagogastroduodenoscopy (EGD) or upper gastrointestinal (GI) study to evaluate for gastro-gastric fistula, gastric pouch dilation or anastomotic dilation. Once a gastro-gastric fistula is ruled out, gastrojejunal anastomosis and/or pouch dilation may underlie weight regain as patients may lose the feeling of early satiety leading to overeating. Indeed, upper endoscopy has revealed that, in patients who regain weight, the size of the stoma or anastomosis is twice the immediate postoperative diameter of 1.0–1.5 cm. If dilatation of the pouch or gastrojejunal anastomosis is the diagnosis, then revisional surgery may be necessary, and issues related to feasibility and safety arise. Recent studies estimate a rate of 5–13 % for major complications with re-operative surgery [60], the most serious of which include anastomotic leaks, wound dehiscence, incisional hernias, and pulmonary complications.

Surgical pouch reduction and anastomotic revision have been described as means to deal with this frustrating problem; however, morbidity and mortality from these operations are significantly higher than primary surgical interventions. Thus, much interest has developed in endoscopic revisional approaches to stomal dilation and pouch enlargement.

Endoscopic Pouch and Anastomotic Reduction

StomaphyX™

The StomaphyX™ (EndoGastric Solutions, Redmond, WA) is an FDA-approved endoscopic device that deploys polypropylene H-fasteners to re-approximate the gastric wall within a dilated pouch or stoma (Fig. 13.8). It can be used in patients who have developed weight gain after gastric bypass. The procedure is performed by first endoscopically measuring the size of both the gastric pouch and the gastrojejunal anastomosis. The device is then mounted over the endoscope and positioned just above the anastomosis. Suction is applied, and an H-fastener is deployed just above the anastomosis. This is repeated in a circular fashion to re-create the stoma, creating a pleat of tissue. A second circular level of fasteners is placed 1 cm proximal to these within the pouch. The residual pouch volume is then measured endoscopically to determine the adequacy of the procedure (see Video 13.1) (Fig. 13.9) [61]. The first reported trial of StomaphyX™ demonstrated mean EWL = 19.5 % at 12 month follow-up [61]. A second trial with similar follow-up period demonstrated mean weight loss = 7.3 kg, with no patients gaining weight after the procedure [62]. Further results of these and other multicenter trials are being conducted to examine long-term outcomes.

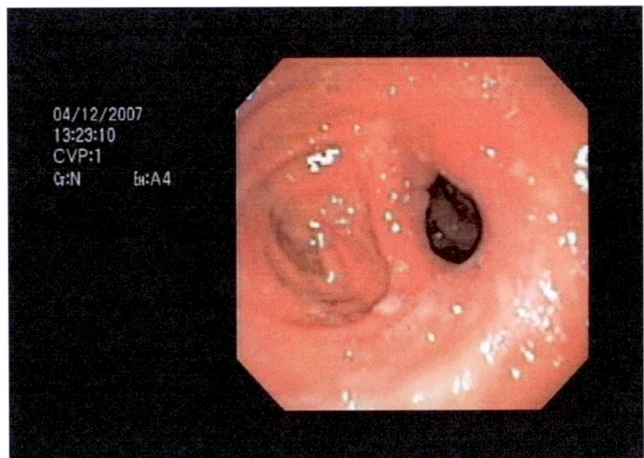

Fig. 13.8 Dilated gastric pouch prior to StomaphyX pouch reduction

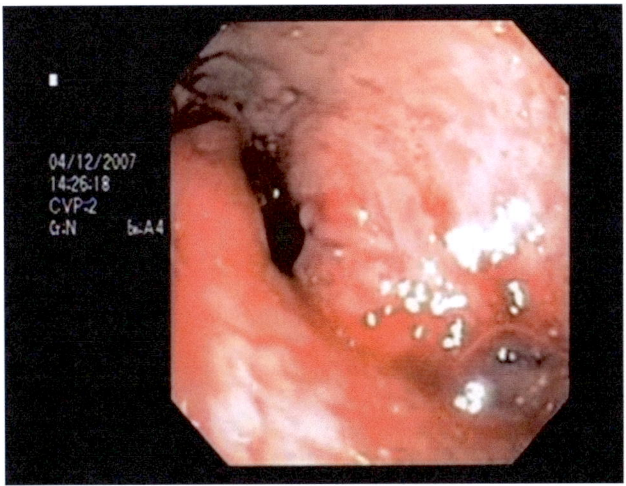

Fig. 13.9 Gastric pouch after StomaphyX pouch reduction

Endoscopic Sclerotherapy

Another approach to gastrojejunal anastomotic or pouch dilation involves endoscopic injection of sodium morrhuate into the gastric mucosa at the level of the pouch or anastomosis (Fig. 13.10). Injection with 10–30 cc can produce fibrosis that reduces stoma size enough to restore satiety in patients with enlarged pouches or anastomoses (Fig. 13.11). Several series describe their results. The procedure is indicated for patients who gain weight 12 months or longer after gastric bypass and whose stoma is greater than 1.2 cm in diameter. Some protocols include an objective evaluation of stomal size with contrast radiography or endoscopy prior to intervention. Loewen reported results of sclerotherapy in 71 patients whose weight had increased significantly from nadir, with a mean stomal diameter of 2.3 cm. Nearly half required a second treatment. Twelve month follow-up demonstrated that only 30 % of the patients continued to gain weight [63]. Catalano described a protocol in which stoma size measurements were obtained

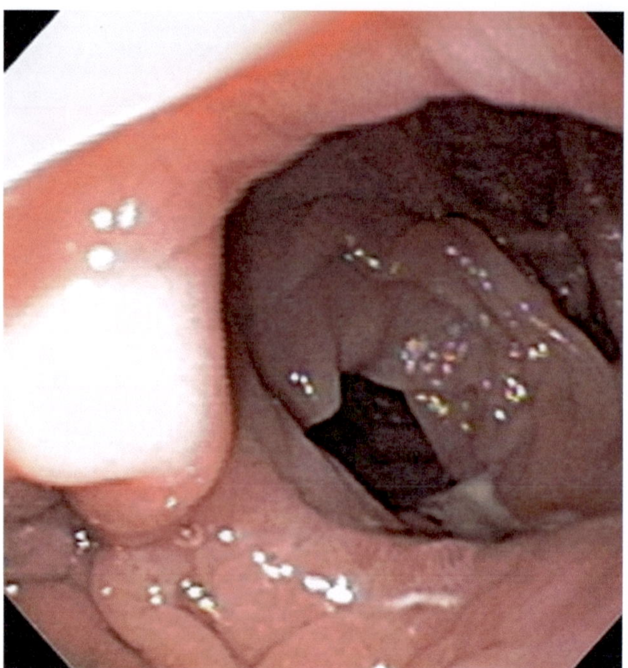

Fig. 13.10 Dilated gastrojejunostomy prior to sclerotherapy injection and treatment

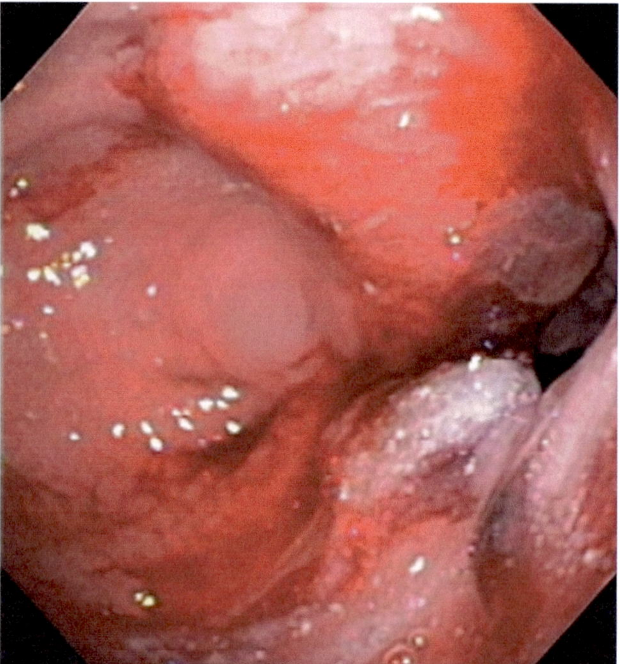

Fig. 13.11 Reduction in cross section of the gastrojejunostomy after sclerotherapy injection and treatment

after sclerosant injection. Twenty-eight patients were treated and followed for mean of 18 months. Criteria for successful treatment included reduction of stoma size to 1.2 cm or less, and loss of 75 % of the weight gained above nadir weight. In this series, 64 % of patients were treated successfully. These

patients had a mean decrease in stoma diameter of 6 mm [64]. In Spaulding's series of 32 patients, over 90 % had either weight loss or stabilization after sclerotherapy, avoiding further weight regain in the majority of patients [65].

Revision Obesity Surgery Endoscopic Procedure

The revision obesity surgery endoscopic (ROSE) procedure is a revisional, endoscopic treatment for weight gain after gastric bypass using the EndoSurgical Operating System (USGI Medical, San Clemente, CA) a prototype suturing and tissue plicating device. First described in porcine models, the ROSE device accommodates an endoscope and three working instruments, and these instruments are used to create a full-thickness plication of the gastric wall. Two anchors are placed on opposite aspects of the pouch, and the suture joining the two anchors is tightened to re-approximate the wall. Multiple approximation sites are created during the procedure, and measurements of the pouch are then taken post reduction [66]. Ryou reported an initial experience with the device in five patients. All patients had significant weight regain, decreased satiety and dilated gastrojejunal anastomosis. All underwent initial endoscopy to estimate pouch size. The procedure was technically successful in all patients, with mean anastomotic diameter reduction of 2.1 cm, and mean pouch reduction of 4.4 cm. Patients were maintained on a restricted diet with frequent follow-up. At 3-month follow-up, mean weight loss of 7.8 kg [66]. An updated series with 20 patients demonstrated successful treatment in 17 patients, with mean weight loss of 8.8 kg. In the three patients unable to undergo ROSE procedure, mean weight gain was 5 kg over the same time period, despite identical dietary restrictions and clinical evaluation (see Video 13.2) [67].

Endoscopic Considerations in Pre- and Post-Roux-en-Y Bypass

Evaluation of the Preoperative Bariatric Patient

The role of upper endoscopy in the preoperative evaluation of bariatric surgery patients is generally based on the presence or absence of symptoms. Patients with symptoms of reflux, dysphagia, and/or dyspepsia are appropriate candidates for preoperative evaluation [68, 69]. However, the threshold for performing preoperative endoscopy in patients undergoing RYGB and DS/BPD procedures should be low. This is due to the fact that postoperatively the distal stomach will be inaccessible via a standard upper endoscope. The rationale for performing an EGD preoperatively is to diagnosis and treat lesions and conditions that might potentially cause complications in the postoperative period [70].

Studies have shown that obesity is a risk factor for GERD, erosive esophagitis, and esophageal adenocarcinoma [71].

Furthermore, the presence of a large hiatal hernia may be a relative contraindication and may require crural tightening at the time of the operation to avoid postoperative complications such as band slippage in LAGB patients [72, 73]. Review of the literature on routine upper endoscopy shows that pathology identified preoperatively can alter the surgical approach and/ or delay the operation [74, 75]. In a study published in 2012, routine preoperative EGD in patients undergoing laparoscopic adjustable band placement revealed an abnormality in 56 % of the 371 patients screened including two occult esophageal adenocarcinomas [76]. In a second study, pathology was identified in 55 % of morbidly obese on routine preoperative EGD [77]. *Helicobacter pylori* infection is present in 30–40 % of bariatric patients and these should be treated preoperatively since these patients are more likely to develop marginal ulcers postoperatively [75].

Guidelines outside the USA recommend routine upper endoscopy in all preoperative bariatric surgery patients regardless of the presence or absence of symptoms [78]. Although an upper endoscopy may reveal lesions in patients without symptoms, there is no data in the literature that evaluates the surgical outcome of these findings. An EGD is not part of the routine work up algorithm in the bariatric population but the threshold for endoscopy should be very low to avoid postoperative complications in this high risk group of patients.

Pre-endoscopic Considerations in a Postoperative Bariatric Patient

Prior to performing any endoscopic evaluation on this group of patients the endoscopist should be aware of the operative procedure and pre-procedure radiological imaging is helpful in delineating the surgical anatomy. Direct communication with the surgeon and access to postoperative notes and information will help in deciding the right equipment needed for the successful completions of any diagnostic or therapeutic procedures [79]. The choice of endoscope depends on the indication and the possible need to access the excluded stomach and duodenum.

Understanding the surgical anatomy of different bariatric procedures is the key to the success of any endoscopic intervention. The expected findings after a RYGB include a normal esophagus and GE junction. The pouch size varies and careful inspection of the gastric suture lines should be done to look for fistulas and ulcerations. The gastrojejunal anastomosis is generally 10–12 mm in diameter. Past the anastomosis is then a short blind afferent limb and alongside is the efferent Roux limb. This limb may vary from 75 to 150 cm in length before the jejunojejunostomy. This is important in determining the type of scope required, if the jejunojejunal anastomosis is to be examined. Of note is that the distal

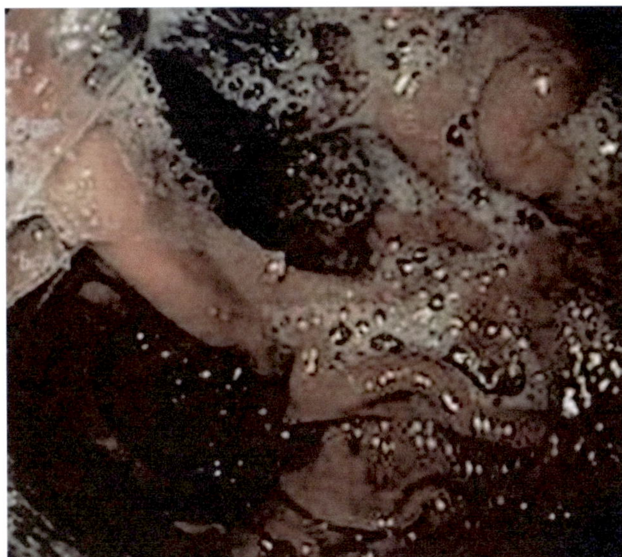

Fig. 13.12 Endoscopic view of vertical banded gastroplasty

stomach and duodenum will not be visualized in this patient. Endoscopic visualization of the jejunojejunostomy can be accomplished with either a pediatric colonoscope or double balloon enteroscopy. On the other hand, a VBG patient has a very similar appearance with a gastric pouch and a banded stoma with a 10–12 mm in diameter (Fig. 13.12). However, in these patients once past the stoma you visualize the unaltered distal stomach and duodenum.

A sleeve gastrectomy is the creation of a long tubular stomach with the long staple line parallel to the lesser curve. The duodenal switch/biliopancreatic diversion (DS/BPD) is often done in conjunction with a sleeve gastrectomy but it also includes a duodeno-jejunal anastomosis distal to the pylorus. Hence, the ampulla may not be accessed via an ERCP. Laparoscopic adjustable gastric bands produce different amounts of extrinsic circumferential compression to limit the opening to the rest of the stomach. This is evident on endoscopy and it is important to assess for band slippage and erosion in this patient population.

Indications for Postoperative Endoscopy

The presence of symptoms is the main indication for postoperative endoscopy. Nausea, vomiting, and abdominal pain are the most commonly encountered symptoms and these may be due to either anatomic or physiologic abnormalities. These include marginal ulcers, GERD, gastro-gastric fistulas, and anastomotic strictures. An endoscopy is preferred unless an anastomotic leak is suspected in which case a water-soluble contrast study is the imaging study of choice. The constellation of symptoms in conjunction with imaging studies can help in the type of investigation needed by the patient.

Abdominal pain, nausea, vomiting, and bloating may suggest strictures, internal hernias and bezoars.

Marginal Ulcers

These can be seen as early as 3 weeks to 6 months out from bariatric surgery. The incidence of marginal ulcers after RYGB is from <1 % up to 36 % [80–82]. These patients present with abdominal pain, bleeding, and nausea. The ulcers are at the gastrojejunotomy anastomosis or just distal to it on the jejunal side. The etiologies vary from staple line disruption and ischemia, presence of sutures and staples to acid exposure to the small intestine mucosa. Smoking, NSAID use and *H. pylori* (HP) colonization are known risk factors for ulcer formation. This is an argument for routine preoperative EGD and testing for HP in patients undergoing gastric bypass. The use of PPI has a protective effect on the intestine.

GERD

As mentioned earlier obesity is a known risk factor for GERD with a prevalence of 30–60 %. Bariatric surgery including RYGB and LAGB have both shown to decrease the symptoms of GERD by 90 % in several studies [83–86], however, other studies show an incidence of reflux esophagitis of up to 56 % [87]. Etiologies may include gastrojejunostomy anastomotic stenosis and worsening of symptoms in patients with motility disorders and laparoscopic gastric banding. Endoscopy is instrumental in the diagnosis and management of these symptoms. Anastomotic strictures can be managed with balloon dilation and non-acid reflux may need adjustment of a tight gastric band.

Fistulas

Incidence of gastric or anastamotic leaks and fistulas after RYGB or sleeve gastrectomy is 1–6 % [88–91]. Gastric leaks present with tachycardia, fever, nausea, vomiting, abdominal pain and renal failure. Most leaks are at the gastrojejunostomy anastomosis or the proximal stomach after sleeve gastrectomy and can be diagnosed via an upper GI contrast study or CT scan. Endoscopy is not recommended in the early postoperative period for leaks and fistulas unless an endoscopic therapy is to be performed, as air insufflation can disrupt the staple line and worsen the problem. Leaks from the jejuno-jejunal anastomosis occur less frequently but require reoperation. Chronic gastro-gastric fistulas, whether from a marginal ulcer or a postoperative leak, can be diagnosed with a contrast study or endoscopy. Endoscopic management of these has been done utilizing fibrin glue, endoscopic clips, reoperation, and covered self-expanding stents [92–94]. Covered plastic and metal stents have been used successfully to treat leaks at the gastrojejunostomy after RYGB or proximal stomach after sleeve gastrectomy definitively managing the leak in up to 72 % of patients. Stenting not only allows

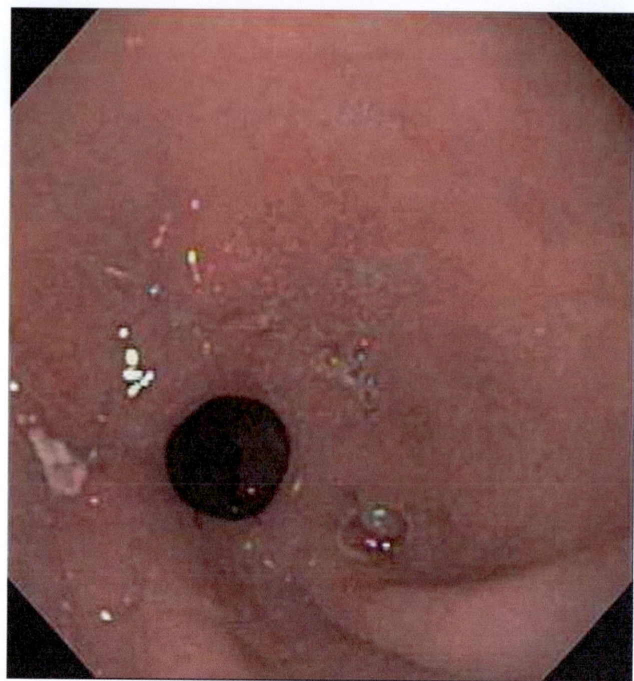

Fig. 13.13 Normal gastrojejunostomy as seen on endoscopy in a postoperative Roux-en-Y gastric bypass patient

resumption of oral intake but symptomatic improvement in up to 89 % of patients [95, 96].

Stenosis

Gastrojejunal anastomotic stricture is a common complication following gastric bypass, occurring in 4–17 % of patients [97, 98]. A normal sized stoma should be approximately 12.5 mm as seen in the figure depicting a normal gastric pouch and stoma (Fig. 13.13). Strictures are defined as a stoma less than 10 mm in diameter, and their symptoms include nausea, vomiting, and inability to maintain adequate oral hydration in the early postoperative period. They can be diagnosed with a contrast study however endoscopic examination is the preferred method for both diagnostic (i.e., marginal ulcerations) and therapeutic intervention. Endoscopic treatment of strictures involves dilatation using either a TTS hydrostatic balloon device or a bougie. If the stenosis cannot be traversed with an endoscope or balloon then fluoroscopy is useful in the passage of the guidewire safely. Care must be taken to ensure a guidewire has not passed extraluminally and this can be confirmed with fluoroscopy with or without injection of contrast through a catheter threaded over the guidewire prior to dilation (Fig. 13.14). Several larger series using balloon dilatation have demonstrated greater than 90 % improvement in symptoms [99, 100]. Many patients will require multiple dilatations prior to symptom relief. Major complications include anastomotic perforation, which may occur in up to 5 % of patients [100].

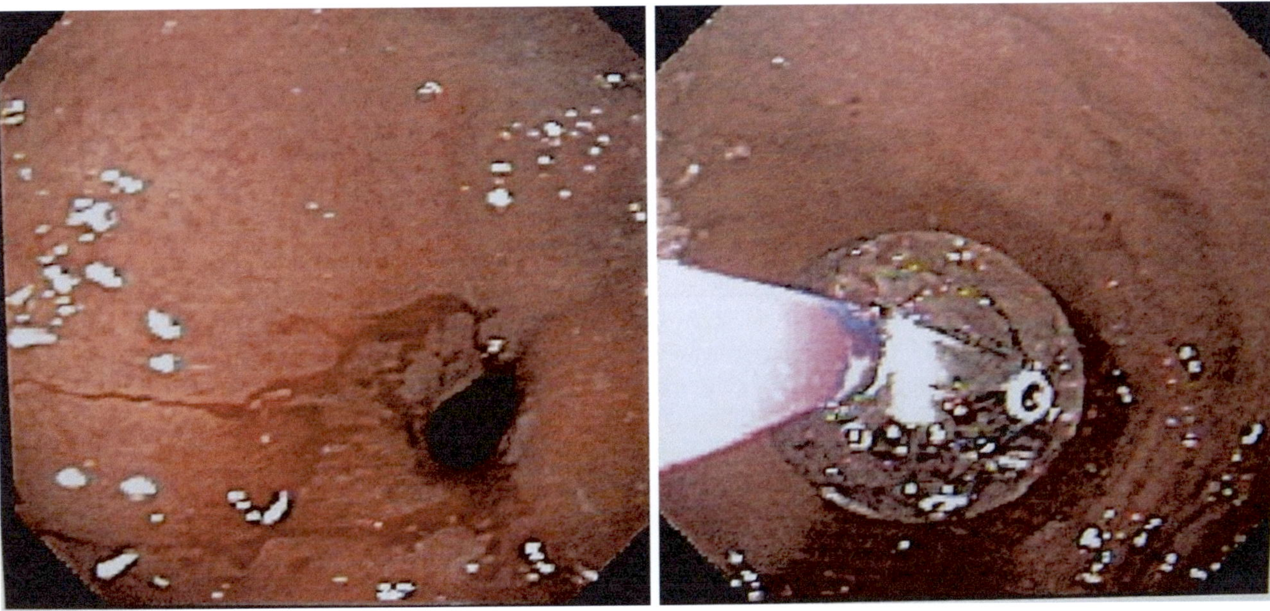

Fig. 13.14 Dilating a strictured gastrojejunal anastomosis in a postoperative Roux-en-Y gastric bypass patient

It is important to remember that the Roux limb can be antecolic or retrocolic. This is important because in retrocolic reconstruction the stricture may be past the gastrojejunostomy in the roux limb. This is the case if the retrocolic tunnel is too tight and the gastrojejunostomy anastomosis is normal on endoscopy. The endoscopist will see the jejunum is dilated to the point at which it traverses the transverse colon mesentery.

Bezoars

Food bezoars can occur both in the early and late postoperative period. They are more common after gastric banding [101, 102]. Presentation includes nausea, vomiting, and dysphagia. Bezoars can be diagnosed and treated endoscopically with fragmentation and removal [103]. If the cause is gastrojejunostomy stenosis, this can be treated endoscopically at the same time.

Band Slippage and Erosion

This is seen in LAGB patients and the incidence of band erosion is 9.5–11 % while pouch dilation and band slippage is 6.3 % [104]. Band erosions are best diagnosed at endoscopy whereas band slippage may be diagnosed with a contrast study. Band erosions may be asymptomatic but can present with nausea, vomiting, abdominal pain and port site infection. Endoscopically band slippage has a large pouch and in severe cases it can lead to gastric necrosis and sepsis [105, 106]. Patients with a VBG have had erosion of the polypropylene mesh in the stomach and this can be removed endoscopically [107, 108]. Upon identification of mesh within the gastric lumen, endoscopic scissors can effectively cut and remove the mesh that has eroded into the gastric lumen.

Bleeding

Bleeding in the bariatric patient may be acute or chronic in nature. This may present as an upper GI bleed in the reconstruction or the bypassed stomach (gastric remnant) in patients undergoing a RYGB. Chronic presentation is that of iron deficiency anemia. In the early postoperative period bleeding can occur along the staple line in 1–4 % of the RYGB patients [109] and only about 0.1 % in LAGB patients [110, 111]. Majority of the time bleeding can be managed identified and managed endoscopically. Bleeding identified at the time of the operation on routine intraoperative endoscopy can be managed with laparoscopic or open suture ligation or endoscopic clip placement. Bleeding noted in the Roux limb may be coming from the jejuno-jejunal anastomosis or the remnant stomach. This presents its own set of challenges to access the remnant stomach endoscopically. Iron deficiency anemia is present in 30–50 % of the patients undergoing RYGB and a varying prevalence in the DS/BPD patients [112–115]. The mechanism is multifactorial but upper endoscopy is crucial as part of the work up algorithm.

Access to Remnant Stomach Postoperatively

Postoperatively, after a RYGB, access to the remnant stomach cannot be accomplished by standard upper endoscopy whether it is a front or side viewing scope. There are multiple ways of accessing the excluded stomach via an endoscopic approach. This is necessary especially in post RYGB patients who are having symptoms of upper GI bleeding, anemia, or choledocholithiasis. The remnant stomach can be accessed via a pediatric colonoscope, percutaneous access, double balloon/single balloon endoscopy (DBE) with or without ERCP, and laparoscopic assisted transgastric endoscopy/ERCP.

Morbid obesity is a known risk factor of gallstone formation and rapid weight loss tends to compound the problem. Preoperative incidence of cholelithiasis is 14 % in bypass patients and 27 % in LAGB patients [116, 117]. Postoperative incidence is reported as high as 22–71 % requiring cholecytectomy and other endoscopic interventions in 7–41 % [118, 119]. However, choledocholithiasis can be managed with a standard ERCP in the LAGB patients. In the RYGB the access to the remnant stomach is technically challenging. The success of the ERCP in this population is dependent on the skill level of the operator in accessing the duodenum, and surgical factors such as afferent and efferent limb length play a role. Both side viewing and front viewing scopes have been used successfully but access to the ampulla typically requires the use of double-balloon enteroscopes. The use of specialized instrumentation is limited when using a double-balloon enteroscope and must be considered when undertaking this type of procedure. A series of 15 patients had successful cannulation of the papilla in 66 % of the cases after placing a guidewire through a colonoscope in the afferent limb and accessing the afferent limb with a duodenoscope [120]. In this series the needle knife sphincterotomy, sphincter of Oddi manometry, stone extraction, and biliary stent placement were done successfully. However, in cases not amenable to standard ERCP, laparoscopic assisted transgastric access has been utilized with success [121, 122].

The technique requires two teams—one surgical and one endoscopic. The surgeon gains access to the remnant stomach and creates a gastrotomy via a 15 mm port placed in the gastric remnant. Following this an adult ERCP scope is passed into the duodenum and the papilla is accessed in the standard fashion. The stones are extracted with biliary sphincterotomy and balloon/basket extraction. Of note, the gastrotomy on the remnant stomach should be made proximal (4–6 cm) to the duodenum to help facilitate accessing the second portion of the duodenum (video included). Patel et al. in his series of eight patients cannulated the papilla after laparoscopic or open access to the remnant stomach in 100 % of the cases [123]. The gastrotomy is then closed laparoscopically using a standard stapling technique or fashioned into a gastrostomy tube to allow for future access to the gastric remnant or enteral feeding.

In another series, percutaneous gastrostomy tubes (PEG) were placed in the remnant stomach either at the time of gastric bypass or by interventional radiology and then a pediatric duodenoscope was advanced in the remnant after dilation of the tract [122]. The other ways to access the remnant stomach percutaneously is to place a silastic ring and anchor it to the abdominal wall. This can then identified radiologically and access with a PEG and followed by duodenoscopy.

DBE with ERCP has been utilized in patients with choledocholithiasis but with little success. There were at least five patients in three series and the rate of reaching the papilla or the bilio-enteric anastomosis was 86–94 % and the success rate of ERCP was 67–89 % [124–126]. The success rate is limited because DBEs are forward viewing endoscopes and do not have an elevator. Similarly, the endoscopic instrumentation and catheters needed to perform ERCP are typically not of adequate length to use through a DBE. Cannulation of the ampulla of Vater via a DBE may require use of instrumentation typically not used for ERCP and limit the ability to cannulate and instrument the common bile duct.

Conclusion

Endoscopic treatments for morbid obesity, including primary treatments and revisional therapies, have rapidly developed over the last 5 years. While they do not yet achieve equivalent efficacy as surgical treatments for obesity, these interventions do provide some degree of weight loss for patients. Further advances in technology and refinement in technique may lead to procedures and devices that provide a greater degree of weight loss. In the future, the addition of endoluminal therapies to the treatment armamentarium of bariatric surgeons may allow us to offer lower risk procedures to the morbidly obese patient. Additional randomize prospective studies are needed to add validity to this ever-growing field.

References

1. World Health Organization. Fact sheet: obesity and overweight. 2008. http://www.who.int/mediacentre/factsheets/fs311/en/print.html. Accessed March 2013.
2. Ogden CL. Disparities in obesity prevalence in the United States: black women at risk. Am J Clin Nutr. 2009;89:1001–2.
3. Ogden CL, Carroll MD, Curtin LR, McDowell MA, Tabak CJ, Flegal KM. Prevalence of overweight and obesity in the United States, 1999–2004. JAMA. 2006;295:1549–55.
4. Ogden CL, Carroll MD, McDowell MA, Flegal KM. Obesity among adults in the United States: no statistically significant change since 2003–2004. NCHS Data Brief. 2007;Nov(1):1–8.
5. Schauer PR, Ikramuddin S, Gourash W, et al. Outcomes after laparoscopic Roux-en-Y gastric bypass for morbid obesity. Ann Surg. 2000;232(4):515–29.
6. DeMaria EJ, Sugerman HJ, Kellum JM, et al. Results of 281 consecutive total laparoscopic Roux-en-Y gastric bypasses to treat morbid obesity. Ann Surg. 2002;235(5):640–5. discussion 645–7.
7. Buchwald H, Estok R, Fahrbach K, Banel D, Sledge I. Trends in mortality in bariatric surgery: a systematic review and meta-analysis. Surgery. 2007;142:621–35.
8. Maggard MA, Shugarman LR, Suttorp M, Maglione M, Sugarman HJ, Livingston EH, et al. Meta-analysis: surgical treatment of obesity. Ann Intern Med. 2005;142:547–59.
9. Allen JW. Laparoscopic gastric band complications. Med Clin North Am. 2009;91:485–97.

10. Colquitt JL, Picot J, Loveman E, Clegg AJ. Surgery for obesity. Cochrane Database Syst Rev 2009; Issue 2. Art. No.: CD003641.

11. Hazey JW, Dunkin BJ, Melvin WS. Changing attitudes toward endolumenal therapy. Surg Endosc. 2007;21:445–8.

12. Rodriguez-Grunert L, Neto MPG, Alamo M, Ramos AC, Baez PB, Tarnoff M. First human experience with endoscopically delivered and retrieved duodenal-jejunal bypass sleeve. Surg Obes Relat Dis. 2008;4:55–9.

13. Tarnoff M, Rodriguez L, Escalona A, Ramos A, Neto M, Alamo M, et al. Open label, prospective, randomized controlled trial of an endoscopic duodenal-jejunal bypass sleeve versus low calorie diet for pre-operative weight loss in bariatric surgery. Surg Endosc. 2009;23:650–6.

14. Escalona A, Yanez R, Pimentel F, et al. Initial human experience with restrictive duodenal-jejunal bypass liner for treatment of morbid obesity. Surg Obes Relat Dis. 2010;6(2):126–31.

15. Schouten R, Rijs CS, Bouvy ND, et al. A multicenter, randomized efficacy study of the EndoBarrier Gastrointestinal Liner for pre-surgical weight loss prior to bariatric surgery. Ann Surg. 2010;251(2):236–43.

16. ValenTx Endo Bypass System: initial trial. 2009. http://www.valentx.com/news-1.php. Accessed 15 Jan 2012.

17. Biertho L, Hould F-S, Lebel S, Biron S. Transoral endoscopic restrictive implant system: a new endoscopic technique for the treatment of obesity. Surg Obes Relat Dis. 2010;6:203–5.

18. Felsher J, Farres H, Chand B, et al. Mucosal apposition in endoscopic suturing. Gastrointest Endosc. 2003;58(6):867–70.

19. Fogel R, De Fogel J, Bonilla Y, De La Fuente R. Clinical experience of transoral suturing for an endoluminal vertical gastroplasty: 1-year follow-up in 64 patients. Gastrointest Endosc. 2008;68(1):51–8.

20. Deviere J, Ojeda Valdes G, Cuevas Herrera L, et al. Safety, feasibility and weight loss after transoral gastroplasty: first human multicenter study. Surg Endosc. 2008;22(3):589–98.

21. Familiari P, Costamagna G, Bléro D, Le Moine O, Perri V, Boskoski I, et al. Transoral gastroplasty for morbid obesity: a multicenter trial with a 1-year outcome. Gastrointest Endosc. 2011;74(6):1248–58.

22. Brethauer SA, Chand B, Schauer PR, Thompson CC. Transoral gastric volume reduction for weight management: technique and feasibility in 18 patients. Surg Obes Relat Dis. 2010;6(6):689–94.

23. Evans JD, Scott MH. Intragastric balloon in the treatment of patients with morbid obesity. Br J Surg. 2001;88(9):1245–8.

24. Cha A, Murayama K. Endolumenal approaches to revisional bariatric surgery. In: Murayama K, editor. Evidence based minimally invasive surgery. Cinemed: Woodbury, CT; 2011.

25. Genco A, Cipriano M, Bacci V, et al. BioEnterics Intragastric Balloon (BIB): a short-term, double-blind, randomised, controlled, crossover study on weight reduction in morbidly obese patients. Int J Obes (Lond). 2006;30(1):129–33.

26. Lopez-Nava G, Rubio MA, Prados S, et al. BioEnterics(R) intragastric balloon (BIB(R)). Single ambulatory center spanish experience with 714 consecutive patients treated with one or two consecutive balloons. Obes Surg. 2011;21(1):5–9.

27. Dastis NS, Francois E, Deviere J, et al. Intragastric balloon for weight loss: results in 100 individuals followed for at least 2.5 years. Endoscopy. 2009;41(7):575–80.

28. Fernandez Jr AZ, Demaria EJ, Tichansky DS, et al. Multivariate analysis of risk factors for death following gastric bypass for treatment of morbid obesity. Ann Surg. 2004;239(5):698–702. discussion 702–3.

29. Fernandez Jr AZ, DeMaria EJ, Tichansky DS, et al. Experience with over 3,000 open and laparoscopic bariatric procedures: multivariate analysis of factors related to leak and resultant mortality. Surg Endosc. 2004;18(2):193–7.

30. Regan JP, Inabnet WB, Gagner M, Pomp A. Early experience with two-stage laparoscopic Roux-en-Y gastric bypass as an alternative in the super-super obese patient. Obes Surg. 2003;13(6):861–4.

31. Spyropoulos C, Katsakoulis E, Mead N, et al. Intragastric balloon for high-risk super-obese patients: a prospective analysis of efficacy. Surg Obes Relat Dis. 2007;3(1):78–83.

32. Gottig S, Daskalakis M, Weiner S, Weiner RA. Analysis of safety and efficacy of intragastric balloon in extremely obese patients. Obes Surg. 2009;19(6):677–83.

33. Milone L, Strong V, Gagner M. Laparoscopic sleeve gastrectomy is superior to endoscopic intragastric balloon as a first stage procedure for super-obese patients (BMI>or =50). Obes Surg. 2005;15(5):612–7.

34. Genco A, Cipriano M, Materia A, et al. Laparoscopic sleeve gastrectomy versus intragastric balloon: a case–control study. Surg Endosc. 2009;23(8):1849–53.

35. Forestieri P, De Palma GD, Formato A, et al. Heliosphere Bag in the treatment of severe obesity: preliminary experience. Obes Surg. 2006;16(5):635–7.

36. De Castro ML, Morales MJ, Del Campo V, et al. Efficacy, safety, and tolerance of two types of intragastric balloons placed in obese subjects: a double-blind comparative study. Obes Surg. 2010;20(12):1642–6.

37. Trande P, Mussetto A, Mirante VG, et al. Efficacy, tolerance and safety of new intragastric air-filled balloon (Heliosphere BAG) for obesity: the experience of 17 cases. Obes Surg. 2008;20(9):1227–30.

38. Lopasso FP, Sakai P, Gazi BM, et al. A pilot study to evaluate the safety, tolerance, and efficacy of a novel stationary antral balloon (SAB) for obesity. J Clin Gastroenterol. 2008;42(1):48–53.

39. Espinet-Coll E, Nebreda-Durán J, Gómez-Valero JA, Muñoz-Navas M, Pujol-Gebelli J, Vila-Lolo C, et al. A current endoscopic techniques in the treatment of obesity. Rev Esp Enferm Dig. 2012;104(2):72–87.

40. Carvalho GL, Barros CB, Moraes CE, et al. The use of an improved intragastric balloon technique to reduce weight in pre-obese patients-preliminary results. Obes Surg. 2009;21(7):924–7.

41. Rossi A, Bersani G, Ricci G, et al. Intragastric balloon insertion increases the frequency of erosive esophagitis in obese patients. Obes Surg. 2007;17(10):1346–9.

42. Zdichavsky M, Beckert S, Kueper M, et al. Mechanical ileus induces surgical intervention due to gastric balloon: a case report and review of the literature. Obes Surg. 2010;20(12):1743–6.

43. del Pozo P, Flores B, Liron R, et al. Gastric perforation during removal of an intragastric balloon. Obes Surg. 2009;19(8):1195–6.

44. Koutelidakis I, Dragoumis D, Papaziogas B, et al. Gastric perforation and death after the insertion of an intragastric balloon. Obes Surg. 2009;19(3):393–6.

45. Gaggiotti G, Tack J, Garrido Jr AB, et al. Adjustable totally implantable intragastric prosthesis (ATIIP)-Endogast for treatment of morbid obesity: one-year follow-up of a multicenter prospective clinical survey. Obes Surg. 2007;17(7):949–56.

46. Shikora S. Implantable gastric stimulation—the surgical procedure: combining safety with simplicity. Obes Surg. 2004;14:S9–13.

47. Hasler WL. Methods of gastric electrical stimulation and pacing: a review of their benefits and mechanisms of action in gastroparesis and obesity. Neurogastroenterol Motil. 2009;21:229–43.

48. Bohdjalian A, Prager G, Aviv R, et al. One year experience with Tantalus: a new surgical approach to treat morbid obesity. Obes Surg. 2006;16:627–34.

49. Deb S, Tang SJ, Abell TL, Rao S, Huang WD, To SD, et al. An endoscopic wireless gastrostimulator (with video). Gastrointest Endosc. 2012;75(2):411–5. 415.e1.

50. Peles S, Peterson J, Aviv R, et al. Enhancement of antral contractions and vagal afferent signaling with synchronized electrical

stimulation. Am J Physiol Gastrointest Liver Physiol. 2003;285: G577–85.

51. Cigaina V. Gastric pacing as therapy for morbid obesity: preliminary results. Obes Surg. 2002;12 Suppl 1:12S–6.

52. Cigaina V. Longterm follow up of gastric stimulation for obesity: the Mestre 8-year experience. Obes Surg. 2004;14 Suppl 1:S14–22.

53. De Luca M, Segato G, Busetto L, et al. Progress in implantable gastric stimulation: summary of results of the European multicenter study. Obes Surg. 2004;14 Suppl 1:S33–9.

54. Shikora SA. "What are the yanks doing?" The US experience implantable gastric stimulation (IGS) for the treatment of obesity—update on the ongoing clinical trials. Obes Surg. 2004;14 Suppl 1:S40–8.

55. D'Argent J. Gastric electrical stimulation as therapy of morbid obesity: preliminary results from the French study. Obes Surg. 2002;12 Suppl 1:21S–5.

56. Buchwald H, Avidor Y, Braunwald E, Jensen MD, Pories W, Fahrbach K, et al. Bariatric surgery. A systematic review and meta-analysis. JAMA. 2004;292(14):1724–37.

57. Yale CE. Gastric surgery for morbid obesity. Complications and long-term weight control. Arch Surg. 1989;124:941–6.

58. Sugerman HJ, Kellum JM, Engle KM, et al. Gastric bypass for treating severe obesity. Am J Clin Nutr. 1992;55 Suppl 2:560S–6.

59. Christou NV, Look D, Maclean LD. Weight gain after short and long limb gastric bypass in patients followed for longer than 10 years. Ann Surg. 2006;244(5):734–40.

60. Martin MJ, Mullenix PS, Steele SR, See CS, Cuadrado DG, Carter PL. A case-match analysis of failed prior bariatric procedures converted to resectional gastric bypass. Am J Surg. 2004;187(5): 666–70.

61. Mikami D, Needleman B, Narula V, Durant J, Melvin WS. Natural orifice surgery: initial US experience utilizing the StomaphyXTM device to reduce gastric pouches after Roux-en-Y gastric bypass. Surg Endosc. 2010;24:223–8.

62. Leitman IM, Virk CS, Averinos DV, Patel R, Lavarias V, Surick B, et al. Early results of trans-oral endoscopic placation and revision of the gastric pouch and stoma following Roux-en-Y gastric bypass surgery. JSLS. 2010;14(2):217–20.

63. Loewen M, Barba C. Endoscopic sclerotherapy for dilated gastrojejunostomy of failed gastric bypass. Surg Obes Relat Dis. 2008;4(4):539–42. discussion 542–3.

64. Catalano MF, Rudic G, Anderson AJ, Chua TY. Weight gain after bariatric surgery as a result of a large gastric stoma: endotherapy with sodium morrhuate may prevent the need for surgical revision. Gastrointest Endosc. 2007;66(2):240–5.

65. Spaulding L, Osler T, Patlak J. Long-term results of sclerotherapy for dilated gastrojejunostomy after gastric bypass. Surg Obes Relat Dis. 2007;3(6):623–6.

66. Ryou M, Mullady DK, Lautz DB, Thompson CC. Pilot study evaluating technical feasibility and early outcomes of second-generation endosurgical platform for treatment of weight regain after gastric bypass surgery. Surg Obes Relat Dis. 2009;5(4): 450–4.

67. Mullady DK, Lautz DB, Thompson CC. Treatment of weight regain after gastric bypass surgery when using a new endoscopic platform: initial experience and early outcomes (with video). Gastrointest Endosc. 2009;70(3):440–4.

68. Ikenberry SO, Harrison ME, Lichtenstein D, et al. American Society of Gastrointestinal Endoscopy. The role of endoscopy in dyspepsia. Gastrointest Endosc. 2007;66:1071–5.

69. Lichtenstien DR, Cash BD, Davilla R, et al. American Society of Gastrointestinal Endoscopy. The role of endoscopy in the management of GERD. Gastrointest Endosc. 2007;66:219–24.

70. Anderson MA, Gan SI, Fanelli RD, Baron TH, et al. Guidelines statement: American Society of Gastrointestinal Endoscopy/ SAGES. Role of endoscopy in the bariatric surgery patient. Gastrointest Endosc. 2008;68:1–10.

71. Hampel H, Abraham NS, El-Serag HB. Meta-analysis: obesity and the risk of GERD and its complications. Ann Intern Med. 2005;143:199–211.

72. Greenstein RJ, Nissan A, Jaffin B. Esophageal anatomy and function in laparoscopic gastric restrictive bariatric surgery. Obes Surg. 1998;8:199–206.

73. Dolan K, Finch R, Fielding G. Laparoscopic gastric banding and crural repair in the obese patient with a hiatal hernia. Obes Surg. 2003;13:772–5.

74. Sharaf RN, Weinshel EH, Bini EJ, et al. Endoscopy plays an important preoperative role in bariatric surgery. Obes Surg. 2004;14:1367–72.

75. Schirmer B, Erenoglu C, Miller A. Flexible endoscopy in the management of patients undergoing RYGB. Obes Surg. 2002;12: 634–8.

76. Humphreys LM, Meredith H, Morgan J, Norton S. Detection of asymptomatic adenocarcinoma at endoscopy prior to gastric banding justifies routine endoscopy. Obes Surg. 2012;22(4):594–6.

77. Csendes A, Burgos AM, Smok G, Beltran M. Endoscopic and histologic findings of the foregut in 426 patients with morbid obesity. Obes Surg. 2007;17(1):28–34.

78. Sauerland S, Angrisani L, Belachew M, et al. European Association for Endoscopic Surgery. Obesity surgery: evidence based guidelines of the EAES. Surg Endosc. 2005;19:200–21.

79. Feitoza AB, Baron TH. Endoscopy and ERCP in the setting of previous upper GI tract surgery. Part I: postsurgical anatomy without alteration of the pancreaticobiliary tree. Gastrointest Endosc. 2001;54:743–9.

80. Wilson JA, Romagnuolo J, Byrne TK, et al. Predictors of endoscopic findings after Roux-en-Y gastric bypass. Am J Gastroenterol. 2006;101:2194–9.

81. Sapala JA, Wood MH, Sapala MA, et al. Marginal ulcer after gastric bypass: a prospective 3-year study of 173 patients. Obes Surg. 1998;8:505–16.

82. MacLean LD, Rhode BM, Nohr C, et al. Stomal ulcer after gastric bypass. J Am Coll Surg. 1997;185:1–7.

83. Nelson LG, Gonzalez R, Haines K, et al. Amelioration of gastroesophageal reflux symptoms following RYGB for clinically significant obesity. Am Surg. 2005;71:950–3.

84. Perry Y, Courcoulas AP, Fernando HC, et al. Laparoscopic RYGB for recalcitrant gastroesophageal reflux disease in morbidly obese patients. JSLS. 2004;8:19–23.

85. Raftopoulos I, Awais O, Courcoulas AP, et al. Laparoscopic gastric bypass after antireflux surgery for the treatment of gastroesophageal reflux in the morbidly obese patients: initial experience. Obes Surg. 2004;14:1373–80.

86. Nguyen NT, Varela JE, Sabio A, et al. Reduction in prescription medication costs after laparoscopic gastric bypass. Am Surg. 2006;72:853–6.

87. Westling A, Bjurling K, Ohrvall M, et al. Silicone—adjustable gastric banding: disappointing results. Obes Surg. 1998;8: 467–74.

88. Filho AJ, Kondo W, Nassif LS, et al. Gastrogastric fistula: a possible complication of RYGB. JSLS. 2006;10:326–31.

89. Carrodeguas L, Szomstein S, Soto F, et al. Management of gastrogastric fistulas after divided RYGB surgery for morbid obesity: analysis of 1292 consecutive patients and review of the literature. Surg Obes Relat Dis. 2005;1:467–74.

90. Gould JC, Garren MJ, Starling JR. Lessons learned from the first 100 cases in a new minimally invasive bariatric surgery program. Obes Surg. 2004;14:618–25.

91. Gumbs AA, Duffy AJ, Bell RL. Management of gastrogastric fistula after laparoscopic RYGB. Surg Obes Relat Dis. 2006;2:117–21.

92. Kriwanek S, Ott N, Ali-Abdullah S, et al. Treatment of gastro-jejunal leakage and fistulization after gastric bypass with coated self expanding stents. Obes Surg. 2006;16:1669–74.

93. Salinas A, Baptista A, Santiago E, et al. Self expanding metal stents to treat gastric leaks. Surg Obes Relat Dis. 2006;2:570–2.

94. Fukumoto R, Orlina J, McGinty J, et al. Use of Polyflex stents in treatment of acute esophageal and gastric leaks after bariatric surgery. Surg Obes Relat Dis. 2007;3:68–71.

95. Freedman J, Jonas E, Näslund E, Nilsson H, Marsk R, Stockeld D. Treatment of leaking gastrojejunostomy after gastric bypass surgery with special emphasis on stenting. Surg Obes Relat Dis. 2012; Mar 20. [Epub ahead of print].

96. Yimcharoen P, Heneghan HM, Tariq N, Brethauer SA, Kroh M, Chand B. Endoscopic stent management of leaks and anastomotic strictures after foregut surgery. Surg Obes Relat Dis. 2011;7(5):628–36. Epub 2011 May 25.

97. Kravetz AJ, Reddy S, Murtaza G, Yenumula P. A comparative study of handsewn versus stapled gastrojejunal anastomosis in laparoscopic Roux-en-Y gastric bypass. Surg Endosc. 2011;25(4):1287–92.

98. Nguyen NT, Dakin G, Needleman B, et al. Effect of staple height on gastrojejunostomy during laparoscopic gastric bypass: a multicenter prospective randomized trial. Surg Obes Relat Dis. 2010;6(5):477–82.

99. Go MR, Muscarella 2nd P, Needleman BJ, et al. Endoscopic management of stomal stenosis after Roux-en-Y gastric bypass. Surg Endosc. 2004;18(1):56–9.

100. Ukleja A, Afonso BB, Pimentel R, et al. Outcome of endoscopic balloon dilation of strictures after laparoscopic gastric bypass. Surg Endosc. 2008;22(8):1746–50.

101. Parameswaran R, Ferrando J, Sigurdsson A. Gastric bezoar complicating laparoscopic adjustable gastric banding with band slippage. Obes Surg. 2006;16:1683–4.

102. Veronelli A, Ranieri R, Laneri M, et al. Gastric bezoars after adjustable gastric banding. Obes Surg. 2004;14:796–7.

103. Pinto D, Carrodeguas L, Soto F, et al. Gastric bezoar after laparoscopic roux-en-Y gastric bypass. Obes Surg. 2006;16:365–8.

104. Frigg A, Peterli R, Zynamon A, et al. Radiologic and endoscopic evaluation for laparoscopic adjustable gastric banding: preoperative and follow-up. Obes Surg. 2001;11:594–9.

105. Iannelli A, Facchiano E, Sejor E, et al. Gastric necrosis: a rare complication of gastric banding. Obes Surg. 2005;15:1211–4.

106. Foletto M, De Marchi F, Bernante P, et al. Late gastric pouch necrosis after Lap-Band, treated by an individualized conservative approach. Obes Surg. 2005;15:1487–90.

107. Evans JA, Williams NN, Chan EP, et al. Endoscopic removal of eroded bands in vertical banded gastroplasty: a novel use of endoscopic scissors (with video). Gastrointest Endosc. 2006;64:801–4.

108. Adams LA, Silva Jr RG, Rizk M, et al. Endoscopic argon plasma coagulation of Marlex mesh erosion after vertical banded gastroplasty. Gastrointest Endosc. 2007;65:337–40.

109. Nguyen NT, Longoria M, Chalifoux S, et al. Gastrintestinal hemorrhage after laparoscopic gastric bypass. Obes Surg. 2004;14:1308–12.

110. Rao AD, Ramalingam G. Exsanguinating hemorrhage following gastric erosion after laparoscopic adjustable gastric banding. Obes Surg. 2006;16:1675–8.

111. Biertho L, Steffan R, Ricklin T, et al. Laparoscopic gastric bypass versus laparoscopic adjustable gastric banding: a comparative study of 1200 cases. J Am Coll Surg. 2003;197:536–44. discussion 544–5.

112. Halverson JD. Micronutrient deficiencies after gastric bypass for morbid obesity. Am Surg. 1986;52:594–8.

113. Amaral JF, Thompson WR, Caldwell MD, et al. Prospective hematologic evaluation of gastric exclusion surgery for morbid obesity. Ann Surg. 1985;201:186–93.

114. Skroubis G, Sakellaropoulos G, Pouggouras K, et al. Comparision of nutritional deficiencies after Roux-en-Y gastric bypass and after biliopancreatic diversion with Roux-en-Y gastric bypass. Obes Surg. 2002;12:551–8.

115. Dolan K, Hatzifotis M, Newbury L, et al. A clinical and nutritional comparision of biliopancreatic diversion with and without duodenal switch. Ann Surg. 2004;240:51–6.

116. Kiewiet RM, Durian MF, van Leersum M, et al. Gallstone formation after weight loss following gastric banding in morbidly obese Dutch patients. Obes Surg. 2006;16:592–6.

117. Villegas L, Schneider B, Provost D, et al. Is routine cholecystectomy required during laproscopic gastric bypass? Obes Surg. 2004;14:60–6.

118. Jr WL, Wright JK, Debelak JP, et al. Prevention of gallstone formation in morbidly obese patients undergoing rapid weight loss: results of a randomized controlled pilot study. J Surg Res. 2002;102:50–6.

119. Puzziferri N, Austrheim-Smith IT, Wolfe BM, et al. Three-year follow-up of a prospective randomized trial comparing laproscopic versus open gastric bypass. Ann Surg. 2006;243:181–8.

120. Wright BE, Cass OW, Freeman ML. ERCP in patients with long limb roué-en-Y gastrojejunostomy and intact papilla. Gastrointest Endosc. 2002;56:225–32.

121. Ceppa FA, Gagne DJ, Papasavas PK, et al. Laparoscopic transgastric endoscopy after RYGB. Surg Obes Relat Dis. 2007;3:21–4.

122. Martinez J, Guerrero L, Byers P, et al. Endoscopic retrograde cholangiopancreatography and gastroduodenoscopy after RYGB. Surg Endosc. 2006;20:1548–50.

123. Patel JA, Patel NA, Shinde T, et al. Endoscopic retrograde cholangippancreatography after laparoscopic Roux-en-Y gastric bypass: a case series and review of the literature. Am Surg. 2008;74:689–94.

124. Aabakken L, Bretthauer M, Line PD. Double balloon enteroscopy for endoscopic retrograde chalagiography in pateints with Roux-en-Y anastomosis. Endoscopy. 2007;39:1068–71.

125. Emmett DS, Mallat DB. Double balloon ERCP in patients who have undergone Roux-en-Y surgery: a case series. Gastrointest Endosc. 2007;66:1038–41.

126. Ryozawa S, Iwamato S, Urayama N, et al. Diagnostic and therapeutic endoscopy using a double balloon endoscope in long limb surgical bypass patients: focusing on ERCP in patients with Roux-en-Y gastrojejunostomy (in Japanese with English abstract). Shokaki Naishikyo (Endoscopia Digestiva). 2007;19:1611–8.

W. Scott Melvin and Jeffrey L. Eakin

History and Background

Gastroesophageal reflux disease (GERD) affects approximately 50 million Americans and some studies estimate the prevalence approaches 20 % of the population in many Western countries. Approximately 50 % of the U.S. population experiences GERD related symptoms once a month, and 1 in 10 Americans experience symptoms of heartburn and bloating every day. This tremendously prevalent condition has had and will continue to have a significant economic impact on the Unites States and other developed Western countries. In view of that, numerous countries expend a considerable amount of resources on direct and indirect costs attributable to the prevention and treatment of reflux disease. GERD has a substantial impact on clinical and financial welfare since patients suffering from this disorder generally report a diminished health-related quality of life (HRQL), reduced work productivity, and depressed psychological health. While it is difficult to quantify or even estimate the comprehensive economic impact of this pervasive illness it is feasible to put the current cost of proton-pump inhibitor (PPI) treatment into financial perspective. In 2009, Hiedelbaugh et al. analyzed cohort of 19 individuals who underwent a supervised clinical step-down treatment algorithm using proton-pump inhibitor therapy. In this study 84 % of individuals were able to decrease their PPI therapy to once daily dosing using strict adherence to actual prescribing recommendations and lifestyle modification [1]. This led to an overall clinical phar-

macy savings of $33,708 for the 19 patient cohort, yielding an average annual cost-savings of $1,774 per patient [1].

GERD leads to a severely diminished quality of life approaching illnesses such as diabetes and chronic heart failure [2]. Whatever the underlying mechanism, GERD results in chronic exposure of acidic gastric contents to the distal esophagus and this eventually can lead to considerable long-term clinical consequences. Chronic esophageal exposure to acid leads to mucosal damage as well as chronic inflammation ultimately resulting in ulceration and eventual metaplasia with a well-documented natural tendency for dysplastic and even malignant transformation.

There are two initial therapies for GERD: lifestyle modification and medical therapy. Proton-pump inhibitors (PPIs) are the foundation of medical management, and this class of drugs includes an assortment of patented, generic, prescription and over-the-counter medications. Unfortunately, there are drawbacks to the medications: (1) they are expensive, (2) they often require life-long therapy and compliance, (3) and they fail to address the underlying anatomical and functional abnormality at the lower esophageal sphincter (LES).

Often individuals fail to respond to lifestyle-modification and acid reduction therapy, and may require a Laparoscopic Nissen fundoplication for symptom control: the most definitive treatment option for medically refractory GERD patients. Rudolph Nissen performed the first fundoplication in 1956 after serendipitously discovering this century's most definitive and efficacious surgical option for GERD. Twenty years earlier, in 1936, Nissen was performing an esophagogastrectomy while repairing a case of peptic ulceration involving the cardia, and he decided to cover his gastric closure line with a cuff of gastric fundus to avoid postoperative anastamotic leakage [3]. More than 15 years later and much to his surprise, the patient failed to develop postoperative reflux symptoms. Following Nissen's discovery, Dallemagne and others surgical innovators developed, enhanced, and popularized the above mentioned fundoplastic procedure

W.S. Melvin, M.D. (✉)
Department of General Surgery, The Ohio State University Hospital,
410 West 10th Ave, N729 Doan Hall, Columbus, OH 43210, USA
e-mail: Scott.Melvin@osumc.edu

J.L. Eakin, M.D., B.A.
Department of General Surgery Center for Minimally Invasive
Surgery, The Ohio State University Medical Center,
Columbus, OH, USA

J.M. Marks and B.J. Dunkin (eds.), *Principles of Flexible Endoscopy for Surgeons*,
DOI 10.1007/978-1-4614-6330-6_14, © Springer Science+Business Media New York 2013

laparoscopically [4]. Complete laparoscopic fundoplication is the gold standard treatment of medically refractory GERD patients who are ready surgical candidates. Ultimately, the goals of reflux treatment are to heal erosive esophagitis, relieve esophageal and extraesophageal symptoms, improve quality of life, and prevent the complications of GERD: ulceration, stricture, Barrett's esophagus with or without dysplasia, and adenocarcinoma.

The laparoscopic Nissen fundoplication remains the gold standard for the treatment of GERD. However, current clinical, socioeconomic, industrial pressures and technologic advancement in combination with rising prescription drug costs have lead to the emergence of endoscopic or natural orifice treatment modalities, thus potentially reducing the trauma of surgery. Terms describing these techniques in the literature include "incisionless," "endoluminal," "trans-luminal," and "natural orifice transluminal endoscopic surgery (NOTES)." Modern surgical and societal pressures desire that surgical innovators find new ways to treat old problems with minimal collateral damage to the patient. These technologies are emerging from a foundation of endoscopic proficiency, which has been accumulating among surgeons and surgical endoscopists over the past few decades.

One of the earliest reports of experiments evaluating endoscopic therapeutic modalities for GERD dates back to the 1980s when Donahue et al. created an experimental therapeutic model in canines in which they performed endoscopic injectional therapy at the gastroesophageal junction (GEJ) [5]. They created permanent esophagostomies and gastrostomies and utilized these stomas for frequent pH monitoring. They performed their sclerosis technique using a sclerotherapy needle through a standard endoscope. Next, Morrhuate sodium, a sodium salt comprised of saturated and unsaturated fats was injected just below the GEJ in the submucosal plain along six separate injection points. This process was completed on four separate occasions. Their study showed that sclerosing the GEJ failed to affect the length or pressure of the LES. In spite of that, it was encouraging to find that sclerosis reduced the percentage of reflux time and frequency of reflux episodes. Since the time of this study, surgeons and endoscopists have witnessed an explosion of endoscopic and surgical technologies aimed at minimizing collateral therapeutic damage while maximizing physiologic restoration of the GEJ valve-mechanism. Two decades following Donahue's canine experiments, the FDA approved the first two endoscopic devices used to treat GERD. Following this initial device approval, translational clinical and nonclinical scientists have been working diligently they have developed three general techniques aimed at improving the efficacy of the valve mechanism at the GEJ: (1) injectional therapy, (2) radiofrequency thermal application, and (3) suturing and plication. Later on in the chapter we provide detailed instructions and descriptions of these various endoscopic techniques and we will summarize the current

scientific literature regarding procedural safety, efficacy and durability of these novel procedures. Nonetheless, we will first provide a review the normal antireflux mechanism and the pathophysiology of GERD as well as generally accepted definitions and modalities used to diagnose it. Clinicians responsible for treating GERD should have a thorough understanding of the epidemiological, diagnostic, pathologic and clinical aspects this disease in order to provide appropriate, effective, and durable treatment options for GERD, regardless of which modality a clinician chooses.

Anatomy, Antireflux Mechanism, and Pathophysiology

Over the past few decades physicians and clinical investigators have made significant advances in esophageal research. And this has led to an enhanced understanding of normal esophageal physiology and the physiologic mechanisms behind pathologic reflux. Indeed, an enhanced understanding coupled with a sudden increase in clinical innovation has been paramount in the development of minimally invasive and endoscopic techniques to treat reflux disease. The normal anatomy of the esophagus is complex and subtle and there is a wealth of knowledge regarding esophageal physiology. Understanding normal esophageal physiology and anatomy is germane to providing treatments aimed at restoring the barrier function of the esophagus.

The esophagus is a 30-cm muscular tube, which provides for the unidirectional flow of materials from the pharynx to the stomach. Most clinicians and researchers agree the paucity of the normal physiological barrier to reflux is usually due to complex interactions at the level of the LES. The LES is a structure resulting from a complex interaction of serous membranes and smooth muscle arising from the distal esophagus, and this sphincter in conjunction with other physiologic mechanisms is responsible for generating the normal barrier to reflux. When this mechanism breaks down, the distal esophagus becomes exposed to harmful gastric contents and the clinical consequences of GERD ensue. Several mechanisms are felt to be responsible for the breakdown of the GEJ valve mechanism: transient lower esophageal relaxations (TLESRs), ineffective esophageal motility and reduced LES tone and efficacy. TLESRs were described in 1980 by Dent and colleagues when they demonstrated that a significant number of gastroesophageal reflux episodes occur during complete relaxations of the LES that are not induced by swallowing [6]. These LES relaxations have been coined TLESRs to distinguish them from swallow-induced LES relaxations. Equally important, the LES tone and function are affected by and dependent on multiple factors: LES resting pressure, LES length and intra-abdominal length of the LES. The previously mentioned factors are well-documented parameters, which affect the normal barrier to reflux, and there are a plethora of external factors, which upset the physiologic balance of this barrier. A small list of aggravating factors would include gastric distension, medications and foods, delayed gastric emptying, neurologic abnormalities (e.g., achalasia) and anatomic abnormalities (e.g., hiatal hernia). Whatever the underlying cause of reflux most experts believe that optimally restoring the physiologic function and structure of the LES is germane to creating an effective durable treatment for GERD.

Diagnosis

Inherent to any diagnostic profile is recognizing historical and physical factors that predispose individuals to reflux disease. These factors include obesity, the presence of a hiatal hernia, use of medications such as nitrates, anticholinergics and the use of tobacco, nicotine or caffeine-containing products. Typically, patients with GERD complain of fundamental symptoms such as regurgitation and pyrosis, and these are often described as feeling of solid or liquid material in the hypopharynx and as severe retrosternal or cervical burning sensation, respectively. GERD is a prevalent illness with a variety of modes of presentation. For example, some individuals suffering from GERD present with endoscopic evidence of esophagitis while others never demonstrate any endoscopic findings of chronic esophageal exposure. In fact, approximately 10–20 % of patients will present with non-erosive esophageal reflux disease (NERD). Some patients may never complain of pyrosis or classic "heartburn" however physiologic testing will reveal severe frequent acidic exposures in the distal esophagus. Thus, the diagnosis can be difficult and in light of the many diagnostic modalities available to modern surgeons there may sometimes be an inappropriate or inadequate diagnosis of GERD. Therefore, clinicians must proceed with caution when interpreting the wide array of testing modalities available to document objective pre-procedural disease presence and or severity.

A great deal controversy exists regarding the best standard for diagnosing GERD. There exists an abundance of diagnostic options (e.g., 24-h pH monitoring, manometry, impedance testing, esophagram, video esophagram and endoscopy, etc.) available to physicians. Ultimately, these studies should be used in conjunction with clinical constellations to make a diagnosis of GERD. Endoscopy can play a major role in diagnosing GERD and it provides surgeons and endoscopists with an abundance of knowledge regarding disease spectrum and anatomical structure. It is extremely important for anyone considering therapeutic modalities for GERD to document pre-procedural motility and LES function with manometry or a video esophagram. There remains ambiguity and argument over the best progression of standardized diagnostic modalities for this illness. However, it is important to remember that anyone with a smoking history who presents with chronic GERD symptoms, weight loss and obstruction deserves an endoscopic evaluation in order to rule out any underlying benign or malignant lesion. In the end, clinicians should utilize consistent and reproducible methods not only to diagnose or document the presence of GERD but also to provide pre-procedural objective data, which can be used to document a failure or response to treatment.

Available Treatment Techniques

Physicians can employ three general categories of endoscopic maneuvers to restore the natural barrier at the GEJ: placing injectable or implantable substances into the GE junction, application of thermal energy and suturing or plication at the GE junction. Many have proposed theoretical mechanisms of how endoluminal therapies work to restore the normal barrier to reflux. Some of the hypothesized mechanisms include alterations in the compliance of the gastric cardia, a reduction in transient LES relaxations (TLESRs), increasing the length of the LES and decreasing the diameter of the distal esophagus. It is important to mention that the type of underlying pre-procedural anatomy can determine the efficacy of the type of therapy being offered. It is important to discern whether or not any patient undergoing endoscopic treatment of GERD has an anatomic defect such as a hiatal hernia, because the presence of a significant hiatal hernia is often a relative to absolute contraindication for many of these endoscopic procedures. In the subsequent section we will discuss some old and some evolving natural orifice techniques, which are evolving and challenging the common surgical paradigm for reflux.

Injectional Therapy

One of the first tactics devised to "fortify" or restore the GE junction relied on the placement of prosthetic materials into the distal esophagus. The Gatekeeper System and the Enteryx® device were built on this technology. A variety of bulking agents were developed and were under investigation in the USA; however, few have made it to clinical trials and clinical use.

Enteryx
Enteryx® is an injectable solution which approved by the Food and Drug Administration for its use in the treatment of GERD. The patented Enteryx® solution is an injectable liquid which is supplied in packets within the Enteryx® procedure kits. Enteryx® is a liquid comprised of 8 % ethylene vinyl alcohol and dimethyl sulfoxide. The solution contains a fluoroscopically

visible radiopaque contrast agent. This solution is injected under endoscopic visualization through a standard sclerotherapy needle into and along the submucosal muscular plane of the distal esophagus. Altogether, 6 mL of fluid is injected circumferentially at the level of the GE junction. Most injections take place at approximately 1–3 mL proximal to the squamocolumnar junction. The exact mechanism of Enteryx® remains unclear. Various opinions have been stated in the literature, but many believe it functions by providing bulk and firmness to the LES and thus it bolsters the lower gastroesophageal barrier to reflux.

Clinical exposure to this device was short-lived but some institutions and individuals were able to evaluate its safety and efficacy prior to market withdrawal. For example, Deviere et al. performed a clinical trial in which 15 patients received four quadrant injections with Enteryx® [7]. At 3 months following treatment only 4 of the 15 patients had resumed PPI use. Their heartburn severity scale (1–4) improved from 3.4 to 1.87 and the average LES pressure increased from 12.2 to 16.7 mmHg. Of note, there were no serious adverse events reported in this small series. In a larger study, Johnson et al. reported a Multicenter clinical trial, which also looked at the safety and efficacy of Enteryx® device in 85 patients who had GERD responsive to PPIs [8]. Seventy-four percent of the patients were able to eliminate their PPI use while another 10 % of the study patients were able to decrease their PPI use by half. Patients also saw improvements in average esophageal acid exposure. Of note, nineteen patients had to undergo repeat injection due to lack of therapeutic response. The most frequent postoperative symptom was chest pain. Ninety-two percent of patients experienced retrosternal chest pain, but 82 % of these individuals experienced symptom resolution in 2 weeks time.

In the end, the Enteryx® system was placed under scrutiny by the FDA due to its long-term consequences (e.g., stenosis and dysphagia) and adverse events related to improper placement of the bulking solution. There were isolated events in which the solution was improperly injected into the mediastinum, pleural cavities, and in one case directly into the aorta. Direct vascular injection was directly responsible for aortoenteric fistulization and renal failure from arterial occlusion. Eventually, the abovementioned reasons led to the voluntary recall of the device and it remains unavailable to the endoscopic surgeon.

The GateKeeper™ Reflux Repair System

The gatekeeper reflux repair system is a technique based on the placement of prosthetic devices, which are expandable bulking agents comprised of bioinert polyacrylonitrile-based hydrogel. These bulking agents are introduced into the distal esophagus in the submucosal plane, and over the first 24 h the LES is augmented as the prosthetic implants expand. Gradual expansion of the hydrogel implants creates folds in the distal esophagus and this is believed to augments reflux in the distal esophagus. The Gatekeeper procedure is performed with patients under conscious sedation. A standard video endoscope is introduced to measure the distance from the incisors to the GE junction. The tip of the overtube is positioned into the distal esophagus and an endoscope is inserted into the distal portion of the overtube. Typically, a guidewire is inserted and the endoscope is removed. Next, under direct vision the markings on the distal portion of the overtube are lined up with a previously chosen landing zone in the distal esophagus. Then an injection needle is introduced through the sheath of the overtube. A vacuum is used to stabilize the esophageal mucosa in the distal portion of the delivery system and sterile saline is injected to blanch the esophageal mucosa. The delivery sheath is then inserted into the submucosal plane and then needle withdrawn. After the needle is removed from the injection sheath, the prostheses are then inserted into the distal portion of the injector sheath and then placed in the submucosal position using a push-rod assembly. The overtube is then rotated circumferentially and the process is repeated to place the additional prosthesis. Typically an endoscopy is performed after withdrawing the scope-device complex to confirm the position of the prosthetic implants and evaluate for any esophageal or gastric injury from the device-overtube complex.

There have been several studies aimed at evaluating the efficacy of the GateKeeper™ Reflux Repair system. For instance, Fockens et al. reported on an early multi-institutional study in which 67 patients underwent 77 procedures with the GateKeeper™ Reflux Repair system [9]. Overall they placed 270 prostheses. Eighty and seventy percent of prostheses were retained at 1 and 6 months respectively. In their study, the median LES pressure and Median GERD heartburn-related quality of life scores improved significantly. More specifically, the mean LES pressure increased from 8.8 mmHg baseline to 13.8 mmHg and median GERD heartburn-related quality of life scores improved significantly from 24 to 5, and both difference (i.e., improvements) were statistically significant. Of note, 10 patients received repeat treatments for failure to respond to therapy in the subacute treatment period. There were two serious adverse events: one patient experienced a pharyngeal perforation, which was successfully treated non-operatively by keeping the patient NPO for several days.

Five years later Fockens et al. was part of a follow-up study, which was a prospective, randomized, sham-controlled, single-blinded, international multicenter study, which had a planned enrollment of 240 individuals. Only 143 patients were enrolled because the trial was closed early due to failure to demonstrate efficacy. There were four major adverse events including two perforations, a pulmonary infiltrate related to a perforation and severe chest pain.

While heartburn symptoms had improved significantly at 6 months, there was no significant difference between the treatment and the sham group. Moreover, esophageal acid exposure was improved significantly in the sham and the treatment arms but there was no statistical difference between the two groups.

All in all, following a 6-month pilot study, a multicenter trial was initiated to evaluate the GateKeeper™, but a lack of improved efficacy over the sham group led to early termination of investigation and failure of widespread adoption of this endoscopic technique.

Radiofrequency Thermal Application

Radiofrequency energy is used for a variety of therapeutic maneuvers: cardiac ablation, tumor ablation and more recently, endoscopic GERD therapy. Dr. David Utley in Sunnyvale California developed the first device approved to use radiofrequency energy to alter the anatomy of the GEJ. Dr. Utley's device, known as Stretta™, gained clinical approval by the Food and Drug Administration in April of 2000. Like others before it, this device was developed for the clinical realm, trialed and has seen market difficulties in its most recent past.

The Stretta™ radiofrequency delivery system exact mechanism of action remains unclear; however, it is hypothesized that the system works in the following manner The radiofrequency energy delivered to the distal esophagus by the Stretta™ device is believed to work by inducing coagulative necrosis which then heals by fibrosis, resulting in hypertrophy and scarring of adjacent muscle and thickening of the gastric cardia. The resultant three-dimensional anatomical alteration in the GE junction is what is thought to be responsible for the reduction of the symptoms associated with GERD patients experience following this procedure. Furthermore, it is hypothesized that the radiofrequency

Energy disrupts the vagal nerve afferent pathways within the myenteric plexus of the upper stomach, which have been implicated in transient LES sphincter relaxations or TLESRs [10]. In the next paragraph we offer a more detailed description of this procedure.

Immediately prior to the procedure, diagnostic endoscopy is performed and the distance from the incisors to the Z-line is measured. Next, (also using a standard endoscope) a guidewire is slipped into the stomach and then a balloon tipped catheter is passed over the guidewire until it is 1 cm above the Z-line. The Stretta™ device relies on a catheter equipped with a balloon. The balloon is inflated at the level of the lower esophagus and the cardia, and after expansion of the balloon a needle electrode that penetrate the muscular layer of the esophagus is deployed. The catheter, comprised of a balloon basket combination and four-needle delivery sheaths is positioned radially around the balloon. The distal portion of the catheter is positioned at the squamocolumnar junction. The needles are deployed at a 45° angle through the mucosa into the smooth muscle into the longitudinal muscle layer of the esophagus and cardia of the stomach. Sterile water is delivered to the base of each needle through the catheter to cool and preserve the overlying mucosa [11]. Radiofrequency energy is delivered for 90 s via a radiofrequency energy generator. The procedure is repeated for the final result of four rings in the distal LES and two in the gastric cardia.

The application of radiofrequency energy at the level of the LOS creates thermal injury, nerve ablation ant tissue remodeling leading to fibrosis, allowing a decrease in the occurrence of TLESRs and a decrease in the compliance of the GE junction as demonstrated by Richards et al. [12].

Clinical evidence of efficacy has been demonstrated. For instance, Corley et al., 2003 completed the first randomized, double-blinded, sham-controlled trial using Stretta™ that involved eight treatment centers. The sham procedure involved balloon inflation at each deployment position without needle deployment or energy delivery. Treatment subjects reported a significantly increased quality of life scores versus sham patients. Nineteen versus seven patients in the treatment and sham group respectively were without daily heartburn. There was not any statistically significant difference in daily use of proton pump inhibitors between groups at 6 months. Thirteen of thirty-five (37 %) treatment and ten out of twenty-nine (34 %) of sham subjects saw a reduction in their daily PPI use. There was no statistical difference between the two groups with respect to this outcome. Additionally, they found no difference in median esophageal acid exposure. At 6 months, 20 of the 25 remaining sham patients crossed over to active treatment and these patients then significantly improved their GERD-HRQL scores. There were no significant adverse events associated with radiofrequency energy in this trial. Moreover, there were no reports of post-procedure perforations, bleeding, or deaths.

Recent data from our institution regarding a systematic review of the literature and we found 1,441 patients, which were evaluated across 20 studies published between 2001 and 2010 [13]. The overall mean follow-up for patients in these studies was 17.1 months. GERD-HRQL scores, quality of life reflux and dyspepsia scores, heartburn and patient satisfaction scores were all improved following the Stretta procedure. Esophageal acid exposure and DeMeester score were also evaluated and overall these two variables were significantly reduced in the treatment groups.

Endoscopic Suturing and Plication

Recent advances in endoscopic suturing technology have generated a great deal of ambition to devise an endoscopic procedure that rivals the physiologic benefit of the gastroplasty created during a Nissen fundoplication. While this has yet to be accomplished there are several instrument platforms that have become available to the US market and we offer an overview of the execution, safety, and efficacy of those devices: the full-thickness Plicator™, the Bard EndoCinch System, and the EsophyX™ device.

The Plicator™

The Plicator™ also referred to in the literature as the full-thickness Plicator™ is currently owned by Ethicon Endosurgery (Sommerville, NJ, USA) and is an over-the-scope device originally created by NDO Surgical (Mansfield, MA, USA). The FDA approved The Plicator™ in 2004 for the treatment of GERD. The system is designed to create a transmural plication 1 cm distal to the GE junction, and this plication is believed to provide an additional barrier to pathologic reflux. Endoscopic full-thickness plication with the NDO can performed on an outpatient basis with minimal conscious sedation. The video endoscope is placed within the gastric lumen after performing a complete esophagogastroduodenoscopy to rule out the presence of a hiatal hernia and placement of an esophageal overtube. Following the endoscopic evaluation the scope is removed over a guidewire, and a 45-French Plicator System is threaded into the stomach over the guidewire. After that the video endoscope is placed down the endoscopic channel. Under endoscopic guidance the Plicator™ is retroflexed towards the GE junction. The Plicator™ arms are then opened and the endoscopic tissue retractor is deployed into the cardia 1 cm below the GE junction and the tissue are pulled in between the jaws. Excess endoscopic air is removed via endoscopic suction and the jaws of the plicator are closed. Lastly, a pre-tied suture is passed between the jaws of the plicator. The NDO is withdrawn from the esophagus and the endoscope is replaced into the stomach to evaluate the fundoplication. Theoretically, this plication stitch attempts to improve (i.e., tighten) or recreate the gastroesophageal valvular mechanism, which enhances the barrier to reflux at the GEJ.

Multicenter trials have evaluated the safety and efficacy of the Plicator. Investigators in a multicenter trial involving four tertiary care centers and 41 patients reported a mean operative time of 27.5 min [14]. Operative time was recorded as the amount of time to complete the plication procedure once the NDO was introduced into the stomach. In an additional multicenter trial of 61 patients, Filipi et al. evaluated the efficacy of the procedure at 3 and 6-month follow-up [15]. They demonstrated that patients had mean 6-month symptom score changes, which demonstrated procedural efficacy. Heartburn severity and frequency and regurgitation all improved significantly and 24-h pH monitoring showed improvement in number of episodes below pH of 4 at 3 and 6 months. In addition, Filipi et al. found that the percentage of total time patients experienced an esophageal pH less than

4 was reduced at 6 months [15]. Patients were randomized to receive two different linear configurations and the type of plication configuration did not affect symptoms or pH monitoring results. One patient had a self-contained gastric perforation that was successfully treated non-surgically with cessation of oral intake and antibiotics.

Pleskow et al. published a multicenter report on 64 patients with follow-up at 1 year [16]. They demonstrated a 62 % median reduction in GERD Health Related Quality of Life (GERD-HRQL) score at 6 months after the procedure when using an intent-to-treat analysis. Similarly, they saw a 61 % median reduction in GERD-HQRL at 12 months after the procedure. Overall, 74 % of patients who were taking a PPI before treatment, and after treatment 74 and 68 % were not taking a PPI at 6 and 12 months follow-up, respectively. Improvements in GERD-specific quality of life questionnaires at 1 year coupled with reduction in PPI dependence suggest that the NDO might have a sustained benefit. Pleskow et al. also analyzed the 5-year post-treatment data on 33 patients who were enrolled in the previously mentioned 12-month multicenter analysis [17]. Thirty of the thirty-three (91 %) patients required baseline daily proton-pump inhibitor pretreatment and at 5 years post-plication, 67 % (20/30) of subjects remained off daily PPI therapy. Complete PPI cessation was achieved in 10/30 (33 %) subjects. Overall treatment effect remained stable between year 3 and year 5 post-procedure, with 11 out of 28 (39 %) subjects requiring daily PPI 3 years post-procedure, compared to 12/30 (40 %) subjects at 60-months. Common post-procedural complaints include sore throat, abdominal pain and chest pain [17]. In the largest multicenter trial reported there were no major adverse events. Nonetheless, reports of gastric perforation exist in the literature. This device has demonstrated moderate clinical efficacy; however, this platform is not currently available for sale in the USA.

EndoCinch

The Bard EndoCinch System is an endoscopic suturing system (Bard Endoscopic Technologies, MA, USA) that like the Plicator™ was approved by the FDA in 2000. The EndoCinch is a device, which can be placed over the top of a standard endoscope. The suturing system includes a knot-pusher, a suturing capsule that fits onto the end of the scope, tags attached to a suture, a tag pusher and a suture cutter. Most authors' description of the Endocinch procedure includes the placement of two plications along the lesser curve of the stomach at 1 and 2 cm below the "Z"-line. The median procedure time for their trial was 45 min, and the most common post-plication complaints were sore throat, emesis, abdominal pain, chest soreness and bloating. Nonetheless, all transient post procedure complaints resolved within 72 h. The mean age for the study was 39 years. At 12 months the mean heartburn symptom score was significantly reduced from 19.22 to 7.5. Similarly, the regurgitation score reduced from a mean of 2.27 at baseline to 0.86 at 12 months. Upright acid exposure and number of reflux episodes were also significantly reduced. Use of PPIs was reduced by 64 % at one year post treatment [18].

Schwartz et al. reported a sham controlled study evaluating the EndoCinch device and at 3 months, "the percentage of patients who had reduced drug use by >50 % was greater in the active treatment group (65 %) than in the sham (25 %) or observation groups (0 %) [19]. In fact, drug use, symptom improvement, and esophageal acid exposure were all improved in the treatment group compared to the control group The active treatment effects persisted after 6 and 12 months of open-label follow-up but approximately one-third (29 %) of patients were retreated in this period. No serious adverse events occurred [19].

While a sham-controlled trial with the EndoCinch has demonstrated statistically significant improvements in GERD symptoms, medication use and quality of life at twelve-months following the procedure there was only modest improvement in esophageal acid exposure that was not statistically significant. Some authors have recommended improved suture durability as a limiting factor for this procedure [19]. One interesting factor that seemed to correlate with post-procedural success was the presence of immediate post-procedural dysphagia. In Schwartz's 12-month analysis 10 out of 60 patients had post-procedural dysphagia and those individuals were more likely to respond to treatment with an odds ratio of 13.5 [19]. Additional long-term data (5 and 10 years) is necessary to comment on the true efficacy and durability of this device and technique. Based on a compilation of the data, the device is not widely used for the treatment of reflux disease, although it is commercially available in the USA.

EsophyX™

The EsophyX™ device is the newest device in the generation of endoscopic devices marketed for the endoscopic treatment GERD (Figs. 14.1–14.3) [20]. The EsophyX™ was developed and is currently manufactured by Endogastric Solutions Inc. (Redmond, WA). The EsophyX™ device is an over the scope device which is used to create a gastroplasty which yields a fundoplication at the GEJ. Guy-Bernard Cadiere of the University of Brussels reported the first use of this device in September 2005 in an experimental clinical trial. The EsophyX™ device was created with the intention to construct a 3–5 cm valve at the GEJ with a 200–300° fundoplication [21]. Essentially, the procedure relies on the devices' ability to intussuscept the distal esophagus into the gastric fundus. Once the positioning is complete, full thickness T-fasteners are used to create a fundoplication.

The EsophyX™ procedure requires a coordinated set of steps and maneuvers, and a team of two physicians is required to operate the endoscope-implant complex. First, the patient

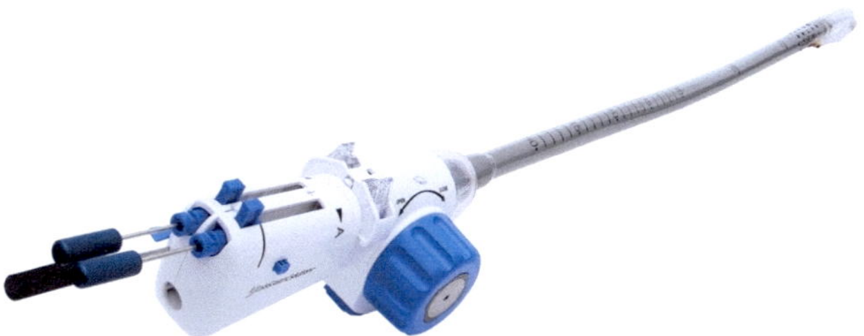

Fig. 14.1 The EsophyX™ device is the newest device in the generation of endoscopic devices marketed for the endoscopic treatment GERD. *With permission from EndoGastric Solutions, Inc.*

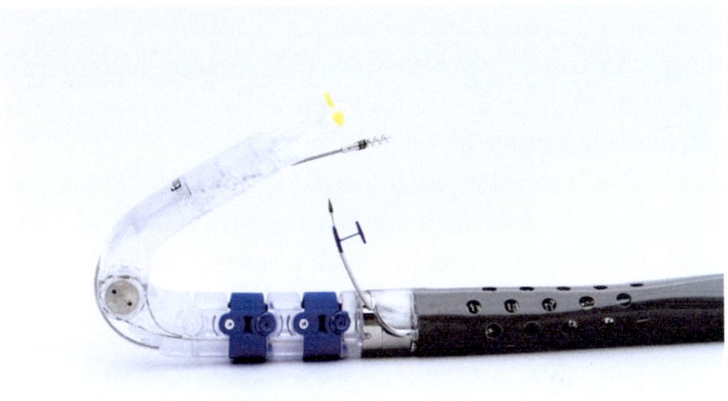

Fig. 14.2 The EsophyX™ device. Stylet. *With permission from EndoGastric Solutions, Inc.*

is placed under general nasotracheal anesthesia and then placed in the left lateral decubitus position. Next, the endoscopist operates the video-endoscope while the surgeon operates the EsophyX™ device (Fig. 14.1). The surgeon operating the EsophyX™ device will be responsible for deploying the full-thickness fasteners. Endoscopy is used to measure the distance from the Z-line to the incisors. Subsequently, the device and scope are mated and lubricated and the scope-device complex is introduced into the gastric lumen. The scope is detached from the device and the scope is retroflexed for the remaining portion of the procedure. This retroflexed position allows the endoscopist to visualize and monitor the plication maneuvers. The plication begins when the device is used to grasp the squamocolumnar junction and invaginate the GE junction using a helical tissue retractor. The gastric fundus is then retracted caudally and the mold flexes and holds tightly this tissue flap, permitting the advancement of a stylet through the flap (Fig. 14.2). Following this, the "H" fastener is deployed and this maneuver approximates the inverted gastric flap (Fig. 14.3). This procedure is repeated in a counter-clockwise fashion in order to construct a 270° omega-shaped gastroesophageal valve, which is 3–5 cm in length. A valve analogous to that created during antireflux surgery is constructed by creating full-thickness plications, semi-circumferentially around the GE junction starting on

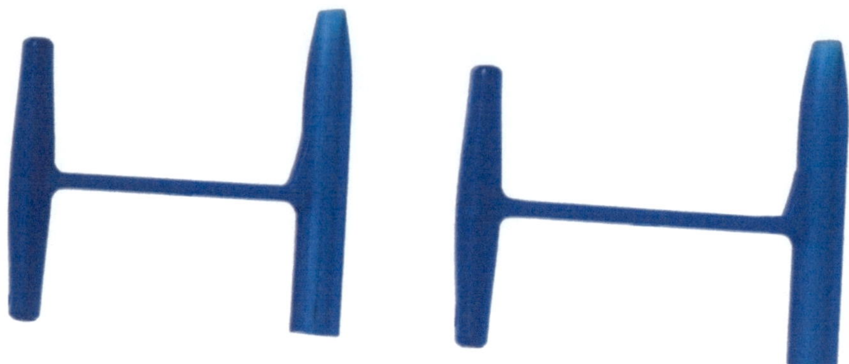

Fig. 14.3 The EsophyX™ device. "H" fasteners. *With permission from EndoGastric Solutions, Inc.*

the greater curve side of the valve [22]. Finally, the scope and device are aligned, the stomach deflated and the esophagus is inspected for iatrogenic injury.

Cadière et al. presented the initial 12-month follow-up data of a multicenter trial involving 86 patients in 2006. There were three major adverse events, which occurred during this trial, which included: two esophageal perforations during device insertion and one case of intraluminal bleeding. At 12 months 79 patients were analyzed and 73 % experienced a 50 % improvement in the GERD HRQL Scores. At one year, 85% of patients had discontinued daily PPI use while 81 % saw complete cessation of PPI use. Cadiere et al. also published 2-year data on a subset of patients from their original feasibility study which revealed a 50 % improvement in GERD-HRQL was sustained by 64 % of patients and transoral incisionless fundoplication (TIF) and that TIF was effective in eliminating heartburn and daily PPI therapy in 93 % and 71 % of patients, respectively [23]. In their analysis, TIF was effective in eliminating esophagitis in 55 % of patients. Other recent experimental clinical trials that have been reported include small series of patients reporting clinical success with few objective endpoints. Oleshlager performed TIF on 23 patients using the EsophyX device [20]. Those subjects saw a reduction in acid exposure and DeMeester scores but 11 out of 19 (57 %) remained on PPI therapy at 6 months follow-up. Demyttenaere et al. reported on the initial experience at our Institution as well, 26 pts were reported with an average follow-up of 10 months. There were significant improvements in GERD related Quality (Velonovich Scores) and symptom scores (Anvari), 65 % of patients remained on PPI [24].

Wendling et al. performed a meta-analysis, identifying 12 qualifying studies involving 358 patients evaluating the efficacy of the EsophyX device. The mean follow-up interval was 8 months and they reported that 9.4 % of patients when on to require another therapeutic procedure and 2 % of patients required PPI therapy at 9 months post-treatment [25]. This evaluation was limited by inconsistency in trial design and a paucity of long-term data regarding efficacy and durability. Significant improvement was seen in GERD related quality of life scores and in reduction of PPI usage in the

combined data. Ongoing evaluations are underway to determine long-term efficacy. A company sponsored multicenter trial is currently in process sponsored by the manufacturer to determine efficacy in GERD patients.

Future Techniques

Currently, there are several undeveloped techniques and prosthetic devices under investigation for the endoscopic/laparoscopic treatment of reflux. Ongoing advancements in technology and the understanding of the path physiology will allow clinicians and scientists the opportunity to pursue pathways that perhaps will decrease the burden of symptomatic GERD on patients.

Recently the US Food and Drug Administration has approved the use of the LINX system (Torax Medical, Minneapolis, MN) for the treatment of GERD (Fig. 14.4a–d). This device is an implantable system of independently linked magnetic beads that form a flexible ring when placed surgically around the distal esophagus. Initial data has demonstrated and excellent safety profile and a high degree of pH normalization at time intervals of one and 2 years. While just recently released for widespread clinical use, it has significant promise for an additional procedure for the treatment of reflux disease eliminating some of the troublesome side effects commonly seen with surgical fundoplication [26].

Summary

A variety of various treatment options have been tried and few are currently available. Individual clinical decisions should be made based on each patients clinical characteristics and the expertise of the treating physician and institution. Currently, Stretta and EsophyX appear to be the most well-studied options for nonsurgical intervention for the treatment of reflux. Ongoing scrutiny and review will allow further conclusions to be made to determine the precise role of various treatments for each patient.

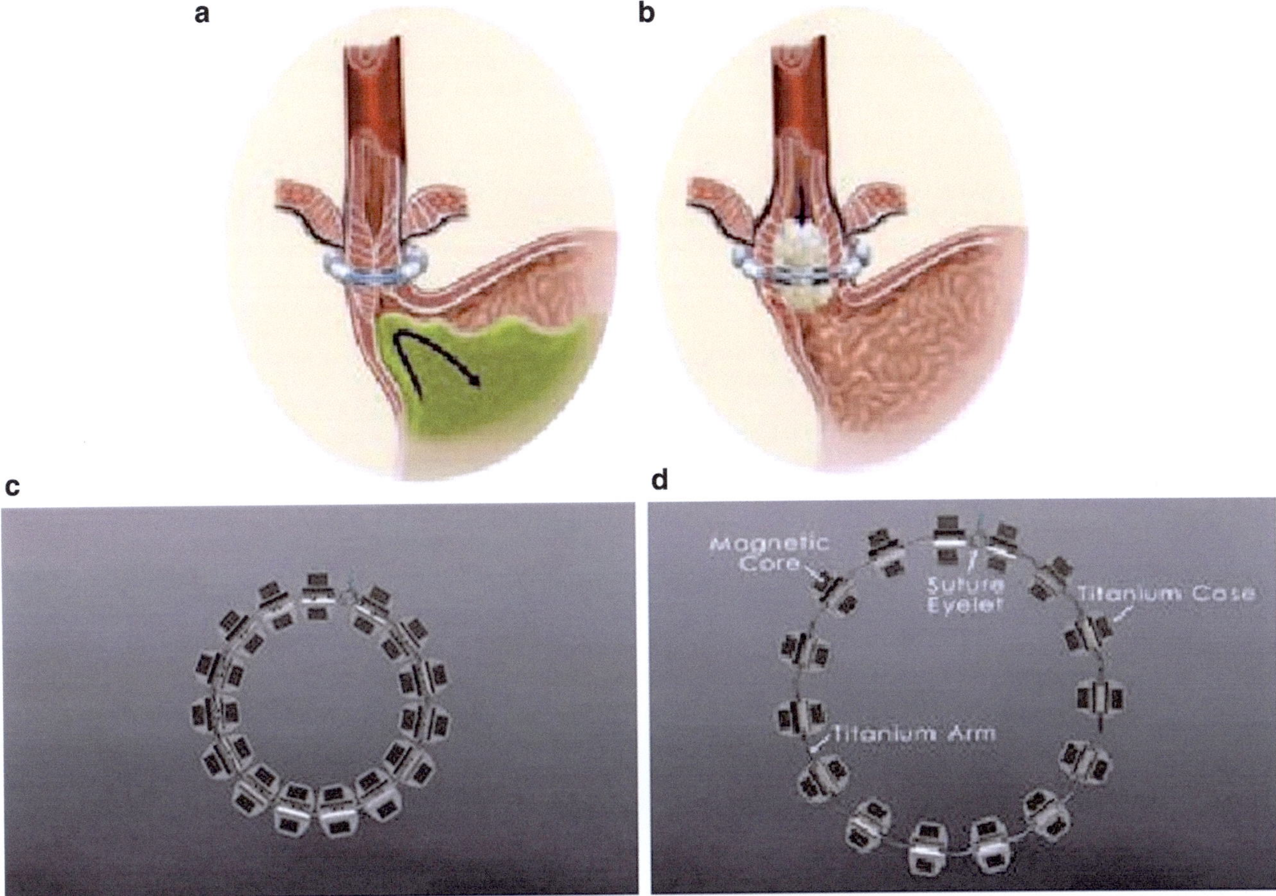

Fig. 14.4 LINX Device, an implantable system of independently linked magnetic beads that form a flexible ring when placed surgically around the distal esophagus. (**a**) LINX animation closed; (**b**) LINX animation open with bolus; (**c**) LINX closed; (**d**) LINX expanded section. *With permission from Torax Medical Inc.*

References

1. Heidelbaugh JJ, Goldberg KL, Inadomi JM. Overutilization of proton pump inhibitors: a review of cost-effectiveness and risk [corrected]. Am J Gastroenterol. 2009;104 Suppl 2:S27–32.
2. Revicki DA, Wood M, Maton PN, Sorenson S. The impact of gastroesophageal reflux disease on health-related quality of life. Am J Med. 1998;104:252–8.
3. Read RC. The contribution of Allison and Nissen to the evolution of hiatus herniorrhaphy. Hernia. 2001;5:200–3.
4. Dallemagne B, Weerts JM, Jehaes C, Markiewicz S, Lombard R. Laparoscopic Nissen fundoplication: preliminary report. Surg Laparosc Endosc. 1991;1(3):138–43.
5. Donahue PE, Carvalho P, Yoshida J, et al. Endoscopic sclerosis of the cardia affects gastroesophageal reflux. Surg Endosc. 1989;3(1):11–2.
6. Dent J, Dodds WJ, Friedman RH. Mechanism of gastroesophageal reflux in recumbent asymptomatic human subjects. J Clin Invest. 1980;65:256–67.
7. Deviere J, Pastorelli A, Louis H, de Maertelaer V, Lehman G, Cicala M, et al. Endoscopic implantation of a biopolymer in the lower esophageal sphincter for gastroesophageal reflux: a pilot study. Gastrointest Endosc. 2002;55(3):335–41.
8. Johnson DA, Ganz R, Aisenberg J, Cohen LB, Deviere J, Foley TR, et al. Endoscopic, deep mural implantation of Enteryx for the treatment of GERD: 6-month follow-up of a multicenter trial. Am J Gastroenterol. 2003;98(92):250–8.
9. Fockens P, Bruno MJ, Gabbrielli A, Odegaard S, Hatlebakk J, Allescher HD, et al. Endoscopic augmentation of the lower esophageal sphincter for the treatment of gastroesophageal reflux disease: multicenter study of the gatekeeper reflux repair system. Endoscopy. 2004;36(8):682–9.
10. Utley DS, Kim M, Vierra MA, Triadafilopoulos G. Augmentation of lower esophageal sphincter pressure and gastric yield pressure after radiofrequency energy delivery to the gastroesophageal junction: a porcine model. Gastrointest Endosc. 2000;52(1):81–6.
11. Richards WO, Houston HL, Torquati A, Khaitan L, Holzman MD, Sharp KW. Paradigm shift in the management of gastroesophageal reflux disease. Ann Surg. 2003;237(5):638–49.
12. Richards WO, Scholz S, Khaitan L, Sharp KW. Holzman Initial experience with the stretta procedure for the treatment of gastroesophageal reflux disease. J Laparoendosc Adv Surg Tech A. 2001;11(5):267–73.
13. Perry KA, Banerjee A, Melvin WS. Radiofrequency energy delivery to the lower esophageal sphincter reduces esophageal acid exposure and improves GERD symptoms: a systematic review and meta-analysis. Surg Laparosc Endosc Percutan Tech. 2012;22(4):283–8.

14. Renteln D, Schiefke I, Fuchs K, et al. Endoscopic full-thickness plication for the treatment of gastroesophageal reflux disease using multiple Plicator implants: 12-month multicenter study results. Surg Endosc. 2009;23(8):1866–75.
15. Filipi CJ, Lehman GA, Rothstein RI, et al. Transoral, flexible endoscopic suturing for treatment of GERD: a multicenter trial. Gastrointest Endosc. 2001;53(4):416–22.
16. Pleskow D, Rothstein R, Lo S, et al. Endoscopic full-thickness plication for the treatment of GERD: 12-month follow-up for the North American open-label trial. Gastrointest Endosc. 2005;61(6):643–9.
17. Pleskow D, Rothstein R, Kozarek R, et al. Endoscopic full-thickness plication for the treatment of GERD: five-year long-term multicenter results. Surg Endosc. 2008;22(2):326–32.
18. Mahmood Z, McMahon B, Arfin Q, et al. Endocinch therapy for gastro-oesophageal reflux disease: a one year prospective follow up. Gut. 2003;52(1):34.
19. Schwartz MP, Wellink H, Gooszen HG, Conchillo JM, Samsom M, Smout AJ. Endoscopic gastroplication for the treatment of gastrooesophageal reflux disease: a randomised, sham-controlled trial. Gut. 2007;56:20–8.
20. Petersen RP, Filippa L, Wassenaar EB, Martin AV, Tatum R, Oelschlager BK. Comprehensive evaluation of endoscopic fundoplication using the EsophyXTM device. Surg Endosc. 2012;26:1021–7.
21. Cadière GB, Rajan A, Rqibate M, Germay O, Dapri G, Himpens J, et al. Endoluminal fundoplication (ELF)—evolution of EsophyXTM, a new surgical device for transoral surgery. Minim Invasive Ther Allied Technol. 2006;15:348–55.
22. Cadière GB, Rajan A, Germay O, Himpens J. Endoluminal fundoplication by a transoral device for the treatment of GERD: a feasibility study. Surg Endosc. 2008;22:333–42.
23. Cadière G-B, Van Sante N, Graves JE, Gawlicka AK, Rajan A. Two-year results of a feasibility study on antireflux transoral incisionless fundoplication using EsophyX. Surg Endosc. 2009;23(5):957–64.
24. Demyttenaere SV, Bergman S, Pham T, Anderson J, Dettorre R, Melvin WS, et al. Transoral incisionless fundoplication for gastroesophageal reflux disease in an unselected patient population. Surg Endosc. 2010;24(4):854–8.
25. Wendling MR MW, Perry K. Impact of transoral incisionless fundoplication on subjective and objective GERD indices: a meta-analysis of the published literature. J Soc Am Gastrointest Endosc Surg (Unpublished data).
26. Bonavina L, DeMeester T, Fockens P, Dunn D, Saino G, Bona D, et al. Laparoscopic sphincter augmentation device eliminates reflux symptoms and normalizes esophageal acid exposure: one and two year results. Ann Surg. 2010;252(5):857–62.

Robert D. Fanelli

Introduction

The intraoperative use of flexible gastrointestinal endoscopes holds significant value for patients and surgeons alike. At its extreme, intraoperative endoscopy serves as the platform that allows for performance of novel procedures like natural orifice surgery, and endoluminal procedures such as transoral fundoplication and gastric volume reduction. While the appeal of performing advanced futuristic procedures may promote an interest in using flexible gastrointestinal endoscopes in the operating room for some surgeons, it is the use of these devices during routine operations on the gastrointestinal tract that will immediately and positively impact patient care.

Gastrointestinal (GI) endoscopy has proven a useful adjunct to abdominal operations, particularly in the setting of laparoscopic surgery. Whether it is the routine use of upper endoscopy during esophageal myotomy that helps ensure that all muscle fibers have been divided and that no perforation has occurred (Video 15.1), using intraoperative enteroscopy to locate a small bowel lesion identified on capsule endoscopy as the likely lead point for recurring intussusception, or using a gastroscope to provide a second field of view from within the stomach during laparoscopic gastric resection, flexible endoscopy has emerged as an essential component of minimally invasive gastrointestinal surgery. Even during traditional open surgery, where most surgeons have employed a variety of methods to check the

security of a newly created colonic anastomosis, intraoperative colonoscopy offers additional diagnostic yield by combining this leak check with a visual inspection of the mucosal surfaces and the anastomosis itself, providing an opportunity to diagnose and treat staple-line hemorrhage, verify the adequacy of resection, and identify retained polyps or additional pathology at a time when definitive action can be taken.

By performing intraoperative endoscopy at the time of abdominal surgery, surgeons are afforded the opportunity to immediately evaluate the surgical reconstruction. Envision performing laparoscopic gastric bypass for morbid obesity, and then relying on a contrast swallow study performed the next day to identify an anastomotic leak that could have been identified immediately using intraoperative upper endoscopy and remedied in minutes at the time of the index operation. It is likely that the routine use of endoscopy during gastrointestinal surgery will improve the clinical outcomes of the operations we perform and improve the safety of our procedures by identifying potential postoperative complications intraoperatively, allowing immediate correction, precluding their postoperative manifestation.

The following pages first outline general considerations important to performing intraoperative endoscopy, such as credentialing, equipment needs, and staff requirements, and then outline specific considerations for each of a variety of endoscopic procedures routinely performed at the time of surgery.

This chapter contains a video segment that can be found by accessing the following link: http://www.springerimages.com/videos/978-1-4614-6329-0.

Robert D. Fanelli, M.D., F.A.C.S., F.A.S.G.E. (✉)
Chief, Minimally Invasive Surgery and Surgical Endoscopy,
Department of Surgery, The Guthrie Clinic Ltd.,
One Guthrie Square, Sayre, PA 18840, USA
e-mail: rfanelli125@gmail.com

General Considerations

Training and Credentialing

Surgeons interested in performing intraoperative endoscopy should pursue education in these techniques. Formal training, whether during surgical residency, fellowship, or through appropriately structured alternative pathways are necessary to convey the knowledge and skills required to perform high quality endoscopy for patients. Complete familiarity with the endoscopic procedure to be performed, and the primary and adjunctive equipment to be utilized, is essential, and it is recommended that the operating room staff be experienced in the setup, use, aftercare, and troubleshooting of endoscopic equipment as well as the surgeon. The surgeon must have a complete understanding of the potential risks and complications of the endoscopic procedure to be performed, and must be prepared to diagnose and treat complications that might arise. Finally, surgeons performing intraoperative endoscopy should be credentialed to perform these procedures, through mechanisms that are consistent with professional society guidelines for credentialing surgeons for the performance of flexible endoscopy.

Patient Preparation and Consent

Informed consent is generally recognized as the process that surgeons use to educate patients about options for treatment and the associated risks, benefits, and alternatives. Whenever intraoperative endoscopy is likely to be used as an adjunct during a surgical procedure, it is incumbent upon the surgeon to educate the patient about the value of intraoperative endoscopy, and its potential hazards, which might include recognized or unrecognized perforation, anastomotic disruption, hemorrhage, unidentified but important lesions, adjacent organ injury, the need for surgery at a site not related to the primary operation, and disability or loss of life, among others. When intraoperative endoscopic retrograde cholangiopancreatography (ERCP) is to be utilized, additional possible risks include pancreatitis, ductal injuries, incomplete stone retrieval, stent migration, sepsis, the need for additional endoscopic, radiologic, and surgical procedures, and inability to perform the intended procedure related to cannulation failure, among others.

Since all but emergency surgical procedures are associated with patients being kept nil per os prior to surgery, it is rare that additional preparatory measures are needed for procedures that will include transoral endoscopy or even transabdominal enteroscopy. Despite an ongoing debate regarding the role of mechanical bowel preparation before colon surgery, there is little controversy that mechanical bowel preparation is necessary if the benefits of intraoperative colonoscopy are to be realized. Any standard bowel preparation typically prescribed for colonoscopy will suffice as long as its directions have been followed and the cleansing is adequate to permit visualization of the mucosal surface of the colon.

Equipment Availability

The equipment needed to perform intraoperative endoscopy generally is available in other areas of the hospital, like the GI Endoscopy unit, but should be readily accessible in the operating room both so that patient care is not delayed while the surgeon waits for the equipment to become available, and so that these additional equipment towers can be positioned appropriately at a time during the procedure that will not be disruptive to the surgeon's concentration or performance of the primary operation. During certain operations, the endoscopic equipment might be needed both at the beginning and the end of the procedure, and in others, it may be utilized during the entirety of the procedure. It is best if the facility acquires dedicated endoscopy equipment intended to service the operating rooms alone if the volume of gastrointestinal surgical procedures is sufficient to justify the cost. As a minimum, a cart outfitted with a central processing unit and video monitor, and an available upper endoscope and colonoscope will be needed to perform diagnostic intraoperative endoscopy (Fig. 15.1). Still image and video capture devices, carbon dioxide insufflation equipment, cautery and argon plasma coagulation units, and a variety of endoscopes and therapeutic accessories will round out a more reasonably outfitted mobile endoscopy unit suitable for therapeutic use in the operating room.

Insufflation

Just as working space during open surgery is created with retractors, and working space during laparoscopic surgery is created with carbon dioxide insufflation, the working space used during flexible endoscopy is created by distending the lumen of the gastrointestinal organ under examination with insufflated gas. Ordinarily, room air is introduced through the endoscope, and this can be used during intraoperative endoscopy as well. However, there has been recent enthusiasm for the use of carbon dioxide insufflation during gastrointestinal endoscopy because of more rapid absorption, less patient discomfort, and proven safety in a wide variety of patient care settings. The use of carbon dioxide insufflation for intraoperative endoscopy is recommended for the same reasons, adding the advantage that rapid absorption of carbon dioxide allows visceral decompression to occur much more rapidly than when air insufflation has been utilized. Distending segments of the gastrointestinal tract during laparoscopic surgery can compromise the laparoscopic working space needed to complete the index operation safely, and has been described as a reason for converting to open surgery. Carbon dioxide insufflation seems to lessen the risk that intestinal organs

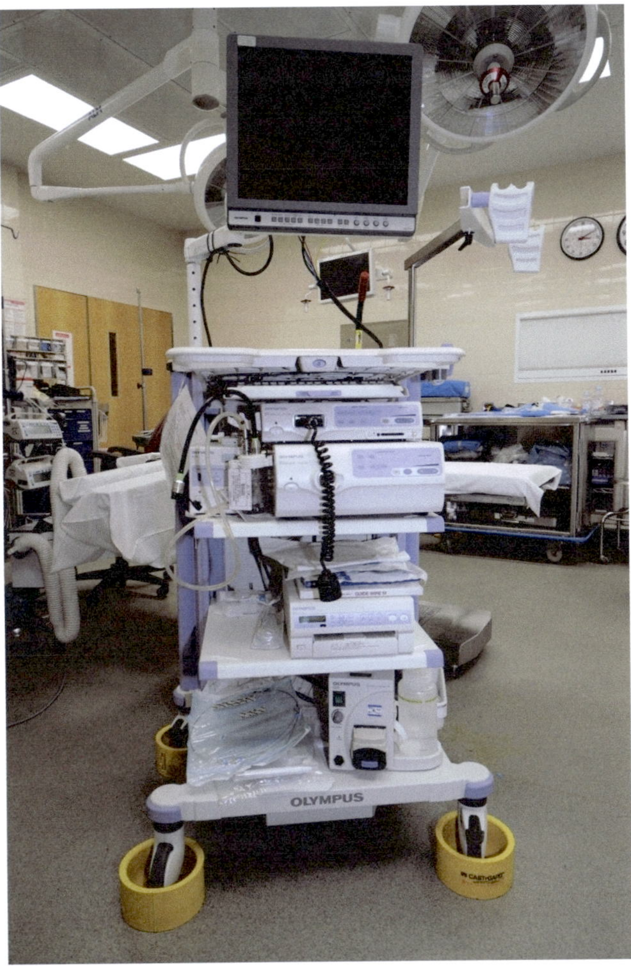

Fig. 15.1 A well appointed mobile endoscopy cart. Modern processing units (*top shelf, right*) facilitate gastrointestinal and biliary endoscopy as well as bronchoscopy. Power irrigation (*bottom shelf*), image printer (*center shelf*), and carbon dioxide insufflators (*top shelf, left*) are useful accessories. The high resolution video monitor mounted to the cart is used when image routing to remote monitors isn't practical. Note the wheel collars, useful in pushing cables and cords out of the way as the cart is advanced into position

will remain distended. Regardless of which gas is used for insufflation, care should be taken to avoid excessive distension of intestinal organs and fresh anastomoses, as high insufflation pressures might result in disruption. The proper amount of insufflation is that which results in gentle distension of an anastomosis, for example, so that when submerged in irrigant, a leak would be manifested by bubbling through the defect.

Regardless of the type of insufflation gas used for intraoperative endoscopy, it is recommended that measures be taken to limit the amount of insufflation gas used. Judicious administration of insufflation gas is always advised, using a light touch on the insufflation control of the endoscope. Mechanical devices are sometimes used to limit the portions of the gastrointestinal tract that can be insufflated. During laparoscopic foregut surgery, for example, the gentle application of a non-crushing instrument across the proximal small bowel effectively limits distal insufflation and prevents even temporary loss of abdominal working space. Some surgeons will use a linear mechanical stapler loaded with a spent cartridge to occlude the bowel. Whichever technique is utilized, care should be taken to support the instrument utilized to prevent injury.

Therapeutic Accessories

Although the majority of intraoperative endoscopy that a surgeon will perform is diagnostic in nature, intended to check an anastomosis for patency, leak, and hemorrhage, there are circumstances where adjunctive therapeutic measures will be required. Such situations include intraoperative colonoscopy intended to inspect an anastomosis, where a previously unrecognized/untreated polyp is identified, or where intraluminal hemorrhage from the anastomosis is discovered. In the former scenario, the surgeon may utilize a biopsy forceps or snare to remove the retained polyp, while in the latter, the surgeon may choose to place an endoscopic clip on the bleeding staple line. Another chapter in this text reviews these adjunctive tools and their uses in great detail, but the surgeon performing intraoperative endoscopy should become familiar with a broad armamentarium of endoscopic devices and be ready to deploy them when necessary. Similarly, operating room staff should maintain a level of practical familiarity as well, and as a minimum, should maintain a ready supply of bite blocks, biopsy forceps, polypectomy snares, endoscopic clips, and injection needles. Surgeons planning to perform intraoperative ERCP and other advanced procedures will need ready access to these devices as well as sphincterotomes, guidewires, dilation balloons, biliary stone balloons, baskets, and stents. Finally, performing intraoperative ERCP, stenting, and other advanced procedures will require ready access to fluoroscopic imaging equipment.

Endoscope Reprocessing

Endoscopes require immediate rinsing and cleansing after use to maintain functionality, ensure a long service life, and limit the transmission of infectious agents to subsequent patients, and those endoscopes used to perform intraoperative endoscopy are no exception. Intraoperative endoscopy often occurs at the end of a surgical procedure, when preparations for closing, instrument counts, anesthetic reversal, rooming arrangements, etc., are commencing. Because flexible endoscopes should be rinsed and cleansed soon after use, it is important to ensure that operating room staff is able to irrigate the endoscope immediately, and that reprocessing procedures will be implemented in a timely manner. After reprocessing, endoscopes should be stored hanging on a specifically designed rack, buttons and caps removed, situated where they are unlikely to become soiled or contaminated. Some guidelines suggest that endoscopes that aren't utilized frequently be reprocessed again before use. Many hospitals find it most efficient to maintain an equipment tower and frequently used supplies in the operating room but to store all endoscopes together in their main endoscopy units, where they are cycled through use, reprocessing, and maintenance routines in aggregate. Calling for an endoscope before the start of the surgical procedure then becomes a routine part of the room setup for surgery.

Physician Staffing

Single Surgeon

Intraoperative endoscopy can most often be performed quite efficiently by the operating surgeon, but there are circumstances where a second surgeon, or a gastroenterologist, might be called to assist with performing intraoperative endoscopy. Generally speaking, when intraoperative endoscopy is used as a checkpoint at the end of the surgical procedure, e.g., during laparoscopic colectomy where colonoscopy is used to verify the integrity of the anastomosis, the operating surgeon will face little difficulty in providing this service alone. After having completed the resection and anastomosis, the surgeon will submerge the intestinal anastomosis in a pool of irrigant, and then have an assistant maintain an appropriate view of this area while the surgeon introduces the colonoscope, inspects the anastomosis visually for hemorrhage and signs of ischemia, and tests its integrity with gentle insufflation. Once satisfied that the anastomosis is proper, the surgeon decompresses the colon as the colonoscope is withdrawn, and the endoscope is rinsed and reprocessed by staff while the surgeon replaces gown and gloves and returns to the operative field to complete the procedure.

Two Surgeons

There are circumstances where it is desirable to have a colleague join the team performing surgery to provide an endoscopic service that will serve as another significant portion of the procedure. For example, during laparoscopic resection of a gastrointestinal stromal tumor (GIST) of the gastric fundus, it is essential to ensure that the gastric resection will not compromise the esophagogastric junction. Having a colleague skilled in flexible endoscopy place the gastroscope

early in the operation enhances surgery since the gastroscope provides a real-time intragastric view of the procedure while the laparoscope provides the extraluminal intraabdominal view of the operation. This coordinated effort affords the surgeon additional information by providing an otherwise unattainable endoluminal view, and provides a mechanism for immediately assessing the completeness of resection, staple line hemorrhage, and leak-free closure all while assuring that the esophagogastric junction is not compromised.

Intraoperative ERCP is a procedure that sometimes is performed by the operating surgeon who is trained in this advanced procedure, but often is performed by another surgeon, or a gastroenterologist, while the primary surgeon maintains operative exposure. Although the technical aspects of rendezvous ERCP are discussed later in this chapter, envision the operating surgeon passing a guidewire through the cystic duct opening created for cholangiography, and the surgeon-endoscopist grasping that guidewire with an instrument deployed through the duodenoscope used for ERCP once the wire exits the duodenum's major papilla. This virtually ensures selective cannulation of the common bile duct, often difficult in a supine patient with an insufflated abdomen, and facilitates sphicterotomy, stone removal, stent placement, and other therapeutic measures. Both roles in such a procedure require unique and complementary skills, and rarely can this procedure be accomplished in this manner by a single surgeon. ERCP or remnant gastroscopy in the setting of prior Roux-en-Y gastric bypass is another example where having a second surgeon involved is useful. In this situation, one surgeon will access the gastric remnant and limit the potential for spillage, while the other performs transabdominal remnant gastroscopy or ERCP.

Residents and Fellows

Intraoperative endoscopy represents an excellent opportunity for residents and fellows to hone their endoscopic skills and supplement the experiences they garner in the inpatient and outpatient endoscopy units. Whether the resident or fellow assigned to the index operation breaks out to perform the endoscopic portion, remains at the field while the attending surgeon performs the endoscopy, or a second resident or fellow is called to the operating room to perform the endoscopic portion of the procedure, the experience gained will ensure that the use of intraoperative endoscopy becomes a standard portion of GI operations performed in that resident or fellow's career.

Specific Considerations

Planning for intraoperative endoscopy begins during the preoperative patient visit, where the approach is discussed and consent obtained. It is helpful to specify the need for the endoscopic tower and scopes, other specialty equipment and dedicated staff, when booking the procedure so that there are no delays in rounding up necessary equipment or preparing OR staff on the day of surgery. As the room is prepared and instrumentation opened for the planned operation, the endoscopic equipment tower should be positioned such that it easily can be rolled into place for use during the appropriate phase of the procedure, minimizing the need to rearrange equipment carts and booms. Given the increasing numbers of cords and cables in today's operating rooms, collars placed around the wheels of the endoscopy cart often prove useful by pushing cords ahead of the wheels as the cart is advanced toward the operative field.

Endoscope selection is based on the anatomical region of the targeted pathology, and the portal of entry that will be used to introduce the endoscope. Table 15.1 lists the range of insertion tube diameters and working lengths for endoscopes manufactured by major suppliers, and suggests appropriate uses for intraoperative endoscopy. For example, a typical gastroscope has a working length of about 100 cm, provides a forward view, and is useful in accessing the esophagus, stomach, and duodenum when introduced transorally. A duodenoscope might seem an interchangeable alternative, but its specialty lens orientation provides a side view useful only during ERCP, essentially limiting its use to this one procedure. When deeper small bowel penetration is needed, the surgeon may select an enteroscope or a pediatric colonoscope for transoral use, or may choose to place an endoscope transabdominally via enterotomy. Familiarity with the equipment available at your institution, and your facility's ability to present a sterile endoscope to your operative field for transabdominal placement, is essential to considering your options in devising an endoscopic access plan for any operation where intraoperative endoscopy is planned.

Proper placement of the flexible endoscopy tower is essential to the smooth performance of intraoperative endoscopy. Equipment placement is eased somewhat in integrated operating rooms, where appropriate cabling and image routing switches present the endoscopic image for display on any monitor in the room, but preserving ergonomics and a functional arrangement remain essential. A final consideration in room setup is patient positioning. The section below reviews equipment placement, patient and endoscopist positioning, unique anesthetic considerations, and other specific concerns related to the endoscopic access route chosen.

Transoral Access Procedures

Transoral access procedures are those where the endoscope will be introduced through the patient's mouth to facilitate thoracic or abdominal gastrointestinal operations. Examples include esophagectomy, myotomy for treatment of Zenker's diverticulum or achalasia, antireflux surgery, weight loss surgery, and cholecystectomy complicated by choledocholithiasis among others.

To facilitate transoral endoscopy, the endoscopy cart should be positioned either at the head, just off the patient's left shoulder where the cart is adjacent to the anesthesia provider, or directly across from the patient's right upper arm when tucked at the side (Fig. 15.2a, b). The former cart position is most useful when an integrated operating room allows image placement on remote monitors, while the latter is preferred when the monitor on top of the endoscopy cart will be viewed by the endoscopist. Although not essential, it is often useful to tuck the patient's arms bilaterally at their sides, in order to create free space for the equipment and the endoscopist.

After the patient is anesthetized, securing the endotrachial tube to the right side of the patient's mouth allows smooth passage of the endoscope from the left, where the endoscopist will stand. The endoscope is then advanced over the tongue into the esophagus under direct vision, and advanced into the esophagus while gentle insufflation is provided. In intubated patients, passage of the endoscope sometimes requires forward flexion of the head and neck, jaw thrust, or partial deflation of the endotrachial tube balloon. Whenever transoral endoscopy is performed in an intubated patient, it is important to ensure that the endotrachial tube remains secure. Additionally, esophageal temperature probes, nasogastric tubes, and other orally or nasally placed devices should be removed before introducing the endoscope whenever feasible. This is especially important in procedures where mechanical stapling devices will be deployed, such as in gastric bypass surgery, where endoscope advancement could displace one of these devices distally, where entrapment within a staple line might occur.

Transoral intraoperative endoscopy can be employed during any foregut procedure. For example, consider laparoscopic Roux-en-Y gastric bypass for weight reduction, where leak testing constitutes an important adjunctive procedure. In the example video, a small staple line defect is identified during leak testing that is easily remedied by placement of a single suture (Video 15.2). However, left undiagnosed, this small leak would have proven troublesome clinically, and would have surely resulted in a return trip to the operating room.

Anastomotic leak testing is conducted by introducing insufflation gas into the area in question while that area is submerged under saline irrigant. If the anastomosis is intact, the viscera will distend and no bubbling will occur. If there is a leak, bubbling will be seen as in the example video, and as the fluid is slowly suctioned away, the area of the leak is exposed so that definitive management strategies can be applied. Insufflation should be applied gently, as overzealous inflation of any freshly created anastomosis will result in bubbling, and could result in mechanical disruption.

Transoral intraoperative endoscopy is used for more than just leak testing, although that one technique alone justifies its use in all foregut operations where an anastomosis is created. During gastric resection, the endoscope provides an

Table 15.1 Insertion tube diameters and working lengths for commonly available endoscopes, with suggested anatomical targets and appropriate uses for intraoperative endoscopy

Type of scope	Typical diameter (mm)	Working length (cm)	Accessible anatomy			Operations where useful
			Transoral	Transabdominal	Transanal	
Choledochoscope	2.8–3.4	190	n/a	Biliary tree	n/a	Common bile duct exploration
Gastroscope	5.1–12.9	92–110	Esophagus Stomach Duodenum	Small bowel, limited to 60–80 cm segments	Rectum Sigmoid colon	Esophageal, gastric surgery; resection, myotomy, fundoplication, weight loss surgery, enteral access
Duodenoscope	10.8–12.1	125	Duodenum	Duodenum	n/a	ERCP
Enteroscope	9.2	200	Esophagus Stomach Duodenum Proximal jejunum	Jejunum Ileum	n/a	Small bowel resection
Pediatric colonoscope	11.5–11.8	130–170	Esophagus Stomach Duodenum Proximal jejunum	Jejunum Ileum	Rectum Entire colon Terminal ileum	Small bowel resection Colon resection Rectal resection
Colonoscope	12.8–13.7	130–170	n/a	n/a	Rectum Entire colon Terminal ileum	Colon resection Rectal resection
Sigmoidoscope	11.3–13.2	70	n/a	n/a	Rectum Sigmoid colon	Rectal resection Sigmoid colon resection

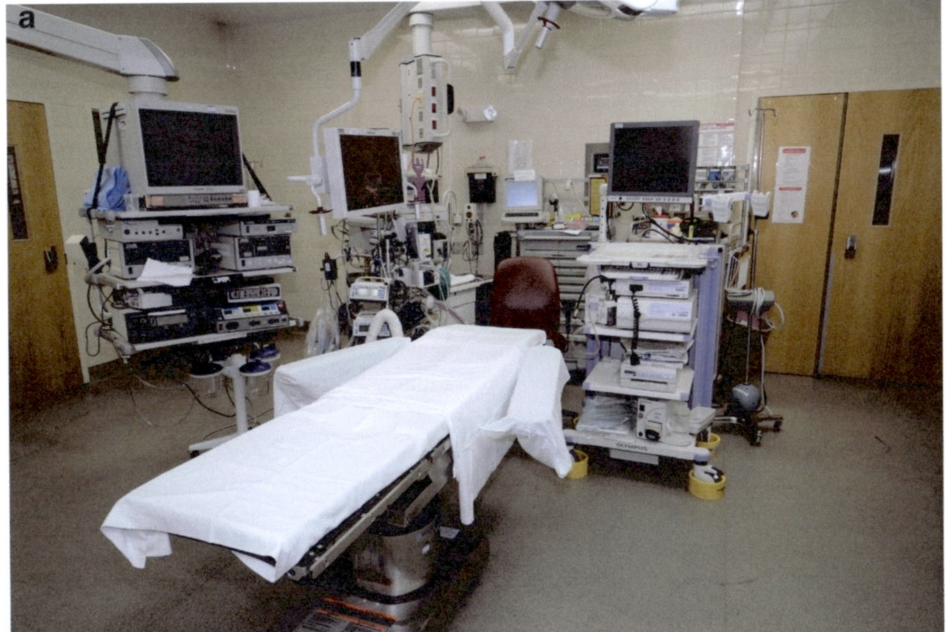

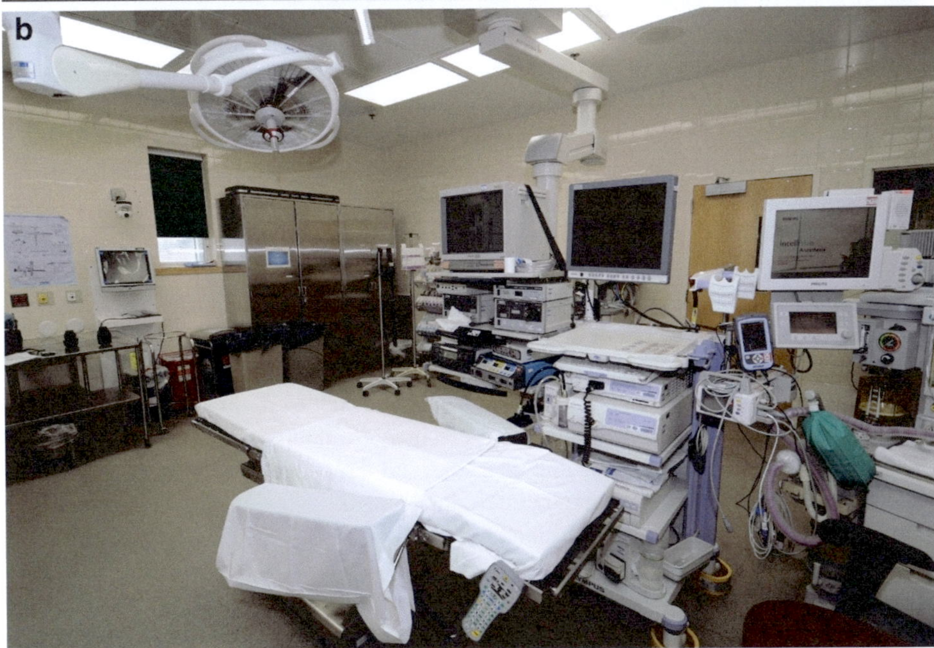

Fig. 15.2 (**a**) Transoral endoscopy. When routing images to remote monitors in an integrated operating room, placing the mobile endoscopy tower left of the patient's head reproduces the same efficiencies of the endoscopy unit. Note the remote monitor above the patient's right arm, visible to the endoscopist standing on the patient's left. (**b**) Transoral endoscopy. When image routing is not available, the mobile endoscopy cart is placed adjacent to the patient's right upper arm, and the endoscope itself is passed across the patient's chest to the endoscopist, standing left of the operating platform

alternate view from within the stomach. When resecting small benign specimens, these can be placed within a laparoscopic specimen retrieval pouch, which is then grasped with an endoscopic snare introduced through the gastroscope, and removed transorally, obviating the need to enlarge an abdominal wall incision for specimen removal. In the case of choledocholithiasis, intraoperative ERCP provides the surgeon with another management option, in addition to intraoperative laparoscopic

endobiliary stenting as a bridge to postoperative ERCP, transabdominal choledochoscopy, laparoscopic common bile duct exploration, conversion to open common bile duct exploration, or expectant management.

In performing intraoperative ERCP, the endoscopic equipment tower is most often placed above the patient's left shoulder, as shown in Fig. 15.2a. ERCP is ordinarily performed with the patient in a left lateral or prone position, but intraoperative ERCP introduces the additional challenges associated with performing ERCP in the supine patient. Experienced biliary endoscopists will notice the subtle changes required in their stance, and their grip of the duodenoscope control head, in order to reproduce a more normal view of the biliary papilla. Cannulation can be achieved freehand, as during ordinary ERCP performed in the endoscopy suite for other patients, where a cannulatome or sphincterotome is used to gain access to the bile duct orifice, and then a guidewire is deployed to maintain access and serve as the route of introduction for stone balloons, baskets, stents, and other instruments commonly advanced over a guidewire.

Alternatively, cannulation can be assisted by using the rendezvous technique, which often improves the time required for transoral intraoperative ERCP. In this method, a 450 cm guidewire is passed through the cystic duct opening that was used for cholangiography by the surgeon, often through the cholangiogram catheter that now has been advanced into the common bile duct. The guidewire is passed across the biliary papilla, into the field of view of the endoscopist who has already placed the transoral duodenoscope in position for ERCP. The endoscopist will then grasp the wire with an endoscopic snare, withdraw the guidewire into the endoscope and out through the cap of the working channel, and will then advance a sphincterotome over the wire until it achieves a secure yet temporary position within the distal common bile duct. At this point, because traditional guidewires have one soft, floppy end that protects the delicate biliary ductal mucosa and bile duct wall from injury, and one end that is stiff and unfinished, the guidewire must be reversed before it can be used for instrument exchanges. Once the sphincterotome has been advanced over the guidewire, the wire itself is withdrawn from the duodenoscope through the sphincterotome and reversed so that the soft flexible tip will now constitute the point of advancement as it is replaced into the common bile duct and advanced into the common hepatic duct to facilitate the remainder of the ERCP. An alternative is the use of double-ended guidewires, specially constructed so that each end is finished with a soft, flexible leader.

Once appropriately positioned, the guidewire serves as the track upon which the sphincterotome and other instruments will be advanced into position. In cases where intraoperative ERCP is intended to facilitate clearance of common bile duct stones, a sphincterotomy is then created, and stone balloons or baskets deployed over the guidewire in exchange for the sphincterotome to remove ductal stones. When ERCP is intended to address a bile leak, and is performed either in recognition of ductal injury during the index operation, or more likely, at the time of laparoscopic washout for a bile leak associated with an incompletely sealed Luschka duct, biliary stenting usually is the primary aim, and sphincterotomy is not typically required. In this case, once the guidewire has been positioned accordingly, the stent assembly is advanced until appropriate positioning has been confirmed endoscopically and fluoroscopically, and stent deployment accomplished. There are many different types of stents on the market, and the endoscopist is advised to arrange that an adequate variety of devices and sizes is made available at the facility where intraoperative ERCP will be performed.

Transoral enteroscopy often is used to inspect the proximal small bowel, in order to localize lesions identified during radiographic studies or during wireless capsule endoscopy. The gastroscope rarely provides visualization beyond the ligament of Treitz, even in the supine, anesthetized patient. Additional lengths of small bowel can be inspected if a dedicated enteroscope or pediatric colonoscope is introduced transorally. Enteroscopes typically are used with an overtube, and many newer enteroscopes utilize single or double balloon techniques for advancement. These devices use one or two balloons, inflated and deflated in sequence to provide traction on the small bowel so that intestinal loops can be straightened and coiled onto the shaft of the overtube and/or endoscope as it is advanced, facilitating deeper inspection. These techniques are often performed using fluoroscopy in the endoscopy suite, but in the operating room, laparoscopic or open visualization affords the endoscopist direct visual feedback that usually is inferred through fluoroscopy. Advancement can stretch the intestinal wall, mesentery, and adjacent ligamentous attachments or adhesions to other viscera, including solid organs, where even normally encountered forces could disrupt capsular or mesenteric structures and result in hemorrhage. As an enteroscope is passed transorally, it can be helpful to have the surgeon gently place the small bowel on to the enteroscope as it is advanced, using atraumatic laparoscopic forceps, to limit the force applied to these tissues (Video 15.3). Despite these techniques, rarely is it possible to advance transoral devices beyond the upper third to upper half of the small intestine's total length.

Transabdominal Access Procedures

Transabdominal placement of endoscopic instruments is useful when the gastrointestinal anatomy has been altered such that oral access to a specific region or structure is no longer possible, or when a portion of the GI tract that cannot be reached endoscopically from the mouth is the target of diagnostic or therapeutic measures. Examples that are discussed include ERCP after gastric bypass or ulcer surgery, choledochoscopy to facilitate common bile duct exploration, and enteroscopy where the targeted region is beyond the proximal third of the small bowel.

The equipment tower most often is placed behind the endoscopist, off his/her right hip, much as it is positioned in the endoscopy suite (Fig. 15.3). When utilizing transabdominal intraoperative endoscopy, the endoscopist will almost

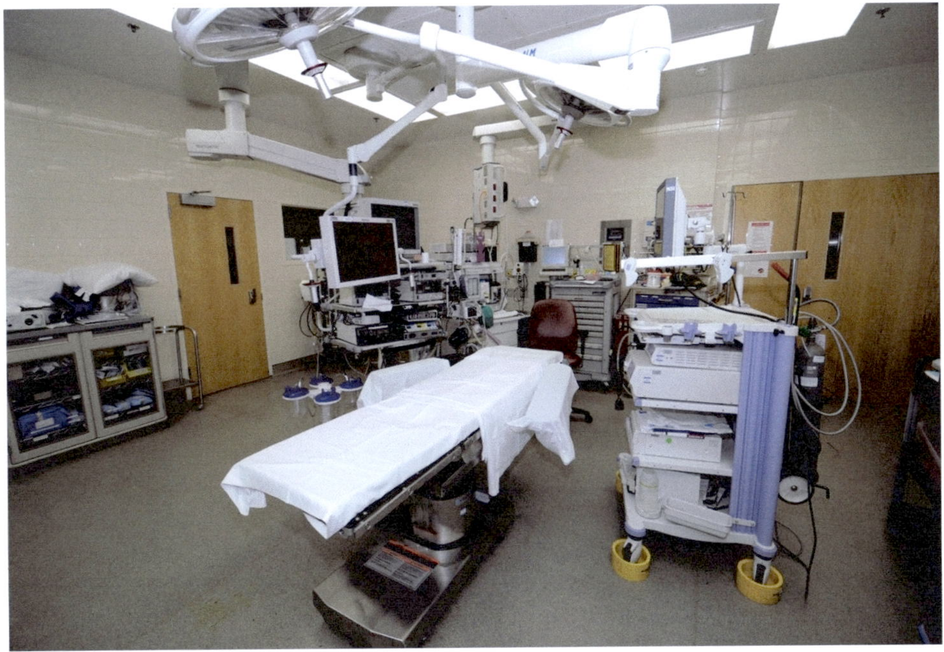

Fig. 15.3 Transabdominal endoscopy. Intraoperative transabdominal endoscopy is facilitated by placing the mobile endoscopy cart left of the patient, just off the endoscopist's hip. Image routing is important during transabdominal procedures, but when unavailable, the endoscopy cart can be rotated to face the endoscopist. Placing the endoscopy cart to the patient's right and delivering the endoscope across the operative field is not recommended

always stand on the supine patient's left side. Routing the image to additional monitors is very useful, as delivering the endoscope across the operative field from a tower placed opposite the endoscopist is cumbersome, and often interferes with proper conduct of the operative portion of the surgical procedure. When image routing isn't an option, positioning the endoscopy cart off the surgeon's left hip, turned slightly to face the endoscopist who rotates his/her stance slightly to the left, facilitates right-handed endoscope advancement.

Transabdominal endoscopy requires no particular anesthetic considerations aside from those germane to the primary surgical procedure. Although it is recommended that carbon dioxide insufflation be considered for use during almost all intraoperative endoscopic procedures, its use is particularly important in transabdominal enteroscopy in order to reduce the likelihood that operative domain will be lost to small bowel distension.

Roux-en-Y reconstruction after gastric bypass surgery, and to a lesser extent Billroth II reconstruction after gastrectomy for benign and malignant diseases, effectively precludes performance of transoral ERCP in all but the most occasional of circumstances. While there are series of successful transoral ERCP in anatomically altered patients reported by expert endoscopists at specialty centers, most surgeons provide access to the GI tract for placement of the duodenoscope, or in rare cases a gastroscope, in patients lacking normal transpyloric access to the biliary papilla.

The most likely scenario where surgeons will assist with intraoperative ERCP is in patients who have undergone Roux-en-Y gastric bypass for weight loss. A common approach to ERCP in this patient population will be for the surgeon to create a gastrotomy centered within a purse-string suture on the anterior gastric wall that permits endoscopic access to the remnant stomach. The sterile duodenoscope can be introduced directly through a skin incision into the gastrotomy, or can be placed through a 15 mm laparoscopic port that traverses both the abdominal and gastric walls, that can also serve to direct this side-viewing endoscope toward the pylorus.

Alternatively, scopes undergoing high level disinfection can be placed into a sterile camera bag affixed to the laparoscopic port to help minimize contamination. Balloon-tipped laparoscopic ports are particularly useful in this setting.

Once ERCP and its adjunctive measures have been performed to address the needs of the patient, the gastrotomy is managed either with stapled or sutured closure, or with the placement of a gastrostomy tube in this location. The former approach, stapling the gastrotomy closed using a linear stapler cutter, is preferred by patients when additional access to the stomach or biliary tree is not likely. Leaving a gastrostomy tube in place, while less acceptable to many patients, provides a reliable portal of entry that can be used for subsequent endoscopic procedures by removing the tube and dilating the tract once it has matured. In patients who undergo ERCP for the treatment of choledocholithiasis, further need for access is unlikely, and definitive closure of the gastrotomy is advantageous. However, if a biliary or pancreatic stent has been placed that will require removal, or if transabdominal endoscopy was undertaken to evaluate and treat GI bleeding from the remnant stomach or duodenal bulb, for example, the placement of a gastrostomy tube is useful in that it permits easier access to this excluded portion of the GI tract during the follow-up endoscopic procedures that likely will be required.

Another approach to ERCP that is useful in some patients after Roux-en-Y reconstruction is placement of the endoscope through an enterotomy in the terminus of the biliopancreatic limb at the jejunojejunostomy. Whereas placing the endoscope transabdominally into the gastric remnant requires an incision high on the left anterior axillary line closely abutting the costal margin, access through the jejunojejunostomy is accomplished with an incision in the left mid-clavicular line, just below the level of the umbilicus. Once a jejunal enterotomy is created within a purse-string suture at the tip of the defunctionalized segment of the biliopancreatic limb, the sterile endoscope can be introduced directly, or through a 15 mm laparoscopic port. When performing ERCP in this fashion, it is sometimes possible to use a forward viewing endoscope, like a standard gastroscope, since the biliary papilla is visualized head-on from this direction, differing from the usual angle encountered with the standard transpyloric approach. While the forward viewing gastroscope lends an ease of insertion with this approach, what is sacrificed is the use of the elevator, a device on the side viewing duodenoscope that affords dynamic control of endoscopic tools through deflection, aiding cannulation. The experienced endoscopist should select the endoscopic devices most likely to yield a successful outcome when assembling a treatment plan for any particular patient.

Historically, the most common method of intraoperative endoscopy employed for visualization of the biliary tree has been choledochoscopy, not intraoperative ERCP. Since the advent of laparoscopic cholecystectomy, and the increasingly reliable results of postoperative ERCP, surgeons have performed fewer common bile duct explorations and have used choledochoscopy much less frequently than when open cholecystectomy was the norm. Still, choledochoscopy remains an important skill for surgeons to master. Choledochoscopes are placed transabdominally, typically through a laparoscopic port in the epigastrium, although advancement through right upper quadrant ports also is useful. Once across the abdominal wall, the choledochoscope is advanced into the biliary tree using one of two available approaches, placement through the cystic duct incision used for cholangiography, or through a choledochotomy. Unlike traditional GI endoscopy that relies on gas insufflation to provide a working space and visualization, the working space of the choledochoscope is provided by the infusion of fluid supplied to the scope by sterile tubing with an on/off roller valve or stopcock attached to a bag of dextrose-free intravenous saline solution suspended near the operative field.

When choledochoscopy is performed through a cystic duct incision, angulation of the cystic duct common bile duct junction often limits inspection to more distal portions of the biliary tree. Access typically requires cystic duct dilation; vascular and biliary dilation balloons are equally useful. Visualized stones may be flushed from the duct. Irrigating the common bile duct with a small volume of 1 % lidocaine without epinephrine, and concomitant intravenous administration of up to 1 mg of glucagon, may improve success by relaxing the papilla. Papillary dilation, using a balloon with a diameter no greater than that of the distal common bile duct itself, may further aid flushing stones into the duodenum but can be associated with postoperative pancreatitis. Common bile duct stones may be removed very efficiently using ureteral stone baskets introduced through the working channel of the choledochoscope, under direct endoscopic vision. In this scenario, the choledochoscope is removed with each stone, and replaced after the stone is cleared from the basket, to be deployed again and again in this fashion until all stones have been cleared.

Transabdominal transcholedochal choledochoscopy is performed by introducing the choledochoscope through a surgical incision in the common bile duct. This approach is reserved for patients with a dilated, distended common bile duct and for surgeons skilled in laparoscopic suturing, required to close the duct securely without narrowing it, or for those choosing conversion to open surgery to remove common bile duct stones. Choledochotomy can be performed with or without the use of lateral stay sutures, but when used, small caliber monofilament suture is advised to reduce the sawing effect of braided suture material as it is pulled through the duct wall. When stay sutures are utilized, delivering them through the abdominal wall rather than through a laparoscopic port is useful, as they may then be suspended by their attachment to the abdominal wall, and their tension adjusted with the application of an externally applied hemostat.

It is often helpful to use a drainage needle, the type used to decompress an acutely inflamed and distended gallbladder, to puncture the anterior wall of the common bile duct at the inferiormost position of the planned choledochotomy, taking care to avoid penetration through the posterior wall of the duct or puncture of vascular structures such as the portal vein. The choledochotomy can then be extended superiorly from that puncture site using endoscopic scissors. The size of the choledochotomy, which is most often oriented along the long axis of the common bile duct, must accommodate removal of the largest stone identified but should be limited to the shortest length possible. Once the choledochoscope is advanced into the common bile duct, the same patterns of use identified above will be applied, although when choledochotomy has been employed for entry, it usually is because the stones identified on cholangiography are too large to be flushed from the ductal system, or retrieved through the cystic duct, require direct stone basket retrieval, or are positioned proximal to the cystic duct common bile duct junction.

Choledochoscopy by either route is often accompanied by intraoperative use of fluoroscopy, and after clearance of ductal stones, a completion cholangiogram should be performed before proceeding with cholecystectomy to ensure that all stones have been recovered. When a cystic duct incision has been utilized for choledochoscopy, standard ductal closure techniques are employed. When choledochotomy has been used for choledochoscopy, monofilament self-resorbing suture closure is performed, ensuring that knots are placed outside the ductal lumen, and that the closure is secure and leak free. Laparoscopically placed endobiliary stents and closed suction drains placed adjacent to the choledochotomy, have been advocated by some while others have reported success without using either when all stones have been cleared.

Widespread use of wireless capsule endoscopy has resulted in increasingly frequent identification of small bowel pathology, some of which requires surgical treatment. Patients diagnosed with small bowel neoplasia, sites of occult blood loss, strictures and stenoses, among others, now more commonly present for surgical treatment. Intraoperative localization of these lesions through liberal use of intraoperative enteroscopy has become a mainstay of GI surgery practices treating patients diagnosed using wireless capsule endoscopy. As discussed above, transoral enteroscopy rarely permits visualization of more than the upper jejunum; transabdominal enteroscopy is often more useful.

When performing transabdominal enteroscopy, it is most useful to introduce the enteroscope through a free portion of the mid small bowel, such as mid-jejunum. While wireless capsule endoscopy rarely identifies the exact location of identified pathology, consulting with the interpreting physician is helpful, as those experienced in reading these studies often can direct surgeons to the general segment of small bowel involved. The enteroscope is usually introduced through an incision in the anterior axillary line, at the level of the umbilicus, on the patient's left. While a 15 mm laparoscopic port can be used, it is often easier to manipulate the enteroscope, gastroscope, or pediatric colonoscope if it is introduced directly through the abdominal wall into the small bowel, through a purse string suture. Carbon dioxide insufflation provides the optimal balance between the visualization and rapid absorption required for intraoperative enteroscopy.

The endoscope selected, often a pediatric colonoscope, is advanced first proximally, and then distally, inspecting for pathology. A non-crushing bowel clamp applied ahead of the endoscope is useful to limit bowel distension with insufflated gas, and can be repositioned as necessary during the procedure. During insertion, laparoscopic instruments can be used to advance loops of small bowel onto the endoscope to facilitate deeper inspection, but care should be exercised both to guard against serosal disruptions from handling the small bowel, and from inadvertent bowel or organ injury from laparoscopically or surgically deployed instruments when the focus shifts to intraoperative endoscopy. Instruments present in the abdominal space, including the laparoscope, can prove hazardous as the bowel distends with insufflation gas and is manipulated, often outside the field of view of the laparoscope, and although uncommon, unrecognized injury could occur. Removing instruments that aren't necessary for this phase of the procedure, diligently inspecting and testing for injuries at the conclusion of the endoscopic phase, maintaining a heightened level of awareness for deviations from the usual postoperative recovery trajectory, and exercising great caution when employing new techniques all are advised to deliver the safe surgical experience expected by patients and surgeons alike.

When pathology is identified, the decision must be made as to whether this will be addressed primarily by using endoscopic measures, such as snare polypectomy or cautery ablation, or by using surgical measures, such as resection or stricturoplasty, for example. Regardless, it is often helpful to place a suture on the serosal surface of the small bowel immediately adjacent to the pathologic lesion identified while decisions are made about definitive therapy. Once polypectomy, cautery, resection, stricturoplasty, or whatever particular technique demanded by the clinical circumstance has been completed, the enteroscope is withdrawn slowly, allowing the loops of small bowel to fall off the scope gently, removing insufflation gas along the way, and inspecting for additional pathology. Once the examination is completed, the enteroscope is removed for reprocessing, and the enterotomy is closed using traditional surgical methods.

Transanal Access Procedures

The transanal endoscopic approach is used during rectal and colonic surgery, or during performance of related surgical procedures like reversal of a diverting ileostomy or colostomy. Procedures where intraoperative colonoscopy is useful include segmental colon resection, anterior resection of the rectum, and other hindgut procedures where an anastomosis is created or the intraoperative localization of pathology is useful. Despite ongoing debate about the necessity of mechanical bowel preparation before colon and rectal surgery, an effective preoperative bowel preparation is required of patients who are considered candidates for intraoperative colonoscopy as a component of their surgical procedure. One notable caveat is the patient with extensive acute gastrointestinal bleeding who presents for emergent colon resection, where the cathartic nature of blood often provides a very

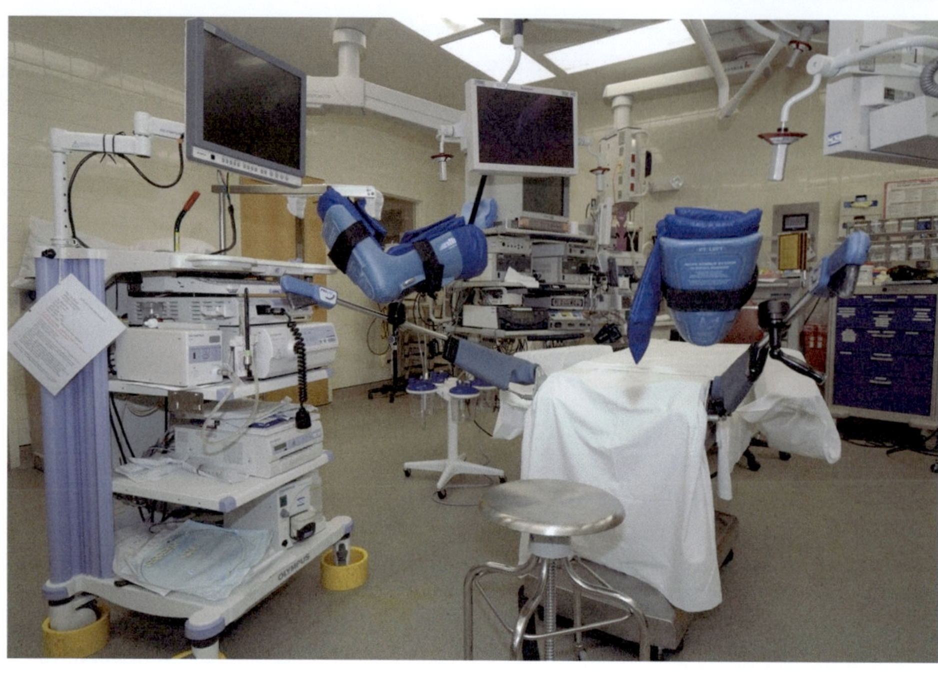

Fig. 15.4 Transanal endoscopy. Intraoperative colonoscopy is facilitated by placing the mobile endoscopy cart lateral to the patient's right foot, in stirrups supporting the lithotomy leg position. While seated at the patient's foot, the endoscopist views the colonoscopic image on the mobile cart monitor while maintaining view of the laparoscopic field displayed on the remote monitor positioned nearby

reasonable clearance of stool. In this situation, if patient condition and time permit, tap water enemas often are useful in clearing blood and improving colonoscopic visualization.

There are no particular anesthetic considerations related to the transanal endoscopic approach, but positioning the patient in low lithotomy on the operating room table so that the anus is in plane with the end edge of the table pad, legs in full support stirrups (Allen type), with the distal platform of the bed removed, is most desirable. The posterior thighs, perineum, and perianal area should be prepared from the outset, and leggings and under buttocks drapes are useful. Although the legs can be left relatively flat to facilitate laparoscopic colon and rectal resections, they often are raised later in the procedure to facilitate transanal stapling techniques and intraoperative colonoscopy. This positioning and preparation sequence, while ordinarily not required for right-sided colon resections, is still advised if intraoperative colonoscopy is to be employed. The mobile endoscopy cart is best placed lateral to the patient's right foot, to the left of the endoscopist when seated on a stool between the stirrups. This provides convenient simultaneous views of the cart-mounted endoscopic video monitor and a laparoscopic monitor positioned near the foot of the table on the patient's right side (Fig. 15.4).

Carbon dioxide insufflation is recommended for use during intraoperative colonoscopy, and is considered vital when colonoscopy is performed to confirm pathology immediately prior to laparoscopic colon and rectal resection. In this situation, judicious insufflation on insertion, and diligent evacuation during withdrawal, accompanied by the rapid absorption of carbon dioxide insufflation from the colon, combine to preserve the laparoscopic working space.

The three most common scenarios where intraoperative colonoscopy is employed are lesion verification immediately prior to resection, assessment of the adequacy of the proposed distal margin during anterior resection of the rectum, and anastomotic inspection and leak testing following resection and reconstruction of the colon or rectum.

It is always more desirable to have marked the location of a colonic lesion preoperatively, during the diagnostic colonoscopy where target pathology was identified and sampled. If the lesion was reported during diagnostic colonoscopy but not labeled with the injection of suspended carbon black, it may be worthwhile to perform colonoscopy at the outset of surgery, before preparing and draping the patient, so that this laparoscopically identifiable tattoo can be placed adjacent to the lesion. Methylene blue and other temporary labels are not recommended, as their persistence is variable and may not last throughout the surgical dissection. Minimal carbon dioxide insufflation during advancement of the colonoscope, and diligent decompression during withdrawal, will lessen the chance that laparoscopic resection will be hampered by colonic distension when colonoscopy is required immediately before resection.

Once the lesion to be resected has been identified, an endoscopic injection needle is used to deliver suspended carbon black to the submucosal space, adjacent to the lesion. Injections should be performed in several locations around the circumference of the colon at the level of the lesion, near enough to guide resection, but injections should not be made through tissue suspected to be malignant. If injections are made through malignant tissue, that injection needle should be discarded and replaced with a fresh needle if additional injections are to be made in areas that will not be removed in continuity with the surgical specimen. Transmural injections should be avoided as well, as this leads to widespread disbursement of carbon particles within the abdominal cavity, sometimes impairing localization of the index lesion. Once the lesion has been confirmed and marked, the endoscope is withdrawn and reprocessed. It is important to reiterate that whenever possible, lesion verification and marking should take place days if not weeks prior to surgery, and colonoscopy immediately prior to surgery should be reserved for unique circumstances.

Margin assessment begins during the preoperative colonoscopy performed for patients with rectal malignancy amenable to resection. In addition to obtaining diagnostic biopsies of the index lesion and eliminating from concern additional benign lesions and synchronous malignant lesions, having marked the distal border of the rectal mass is often quite useful when surgery is performed. By marking the distal extent of the lesion, one can more easily assess the depth of dissection during laparoscopic or open anterior resection, by visualizing the previously applied intramural tattoo. When it is unclear that the distal margin will be adequate, introducing the colonoscope intraoperatively allows the surgeon to visualize the distal extent of the tumor, the segment of rectum impinged by trial closure of the stapling device or bowel clamp, and to make operative adjustments based on these findings. Often, the endoscopist will place the tip of the colonoscope at the region where distal division is desired, to illuminate for the surgical team the further extent of dissection required. In some instances, this use of the colonoscope represents an essential adjunct in determining whether an ultralow anastomosis will be possible, or if abdominoperineal resection will be necessary. In the event of resection with anastomosis, additional evaluation as described below will prove useful.

The vast majority of intraoperative colonoscopy will be used to assess a freshly created anastomosis, evaluating its mucosal integrity, hemostasis, and testing for leaks through suture and staple lines. After completion, the anastomosis is flooded with irrigation fluid and kept submerged. Open or laparoscopic visualization of the anastomosis is maintained as the colonoscope is introduced transanally, using direct visualization during advancement (Video 15.4). Once reached, the anastomosis is inspected for signs of adequate mucosal perfusion, staple-line hemostasis, and patency. Occlusion of the bowel proximal to the anastomosis can be used to avoid loss of surgical domain as the colon becomes distended with carbon dioxide. Insufflation is administered within the lumen of the colon or rectum until the bowel segment immediately proximal to the anastomosis distends; overdistension is avoided as this may disrupt the anastomo-

sis. The serosal aspect of the anastomosis is inspected for bubbles escaping through defects as the insufflated gas is introduced through the colonoscope. Adequate anastomoses will be airtight; no bubbles will be seen. If bubbling is identified, slowly suctioning irrigation fluid while tracing the bubbles back to their source is useful in localizing the disrupted segment of the anastomosis. Repair, reconstruction, or diversion should be chosen according to standard surgical principles, and the anastomosis retested as needed.

Laparoscopic insufflation, or atmospheric air in the case of open surgery, can become trapped beneath the mesentery during colon resection, particularly during anterior resections of the rectum. When the abdomen and pelvis are first filled with irrigant, large bubbles might be seen escaping from these sequestered pockets as the colon and rectum are initially manipulated with the colonoscope. To avoid such false positive findings, it is advised that surgeons gently agitate the intestinal and mesenteric tissues after irrigant is used to submerge the anastomosis, dislodging such trapped collections of gas.

False negative findings appear to be uncommon; this author has not identified any false negatives in his large personal experience using intraoperative endoscopy during gastrointestinal surgical procedures. While intraoperative endoscopy is believed to improve operative outcomes by identifying mechanical defects during the index operation when they are most easily addressed, rather than allowing them to manifest as postoperative complications, anastomotic failure still could develop postoperatively in some patients. It is important to maintain a high index of suspicion when postoperative patients do not follow the typical course, or are delayed in achieving the expected milestones of recovery.

Although direct visual inspection of the anastomosis will provide immediate feedback regarding mucosal integrity and hemostasis, it is possible to perform leak testing without inserting the colonoscope to the level of the anastomosis in select situations, for example, after ileocolonic reconstruction. When this approach becomes necessary, the colonoscope is advanced into the left colon, or to the extent deemed appropriate by the endoscopist, and carbon dioxide insufflation administered to the extent necessary to distend the submerged, more proximal anastomosis. It may not be possible to evacuate as much insufflation gas using this technique, and direct visualization is recommended whenever feasible.

Reporting Intraoperative Endoscopy

The use of intraoperative endoscopy should be documented in the patient record. When performed by the primary surgeon, the endoscopic technique can be listed in the main operative note's procedure list, and the technique and findings described in the narrative section. When a second endoscopist performs the procedure, a separate endoscopic procedure note should be created. In this situation, it is useful to reference the separately available endoscopic report in the primary operative record.

Suggested Reading

1. Cingi A, Yavuz Y. Intraoperative endoscopic assessment of the pouch and anastomosis during laparoscopic Roux-en-Y gastric bypass. Obes Surg. 2011;21(10):1530–4.
2. Del Rio P, Dell'Abate P, Labonia D, et al. Choledocholithiasis and endo-laparoscopic rendezvous. Analysis of 59 consecutive cases. Ann Ital Chir. 2011;82(3):221–4.
3. Alfa MJ, Sepehri S, Olson N, Wald A. Establishing a clinically relevant bioburden benchmark: a quality indicator for adequate reprocessing and storage of flexible gastrointestinal endoscopes. Am J Infect Control. 2012;40(3):233–6.
4. Alasfar F, Chand B. Intraoperative endoscopy for laparoscopic Roux-en-Y gastric bypass: leak test and beyond. Surg Laparosc Endosc Percutan Tech. 2010;20(6):424–7.
5. Borzellino G, Rodella L, Saladino E, et al. Treatment for retained [corrected] common bile duct stones during laparoscopic cholecystectomy: the rendezvous technique. Arch Surg. 2010;145(12): 1145–9.
6. Nishikawa K, Yanaga K, Kashiwagi H, Hanyuu N, Iwabuchi S. Significance of intraoperative endoscopy in total gastrectomy for gastric cancer. Surg Endosc. 2010;24(10):2633–6.
7. Levitzky BE, Wassef WY. Endoscopic management in the bariatric surgical patient. Curr Opin Gastroenterol. 2010;26(6):632–9.
8. Borzellino G, Rodella L, Saladino E, et al. Treatment for retained [corrected] common bile duct stones during laparoscopic cholecystectomy: the rendezvous technique. Arch Surg. 2010;145(12): 1145–9.
9. Tzovaras G, Baloyiannis I, Kapsoritakis A, Psychos A, Paroutoglou G, Potamianos S. Laparoendoscopic rendezvous: an effective alternative to a failed preoperative ERCP in patients with cholecystocholedocholithiasis. Surg Endosc. 2010;24(10):2603–6.
10. Greenwald D. Reducing infection risk in colonoscopy. Gastrointest Endosc Clin N Am. 2010;20(4):603–14.
11. Ferenc J. Endoscopes require constant care. Hospitals must remain vigilant: ECRI institute. Mater Manag Health Care. 2010;19(2): 24–5.
12. Adikibi BT, MacKinlay GA, Munro FD, Khan LR, Gillett PM. Intraoperative upper GI endoscopy ensures an adequate laparoscopic Heller's myotomy. J Laparoendosc Adv Surg Tech A. 2009;19(5):687–9.
13. Alaedeen D, Madan AK, Ro CY, Khan KA, Martinez JM, Tichansky DS. Intraoperative endoscopy and leaks after laparoscopic Roux-en-Y gastric bypass. Am Surg. 2009;75(6):485–8; discussion 488.
14. DiMaggio V, Hoffman K, Baxter R, Cekic V, Nasar A, Whelan RL. Increased utilization of flexible endoscopic methods during colorectal resection over a 3-year period. Surg Innov. 2009;16(4):293–8.
15. Eisenberg D, Bell R. Intraoperative endoscopy: a requisite tool for laparoscopic resection of unusual gastrointestinal lesions—a case series. J Surg Res. 2009;155(2):318–20.
16. Souma Y, Nakajima K, Takahashi T, et al. The role of intraoperative carbon dioxide insufflating upper gastrointestinal endoscopy during laparoscopic surgery. Surg Endosc. 2009;23(10):2279–85.
17. Li VK, Wexner SD, Pulido N, et al. Use of routine intraoperative endoscopy in elective laparoscopic colorectal surgery: can it further avoid anastomotic failure? Surg Endosc. 2009;23(11): 2459–65.
18. Ghazal AH, Sorour MA, El-Riwini M, El-Bahrawy H. Single-step treatment of gall bladder and bile duct stones: a combined endoscopic-laparoscopic technique. Int J Surg. 2009;7(4):338–46.
19. Wilhelm D, von Delius S, Burian M, et al. Simultaneous use of laparoscopy and endoscopy for minimally invasive resection of gastric subepithelial masses—analysis of 93 interventions. World J Surg. 2008;32(6):1021–8.
20. Banerjee S, Shen B, Baron TH, et al. Antibiotic prophylaxis for GI endoscopy. Gastrointest Endosc. 2008;67(6):791–8.
21. Banerjee S, Shen B, Nelson DB, et al. Infection control during GI endoscopy. Gastrointest Endosc. 2008;67(6):781–90.
22. Dominitz JA, Ikenberry SO, Anderson MA, et al. Renewal of and proctoring for endoscopic privileges. Gastrointest Endosc. 2008;67(1):10–6.
23. SAGES. Granting of privilege for gastrointestinal endoscopy. Surg Endosc. 2008;22(5):1349–52.
24. del Genio G, Rossetti G, Brusciano L, et al. Laparoscopic Nissen-Rossetti fundoplication with routine use of intraoperative endoscopy and manometry: technical aspects of a standardized technique. World J Surg. 2007;31(5):1099–106.
25. Osborne S, Reynolds S, George N, Lindemayer F, Gill A, Chalmers M. Challenging endoscopy reprocessing guidelines: a prospective study investigating the safe shelf life of flexible endoscopes in a tertiary gastroenterology unit. Endoscopy. 2007;39(9):825–30.
26. Zuckerman MJ, Shen B, Harrison 3rd ME, et al. Informed consent for GI endoscopy. Gastrointest Endosc. 2007;66(2):213–8.
27. Lyass S, Phillips EH. Laparoscopic transcystic duct common bile duct exploration. Surg Endosc. 2006;20 Suppl 2:S441–5.
28. Morino M, Baracchi F, Miglietta C, Furlan N, Ragona R, Garbarini A. Preoperative endoscopic sphincterotomy versus laparoendoscopic rendezvous in patients with gallbladder and bile duct stones. Ann Surg. 2006;244(6):889–93; discussion 893–886.
29. Rabago LR, Vicente C, Soler F, et al. Two-stage treatment with preoperative endoscopic retrograde cholangiopancreatography (ERCP) compared with single-stage treatment with intraoperative ERCP for patients with symptomatic cholelithiasis with possible choledocholithiasis. Endoscopy. 2006;38(8):779–86.
30. Alimoglu O, Sahin M, Cefle K, Celik O, Eryilmaz R, Palanduz S. Peutz-Jeghers syndrome: report of 6 cases in a family and management of polyps with intraoperative endoscopy. Turk J Gastroenterol. 2004;15(3):164–8.
31. Bloomston M, Brady P, Rosemurgy AS. Videoscopic Heller myotomy with intraoperative endoscopy promotes optimal outcomes. JSLS. 2002;6(2):133–8.
32. Fanelli RD, Gersin KS, Mainella MT. Laparoscopic endobiliary stenting significantly improves success of postoperative endoscopic retrograde cholangiopancreatography in low-volume centers. Surg Endosc. 2002;16(3):487–91.
33. Wexner SD, Eisen GM, Simmang C. Principles of privileging and credentialing for endoscopy and colonoscopy. Surg Endosc. 2002;16(2):367–9.
34. Eisen GM, Baron TH, Dominitz JA, et al. Methods of granting hospital privileges to perform gastrointestinal endoscopy. Gastrointest Endosc. 2002;55(7):780–3.
35. Fanelli RD, Gersin KS. Laparoscopic endobiliary stenting: a simplified approach to the management of occult common bile duct stones. J Gastrointest Surg. 2001;5(1):74–80.
36. Wexner SD, Garbus JE, Singh JJ. A prospective analysis of 13,580 colonoscopies. Reevaluation of credentialing guidelines. Surg Endosc. 2001;15(3):251–61.
37. Himal HS. Common bile duct stones: the role of preoperative, intraoperative, and postoperative ERCP. Semin Laparosc Surg. 2000;7(4):237–45.
38. Park AE, Mastrangelo Jr MJ. Endoscopic retrograde cholangiopancreatography in the management of choledocholithiasis. Surg Endosc. 2000;14(3):219–26.

39. Walter VA, DiMarino Jr AJ. American Society for Gastrointestinal Endoscopy-Society of Gastroenterology Nurses and Associates Endoscope Reprocessing Guidelines. Gastrointest Endosc Clin N Am. 2000;10(2):265–73.

40. Alvarado A. Intraoperative endoscopy during colorectal surgery. Surg Laparosc Endosc Percutan Tech. 1999;9(2):165.

41. Alves A, Perniceni T, Godeberge P, Mal F, Levy P, Gayet B. Laparoscopic Heller's cardiomyotomy in achalasia. Is intraoperative endoscopy useful, and why? Surg Endosc. 1999;13(6):600–3.

42. Delmotte JS, Gay GJ, Houcke PH, Mesnard Y. Intraoperative endoscopy. Gastrointest Endosc Clin N Am. 1999;9(1):61–9.

43. Crawford DL, Phillips EH. Laparoscopic common bile duct exploration. World J Surg. 1999;23(4):343–9.

44. Forde KA. Intraoperative endoscopy: a continuing need in colorectal surgery. Cancer Invest. 1998;16(1):62–3.

45. Phillips EH. Laparoscopic transcystic duct common bile duct exploration. Surg Endosc. 1998;12(4):365–6.

46. Wexner SD, Forde KA, Sellers G, et al. How well can surgeons perform colonoscopy? Surg Endosc. 1998;12(12):1410–4.

47. Phillips EH, Rosenthal RJ, Carroll BJ, Fallas MJ. Laparoscopic trans-cystic-duct common-bile-duct exploration. Surg Endosc. 1994;8(12):1389–93; discussion 1393–1384.

48. Bombeck CT. Intraoperative esophagoscopy, gastroscopy, colonoscopy, and endoscopy of the small bowel. Surg Clin North Am. 1975;55(1):135–42.

Techniques of Upper Endoscopy

16

Thadeus L. Trus

Introduction

An increasingly central component to the practice of general surgery is flexible endoscopy. At least half of the practicing surgeons in the USA depend on basic upper and lower endoscopy for a substantial portion of their practice. In fact, outside of most urban centers, the burden of providing endoscopy falls entirely on the general surgeon.

Many common surgical disease treatments have already shifted, or are rapidly shifting towards less invasive approaches which increasingly include interventional flexible endoscopic procedures. A brief look in the recent past underlines this fact. Common bile duct exploration, pancreatic pseudocyst drainage, colectomy for benign or early neoplasia, and esophagectomy for Barrett's disease are but a few of the conditions that are now treated endoscopically instead of surgically.

As this trend continues, surgeons unskilled in flexible endoscopy will find themselves increasingly cut out of the treatment of these diseases. The following outlines the basic technique and tips of upper endoscopy.

Indications

Esophagogastroduodenoscopy (EGD) provides excellent visualization of the mucosal surfaces of the entire esophagus, stomach, and proximal duodenum. In general, endo-

scopic examination is indicated in patients whose symptoms are unresponsive to simple conservative treatment, if a change in management is likely based on the endoscopic findings, as a method of evaluation instead of contrast studies and where a therapeutic procedure is considered. Other indications include the evaluation of alarm symptoms such as bleeding, weight loss, or anemia, surveillance of esophageal dysplasia, or other premalignant conditions such as familial polyposis and to assess gastric ulcer healing.

An all-encompassing list of indications is dictated by the local resources and the experience of the endoscopist. Advanced procedures such as enteral access [i.e., percutaneous endoscopic gastrostomy (PEG)], stricture dilation, EMR, ESD, and Barrett's ablation among others are covered in other areas in this book and are beyond the scope of this chapter. All of these advanced procedures have specific indications and contraindications to consider. Table 16.1 provides the specific American Society of Gastrointestinal Endoscopy (ASGE) recommendations for EGD [1].

Safe endoscopic examination requires the cooperation of the patient. A combative, unwilling patient should not undergo endoscopic examination unless adequate anesthesia can be achieved which usually requires deep sedation or general anesthesia in these situations. Other contraindications include a suspected perforation or hemodynamic or respiratory instability. Relative contraindications include the presence of a pharyngeal diverticulum, or head and neck surgery. In these situations, endoscopy should be performed by an experienced endoscopist.

Anticoagulation is not always a contraindication to EGD. Diagnostic EGD is a relatively low bleeding risk procedure in the anticoagulated patient and therefore can be performed without anticoagulant reversal or adjustment (see Chap. 4). Rarely, retropharyngeal hematoma may occur in patients with severe coagulation abnormalities. Therapeutic procedures,

This chapter contains a video segment that can be found by accessing the following link: http://www.springerimages.com/videos/978-1-4614-6329-0.

T.L. Trus, M.D. (✉)
Dartmouth Hitchcock Medical Center, 1 Medical Center Drive,
Lebanon, NH 03756, USA
e-mail: Thadeus.Trus@Hitchcock.org

J.M. Marks and B.J. Dunkin (eds.), *Principles of Flexible Endoscopy for Surgeons*,
DOI 10.1007/978-1-4614-6330-6_16, © Springer Science+Business Media New York 2013

Table 16.1 American society for gastrointestinal endoscopy (ASGE) indications for endoscopy

Upper abdominal symptoms that persist despite an appropriate trial of therapy	To assess diarrhea in patients suspected of having small-bowel disease (i.e., celiac disease)
Upper abdominal symptoms associated with other symptoms or signs suggesting structural disease (e.g., anorexia and weight loss) or new-onset symptoms in patients older than 50 years of age	Treatment of bleeding lesions such as ulcers, tumors, vascular abnormalities (i.e., electrocoagulation, heater probe, laser photocoagulation, or injection therapy)
Dysphagia or odynophagia	Removal of foreign bodies
Esophageal reflux symptoms that persist or recur despite appropriate therapy	Removal of selected lesions
Persistent vomiting of unknown cause	Placement of feeding or drainage tubes (i.e., peroral, percutaneous endoscopic gastrostomy, percutaneous endoscopic jejunostomy)
Other diseases in which the presence of upper GI pathology might modify other planned management *Examples include patients who have a history of ulcer or GI bleeding who are scheduled for organ transplantation, long-term anticoagulation or nonsteroidal anti-inflammatory drug therapy for arthritis and those with cancer of the head and neck*	Dilation and stenting of stenotic lesions (i.e., with transendoscopic balloon dilators or dilation systems using guidewires)
Familial adenomatous polyposis syndromes	Management of achalasia (i.e., botulinum toxin, balloon dilation)
For confirmation and specific histologic diagnosis of radiologically demonstrated lesions: 1. Suspected neoplastic lesion 2. Gastric or esophageal ulcer 3. Upper tract stricture or obstruction	Palliative treatment of stenosing neoplasms (i.e., laser, multipolar electrocoagulation, stent placement)
Gastrointestinal bleeding: 1. In patients with active or recent bleeding 2. For presumed chronic blood loss and for iron deficiency anemia when the clinical situation suggests an upper gastrointestinal source or when colonoscopy does not provide an explanation	Endoscopic therapy of intestinal metaplasia
When sampling of tissue or fluid is indicated	Intraoperative evaluation of anatomic reconstructions typical of modern foregut surgery (i.e., evaluation of anastomotic leak and patency, fundoplication formation, pouch configuration during bariatric surgery)
Selected patients with suspected portal hypertension to document or treat esophageal varices	Management of operative complications (i.e., dilation of anastomotic strictures, stenting of anastomotic disruption, fistula, or leak in selected circumstances)
To assess acute injury after caustic ingestion	Sequential or periodic EGD may be indicated for surveillance for malignancy in patients with premalignant conditions (i.e., Barrett's esophagus, polyposis syndromes, gastric adenomas, tylosis, or previous caustic ingestion)

EGD esophagogastroduodenoscopy

such as dilations, PEG, polypectomy, endoscopic sphincterotomy, endoscopic ultrasound (EUS)-guided fine-needle aspiration, and laser ablation carry a much higher risk for bleeding, and adjustment of anticoagulation should be undertaken prior to the procedure [2–4].

EGD is not indicated for patients whose symptoms are functional other than to rule out an organic disease or evaluate a new or alarm symptom. It is also not indicated in the setting of metastatic disease unless the results will change the management of the disease or a complication symptom. There is no role for diagnostic EGD to confirm a benign radiographic finding such as a sliding hiatal hernia or duodenal diverticulum. There is also no role for endoscopic reexamination of a duodenal ulcer that has responded to treatment. Sequential EGD is also not indicated for malignancy surveillance in patients with gastric atrophy, pernicious anemia, hyperplastic or fundic gland polyps, or gastric intestinal metaplasia of the stomach.

Upper Endoscopy Technique

Most upper endoscopy can be successfully performed with a standard forward viewing endoscope. Occasionally, a larger therapeutic endoscope is necessary for certain therapeutic procedures. Larger channels (3.7 mm vs. standard 2.8 mm) allow for passage of more substantial tools and facilitate suction of clot and debris. Smaller endoscopes have a much smaller channel and can sometimes be more difficult to pass through the pharynx since they are more floppy. In recent years, transnasal endoscopy has allowed simple diagnostic endoscopic examination without sedation (see Chap. 18).

Endoscopy Basics

Prior to performing any endoscopy, the equipment should be inspected and tested. The image should be clear and crisp with proper color balance. Suction, irrigation and air insufflation should be tested before beginning the procedure. It is best to troubleshoot problems with the system before the procedure rather than during it. Adequate sedation, antibiotic prophylaxis, and monitoring are discussed in the previous chapters on pre-procedural and intra-procedural care [5, 6].

The endoscopist should stand facing the patient who is positioned comfortably in a lateral decubitus position. The head of the endoscope is cradled in the left hand with the thumb behind for wheel control and the first and second fingers free in front to control the insufflation, suction and irrigation buttons (Fig. 16.1). The right hand is thus free to advance, withdraw, and torque the scope as well as introduce instruments through the working channel. The short length of the upper endoscope allows one to torque the scope by changing the position of the control head with the wrist of the left hand instead of torqueing with the right hand as in colonoscopy.

The safest and most common way to insert the endoscope is under direct vision. Many endoscopists like to "lock" the "little" wheel and use only the "big wheel" control for esophageal intubation. The big wheel is used to form a downward curve of the endoscope tip. The scope is then fed over the tongue and straightened slightly as one enters the pharynx. It is important to stay behind the epiglottis. Entry into the esophagus is immediately posterior to the cricoarytenoid cartilage in the midline, posterior to the vocal cords (Fig. 16.2). Passage is best achieved to the right or left of this cartilage and then gently guiding the tip towards the midline with gentle pressure and insufflation. Usually the tip will glide into the proximal esophagus. Asking the patient to swallow often opens the cricopharyngeal sphincter briefly allowing easy passage of the scope (Video 16.1). Although some endoscopists use blind intubation, direct visualization is recommended.

Intubation is best achieved in a calm, cooperative patient. The endoscopy nurse is often very helpful in calming a nervous patient during this critical portion of the endoscopy. Patients who are combative, restless or gag excessively are at much higher risk of injury to the esophagus or piriform sinus. Tilting the chin forward towards the chest also helps with intubation with the patient in a decubitus position.

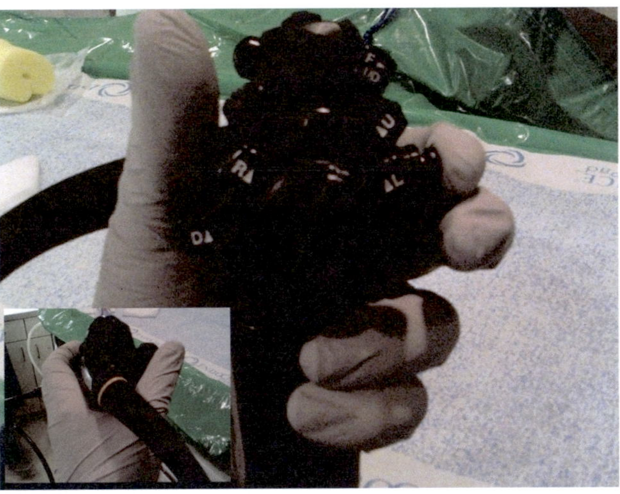

Fig. 16.1 The head of the scope should be cradled between the thumb and forefinger of the left hand. This allows the endoscopist control of both control wheels and the suction, air insufflation and irrigation buttons with one hand

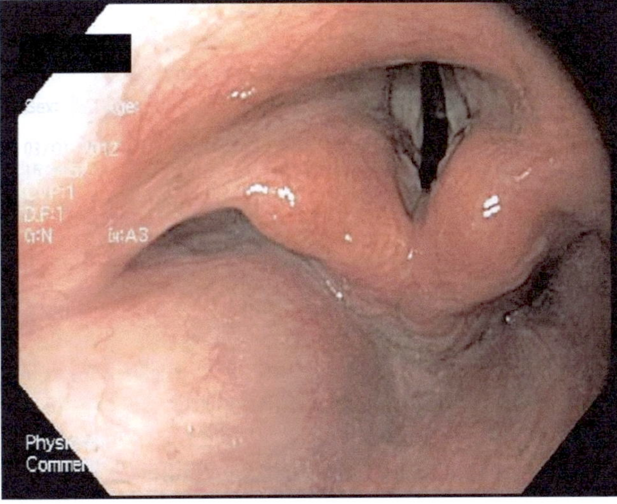

Fig. 16.2 The vocal cords are seen directly anterior to the esophageal entry point

Endotracheal tubes do not usually hinder passage of the endoscope. Occasionally deflation of the cuff is necessary to facilitate passage. Endoscopic entry into the esophagus in intubated patients in the supine position is more challenging. Using a finger to guide the scope and lifting the jaw will ease esophageal intubation. Nasogastric tubes can be left in place and will act as a guide into the esophagus. To allow for adequate insufflation and visualization, the nasogastric tube must often be removed during the procedure.

Once esophageal intubation is achieved, a routine, systematic examination is critical. Insufflation will open the lumen and allow inspection and scope advancement. Blind scope advancement should not be performed. If visualization is lost, it is best to pull back and insufflate. This will allow you to find the lumen again and allow scope advancement under direct vision. Although mucosal inspection is usually done more thoroughly on scope withdrawal with an inflated organ, careful esophageal mucosal inspection on the way in is critical since "false lesions" from scope trauma may occur.

The esophageal landmarks include an indentation from the left main bronchus and obvious pulsation from the aorta and left atrium. The esophageal mucosa should appear smooth and pink all the way to the Z-line, which is usually found approximately 36–42 cm from the incisors. Distal to the Z-line, the mucosa darkens as it changes from squamous esophageal mucosa to gastric. In most patients, this is seen approximately 1 cm above the crural "pinch." Asking the patient to sniff accentuates the crura. Hiatal hernia size (distance from Z-line to crus) is roughly measured from this point (Video 16.2). The esophageal lumen diameter and contractions are important to note during the examination particularly in patients with dysphagia where a motility disorder is suspected. The lower esophageal sphincter is easily seen as a concentric narrowing of the distal esophagus (Fig. 16.3). Scope passage should be effortless. A patulous LES is not normal. Conversely, a sphincter that presents some resistance to passage hallmarked by a "popping" sensation upon traversal is a characteristic finding in achalasia patients.

Upon entering the stomach the endoscopist must insufflate to allow for proper evaluation. As the stomach distends, the lesser curve is visualized on the right side of the monitor image (Fig. 16.4). The tip may be deflected slightly up to achieve this view. The incisura is seen as a fold on the right side of the image distally. The lesser curve should be "hugged" by the scope as one advances towards this landmark which leads the endoscopist towards the antrum and pylorus (Fig. 16.5; Video 16.3). As the scope is advanced it usually assumes a "long position" where it bows out along the greater curve giving the impression that one is not advancing. Excessive gastric fluid should be aspirated and care should be taken not to suction the mucosa directly, creating "suction polyps" which may be misinterpreted as pathology by the inexperienced observer. Excess bubbles can easily be eliminated by irrigating with a solution of simethicone through the working channel.

Motor activity of the stomach is quite obvious in the antrum and pylorus. Here it is important to be patient and advance the scope slowly to allow for complete mucosal inspection during vigorous gastric contractions. The scope is then retroflexed by turning the larger wheel all the way back and the smaller wheel all the way to the left, deflecting the scope in an upward fashion. This is best performed with the stomach well insufflated to distend the fundus. The scope can be seen entering the stomach through the gastroesophageal junction. This view offers an excellent assessment of the GE junction from inside the stomach (Fig. 16.6). Hiatal hernias

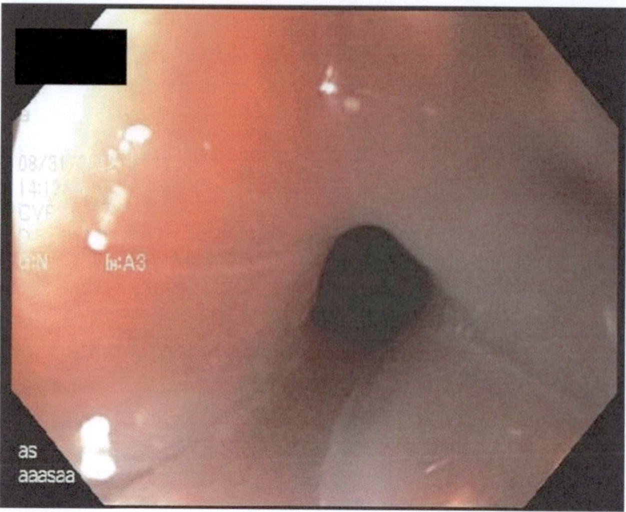

Fig. 16.3 The esophagus ends as a concentric narrowing at the lower esophageal sphincter. Gentle pressure and mild insufflation will result in sphincter relaxation and allow scope passage

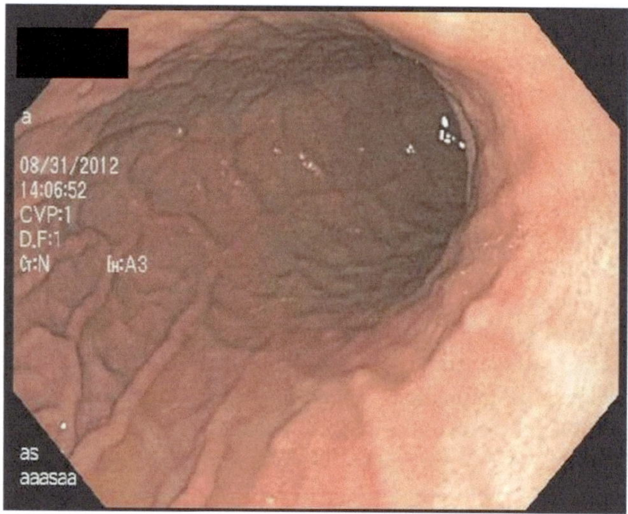

Fig. 16.4 The lesser curve of the stomach is seen on the right hand side of the screen. Following the lesser curve down will place the scope in a "long" position and lead into the antrum

are easily seen in this view and it is critical in evaluating fundoplication integrity (Fig. 16.7; Video 16.4).

The scope should be rotated clockwise and counter clockwise in this retroflexed position to obtain a full 360° assessment of the fundus and proximal stomach. Close up assessment is achieved by withdrawing the scope in a retroflexed position thus bringing the tip closer to the gastroesophageal junction.

The scope is then returned to the neutral position and advanced to the pylorus. Pyloric cannulation can be challenging given the amount of peristaltic activity in the prepyloric region. The pylorus should be lined up in the center of

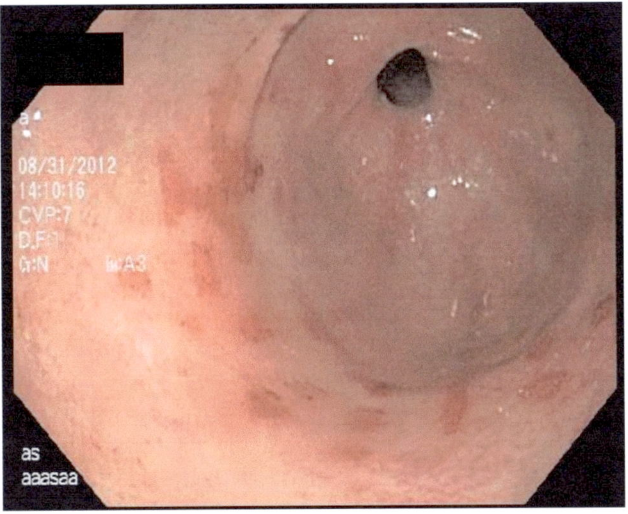

Fig. 16.5 The pylorus is clearly seen as a small opening at the end of the antrum. Often the folds of the antrum coalesce at the pylorus when it is not widely open. This example also has some gastritis of mild GAVE

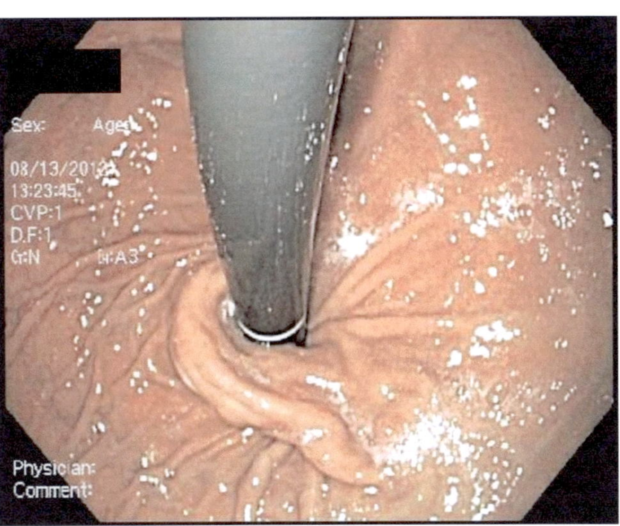

Fig. 16.7 A Nissen fundoplication is seen here in a retroflexed view. The thickened swirl of gastric mucosa is the fundoplication which appears to hug the scope

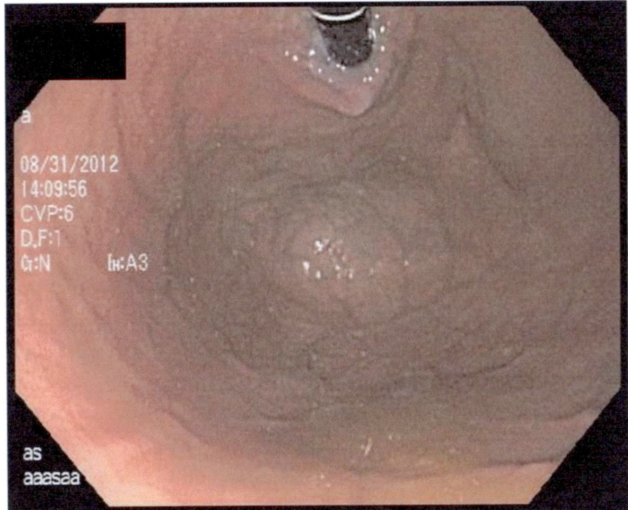

Fig. 16.6 The scope can be seen entering the stomach in this retroflexed view. A normal gastroesophageal junction should appear to snugly hug the scope

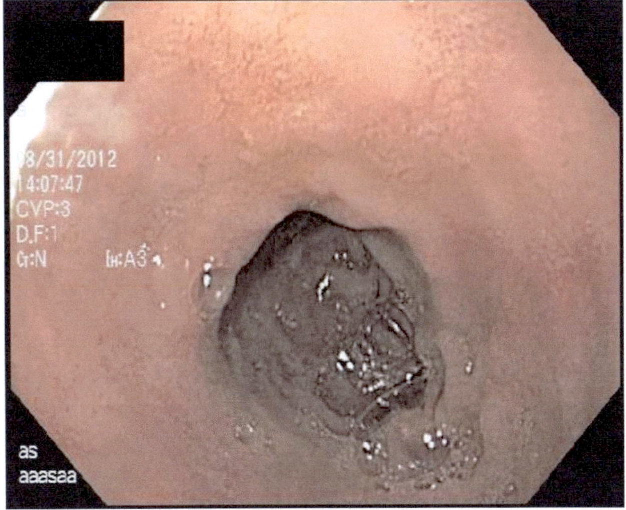

Fig. 16.8 The duodenal bulb is best viewed by slight scope withdrawal after passing through the pylorus. The lumen of the beginning of the duodenal sweep is slightly down and to the right

the visual field. As the peristaltic wave crosses the pylorus, it opens slightly. Gentle pressure is applied and the scope should pass if lined up properly. If one "rolls off" the pylorus, slight scope withdrawal and realignment will reorient the scope for another attempt at cannulation.

Once in the duodenal bulb the scope can be pulled back slightly to visualize the whole bulb (Fig. 16.8). To get beyond the bulb, the scope is advanced and simultaneously rotated clockwise with the tip deflected upwards (big wheel back). This usually results in the scope advancing into the second part. The scope is then slowly withdrawn to place it into a short position, releasing the bow of the scope. The duodenum can be carefully inspected during slow withdrawal (Fig. 16.9; Video 16.5).

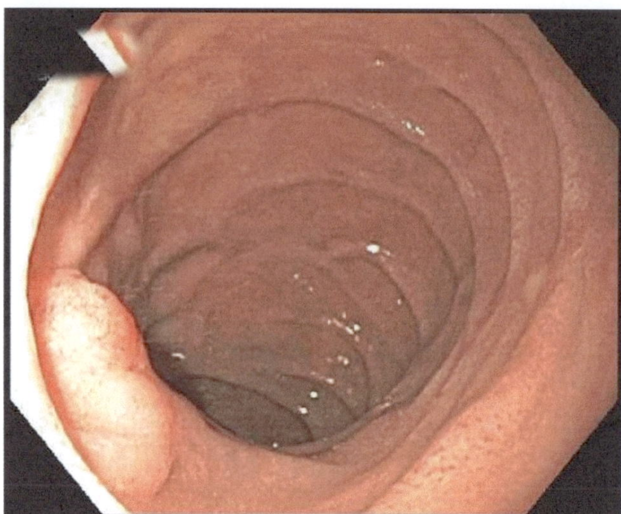

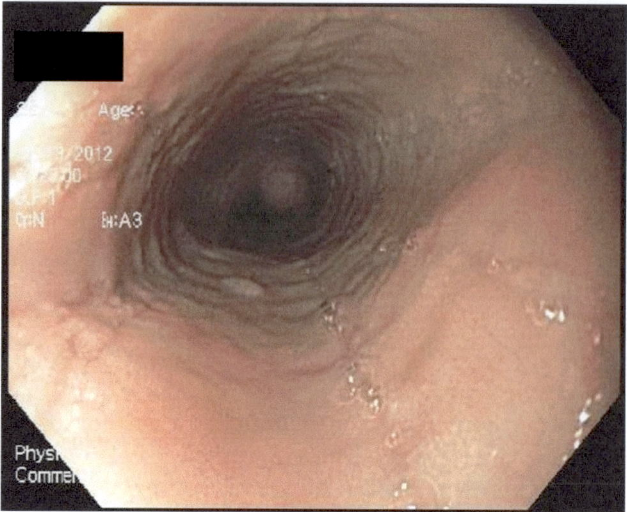

Fig. 16.9 The second part of the duodenum is best cannulated by advancing the scope and simultaneously rotating the scope 90° clockwise while directing the "big wheel" back. The ampulla of Vater is seen at approximately the 7 o'clock position in this image

Fig. 16.10 The concentric rings are a classic appearance of eosinophilic esophagitis

Upper GI Anatomy/Pathology

This final section is meant to familiarize the reader with common pathology found during upper endoscopy but does not constitute a complete review of all upper GI pathology. The reader is encouraged to review specific sections within this text in addition to an endoscopic atlas.

Esophagus

By far the most common pathology found during endoscopic esophageal examination is esophagitis. The most common cause of esophagitis is acid reflux but other causes include infection (candida or less commonly CMV), inflammatory bowel disease, caustic injection, foreign body (NG tube, pill erosion) and rarely eosinophilic esophagitis, which is thought to be allergy mediated.

The most common symptom of eosinophilic esophagitis is solid food dysphagia. Less common symptoms also include heartburn and chest pain. The esophageal mucosa is normally pink and smooth with a clear somewhat jagged demarcation at the Z line as the esophageal mucosa transitions to gastric mucosa, which is somewhat darker in color and rougher appearing texture. Endoscopically, eosinophilic esophagitis may appear as horizontal rings, vertical furrows, strictures and/or white spots (Fig. 16.10). Conversely, the esophageal mucosa may appear relatively normal or only mildly inflamed. Diagnosis is made definitively by biopsy. Intraepithelial eosinophils must number at least 15/HPF in any one field of the biopsy specimen. Fields containing 6–14 eosinophils/HPF are indeterminate. Eosinophils are often

Table 16.2 Los Angeles classification of esophagitis

Grade A	One or more mucosal breaks <5 mm in maximal length
Grade B	One or more mucosal breaks >5 mm, but without continuity across mucosal folds
Grade C	Mucosal breaks continuous between >2 mucosal folds, but involving less than 75 % of the esophageal circumference
Grade D	Mucosal breaks involving more than 75 % of esophageal circumference

located in superficial layers of mucosa and may be diffused or in clusters (clusters of four or more are defined as microabscess) Eosinophilic infiltrates are confined to the esophagus and must not be present in rest of GI tract to make the diagnosis of eosinophilic esophagitis.

The degree of esophagitis is classified by its extent and severity. The most common classification is the Los Angeles classification (Table 16.2). Barrett's esophagus is often seen in the setting of reflux esophagitis. Barrett's dysplasia cannot be reliably diagnosed in severe esophagitis, which is why many endoscopists will forgo biopsy in this setting and repeat the endoscopic examination after a period of high dose acid suppression to resolve the esophagitis. Barrett's esophagus is frequently seen as tongues and/or islands of salmon colored mucosa extending towards the proximal esophagus (Figs. 16.11 and 16.12). Biopsies should be performed using large, spiked biopsy forceps. Mucosal irregularities, (nodules, areas of friability, erosions, ulcers, strictures, or areas where the esophagus seems fixed or less distensible) should be areas of biopsy. If Barrett's is established without dysplasia, 4-quadrant biopsy specimens every 2 cm should be obtained. In patients with known or suspected dysplasia, 4-quadrant biopsy specimens every 1 cm should be obtained.

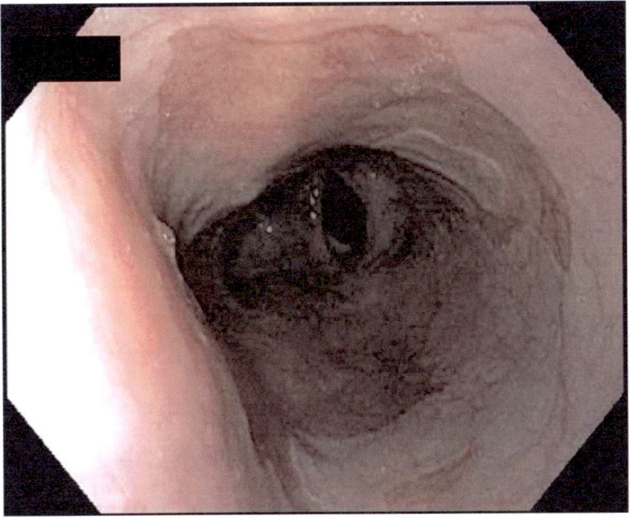

Fig. 16.11 The irregular tongues and islands of darker mucosal represent intestinal metaplasia (Barrett's Esophagus)

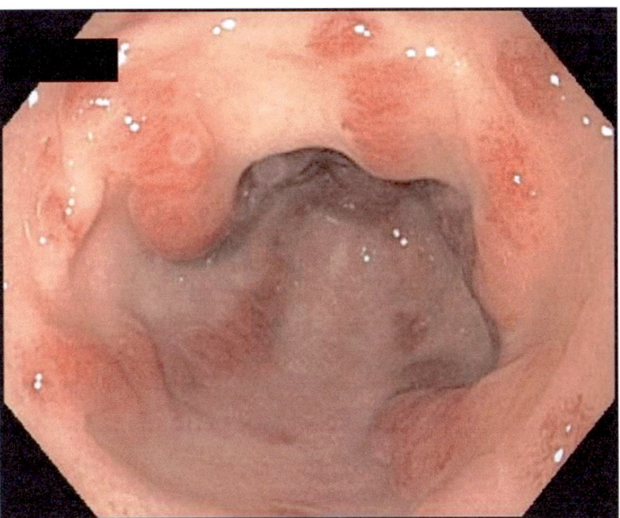

Fig. 16.13 Gastric antral vascular ectasia (GAVE) is often referred to as watermelon stomach because of streaky long red areas in the stomach resembling the markings on watermelon

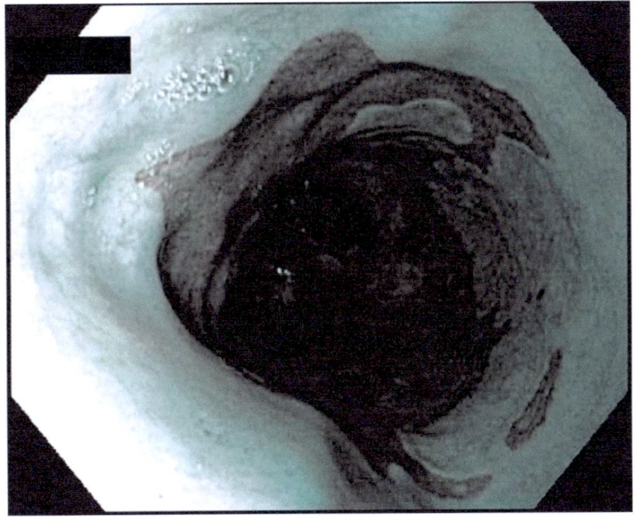

Fig. 16.12 Barrett's esophagus visualization is often enhanced by switching to narrow band imaging (NBI)

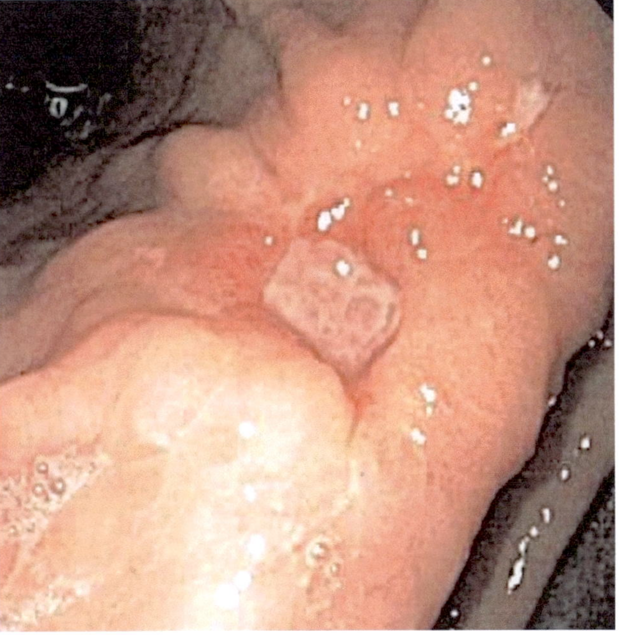

Fig. 16.14 The gastric ulcer will often have raised erythematous borders with a central crater. This particular ulcer is located on the incisura and is seen in a retroflexed position

Stomach

Gastritis is the most common pathology found at upper endoscopy. It is characterized by superficial erosions and redness and often streaks of redness are seen in the pre-pyloric region. Gastric antral vascular ectasia (GAVE) is an uncommon cause of chronic gastrointestinal (GI) bleeding. It is often referred to as watermelon stomach because of streaky long red areas in the stomach resembling the markings on watermelon. This is due to dilated small blood vessels in the antrum, or distal stomach (Fig. 16.13). Chronic gastritis may appear more "speckled" in appearance. The etiology is extensive and includes NSAID use, hyperacidity, alcohol, infection

(*Helicobacter pylori*, candida, CMV), inflammatory bowel disease or often idiopathic. Deeper ulceration in the pre-pyloric region is usually related to acid whereas ulcers in the body are more worrisome for malignancy and mandate biopsy and confirmation of healing on repeat endoscopy (Fig. 16.14).

Gastric polyps have become quite commonplace with the widespread use of proton pump inhibitors. These fundic gland polyps are benign and are frequently multiple, non-ulcerated, and smooth. Ulcerated submucosal masses are more likely to represent a GI stromal tumor (GIST).

Duodenum

An ulcer is among the most common lesions seen in the duodenum. The wide variety of therapeutic options for treatment of bleeding duodenal ulcers is covered elsewhere in this book. The ampulla of Vater is frequently seen through an end viewing scope in the second portion of the duodenum. It is important to familiarize oneself with the normal appearance of the papilla so as not to mistaken it for pathology and biopsy or attempt to snare it. Loss of the velvety, villous appearance of the duodenal mucosa can be seen in celiac disease and warrants biopsy.

Summary

Endoscopy of the upper GI tract has evolved from a diagnostic tool to an invaluable instrument for physicians treating both surgical and nonsurgical disorders of the GI tract. An increasing number of therapeutic tools and techniques continue to develop, supplementing and often replacing traditional surgical treatments. It is imperative that one becomes facile at upper endoscopy and incorporates into practice.

Learning the technique of safe endoscopy is critical, but even more so is need for the endoscopist to differentiate between normal and abnormal, benign and malignant processes.

References

1. ASGE Guideline. Appropriate use of GI endoscopy. Gastrointest Endosc. 2012;75(6):1127–31.
2. Guideline ASGE. Complications of upper GI endoscopy. Gastrointest Endosc. 2002;55(7):784–93.
3. Lieberman DA, Wuerker CK, Katon RM. Cardiopulmonary risk of esophagogastroduodenoscopy: role of endoscope diameter and systemic sedation. Gastroenterology. 1985;88:468–72.
4. Hart R, Classen M. Complications of diagnostic gastrointestinal endoscopy. Endoscopy. 1990;22:229–33.
5. Bell GD. Premedication and intravenous sedation for upper gastrointestinal endoscopy. Aliment Pharmacol Ther. 1990;4:103–22.
6. Scott-Coombes DM, Thompson JN. Hypoxia during upper gastrointestinal endoscopy is caused by sedation. Endoscopy. 1993;25:308–9.

Joanne Favuzza and Conor Delaney

Indications

Colonoscopy has become the method of choice for visualization of the entire colonic mucosa and distal small bowel. The indications for colonoscopy include screening and surveillance as well as for the diagnosis and treatment of many colonic disorders [1].

The majority of colonoscopies are performed for screening or surveillance of colorectal cancer, which occurs in approximately 140,000 cases per year in the USA [2]. Screening endoscopy with polypectomy has lead to a decreased colorectal cancer incidence over the years along with decreased mortality [3]. In the National Polyp Study a cohort of 1,400 patients were followed after colonoscopic removal of adenomas. A followup of 6 years showed a decreased incidence of colorectal cancer [4].

The Joint Guideline from the American Cancer Society, the US Multi-Society Task Force on Colorectal Cancer and American College of Radiology recommend screening colonoscopy every 10 years, beginning at age 50 for average risk patients [5–7]. Patients at higher risk for developing colorectal cancer require more frequent examinations at an earlier age. For example patients with a colorectal cancer or adenomatous polyps in a first degree relative greater than age 60 or in second degree relative with colorectal cancer should begin colonoscopy screening at age 40 [8]. Familial adenomatous polyposis (FAP) patients should begin evaluation at 10–12

years old; while hereditary nonpolyposis colon cancer (HNPCC) patients should begin at 20–25 years of age [8]. Patients with inflammatory bowel disease, chronic ulcerative colitis, or Crohn's disease have an increased cancer risk 8 years after onset of pancolitis or 12–15 years after the onset of left sided colitis. These patients should undergo screening every 1–2 years at that time [8]. Table 17.1 lists the current screening recommendations for colonoscopy.

Colonoscopy is also used as a surveillance tool for patients with a resected colorectal cancer. The American Cancer Society and US Multi-Society Task Force on Colorectal Cancer recommend that a complete colonoscopy be performed to rule out synchronous disease within the first 3–6 months after resection, but ideally pre-operatively for non-obstructing lesions. Metachronous disease is evaluated 1 year after resection followed by every 3 years if negative [6]. Patients must undergo surveillance after polypectomy. Guidelines have been established by the US Multisociety Task Force and American Cancer Society. Patients with 3–10 adenomas or adenomas >1 cm and high grade dysplasia or villous nature should have a colonoscopy every 3 years. If patients have >10 adenomas then surveillance should be less than 3 years. Piecemeal excision requires follow-up at 3–6 months intervals until no residual adenoma is found [5, 6, 9]. Patients with ulcerative colitis and Crohn's disease undergo colonoscopy every 2 years until 20 years after disease onset and then yearly to determine evidence of dysplasia or cancer [5]. Table 17.2 lists surveillance guidelines [5, 6].

Colonoscopy is also used to diagnose and treat common disorders of the colon and rectum [9, 10]. These entities include inflammatory bowel disease, lower gastrointestinal bleeding, change of bowel habits, and acute colonic pseudoobstruction or volvulus. Patients with inflammatory bowel disease may undergo colonoscopy to determine the extent of disease and the need for surgical intervention as well as surveillance due to risk of cancer. In order to differentiate ulcer-

This chapter contains a video segment that can be found by accessing the following link: http://www.springerimages.com/videos/978-1-4614-6329-0.

J. Favuzza, D.O. • C. Delaney, M.D., Ph.D. (☒)
Division of Colorectal Surgery, University Hospitals Case Medical Center, Cleveland, OH 44106-5047, USA
e-mail: conor.delaney@uhhospitals.org

Table 17.1 Recommended colonoscopy screening [5, 8]

Patient population	Recommended age for screening colonoscopy
Average risk	50, then q 10 years if normal colonoscopy
History of colorectal cancer or adenomatous polyps in first degree relative >60 or second degree relative	40
FAP	10–12
HNPCC	20–25
IBD, Crohn's, chronic UC	8 years after pancolitis or 12–15 years after left sided colitis then q 1–2 years

FAP familial adenomatous polyposis, *HNPCC* hereditary non-polyposis colorectcal cancer, *IBD* inflammatory bowel disease, *UC* ulcerative colitis

Table 17.2 Guidelines for surveillance colonoscopy [5, 6]

Patient population	Surveillance colonoscopy
Resected colorectal cancer	1 year after resection, then q 3 years if negative
3–10 adenomas, adenomas >1 cm and high grade dysplasia or villous	q 3 years
>10 adenomas	Less than 3 years
Piecemeal excision	q 3–6 months until no residual adenoma found
UC, Crohn's disease	q 2 years until 20 years after disease onset then yearly

UC ulcerative colitis

Table 17.3 Other indications for colonoscopy [9, 10]

Indications
Lower gastrointestinal bleeding or positive fecal occult blood test
Hematochezia, melena, or unexplained iron deficiency anemia
Inflammatory bowel disease
Change bowel habits
Colonic Pseudoobstruction
Volvulus
Constipation or diarrhea (not acute in nature)
Abnormal CT or barium enema
Adenomas on sigmoidoscopy
Foreign body removal
Balloon dilatation for colonic stricture
Coagulation of bleeding lesions
Marking neoplastic lesions for resection

CT computed tomography

ative colitis from Crohn's disease, terminal ileum intubation and biopsy may be performed colonoscopically. A positive fecal occult blood test is associated with a high prevalence of cancer and thus warrants colonoscopy [11]. Patients with hematochezia, melena, or unexplained iron deficiency anemia should undergo colonoscopy. Evaluation of patients with constipation or diarrhea which is not acute in nature, warrants evaluation to determine etiology of symptoms and exclude neoplasm. Any abnormal barium enema studies or computed tomography (CT) scans or adenomas noted on sigmoidoscopy require colonoscopy [10]. Other therapeutic indications from the American Society for Gastrointestinal Endoscopy include decompression of colon from pseudoobstruction or sigmoid volvulus, foreign body removal, balloon dilation for stricture, coagulation of bleeding lesions, and marking neoplastic lesions for resection. See Table 17.3 for a complete list of other indications for colonoscopy [10, 11].

Contraindications

Colonoscopy is not without risk; contraindications include evidence of perforation or toxic megacolon. There are many relative contraindications; patients with severe colitis, acute diverticulitis due to the risk of perforation or those in the immediate postoperative period due to the risk of anastamotic breakdown. Other contraindications include patients who have had a myocardial infarction within 3 months or following a recent pulmonary embolus, or those who would not tolerate the risks of moderate sedation. Patients who are hemodynamically unstable or with a severe coagulopathy should generally not undergo a colonoscopy unless it is for evaluation of a source of bleeding. Patients who are pregnant, have an anal fissure or large or symptomatic abdominal aortic aneurysm should not undergo a colonoscopy [7].

Lower GI Anatomy

The colonoscopy starts with a thorough digital rectal exam followed by the inspection of the large intestine which extends from the terminal ileum to the anus. The large intestine is about 1.5 m long and includes the cecum, colon, rectum, and anal canal [12]. The colon is further divided into the ascending, transverse, descending, and sigmoid colon. The majority of the length of the colon is occupied by the sigmoid and transverse colon, each approximately 50 cm long. The remainder of the large intestine is divided into 5 cm of cecum, 10 cm each of ascending and descending colon, 15 cm of rectum, and 4 cm of anus [13].

The colonoscope is inserted in a retrograde fashion (Video 17.1). The rectum lies anterior to the sacrum for about 15 cm from the anal verge. Three or more folds known as the valves of Houston are visualized while in rectum (Fig. 17.1). Typically the proximal and distal valves are on

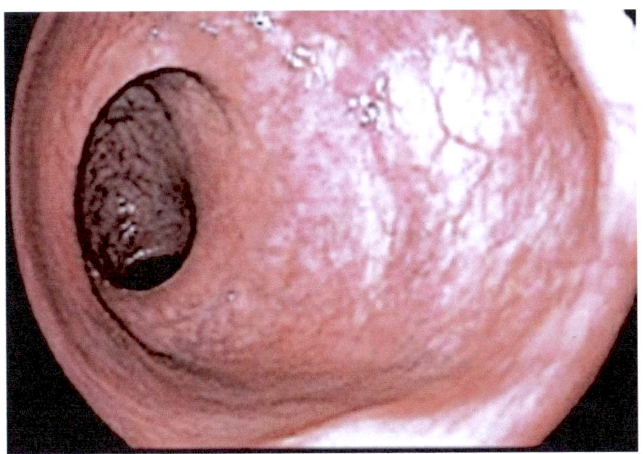

Fig. 17.1 Rectum

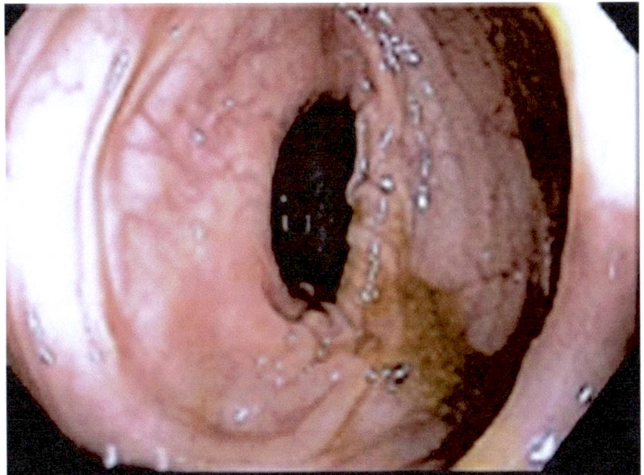

Fig. 17.2 Rectosigmoid junction

the right side and the middle valve on the left [14]. As the rectum joins the sigmoid at the peritoneal reflection, a sharp bend projects anteriorly and toward the left (Fig. 17.2). The colon has three longitudinal folds known as teniae coli which can be visible on colonoscopy. In addition, the interior of the colon is segmented by haustral folds [7]. The distal colon where more formed stool exists has a thicker musculature than the proximal colon [7]. The descending colon is usually straight and allows for easy passage through the colon. As the colonoscope approaches the splenic flexure there is another sharp bend anteriorly and to the right which is due to the tethering from the phrenocolic or splenocolic ligament (Fig. 17.3). As the splenic and hepatic flexures are encountered, blue grey appearance is often noted through the colon (Fig. 17.4) [7]. The transverse colon is triangular in appearance due to the tension in the 3 longitudinal teniae coli (Fig. 17.5). Cardiac pulsations are often seen when the colonoscope is traversing the transverse colon. The hepatic flexure has an acute almost 180 angle which tracks posterior and inferior, leading to the ascending colon and cecum. The ascending colon is usually a straight line. The cecum is marked by a "crow's foot" or "Mercedes Benz sign" which is where the three teniae coli converge around the appendix [15]. For most endoscopists the cecum is reached within 70–80 cm of the colonoscope, after appropriate shortening of the endoscope to straighten the colon. The appendiceal orifice is typically folded under the cecum and is seen as a slit (Fig. 17.6). The ileocecal valve is difficult to visualize endoscopically but may be seen as a bulge about 5 cm from the ileocecal fold (Fig. 17.7) [7]. Once the cecum is reached, careful withdrawal of the colonoscope is performed to allow for endoscopic examination of the colon (Video 17.2). The hepatic and splenic flexures as well as the rectosigmoid junction are particularly difficult due their acute angulations and potential blind spots. Gentle withdrawal, reinsertion, and rotation of the colonoscope is often necessary to visualize the entire mucosa.

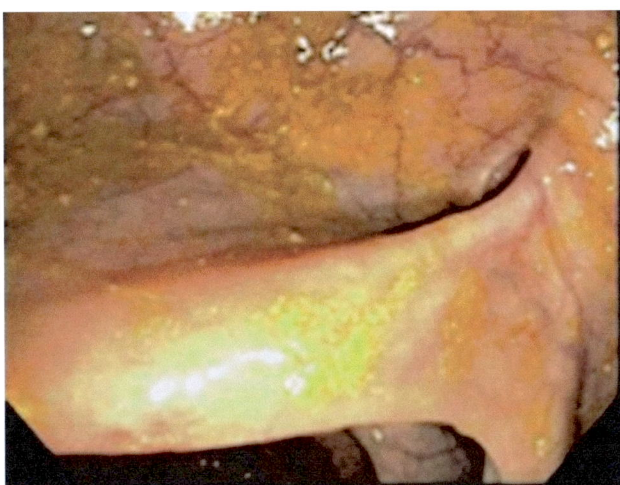

Fig. 17.3 Splenic flexure

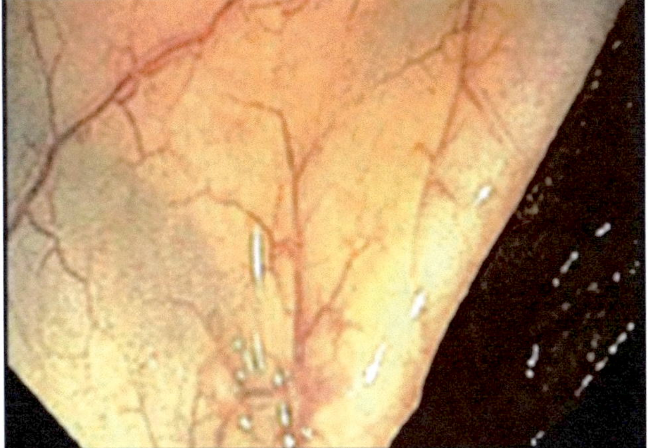

Fig. 17.4 Hepatic flexure

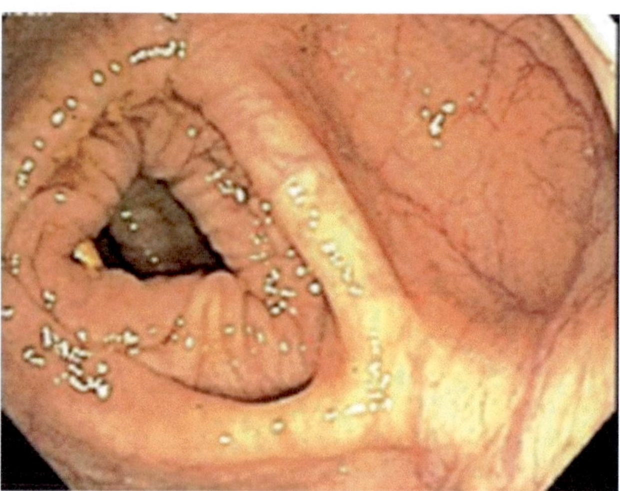

Fig. 17.5 Transverse colon

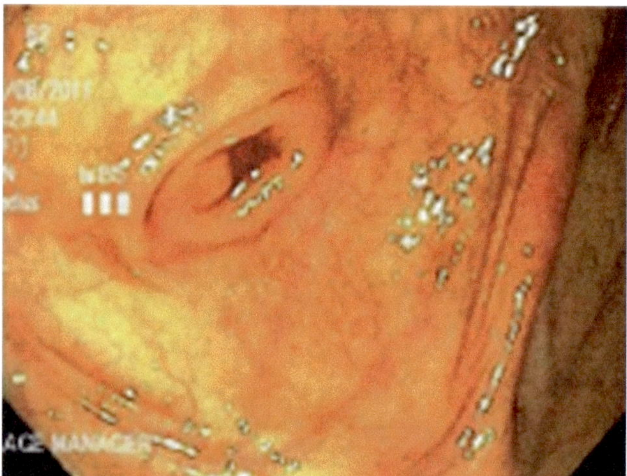

Fig. 17.6 Appendiceal orifice

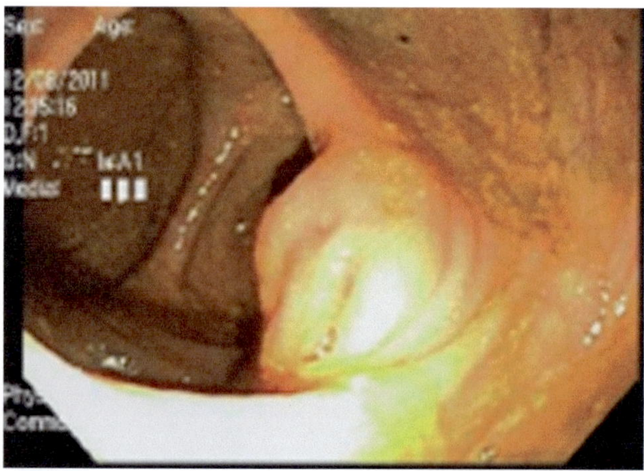

Fig. 17.7 Ileocecal valve

Lower GI Pathology

The colonic mucosa is salmon colored and transparent except when at the hepatic or splenic flexures where the mucosa has a bluish color due to the adjacent solid organs. A vascular network is visible throughout the entire colon and especially prominent in the rectum. In a normal colon, the mucosa should be smooth and regular without evidence of bleeding, pus or mucus [14].

Colonic lesions can be divided into epithelial and nonepithelial lesions. Epithelial lesions are subdivided into polyps (hyperplastic, juvenile, hamartoma, inflammatory), adenomas (tubular, tubulovillous, villous), and carcinomas. Nonepithelial lesions, which include lipomas, leiomyomas, carcinoids, and lymphoma arise from the submucosa, muscularis propria or serosa of colonic wall [16].

Wart-like elevations of the mucosa, known as polyps, are seen in approximately 30 % of patients undergoing screening colonoscopy. Hyperplastic polyps are classically pale sessile lesions, typically 2–3 mm in size, that often disappear with insufflation [17]. These insignificant polyps are usually found in the rectum or distal sigmoid with no benefit for removal as they are of no clinical consequence. Usual practice is to perform biopsy that hyperplastic polyps are noted to confirm diagnosis [18]. Adenomas are typically larger and redder compared to hyperplastic polyps and found throughout the entire colon [15]. More specifically, tubular adenomas are redder, vascular, >5 mm, often pedunculated and homogenous; while villous adenomas are large, sessile, multinodular and friable [19]. Cancers are more likely to be present as the size of the polyp increases. They are classically irregular, fungating and hard. Invasive cancers are also ulcerating, friable, adherent to the mucosa and often tethered. An invasive lesion may be injected with submucosal saline to determine if the lesion can be lifted off the mucosa. The colonoscopic "nonlifting sign" has a positive predictive value of 83 % of cancer, although one may find a false positive in patients with prior attempts at polypectomy which have caused scarring through the muscularis [20].

Submucosal lesions are often difficult to diagnose. Lipomas, which appear as yellowish submucosal bulges into the lumen, are soft lesions that do not require biopsy. Angiodysplasia, mostly seen in the cecum and ascending colon, is characterized by bright red vascular plaques, often with telangiectases, solitary or multiple. Hemangiomas are rarely seen and variable in appearance; they may appear with submucosal discoloration with small telangiectases to massive visible vessels [21]. Diverticular disease is another entity visualized as bulges or pockets out of the colon, usually seen in the descending and sigmoid colon, from couple of millimeters to several centimeters (Fig. 17.8).

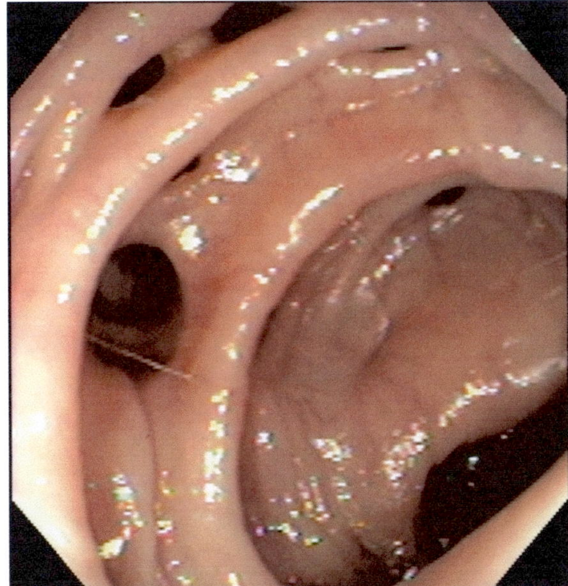

Fig. 17.8 Diverticuli

Colonoscopy can be used to differentiate between inflammatory, infectious or ischemic processes. Crohn's disease and ulcerative colitis is often difficult to distinguish. Crohn's disease, which involves the submucosa and mucosa, present early with small apthous ulcers and surrounding erythema. Cobblestoning, uniform nodules from submucosal edema, discontinuous involvement and anal lesions are typically characteristic of Crohn's disease. Ulcerative colitis, which involves the mucosal layer only, has continuous involvement of the colon. Early findings for ulcerative colitis colonoscopically include increased mucosal erythema, friability and granular appearance. Ulcerations usually indicate more severe disease. An infectious etiology whether bacterial, viral or idiopathic may be suspected if yellowish thick exudate or pus is noted. Ischemia may have a similar appearance to colitis with erythema. In severe cases of ischemia, the mucosa appears white, green or even black [7, 10].

Bowel Preparation

Prior to colonoscopic examination patients should undergo a bowel preparation for adequate visualization of the colonic mucosa. The colonoscopy preparations available to patients include osmotic cathartics and nonabsorbed osmotic agents. The osmotic cathartics, such as sodium phosphate, consist of 20 tablets the evening before the colonoscopy followed by at least 12 tablets about 10–12 h later. The nonabsorbed osmotic agents like polyethylene glycol consist of 4 and 2 L preparations with or without bisacodyl tablets [22]. Many studies have compared the 4 L solutions versus the 2 L solutions. Low volume polyethylene glycol solutions (2 L) along with bisacodyl tablets has

been shown to have equivalent efficacy compared to 4 L preparations with improved patient tolerance [23]. Many physicians are avoiding phosphate based oral preparations, because of concerns about impairment of renal function in some patients.

Colonoscope Setup and Preparation

Colonoscopy may be performed with adult or pediatric scopes. Scopes have varying lengths, either 130 or 160 cm. Prior to starting a colonoscopy, the colonoscope should be checked for insufflation and lens washing checks. The water-wash valve can be depressed to check for water from the scope tip. Air insufflation may be checked by submerging the colonoscope tip in water and looking for bubbles. Ensuring that the light source is turned on and all connections are properly attached and secure is also important. Once these checks are performed, the patient is rolled on to their left side, and visual inspection of the anus followed digital examination is performed with a lubricated finger. The lubricated colonoscope is next gently inserted through the anus under direct visualization with finger support at the tip of the scope. Alternatively with the anus lubricated with copious amounts of jelly, the scope may be directly inserted through the jelly insufflating air while entering the anal canal [7]. With a single person technique, the left hand is used for controlling the insufflation, irrigation, suction and tip deflection while the right hand maneuvers the scope shaft. A two-person technique may also be employed with the endoscopist utilizing both hands for dials and the assistant handling the scope shaft. A single person colonoscopy is preferred but an assistant may be needed for tortuous colons or when performing polypectomy [7].

With the scope within the anus, the right hand of the endoscopist should hold the shaft of the scope about 25–30 cm from the anus with a single gauze pad between the thumb and fingers. At the same time the left index finger manipulates the air, water and suction valves while the thumb drives the right and left valve. As the scope is traversed throughout the colon the movements should be slow and deliberate; rapid movements usually result in loss of visualization. The goal should always be to have the lumen in view. Fluid suctioning along the way will help with this visualization. Air insufflation is necessary for an adequate view of the lumen but overdistension will result in difficulty managing the scope as well as discomfort to the patient.

Colonoscopy Techniques

Many techniques, such as torque steering, pulling back, position change and abdominal hand pressure, may be necessary to navigate by the rectosigmoid, splenic and hepatic flexures.

Torque steering involves using the up and down control with rotation of the shaft of the scope clockwise or counterclockwise. When the scope is angulated up (left hand) with a clockwise rotation (right hand), the scope tip will move to the right. For left movement the scope is angulated down (left hand) with clockwise rotation (right hand), or kept up (left hand) with anti-clockwise rotation. Pulling back is useful when the view is lost to visualize the mucosa and allow for forward motion. This maneuver is also useful with a sharp bend, especially with the rectosigmoid junction, which often results in an N-shaped loop. The key to manipulating an N- loop involves rotating the shaft of the scope with the right hand, while pulling back so as to accordion the sigmoid colon onto the scope. This rotation and pulling back is continued until the lumen is visualized. Once this occurs, forward motion is possible. Usually suction of any air in the lumen will facilitate progress. If no progress is being made, the patient may be repositioned to supine (with knees flexed to permit access to the perineum) or right lateral position to allow for the descending colon to fall into a more favorable orientation to allow for passage of the scope. Applying abdominal pressure may also help by reducing a loop, or holding it in position so it will not re-form as the scope is introduced. Similar techniques of straightening the scope by pulling back and hand pressure may also be necessary for the splenic and hepatic flexures. Furthermore, scope stiffening may be useful at the splenic flexure to prevent looping of the sigmoid. Once at the transverse colon, the scope stiffness is released [7].

Polypectomy Techniques

Colonoscopic polypectomy is the most effective method of preventing colorectal cancer as shown by the National Polyp Study [4]. When a polyp is visualized on colonoscopy various methods are available for removal: forceps (hot or cold), snare (hot or cold) or combined methods. Forceps in general are more useful for small flat polyps than snares. For smaller polyps, 1–3 mm, cold forceps may be used (Fig. 17.9). Cold forceps have minimal risk except for the possibility of leaving residual polyp [18]. The forceps are passed through the endoscope channel and the polyp positioned at the 6 o'clock position, since that is the location of the forceps exit from the scope tip. The forceps grasps the polyp and forceps wire is pulled back gently. Careful inspection is necessary to ensure complete polyp removal from the mucosa. When hot forceps are used, only the tip of the polyp should be grasped and tented up so as to avoid cautery injury. Minimal current is used [24]. Larger polyps, greater than 6–8 mm are often removed with a snare technique (Fig. 17.10) [17]. The snare is passed through the endoscope channel, opened over the polyp at about the 6 o'clock position and closed under the polyp.

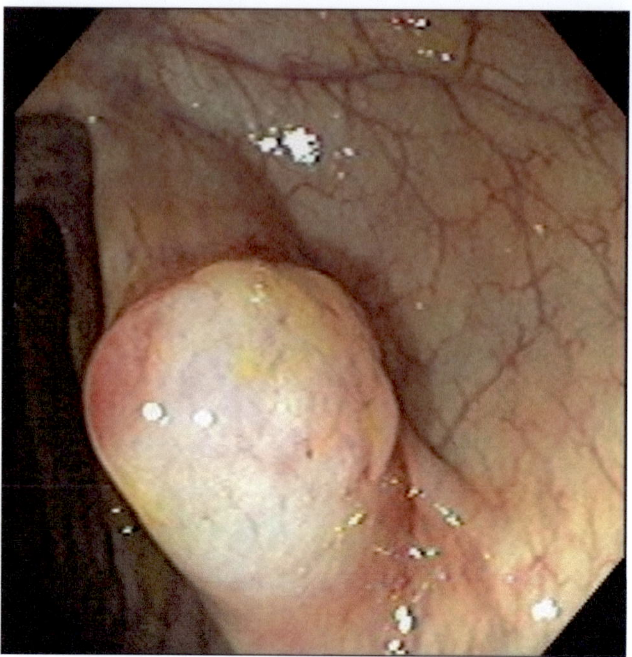

Fig. 17.9 Small polyp

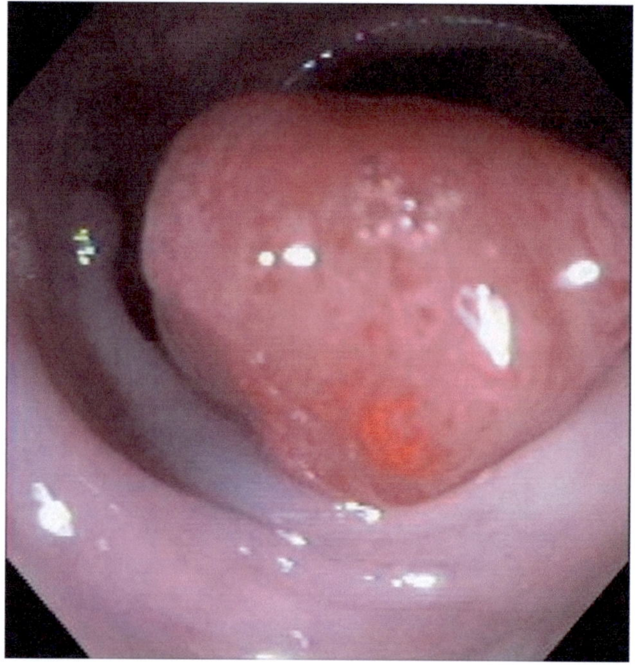

Fig. 17.10 Large polyp

When a hot snare polypectomy is performed the polyp should be tented up from the mucosa so as to avoid thermal injury (Fig. 17.11). The snare is then pulled out of the endoscope channel and the area snared examined for residual polyp [24].

For sessile polyps, endoscopic mucosal resection (EMR) may be performed (Fig. 17.12). With this procedure, saline is injected into the submucosa to elevate the polyp off the muscular

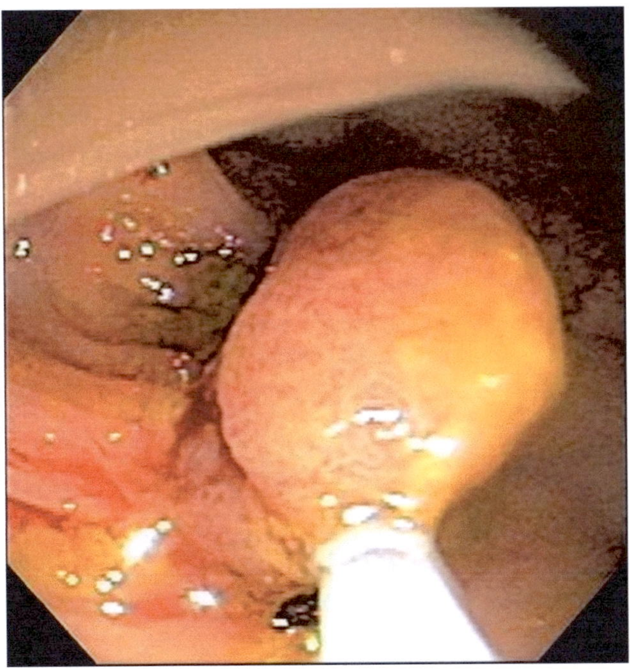

Fig. 17.11 Snare polypectomy

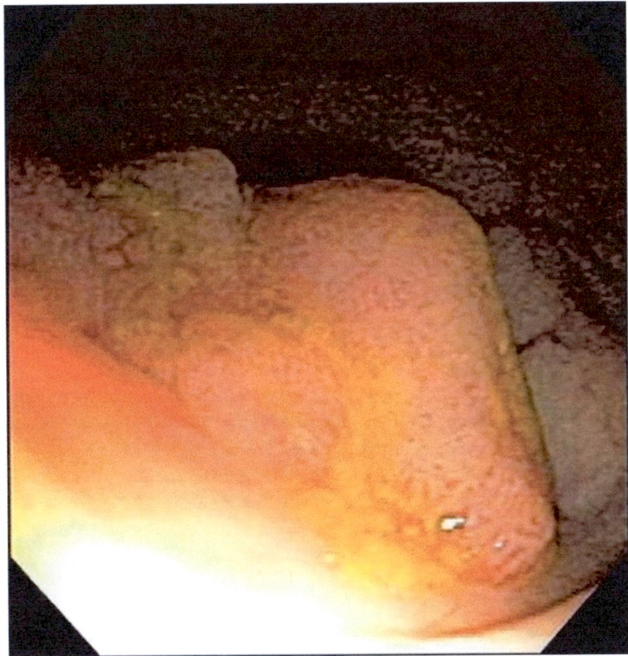

Fig. 17.12 Endoscopic mucosal resection (EMR) may be performed for sessile polyps

wall of the colon and facilitate polypectomy using the snare technique mentioned above [24]. This technique can be used even on large polyps up to 6 or 8 cm in size. Another technique that has been used is endoscopic submucosal dissection (ESD) for en bloc resection of flat polyps, usually greater than 2 cm. The base of the polyp is injected submucosally with saline. Using chromoendoscopy, the lesion may be marked with indigo carmine solution [25]. Following this, a special endoscopic electrocautery instrument, such as a flex, flush or insulated tip knife, is used to incise the mucosa around the polyp circumferentially [26]. The endoscopic knife is then used to dissect under the polyp submucosally to completely excise the specimen [26]. The advantage of ESD over EMR is the ability to obtain an en bloc resection which has been shown to result in a decrease in local recurrence [25, 27]. Both procedures may be complicated by bleeding; perforation rate is higher with ESD [27]. Colonoscopic surveillance is necessary following EMR and ESD.

Polyp retrieval can be achieved in several ways. Small polyps are suctioned through the scope. Larger polyps or multiple fragments can be removed in a Roth net. Other polyps may be fragmented with the snare and suctioned out. Certain larger polyps may be suctioned onto the tip of the scope, and removed by withdrawing the endoscope [28].

Transanal Endoscopic Techniques

Transanal excision involves removal of lesions in the lower third of the rectum. The advantage of transanal approach is that patients are spared an abdominal operation, and offered faster recovery and sphincter preservation. A new technique, transanal endoscopic microsurgery (TEM), utilizes a proctoscope with similar advantages to standard transanal excision.

TEM was first introduced by Buess et al. in the 1980s for local excision of rectal tumors up to 20 cm from the anal verge using a proctoscope with an attached microscope [29]. A 40 mm rectoscope is placed within the rectum to the lesion and is sealed with an airtight device for carbon dioxide insufflation. Entry ports allow for the use of various tissue graspers, scissors, suction, knife and binocular stereoscopic eyepiece with an accessory scope for video [30]. The indications include unresectable polyp by colonoscopy, early stage rectal carcinoma or carcinoid, other benign and malignant lesions of the rectum and anastamotic stenosis. Those who support the use of TEM suggest that the major advantage includes better exposure for lesions in the proximal rectum, and an improved ability to close any defect in the rectal wall [31].

Flexible Sigmoidoscopy

Flexible sigmoidoscopy involves the examination of the rectum, sigmoid and descending colon up to about 55–60 cm. The indications for flexible sigmoidoscopy include screening, young patients with colonic disease and those with fulminant colitis [1]. The sensitivity and specificity of colorectal cancer and large polyps is 96 % and 94 % respectively [3]. Flexible sigmoidoscopy has shown a reduction in death from rectosigmoid cancers [32]. As far as screening, the American Cancer

Society recommends that patients over age 50 have a flexible sigmoidoscopy every 5 years. If a polyp is found, then a colonoscopy is recommended. The advantage of using this modality is that no preparation is needed. Flexible sigmoidoscopy is tolerated by patients better than a rigid sigmoidoscope. There are few contraindications to flexible sigmoidoscopy but high risk of perforation is possible in patients with peritonitis, toxic megacolon or severe colitis, ischemia or diverticulitis. If a sigmoidoscopy is necessary, the examination should be performed with little air insufflation and minimal force and torquing [14]. The rate of perforation has been reported by Marks and Borenstein as 0.1 % [33].

Rigid Sigmoidoscopy and Anoscopy

Rigid sigmoidoscopy allows for the examination of the anus, rectum and distal colon while the anoscope allows for visualization of the anal canal. The advantage of the both procedures is that they may be performed in the office setting. Most commonly the patient is placed at the edge of the table in the left lateral decubitus position with knees drawn forward. Alternatively the patient may be placed on special tilting proctosigmoidoscopy table which allows the chest and abdomen to be flexed forward. This position is typically more uncomfortable for the patient and thus left lateral Sims position is preferred by most clinicians. Since this procedure is usually performed in the office setting, conscious sedation is not offered and therefore the patient should be warned that they may experience some discomfort with examination [14].

With a rigid proctoscope the patient is instructed to take a fleet enema prior to the examination. Insertion of an anoscope and proctoscope is similar with a lubricated scope passed into the anal canal toward the patient's umbilicus for about 4 cm and rotated into the rectal vault. The anoscope allows for the best view of the anal canal permitting examination of hemorrhoids and other pathology. With a proctoscope, once inserted the obturator may be removed and the lens cap secured. Gentle insufflation may be performed with the attached hand pump to allow the proctoscope to be inserted up to 25 cm to the distal colon. Air insufflation allows for visualization of the mucosa examined carefully for any pathology upon withdrawal.

Stoma Endoscopy

A colonoscope may also be used through an ileostomy or colostomy. Prior to performing this procedure the ileostomy or colostomy should be digitalized with a lubricated finger about the size of the colonoscope to be used to ensure no evidence of stenosis. Colonoscopy is usually performed with the patient in a supine position [14].

The preparation for an ileostomy usually consists of clear liquid diet and few hours of fasting [7]. For ileostomy, a pediatric scope may be necessary. During examination through an ileostomy, the scope must be pulled back often to create an accordion allowing for forward advancement.

For a colostomy, an oral bowel preparation and a lavage regimen should be performed. In addition, if attempting to pass a colonoscope through a defunctionalized bowel, tap water or saline enemas are necessary to lavage through the colostomy [7]. Once prepared colonoscopy is generally easier through a colostomy since the sigmoid colon is often removed.

References

1. Nguyen VX, Nguyen VTL, Nguyen CC. Appropriate use of endoscopy in the diagnosis and treatment of gastrointestinal diseases: up-to-date indications for primary care physicians. Int J Intern Med. 2010;3:345–57.
2. National Cancer Instutite. http://www.cancer.gov/cancertopics/types/colon-and-rectal
3. Gollub MJ, Schwartz LH, Akhurst T. Update on Colorectal Cancer Imaging. Radiol Clin North Am. 2007;45:85–118.
4. Winawer SJ, Zauber AG, Ho MN, et al. Prevention of colorectal cancer by colonoscopic polypectomy: The National Polyp Study Workgroup. N Engl J Med. 1993;329:1977–81.
5. Levin B, Lieberman DA, McFarland B, Andrews KS, et al. Screening and surveillance for the early detection of colorectal cancer and adenomatous polyps, 2008: a joint guideline from the American cancer society, the US multi-society task force on colorectal cancer, and the American college of radiology. Gastroenterology. 2008;134:1570–95.
6. Rex DK, Kahi CJ, Levin B, Smith RA, et al. Guidelines for colonoscopy surveillance after cancer resection: a consensus update by the American cancer society and the US multi-society task force on colorectal cancer. Gastroenterology. 2006;130:1865–71.
7. Cotton PB, Williams CB. Practical gastrointestinal endoscopy. 6th ed. Oxford: Blackwell Publishing Ltd; 2008. p. 87–207.
8. Winawer S, Fletcher R, Rex D, et al. Colorectal cancer screening and surveillance: clinical guidelines and rationale—update based on new evidence. Gastroenterology. 2003;124:544–60.
9. Winawer SJ, Zauber AG, Fletcher RH, et al. Guidelines for colonoscopy surveillance after polypectomy: a consensus update by the US Multi-Society Task Force on Colorectal Cancer and American Cancer Society. Gastroenterology. 2006;130:1872–85.
10. Waye JD, Rex DK, Williams CB. Colonoscopy: principles and practice. 2nd ed. Oxford: Blackwell Publishing; 2009.
11. Scholefield JH, Moss S, Sufi F, Mangham CM, Hardcastle JD. Effect of faecal occult blood screening on mortality from colorectal cancer: results from a randomized controlled trial. Gut. 2002;50:840–4.
12. Gray H. Anatomy of the human body. Philadelphia: Lea & Febiger; 1918. Bartleby.com, 2000. www.bartleby.com/107/.
13. Skandalakis JE, Colborn GL, Weidman TA et al. Skandalakis' surgical anatomy: http://www.accesssurgery.com.
14. Sivak MV, editor. Gastroenterologic endoscopy. 2nd ed. Philadelphia, PA: WB Saunders; 2000.
15. Cappell MS. Reducing the incidence and mortality of colon cancer: mass screening and colonoscopic polypectomy. Gastroenterol Clin North Am. 2008;37:129–60.
16. Ginsberg GG, Kochman ML, Norton I, Gostout CJ. Clinical gastrointestinal endoscopy. Philadelphia, PA: Elsevier Inc.; 2005.

17. Cappell MS, Friedel D. The role of sigmoidoscopy and colonoscopy in the diagnosis and management of lower gastrointestinal disorders: endoscopic findings, therapy and complications. Med Clin North Am. 2002;86:1253–88.
18. Tolliver KA, Rex DK. Colonoscopic polypectomy. Gastroenterol Clin North Am. 2008;37:229–51.
19. Cappell MS. From colonic polyps to colon cancer: pathophysiology, clinical presentation, and diagnosis. Clin Lab Med. 2005;25:135–77.
20. Ishiguro A, Uno Y, Ischiguro Y, et al. Correlation of lifting versus nonlifting and microscopic depth of invasion in early colorectal cancer. Gastrointest Endosc. 1999;50:329–33.
21. Hasegawa K, Lee W, Noguchi T, Yaguchi T, Sasaki H, Nagasako K. Colonoscopic Removal of Hemangiomas. Dis Colon Rectum. 1981;24(2):85–9.
22. Beck DE. Bowel preparation for colonoscopy. Clin Colon Rectal Surg. 2010;23:10–3.
23. Wexner SD, Beck DE, Baron TH, Fanelli RD, Hyman N, Shen B, et al. A consensus document on bowel preparation before colonoscopy: prepared by a task force from the American Society of Colon and Rectal Surgeons (ASCRS), the American Society for Gastrointestinal Endoscopy (ASGE), and the Society of American Gastrointestinal and Endoscopic Surgeons (SAGES). Dis Colon Rectum. 2006;49:792–809.
24. Fyock CJ, Draganov PV. Colonoscopic polypectomy and associated techniques. World J Gastroenterol. 2010;16(29):3630–7.
25. Nishiyama H, Isomoto H, Yamaguchi N, Fukuda A, Ikeda K, Ohnita K, et al. Endoscopic Submucosal Dissection for Colorectal Epithelial Neoplasms. Dis Colon Rectum. 2010;53:161–8.
26. Kantsevoy SV, Adler DG, Conway JD, Diehl DL, Farraye FA, Kwon R, et al. Endoscopic mucosal resection and endoscopic submucosal dissection. Gastrointest Endosc. 2008;68:11–8.
27. Tajika M, Niwa Y, Bhatia V, Kondo S, Tanaka T, Mizuno N, et al. Comparison of endoscopic submucosal dissection and endoscopic mucosal resection for large colorectal tumors. Eur J Gastroenterol Hepatol. 2011;23(11):1042–9.
28. Church JM. Experience in the endoscopic management of large colonic polyps. ANZ J Surg. 2003;73:988–95.
29. Lindsetmo R, Joh Y, Delaney CP. Surgical treatment for rectal cancer: an international perspective on what the medical gastroenterologist needs to know. World J Gastroenterol. 2008;14(21):3281–9.
30. Saclarides TJ. Transanal endoscopic microsurgery: a single surgeon's experience. Arch Surg. 1998;133:595–9.
31. Cataldo PA, O'Brien S, Osler T. Transanal endoscopic microsurgery: a prospective evaluation of functional results. Dis Colon Rectum. 2005;48:1366–71.
32. Selby JV, Friedman GD, Queendberry Jr CP, et al. A case–control study of screening sigmoidoscopy and mortality from colorectal cancer. N Engl J Med. 1992;326:653–7.
33. Marks G, Borenstein BD. Complications of flexible fiberoptic sigmoidoscopy. A conceptual approach. Surg Endosc. 1987;1:59–62.

Toshitaka Hoppo and Blair A. Jobe

Introduction

Esophagogastroduodenoscopy (EGD) has been widely accepted as a diagnostic and therapeutic tool for the evaluation and management of foregut disease. Most of procedures are currently performed under conscious sedation in an outpatient setting to reduce patient discomfort. Conscious sedation, commonly achieved by moderate sedation with analgesia such as fentanyl and midazolam, is a depressed level of consciousness that allows patients to respond purposefully to verbal commands while continuously maintaining their own airway [1]. However, most of the morbidity associated with EGD is related to sedation with narcotics and sedative agents (especially in older patients with cardiopulmonary disease), potentially leading to hypoxia, hypotension, cardiac arrhythmia and respiratory failure [2–4]. Sedation also requires the infrastructure and resources of specialized facilities and monitoring both during and after the procedure, which lead to significant associated cost and resource expenditure (direct costs). Furthermore, patients who undergo conventional EGD usually miss an entire day of work and must arrange for post-procedure transportation by a third party (indirect costs) (Table 18.1). Therefore, alternatives to sedated conventional EGD have been sought particularly for the purpose of large-scale screening and surveillance of pre-malignancy and/or malignancy in the upper gastrointestinal (GI) tract. Such alternatives should be well tolerated (patient-friendly), sensitive, cheap, safe and office-based, and be performed quickly. In addition, it would be desirable that a single examination provides information on the status of the larynx and pharynx in the same setting as esophagoscopy. Unsedated transnasal endoscopy (TNE) using a small-caliber endoscope (SCE) has been explored and introduced, expecting reduction of sedation-related complications and costs. In this chapter, the current status of SCE is reviewed, and its indications and applications are summarized.

Overview of the Small-Caliber Endoscope

Dimension of SCE

SCE (outer diameter <6 mm) was initially designed for use in pediatric patients and has been refined for the aim of reducing patient discomfort so that it can be performed without sedation. Since unsedated TNE was first described by Shaker in 1994, [5] unsedated TNE has been widely performed internationally. However, unsedated TNE has not gained widespread acceptance in the USA most likely because of a misperception that the approach is associated with increased patient anxiety and discomfort, and unfamiliarity of nasal anatomy on the part of GI endoscopist [6]. Potential benefits of unsedated TNE include reduced risk of cardiopulmonary complications, reduced recovery time and costs, minimized time lost from work, the ability to provide patient feedback on exam findings, direct examination of nasopharynx and larynx, and no need for a third-party transportation (Table 18.2).

The currently available SCEs were summarized in Table 18.3 [7]. SCEs have a design similar to standard endoscopes, with a control section containing tip deflection dials, an air/water channel, and a coaxial accessory channel (Fig. 18.1, upper left) [8]. A high-quality color image is generated by a charge coupled device (CCD) chip built in

This chapter contains a video segment that can be found by accessing the following link: http://www.springerimages.com/videos/978-1-4614-6329-0.

T. Hoppo, M.D., Ph.D. • B.A. Jobe, M.D., F.A.C.S. (✉)
Department of Surgery, Institute for the Treatment of Esophageal & Thoracic Disease, West Penn Allegheny Health System, North Tower, 4800 Friendship, Suite 4600, Pittsbrugh, PA 15224, USA
e-mail: jobeba@upmc.edu

J.M. Marks and B.J. Dunkin (eds.), *Principles of Flexible Endoscopy for Surgeons*,
DOI 10.1007/978-1-4614-6330-6_18, © Springer Science+Business Media New York 2013

Table 18.1 Direct and indirect costs associated with sedated conventional endoscopy

Sedated endoscopy
Direct costs
Specialized endoscopy suite
Personnel (2 assistants and recovery nurse)
Equipment for monitoring
IV medications
Indirect costs
Loss of work
Third-party transportation
Time-consuming
Risks
Sedation related complications (hypoxia, arrhythmia, respiratory failure, etc.)

Table 18.2 Potential benefits of unsedated transnasal endoscopy

Potential benefits of small-caliber endoscopy
Less cardiopulmonary complications
Less expensive
Less time consuming
Office-based
Direct patient feedback
Lower threshold to perform screening
Less time lost from work
No need for a third-party transportation
Examination of nasopharynx and direct laryngoscopy

the tip of the scope. Some models have advanced image enhancement function such as narrow-band imaging. Most SCEs are compatible with a standard light source and processor. One model (Vision-Sciences, Orangeburg, NY) has a portable "lap-top-like" processor and built-in light and insufflation source for in-office use. Currently available SCE have an outer diameter range of 4.9–6 mm and a working length range of 600–1,100 mm. The scopes with 600–650 mm length are designed for the examination of nasopharyngeal passages and esophagus. The accessory channel for the majority of SCE is 2 mm, which accommodates passage of small-caliber instruments such as pediatric biopsy forceps (Fig. 18.1, upper right). All SCE have either 2-way (up/down) or 4-way angulation (up/down and right/left) at the insertion tube and imaging element. The smallest diameter SCE with 4-way angulation has an outer diameter of 5.3 mm (Pentax, Montvale, NJ). A recent randomized trial demonstrated that SCE with 4-way angulation shortened examination time while providing easy transnasal insertion and improving patient tolerability, although the examination time without biopsy was not significantly different between 2-way (5.2 mm diameter) and 4-way (5.5 mm diameter) models [9]. Similar to standard EGD, most SCEs have a circular cross-sectional configuration. One model (Vision-Sciences, Orangeburg, NY) has an oval configuration and a disposable plastic sheath that contains

Table 18.3 Small-caliber endoscopes available in the USA [7]

Model	Angulation (°)	Field of view (°)	Features	Shaft diameter (mm)	Accessory channel diameter (mm)	Working length (mm)	Cost ($)
Olympus (Center Valley, PA)							
GIF-XP 180N	210 up/90 down 100 left/100 right	120	NB1	5.5	2	1,100	30,000
GIF N180	210 up/120 down	120	NB1	4.9	2	1,100	28,675
PEF-V	180 up/130 down	120	N/A	5.3	2	650	21,400
Fujinon (Wayne, NJ)							
EG-530N	210 up/90 down 100 left/100 right	120	FICE	5.9	2	1,100	26,800
EG-530NP	210 up/120 down	120	FICE	4.9	2	1,100	26,700
EG-270NS	210 up/120 down 100 left/100 right	120	N/A	5.9	2	1,100	
Vision-Sciences (Orangeburg, NJ)							
TNE-5000	145 up/215 down	120	N/A	4.7/5.4 (oval shaft)	1.5	650	25,000
				4.7/5.8 (oval shaft)	2.1		Includes processor, disposable endosheath $40 each
Pentax (Montvale, NJ)							
EG 1580K	210 up/120 down	140	ISCAN[a]	5.1	2	1,050	25,200
EG 1690K	210 up/120 down 120 left/120 right	120	ISCAN	5.4	2	1,100	26,500
EG 1870K	210 up/120 down 120 right/120 left	140	ISCAN	6	2	1,050	24,885
EE 1580K	210 up/120 down	140	ISCAN	5.5 tip, 5.1 shaft	2	600	18,900
FG-16V	180 up/180 down 160 right/160 left	125	Fiberoptic	5.3	2	925	15,750

FICE Fuji intelligent color enhancement, *N/A* not applicable, *NBI* narrow-band imaging

[a]Pentax proprietary image enhancement

Fig. 18.1 *Upper left panel*: Small-caliber endoscope. *Upper right panel*: Biopsy forceps place through the working channel of a small-caliber endoscope. *Lower panel*: Transnasal endoscopy is performed with a patient in the sitting position (reproduced from Kim et al. *Surg Innov* 2006;13(1):31–39)

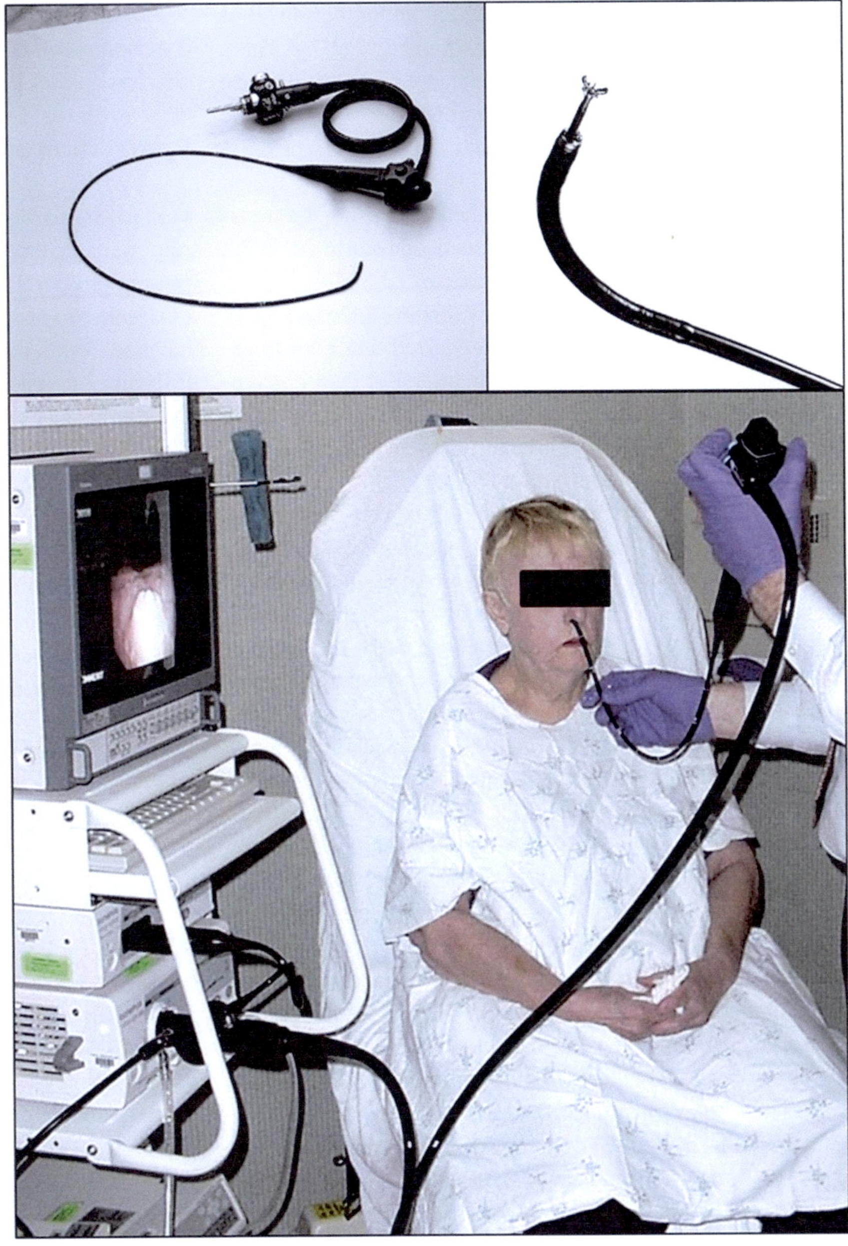

the accessory channel so that none of the endoscope comes into contact with the patient. This disposable sleeve concept has the distinct advantage of eliminating the time and expense of reprocessing which makes it particularly attractive for in-office use.

Transnasal vs. Per-Oral

It remains debatable what is the best route for insertion of SCE, the transnasal or the peroral route. It is thought that the transnasal route results in less nausea and choking probably because the posterior part of tongue is not touched by the endoscope [10]. Although some randomized trials conducted in the late 1990s and early 2000s suggested that the peroral route may be easier to perform and slightly preferred by both patients and endoscopists, [11–14] the following randomized trials that compare two distinct routes have demonstrated considerable benefits of the transnasal routes and these findings are consistent within our practice. In a randomized trial of TNE versus conventional EGD involving 150 patients, Preiss et al. demonstrated that TNE was tolerated better and required less sedation than conventional EGD; additionally, TNE was associated with less gagging compared to the conventional approach and a high level of patient satisfaction [15]. In a randomized trial by Thota et al., 90 patients underwent unsedated SCE via either the transnasal route ($n=44$) or the peroral route ($n=46$), and the transnasal route was better tolerated with equivalent diagnostic accuracy to standard EGD [16]. In the most recent randomized trial to compare unsedated SCE using the transnasal and peroral routes with sedated conventional EGD, Trevisani et al. demonstrated that transnasal SCE is associated with less discomfort and is better tolerated [17]. Additionally, univariate analysis suggested that both transnasal and peroral SCE were better tolerated than conventional EGD, but multivariate analysis indicated that only transnasal SCE showed significantly lower discomfort and higher tolerance than conventional EGD [17].

TNE is likely to be an extremely useful modality to examine the esophagus and gastroesophageal junction (GEJ) because it may result in less gagging and patient discomfort than the unsedated peroral or conventional approaches. In a recent prospective observational study to evaluate the diagnostic yield of unsedated SCE in patients with symptoms of gastroesophageal reflux disease (GERD), patients underwent transnasal SCE ($n=752$), peroral SCE ($n=572$), or conventional EGD ($n=254$), and endoscopic observations and measurements were compared. The results of this work demonstrated that the size of hiatal hernia was smaller in the transnasal route than in the peroral route suggesting that gagging induced by the peroral approach may have caused an overestimation of hiatal hernia. The authors concluded that the transnasal route with less gagging reflex and better-controlled breathing is more beneficial especially for the evaluation of hiatal hernia [18]. Furthermore, TNE has been shown to induce parasympathetic inhibition with less sympathetic stimulation than peroral EGD, thus reducing peristalsis, so that the endoscopists can exam the lumen and anatomical structure of the esophagus and GEJ more accurately without the effect of peristalsis [19]. This is also a potential benefit of TNE for the observation of native GEJ, which may be affected by peristalsis.

GI endoscopists may not be familiar with nasal anatomy and may require additional training for TNE (Fig. 18.2). In fact, this is one of the reasons why transnasal SCE has not been widely accepted. It is noted that the transnasal route is anatomically straighter to the esophageal opening than the peroral route which requires steeper angulation of the insertion tube and results in a fulcrum effect at the base of the tongue; the end result is more gagging and an uncomfortable and/or compromised examination for the patient and endoscopist. Interestingly, a study of the learning curve for TNE demonstrated that skilled endoscopists successfully performed this procedure from their first attempts and could be easily self-trained [20].

Techniques of Unsedated Transnasal Endoscopy (Video 18.1)

Preparation and Anesthesia

Patients should fast at least 4 h prior to undergoing TNE. It is important to obtain a history of epistaxis, nasal or laryngeal trauma or operation, prior difficult nasal intubation, history of Zenker's or epiphrenic diverticulum and allergies or adverse events related to topical or local anesthetic such as lidocaine toxicity and methemoglobinemia. A physical examination is performed, including a careful examination of the oral cavity and nasal passage with a speculum to exclude possible deviated septum or an oropharyngeal lesion that may cause difficulty introducing the SCE. Patients should be asked to identify the more patent side of the nose. In the case of a deviated septum, the SCE should be introduced on the side opposite the deviation.

Unsedated TNE is performed with the patient in the sitting position (Fig. 18.1, lower panel). Successful TNE is highly dependent on adequate topical anesthesia. Complete anesthesia of the nasopharynx, orophayrnx and hypopharynx is critical for the comfortable passage of the endoscope. First, 7 mL of aerosolized 4% liquid lidocaine and 0.05% oxymetazoline hydrochloride (vasoconstricting agent) 50% by volume is instilled into the most patent naris over a 5-min period by using an atomizer (Wolfe Tory Medical, Salt Lake City, UT) (Fig. 18.3a). A single 3-s instillation of aerosolized 14% benzocaine is introduced into the oropharynx followed by the insertion of 5 mL of 2% lidocaine jelly into the nares. Aspiration of a small amount of the anesthetic agent can occur and may cause temporary coughing and cervical dysphagia; when this occurs, the patient should be reassured that the symptoms will subside within 15 min. The anesthetic preparation for TNE takes approximately 10 min. Based on our experience, 7 mL of aerosolized 4% lidocaine instilled using an atomizer into bilateral naris over a 5-min period should be adequate to achieve complete anesthesia of the transnasal and hypopharyngeal route for successful TNE.

Insertion and Withdrawal

We currently use a flexible endoscope (TNE-5000, Vision-Sciences, Inc., Orangeburg, NY) with 2-way angulation (145 up/215 down), 4.7 mm diameter and 65 cm in length (Fig. 18.3b, c). This scope is placed inside a sterile disposable sheath (EndoSheath®, Vision-Sciences, Inc., Orangeburg, NY), which provides a durable, one-use protective barrier as well as a coaxial 2.1 mm biopsy channel, so that none of the endoscope comes into contact with the patient and the time required for scope processing can be eliminated (Fig. 18.3d).

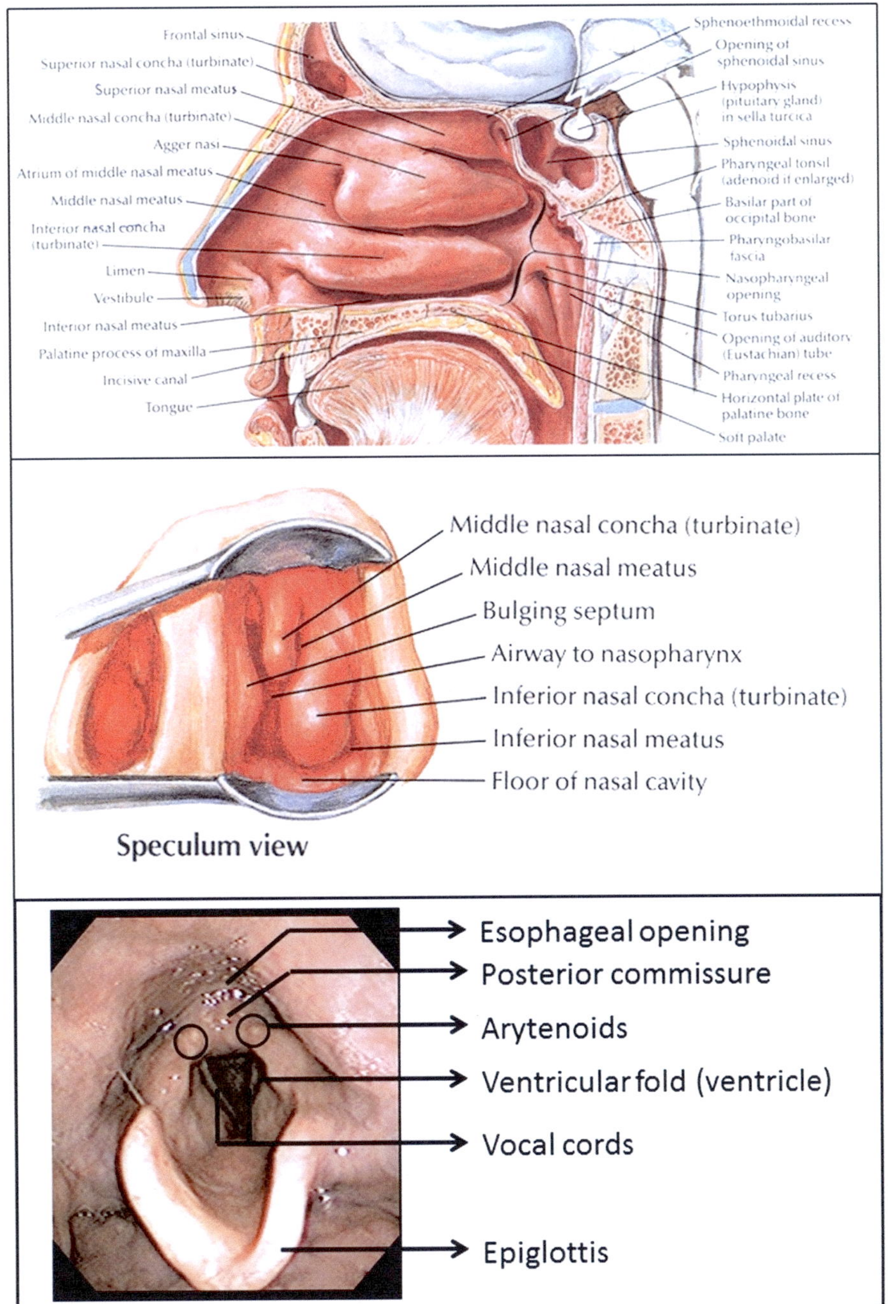

Fig. 18.2 Anatomy of the nasal cavity. *Upper panel*: the sagittal view of the nasal cavity. *Middle panel*: the speculum view of the nasal cavity. *Lower panel*: Appearance of normal larynx

The scope is then inserted transnasally along the floor of the nasal cavity under direct visualization into the posterior pharynx. If access to the nasopharynx is not possible below the inferior turbinate, the endoscopist should attempt to enter between inferior and middle turbinates. Because the insertion tubes of most endoscopes is slightly larger than the endoscope shaft, the most resistance and patient discomfort may be encountered during initial insertion. It is important to apply gentle downward pressure on the shaft as it enters the nose to minimize pressure on the nares and avoid sudden movements of the shaft, which can cause patient discomfort. The mucosa of the nasopharynx, oropharynx and hypopharynx is examined and direct laryngoscopy is performed. With the neck in flexion, the endoscope is passed into the esophagus in coordination with a swallow. Once the esophagus is intubated, upper endoscopy is performed in the standard fashion.

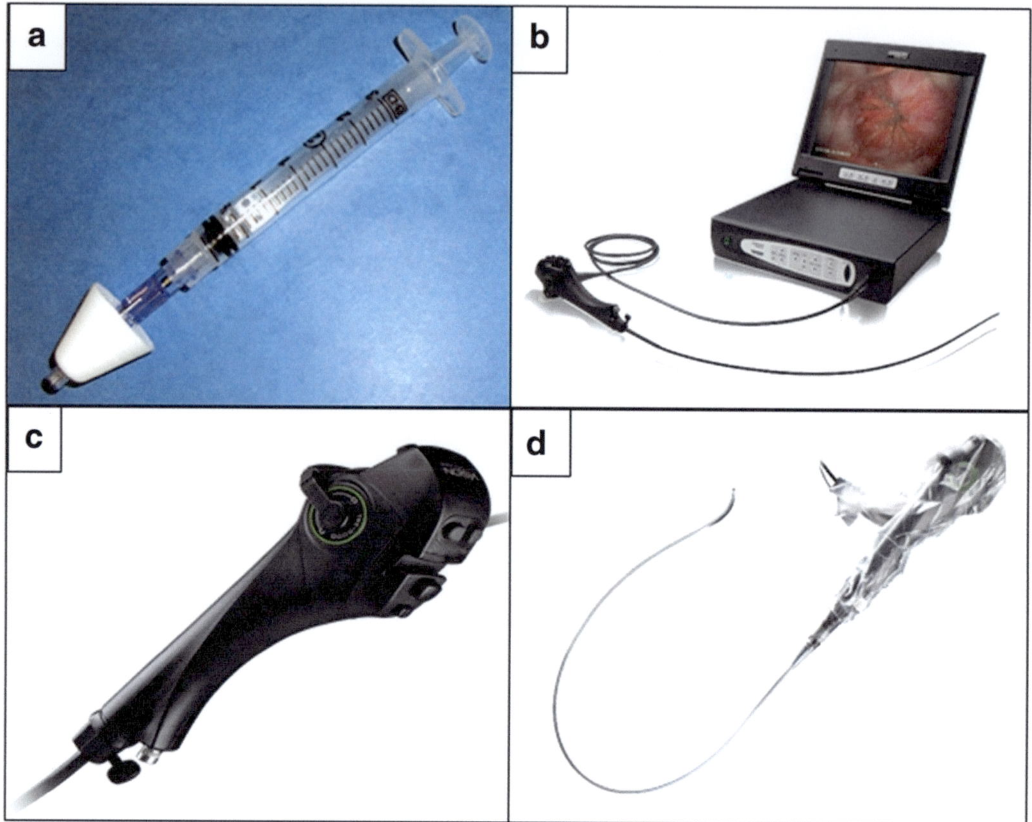

Fig. 18.3 (**a**) Atomizer (Wolfe Tory Medical). (**b** and **c**) TNE-5000 system (Vision-Sciences, Inc.) includes a flexible endoscope with 2-way angulation, 4.7 mm diameter and 65 cm in length, and a portable processor with built-in light source for in-office use. (**d**) The scope is placed inside a sterile disposable sheath (EndoSheath®, Vision-Sciences, Inc.) which provides a durable, protective barrier as well as a coaxial 2.1 mm biopsy channel, so that none of reusable portions in the endoscope contact the patient. (Images of TNE-5000 system, permission for use granted by Vision-Sciences, Inc., Orangeburg, NY)

Unlike conventional EGD, the SCE has less stiffness of the shaft. It is therefore extremely important to avoid any bend or looping of the SCE on the outside of the patient so as to transmit adequate torque along the entire length of the endoscope and thereby deliver 1:1 movements from the provider's hand to the insertion tube; the end result is preservation of all degrees of freedom using a one-knob 2-way deflection device. When SCE is removed through the nose, it should be ensured that the tip of the scope stays in the center of lumen to avoid injury to the nasal septum and turbinates. The peroral route can be used when the scope cannot be passed transnasally; however, in our experience this approach is associated with significantly more patient discomfort and gagging.

It is well known that anxiety decreases patient compliance, making the procedure more difficult [21, 22]. Patients who undergo unsedated TNE may have anxiety and it is therefore important to maintain conversation and reassurance during the procedure, thus significantly reducing patient's anxiety and allowing the thorough examination. The endoscopy room should be dimly lit and quiet, and the patient directed through relaxing imagery prior to insertion.

Endoscopic Examination

A significant advantage of TNE compared with conventional EGD is that complete examination of the nasopharynx and hypopharynx as well as direct laryngoscopy can be performed. The following structures should be carefully examined for edema, erythema, ulceration, granulation tissue formation or masses: the soft palate, sinus and eustachian tube openings, base of tongue, epiglottis, valleculae, piriform recesses, posterior commissure, vocal folds, ventricles, and subglottic region. The findings of laryngeal inflammation such as arytenoid erythema and edema, vocal-cord erythema and edema [23, 24], posterior commissure hypertrophy (pachydermia) [25], and pseudosulcus (diffuse subglottic edema) [26, 27] may be associated with laryngopharyngeal reflux (LPR) (Table 18.4, Fig. 18.4). Vocal cord mobility and medialization with phonation are examined and documented. Vocal-cord dysfunction may be caused by chronic laryngeal irritation via LPR [28].

In a manner identical to conventional EGD, the entire esophagus, stomach and duodenum are examined.

Table 18.4 Laryngoscopic findings of laryngeal inflammation via laryngopharyngeal reflux

Laryngopharyngeal findings of suspicious LPR
Arytenoids erythema and edema
Vocal-cord erythema and edema
Posterior commissure hypertrophy (Pachydermia)
Pseudosulcus (diffuse subglottic edema)
Vocal-cord dysfunction

Esophagogastroscopy can be performed using a shorter length SCE. Retroflexion is performed to evaluate the appearance of the gastric cardia. High-quality images equivalent to standard EGD can be obtained with SCE (Fig. 18.5). A solution of water and simethicone (Gold-line Laboratories Inc., Miami, FL) is used and patients are instructed to swallow sips of water to clear the field and obtain optimal exposure during the procedure. Any questionable lesions should be biopsied by using pediatric biopsy forceps via the accessory working channel.

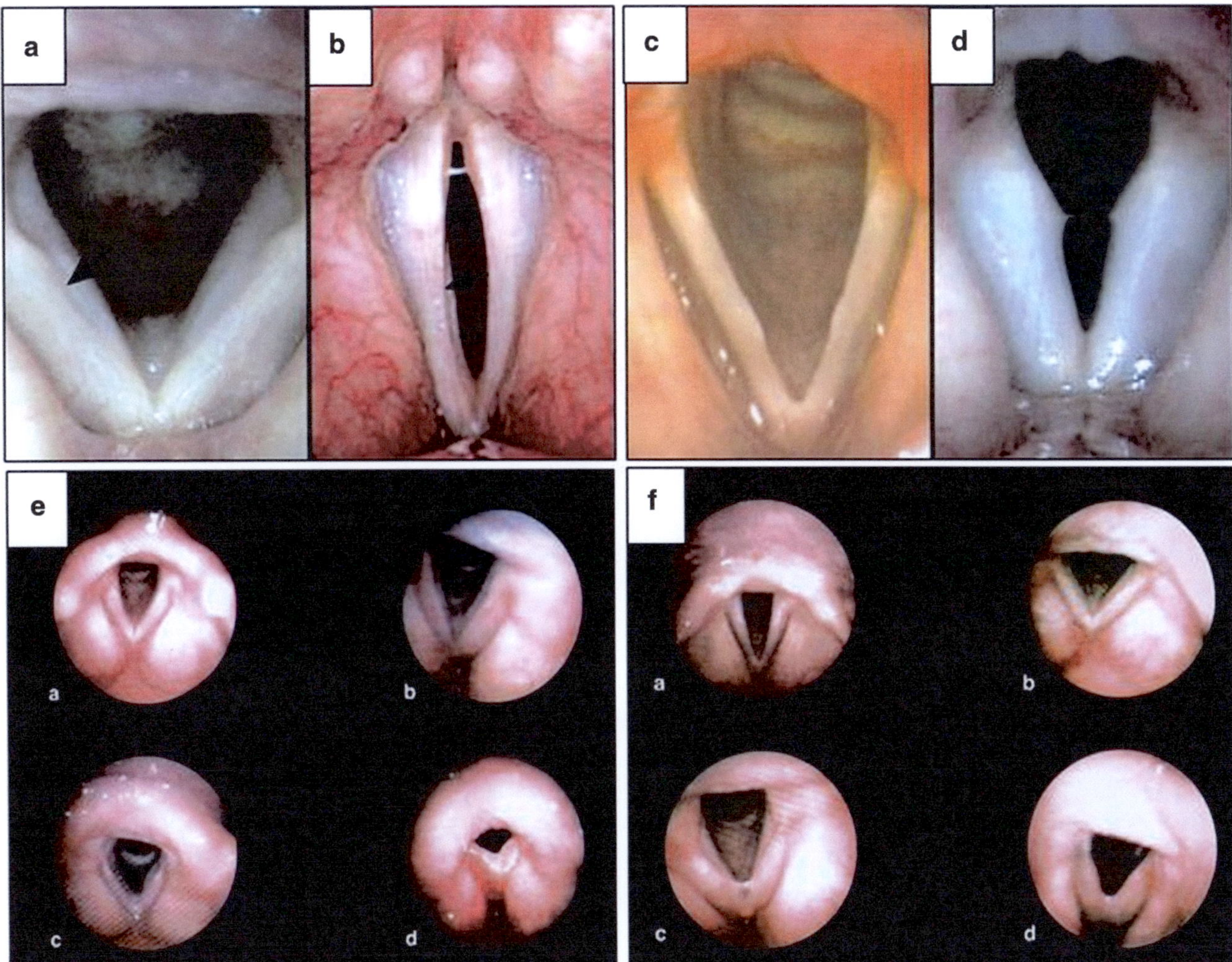

Fig. 18.4 Endoscopic findings of laryngeal inflammation. (**A**) Bilateral pseudosulcus vocalis (*arrow*) (*abnormal*). The subglottic edema extends past the vocal process all the way to the posterior larynx in conjunction with the presence of posterior commissure hypertrophy, vocal fold edema, diffuse laryngeal edema and partial ventricular obliteration. (**B**) *Normal* (*true*) sulcus vocalis (*arrow*). The sulcus is present in the midportion of the striking zone and stops at the vocal process of the arytenoids. (**C**) *Normal* open laryngeal ventricles. The sharp ventricular bands and the open space between the true and false vocal folds are present. (**D**) Ventricular obliteration (*abnormal*). Both the true and false vocal folds are swollen, thus obliterating the ventricles. (**E**) Vocal-cord edema. (*a*) Mild vocal-cord edema. (*b*) Moderate vocal-cord edema. (*c*) Severe vocal-cord edema. Sessile changes are noted. (*d*) Polypoid degeneration of the true vocal folds with the presence of severe posterior commissure hypertrophy, total ventricular obliteration and diffuse laryngeal edema. (**F**) Posterior commissure hypertrophy. (*a*) Normal commissure. Cuneiform cartilages can still be visualized. (*b*) Mild posterior commissure hypertrophy. Slight mustache-like configuration of posterior commissure can be seen. (*c*) Moderate posterior commissure hypertrophy. Straight line across the posterior larynx can be seen. (*d*) Severe posterior commissure hypertrophy (reproduced from Belafsky et al. *Laryngoscope* 2001;111:1313–1317)

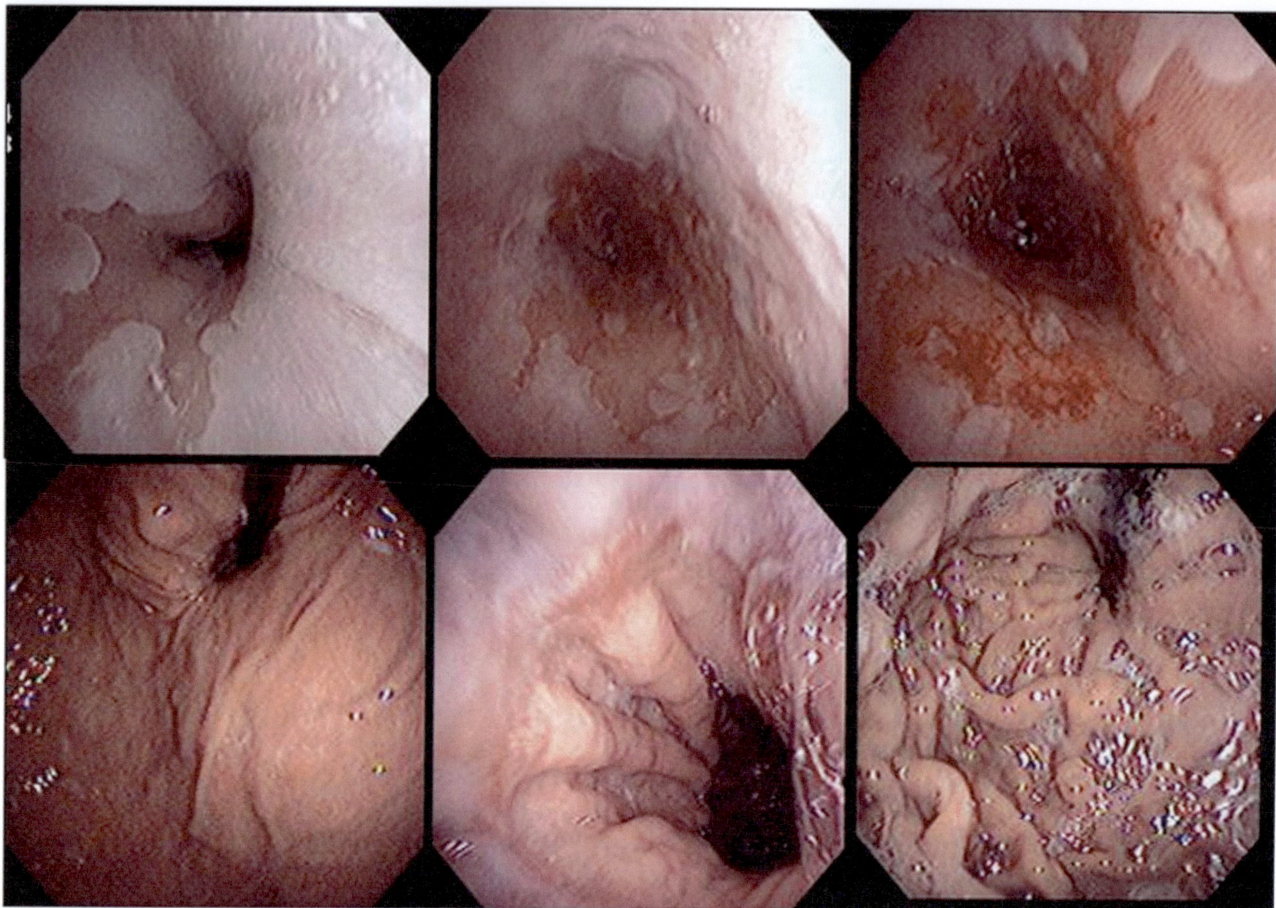

Fig. 18.5 Endoscopic views with small-caliber endoscope. *Upper panels*: Barrett's esophagus. *Lower panels*: Hiatal hernia

Feasibility and Tolerability

In the largest series to evaluate the feasibility and tolerability of TNE involving 1,100 consecutive patients, unsedated TNE was successfully completed in 94% [13]. Causes of failure included the inability to pass the endoscope transnasally (63%), patient refusal (19%) and nasal pain (18%). Factors associated with failed transnasal passage included female gender, age younger than 35 years, and larger endoscope diameter. As this series demonstrated, the diameter of the endoscope has been identified as one of the main factors for successful TNE. The diameter ≤5.3 mm is associated with successful transnasal intubation in 90–100% of cases, as compared to 78–100% with a larger diameter [11, 29]. Based on an amalgam of published series, the inability to pass the endoscope transnasally has been reported in 3–8% of total cases [13, 15, 17]. Furthermore, a higher proportion of patients were willing to repeat TNE compared to conventional sedated endoscopy (82% TNE vs. 60% conventional sedated endoscopy), [15, 30–32] and 57–100% of patients who had undergone both procedures preferred unsedated TNE over conventional EGD [9, 11, 13, 33, 34].

Indications for Unsedated TNE

With recent advances in imaging technology, SCE can provide equivalent image quality to conventional EGD [17, 34]. Unsedated TNE can be performed in a wide range of environments, including the office setting, operating room, outpatient endoscopy suite or at the bedside. The indications for unsedated TNE are essentially the same as for conventional sedated EGD; however, the advanced therapeutic applications are significantly more limited. Unsedated TNE is beneficial especially for the large-scale screening and surveillance of foregut disease because of its potential benefits such as reduced invasiveness and increased cost-effectiveness [34]. Unsedated TNE is suitable for the examination of patients who do not want sedation or cannot tolerate it because of cardiopulmonary disease, or those who cannot tolerate the peroral route [35]. Unsedated TNE is particularly advantageous in the evaluation of critically ill or hemodynamically unstable patients who cannot tolerate narcotics and other sedative agents that may have an impact on blood pressure and cardiac output [6]. SCE is also useful to traverse stenosis within the GI tract, which cannot be passed with standard-caliber EGD [36].

On the other hand, it may be difficult to perform targeted biopsies or endoscopic procedures especially when using SCE with 2-way angulation [9]. Therefore, SCE may be less suitable when a prolonged examination is required (i.e., long-segment Barrett's esophagus).

Diagnostic Applications of Unsedated TNE

Screening and Surveillance

Unsedated TNE is particularly advantageous for the large-scale screening and surveillance of upper GI premalignancies and/or malignancies. For this purpose, image quality and diagnostic accuracy must be equivalent to conventional EGD. With the significant advances in CCD technology, the initial drawback of SCE such as inferior image quality has been overcome and imaging enhancements have been successfully applied (e.g., narrow band imaging, magnification, high-resolution). Several comparison studies have demonstrated that SCE is equivalent in terms of diagnostic accuracy with equivalent image quality [17, 34, 37]. Some authors have suggested that the ability of SCE to detect small malignant lesions within the proximal stomach and along the lesser curvature may be more difficult to observe and take biopsies with SCE [38, 39]. Furthermore, it has been suggested that because SCE is associated with less illumination and air/water pressure for lens washing compared to conventional endoscopy that meticulous examination to detect subtle mucosal abnormalities may be less effective [38–40].

SCEs have a 2-mm working channel, which enables passage of biopsy forceps. Several studies have demonstrated that while the sample size is smaller with TNE obtained biopsies, there is an equivalent histologic yield compared to biopsies obtained with the conventional sedated approach [10, 11].

Barrett's Esophagus

Given the relatively low incidence of esophageal adenocarcinoma compared to the high prevalence of GERD (up to 20% of the general population in the USA) and Barrett's esophagus (6–12% of those with chronic GERD symptoms), [41–43] unsedated TNE can greatly contribute to the cost-effective, large-scale screening and surveillance strategy. Previous studies have demonstrated that SCE can correctly identify the presence of Barrett's esophagus and biopsies through SCE are equivalent to conventional EGD with regard to histopathologic confirmation of Barrett's esophagus and dysplasia in patients with known disease [44]. More recently, in a randomized crossover trial of 121 patients undergoing both unsedated TNE and conventional EGD for screening and surveillance of Barrett's esophagus, Jobe at al. demonstrated that unsedated TNE has equivalent diagnostic accuracy for the detection of Barrett's esophagus and dysplasia, despite the smaller tissue specimens obtained with unsedated TNE [34].

Gastric Cancer

The role of unsedated TNE for the screening of early gastric cancer remains relatively unexplored in the USA. In a recent comparison study for the diagnosis of early gastric cancer, Hayashi et al. demonstrated that the diagnostic yield of unsedated TNE is inferior to that of standard EGD and noted that six lesions larger than 20 mm were not detected [38]. In another study to compare SCE with an equivalent resolution to standard EGD (GIF-XP260N; Olympus Medical Systems, Tokyo, Japan) with a high-resolution EGD (GIF-H260Z; Olympus Medical Systems) involving 57 patients with or without early gastric cancer, all of whom were sedated, the sensitivity of SCE was significantly lower than that of a high-resolution endoscopy for the diagnosis of early neoplasia (58.5% vs. 78%, $p = 0.021$). The miss rate for neoplasia was most pronounced in the proximal stomach for SCE vs. high-resolution endoscopy (29% vs. 7%, $p = 0.002$) [39].

Esophageal Varices

Conscious sedation may be problematic in patients with severe liver cirrhosis because of risk of encephalopathy. Unsedated TNE may be beneficial in evaluating and tracking esophageal varices in cirrhotic patients. In a comparative study involving 15 patients with liver cirrhosis, Saeian et al. demonstrated that the detection and grading of esophageal and gastric varices were equivalent in unsedated TNE and standard EGD [45].

Therapeutic Applications of Unsedated TNE

Feeding Tube Placement

The therapeutic role of TNE has been expanding in the care of patients with foregut diseases. Two main therapeutic applications of TNE have emerged: nasoenteral feeding tube placement and percutaneous endoscopic gastrostomy (PEG). Patients requiring a feeding tube are usually ill, and may not tolerate sedation or sedation-related complications. Numerous studies have demonstrated that TNE provides a good (74–99%) success rate for the placement of nasogastric or nasoenteral feeding tubes [46–54]. Following local anesthesia, a guidewire is placed into the duodenum through the working channel under direct visualization and the SCE is removed while the guidewire is left in place. The feeding tube is then place over the guidewire. The benefits of this

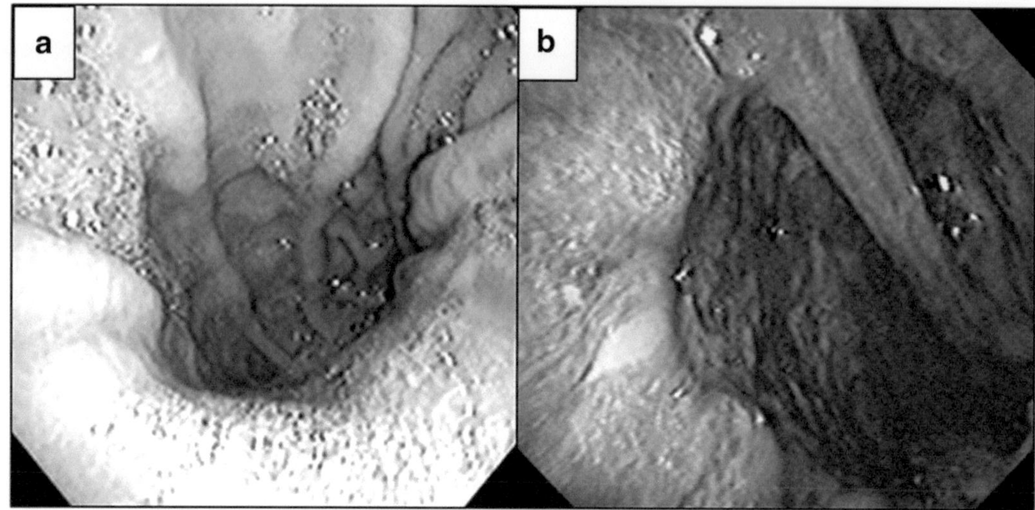

Fig. 18.6 Unsedated transnasal endoscopy is performed to assess the status of gastric conduit after esophagectomy, demonstrating (*left panel*) a viable freshly made conduit, and (*right panel*) a necrotic conduit (reproduced from Kim et al. *Surg Innov* 2006;13(1):31–39)

approach include expediency, reduced risk of cardiopulmonary complications and the absence of radiation exposure. This approach is particularly advantageous for patients who have fresh anastomosis following upper GI surgery such as esophagectomy and gastrectomy because the feeding tube can be placed under direct visualization rather than blind placement [6].

The PEG procedure can be performed transnasally using the "pull" technique if a gastrostomy tube with a collapsible bumper is used, which can be passed through the nasal cavity. Vitale et al. reported that the PEG tube with a collapsible bumper was successfully placed without complications in two patients [55]. In patients with a malignant esophageal stricture, the "push" PEG technique under TNE can be performed to avoid malignant seeding at the PEG site [56]. In this procedure, the PEG tube is directly inserted into the stomach after localization of the puncture site using endoscopic transillumination. Further procedures are being investigated, including cholangioscopy and biliary drainage in septic patients [57, 58].

Perioperative Evaluation at Bedside

Unsedated TNE can be performed at the bedside with minimal equipment and personnel. Therefore, unsedated TNE is extremely useful to evaluate patients who become ill due to possible anastomotic leak or necrotic conduit after upper GI surgery such as esophagectomy, Roux-en-Y gastric bypass and gastrectomy. Kim et al. reported that unsedated TNE enabled direct examination of the mucosa, allowing the accurate diagnosis of an ischemic gastric conduit on seven patients who had undergone esophagectomy (Fig. 18.6), and

showed significant advantages over other diagnostic modalities such as computed tomography and esophagram. The authors further reported that unsedated TNE is useful to evaluate patients with suspicious gastric outlet obstruction and to identify the source of upper GI hemorrhage such as gastric stress ulcers [6].

Positioning of pH and Impedance Catheters

In patients with symptoms suspicious for laryngopharyngeal reflux, TNE is tremendously useful to examine the oropharynx and hypopharynx, and ensure the accurate positioning of pH and impedance catheter [6]. Following TNE with local anesthesia, the SCE is maintained in the oropharynx, and the catheter is transnasally passed under direct visualization. With the hypopharynx in view, the catheter is properly positioned and secured on to the patient's face and neck with a transparent adhesive covering (Fig. 18.7).

Complications of TNE

Because TNE is performed without sedation, most of sedation-related complications can be eliminated. The most frequent complication of TNE is epistaxis, although it is self-limited in most cases. When epistaxis does occur, it requires tamponade with a cotton swab in up to 6% of cases [9]. The two largest series of TNE involving a total of 1,700 patients have demonstrated low rates of complications such as self-limited epistaxis (0.85–2%) and vasovagal events (0.3%) [13, 59]. A single esophageal perforation was reported [14]. The thinner endoscopes have been shown to

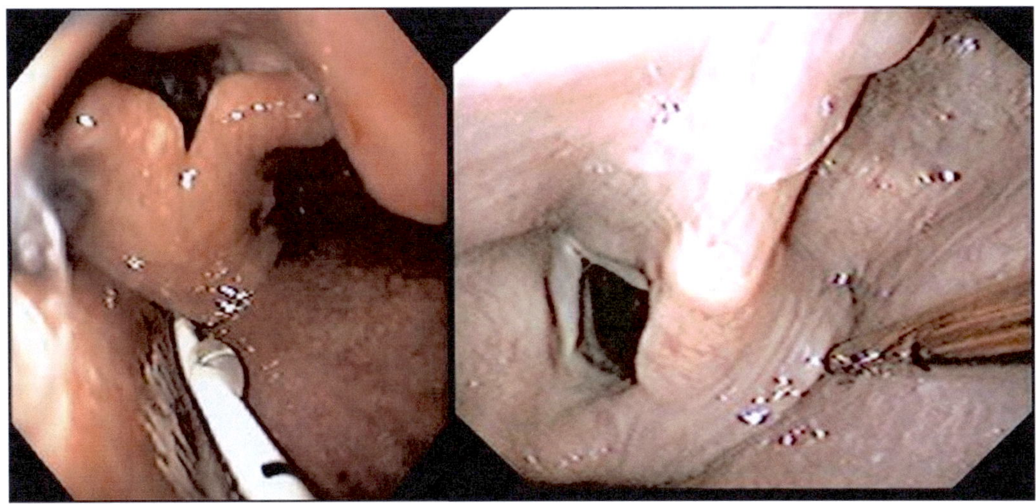

Fig. 18.7 *Right panel*: Placement of a pH probe catheter. *Left panel*: Placement of pH-impedance catheter in a patient with laryngopharyngeal reflux symptoms. The small-caliber endoscope demonstrates the position of the upper impedance electrode pair just proximal to the cricopharyngeus (reproduced from Kim et al. *Surg Innov* 2006;13(1): 31–39)

be associated with less epistaxis compared to SCE with a diameter >5.3 mm (mean incidence, 3% [0–12%] vs. 5% [0–43%], respectively). Patients with coagulopathy (platelet count <50,000/mm³, prothrombin rate <50%) and a history of nasal trauma or surgery should be thoroughly assessed prior to attempting TNE.

Topical anesthesia may cause methemoglobinemia and systemic effects such as arrhythmias and seizures due to absorption of the topical agent, although such events are extremely uncommon [60, 61]. To prevent the development of methemoglobinemia, topical anesthetics (benzocaine > lidocaine) should be avoided in patients with a previous history of methemoglobinemia or known glucose-6-phosphate dehydrogenase deficiency. Methemoglobinemia may be clinically suspected by the presence of clinical cyanosis in the face with a normal arterial PO_2 (PaO_2) as obtained by arterial blood gas measurement. Pulse oximetry is inaccurate in monitoring oxygen saturation in the presence of methemoglobinemia. Methemoglobinemia is suspected when the oxygen saturation as measured by pulse oximetry is significantly different from the oxygen saturation calculated from arterial blood gas analysis ("saturation gap"). The co-oximeter with Evelyn-Malloy method is a reliable diagnostic tool to confirm methemoglobinemia. The treatment varies depending on the severity of methemoglobinemia. Asymptomatic patients with a methemoglobin level <20% require no therapy other than discontinuation of the causative agents. Therapy with methylene blue should be considered for symptomatic patients with a methemoglobin level >20%. Blood transfusion or exchange transfusion may be required in severe cases (i.e., shock). Methylene blue, which is given intravenously in a dose of 1–2 mg/kg over 5 min, acts as an artificial electron transporter, ultimately reducing methemoglobin via the NADPH-dependent pathway [62]. The response to methylene blue is rapid; however, rebound methemoglobinemia may occur in as high as 60% of patients up to 18 h after the initial therapy [62]. Therefore, serial measurements of methemoglobin levels should be performed to evaluate the patient for subsequent worsening.

Cost-Effectiveness

Since TNE can be performed without sedation, there is no need for IV medications and post-procedure observation in a recovery room, which accounts for 70% of the total procedure time [63–65]. Additionally, sedation-related complications should be eliminated, reducing significant direct costs. Finally, the indirect costs are significantly reduced because the patient can drive herself to and from the procedure and can return to work immediately following the procedure. The two studies calculated the total costs of TNE and sedated conventional EGD, and demonstrated that unsedated TNE allows a 20–36% cost reduction as compared to sedated conventional EGD [64–66]. The cost savings is related primarily to the reductions and/or elimination of staff and physical resources required to care for patients after sedation. Furthermore, unsedated TNE reduces total procedure time including recovery time by 1.5 h compared with conventional sedated EGD [64]. However, this assessment did not include indirect costs such as time off work and a third-party transportation, which may be even more important to evaluate when examining total cost savings.

Conclusion

TNE is a novel technology with potentially widespread applications in the evaluation and management of foregut disease. Compared to conventional EGD, TNE appears to have an equivalent diagnostic yield and can be performed with a lower morbidity, less personnel and equipment, and less costs. Office-based unsedated TNE may represent one of the most important future roles of SCE and potentially facilitate the large-scale screening and surveillance of foregut premalignancies and/or malignancies. There may be a lower threshold to perform TNE because of the elimination of sedation, and unsedated TNE could be incorporated as part of standard physical examination in the practices of surgeons and gastroenterologists.

References

1. Bell GD. Premedication, preparation, and surveillance. Endoscopy. 2002;34(1):2–12.
2. Conlong P, Rees W. The use of hypnosis in gastroscopy: a comparison with intravenous sedation. Postgrad Med J. 1999;75(882):223–5.
3. Gattuso SM, Litt MD, Fitzgerald TE. Coping with gastrointestinal endoscopy: self-efficacy enhancement and coping style. J Consult Clin Psychol. 1992;60(1):133–9.
4. Woloshynowych M, Oakley DA, Saunders BP, Williams CB. Psychological aspects of gastrointestinal endoscopy: a review. Endoscopy. 1996;28(9):763–7.
5. Shaker R. Unsedated trans-nasal pharyngoesophagogastroduodenoscopy (T-EGD): technique. Gastrointest Endosc. 1994;40(3):346–8.
6. Kim CY, O'Rourke RW, Chang EY, Jobe BA. Unsedated small-caliber upper endoscopy: an emerging diagnostic and therapeutic technology. Surg Innov. 2006;13(1):31–9.
7. Rodriguez SA, Banerjee S, Desilets D, et al. Ultrathin endoscopes. Gastrointest Endosc. 2010;71(6):893–8.
8. Bosco JJ, Barkun AN, Isenberg GA, et al. Gastrointestinal endoscopes: May 2003. Gastrointest Endosc. 2003;58(6):822–30.
9. Tatsumi Y, Harada A, Matsumoto T, Tani T, Nishida H. Feasibility and tolerance of 2-way and 4-way angulation videoscopes for unsedated patients undergoing transnasal EGD in GI cancer screening. Gastrointest Endosc. 2008;67(7):1021–7.
10. Dumortier J, Ponchon T, Scoazec JY, et al. Prospective evaluation of transnasal esophagogastroduodenoscopy: feasibility and study on performance and tolerance. Gastrointest Endosc. 1999;49(3 Pt 1): 285–91.
11. Craig A, Hanlon J, Dent J, Schoeman M. A comparison of transnasal and transoral endoscopy with small-diameter endoscopes in unsedated patients. Gastrointest Endosc. 1999;49(3 Pt 1):292–6.
12. Dean R, Dua K, Massey B, Berger W, Hogan WJ, Shaker R. A comparative study of unsedated transnasal esophagogastroduodenoscopy and conventional EGD. Gastrointest Endosc. 1996; 44(4):422–4.
13. Dumortier J, Napoleon B, Hedelius F, et al. Unsedated transnasal EGD in daily practice: results with 1100 consecutive patients. Gastrointest Endosc. 2003;57(2):198–204.
14. Zaman A, Hahn M, Hapke R, Knigge K, Fennerty MB, Katon RM. A randomized trial of peroral versus transnasal unsedated endoscopy using an ultrathin videoendoscope. Gastrointest Endosc. 1999;49 (3 Pt 1):279–84.
15. Preiss C, Charton JP, Schumacher B, Neuhaus H. A randomized trial of unsedated transnasal small-caliber esophagogastroduodenoscopy (EGD) versus peroral small-caliber EGD versus conventional EGD. Endoscopy. 2003;35(8):641–6.
16. Thota PN, Zuccaro Jr G, Vargo 2nd JJ, Conwell DL, Dumot JA, Xu M. A randomized prospective trial comparing unsedated esophagoscopy via transnasal and transoral routes using a 4-mm video endoscope with conventional endoscopy with sedation. Endoscopy. 2005;37(6):559–65.
17. Trevisani L, Cifala V, Sartori S, Gilli G, Matarese G, Abbasciano V. Unsedated ultrathin upper endoscopy is better than conventional endoscopy in routine outpatient gastroenterology practice: a randomized trial. World J Gastroenterol. 2007;13(6): 906–11.
18. Mori A, Ohashi N, Yoshida A, et al. Unsedated transnasal ultrathin esophagogastroduodenoscopy may provide better diagnostic performance in gastroesophageal reflux disease. Dis Esophagus. 2011;24(2):92–8.
19. Mori A, Ohashi N, Tatebe H, et al. Autonomic nervous function in upper gastrointestinal endoscopy: a prospective randomized comparison between transnasal and oral procedures. J Gastroenterol. 2008;43(1):38–44.
20. Maffei M, Dumortier J, Dumonceau JM. Self-training in unsedated transnasal EGD by endoscopists competent in standard peroral EGD: prospective assessment of the learning curve. Gastrointest Endosc. 2008;67(3):410–8.
21. Campo R, Brullet E, Montserrat A, et al. Identification of factors that influence tolerance of upper gastrointestinal endoscopy. Eur J Gastroenterol Hepatol. 1999;11(2):201–4.
22. Trevisani L, Sartori S, Gaudenzi P, et al. Upper gastrointestinal endoscopy: are preparatory interventions or conscious sedation effective? A randomized trial. World J Gastroenterol. 2004;10(22): 3313–7.
23. Book DT, Rhee JS, Toohill RJ, Smith TL. Perspectives in laryngopharyngeal reflux: an international survey. Laryngoscope. 2002; 112(8 Pt 1):1399–406.
24. Yorulmaz I, Ozlugedik S, Kucuk B. Gastroesophageal reflux disease: symptoms versus pH monitoring results. Otolaryngol Head Neck Surg. 2003;129(5):582–6.
25. Hill RK, Simpson CB, Velazquez R, Larson N. Pachydermia is not diagnostic of active laryngopharyngeal reflux disease. Laryngoscope. 2004;114(9):1557–61.
26. Hickson C, Simpson CB, Falcon R. Laryngeal pseudosulcus as a predictor of laryngopharyngeal reflux. Laryngoscope. 2001;111(10): 1742–5.
27. Ylitalo R, Lindestad PA, Hertegard S. Is pseudosulcus alone a reliable sign of gastroesophago-pharyngeal reflux? Clin Otolaryngol Allied Sci. 2004;29(1):47–50.
28. Kendall KA, Louie S. Severe obstructive airway disorders and diseases: vocal fold dysfunction. Clin Rev Allergy Immunol. 2003; 25(3):221–31.
29. Maffei M, Dumonceau JM. Transnasal esogastroduodenoscopy (EGD): comparison with conventional EGD and new applications. Swiss Med Wkly. 2008;138(45–46):658–64.
30. Birkner B, Fritz N, Schatke W, Hasford J. A prospective randomized comparison of unsedated ultrathin versus standard esophagogastroduodenoscopy in routine outpatient gastroenterology practice: does it work better through the nose? Endoscopy. 2003;35(8): 647–51.
31. Campo R, Montserrat A, Brullet E. Transnasal gastroscopy compared to conventional gastroscopy: a randomized study of feasibility, safety, and tolerance. Endoscopy. 1998;30(5):448–52.
32. Kawai T, Miyazaki I, Yagi K, et al. Comparison of the effects on cardiopulmonary function of ultrathin transnasal versus normal diameter transoral esophagogastroduodenoscopy in Japan. Hepatogastroenterology. 2007;54(75):770–4.

33. Stroppa I, Grasso E, Paoluzi OA, et al. Unsedated transnasal versus transoral sedated upper gastrointestinal endoscopy: a one-series prospective study on safety and patient acceptability. Dig Liver Dis. 2008;40(9):767–75.

34. Jobe BA, Hunter JG, Chang EY, et al. Office-based unsedated small-caliber endoscopy is equivalent to conventional sedated endoscopy in screening and surveillance for Barrett's esophagus: a randomized and blinded comparison. Am J Gastroenterol. 2006; 101(12):2693–703.

35. Gopal DV, Zaman A, Katon RM. A role for transnasal esophago-gastroduodenoscopy in patients intolerant to the oral route: report of two cases. Gastrointest Endosc. 1999;49(3 Pt 1):379–81.

36. Mulcahy HE, Fairclough PD. Ultrathin endoscopy in the assessment and treatment of upper and lower gastrointestinal tract strictures. Gastrointest Endosc. 1998;48(6):618–20.

37. Sorbi D, Gostout CJ, Henry J, Lindor KD. Unsedated small-caliber esophagogastroduodenoscopy (EGD) versus conventional EGD: a comparative study. Gastroenterology. 1999;117(6):1301–7.

38. Hayashi Y, Yamamoto Y, Suganuma T, et al. Comparison of the diagnostic utility of the ultrathin endoscope and the conventional endoscope in early gastric cancer screening. Dig Endosc. 2009; 21(2):116–21.

39. Toyoizumi H, Kaise M, Arakawa H, et al. Ultrathin endoscopy versus high-resolution endoscopy for diagnosing superficial gastric neoplasia. Gastrointest Endosc. 2009;70(2):240–5.

40. Horiuchi A, Nakayama Y, Hidaka N, Ichise Y, Kajiyama M, Tanaka N. Prospective comparison between sedated high-definition oral and unsedated ultrathin transnasal esophagogastroduodenoscopy in the same subjects: pilot study. Dig Endosc. 2009;21(1):24–8.

41. Eisen GM, Lieberman D, Fennerty MB, Sonnenberg A. Screening and surveillance in Barrett's esophagus: a call to action. Clin Gastroenterol Hepatol. 2004;2(10):861–4.

42. Provenzale D, Schmitt C, Wong JB. Barrett's esophagus: a new look at surveillance based on emerging estimates of cancer risk. Am J Gastroenterol. 1999;94(8):2043–53.

43. Shaheen NJ, Provenzale D, Sandler RS. Upper endoscopy as a screening and surveillance tool in esophageal adenocarcinoma: a review of the evidence. Am J Gastroenterol. 2002;97(6):1319–27.

44. Saeian K, Staff DM, Vasilopoulos S, et al. Unsedated transnasal endoscopy accurately detects Barrett's metaplasia and dysplasia. Gastrointest Endosc. 2002;56(4):472–8.

45. Saeian K, Staff D, Knox J, et al. Unsedated transnasal endoscopy: a new technique for accurately detecting and grading esophageal varices in cirrhotic patients. Am J Gastroenterol. 2002;97(9):2246–9.

46. Dranoff JA, Angood PJ, Topazian M. Transnasal endoscopy for enteral feeding tube placement in critically ill patients. Am J Gastroenterol. 1999;94(10):2902–4.

47. Fang JC, Hilden K, Holubkov R, DiSario JA. Transnasal endoscopy vs. fluoroscopy for the placement of nasoenteric feeding tubes in critically ill patients. Gastrointest Endosc. 2005;62(5):661–6.

48. Kulling D, Bauerfeind P, Fried M. Transnasal versus transoral endoscopy for the placement of nasoenteral feeding tubes in critically ill patients. Gastrointest Endosc. 2000;52(4):506–10.

49. Lin CH, Liu NJ, Lee CS, et al. Nasogastric feeding tube placement in patients with esophageal cancer: application of ultrathin transnasal endoscopy. Gastrointest Endosc. 2006;64(1):104–7.

50. Mahadeva S, Malik A, Hilmi I, Qua CS, Wong CH, Goh KL. Transnasal endoscopic placement of nasoenteric feeding tubes: outcomes and limitations in non-critically ill patients. Nutr Clin Pract. 2008;23(2): 176–81.

51. Mitchell RG, Kerr RM, Ott DJ, Chen M. Transnasal endoscopic technique for feeding tube placement. Gastrointest Endosc. 1992; 38(5):596–7.

52. Sato R, Watari J, Tanabe H, et al. Transnasal ultrathin endoscopy for placement of a long intestinal tube in patients with intestinal obstruction. Gastrointest Endosc. 2008;67(6):953–7.

53. Wildi SM, Gubler C, Vavricka SR, Fried M, Bauerfeind P. Transnasal endoscopy for the placement of nasoenteral feeding tubes: does the working length of the endoscope matter? Gastrointest Endosc. 2007;66(2):225–9.

54. O'Keefe SJ, Foody W, Gill S. Transnasal endoscopic placement of feeding tubes in the intensive care unit. JPEN J Parenter Enteral Nutr. 2003;27(5):349–54.

55. Vitale MA, Villotti G, D'Alba L, De Cesare MA, Frontespezi S, Iacopini G. Unsedated transnasal percutaneous endoscopic gastrostomy placement in selected patients. Endoscopy. 2005;37(1): 48–51.

56. Cappell MS. Risk factors and risk reduction of malignant seeding of the percutaneous endoscopic gastrostomy track from pharyngoesophageal malignancy: a review of all 44 known reported cases. Am J Gastroenterol. 2007;102(6):1307–11.

57. Itoi T, Kawai T, Sofuni A, et al. Efficacy and safety of 1-step transnasal endoscopic nasobiliary drainage for the treatment of acute cholangitis in patients with previous endoscopic sphincterotomy (with videos). Gastrointest Endosc. 2008;68(1):84–90.

58. Mori A, Ohashi N, Maruyama T, et al. Transnasal endoscopic retrograde chalangiopancreatography using an ultrathin endoscope: a prospective comparison with a routine oral procedure. World J Gastroenterol. 2008;14(10):1514–20.

59. Postma GN, Cohen JT, Belafsky PC, et al. Transnasal esophagoscopy: revisited (over 700 consecutive cases). Laryngoscope. 2005; 115(2):321–3.

60. Ash-Bernal R, Wise R, Wright SM. Acquired methemoglobinemia: a retrospective series of 138 cases at 2 teaching hospitals. Medicine (Baltimore). 2004;83(5):265–73.

61. Kane GC, Hoehn SM, Behrenbeck TR, Mulvagh SL. Benzocaine-induced methemoglobinemia based on the Mayo Clinic experience from 28 478 transesophageal echocardiograms: incidence, outcomes, and predisposing factors. Arch Intern Med. 2007;167(18): 1977–82.

62. Guay J. Methemoglobinemia related to local anesthetics: a summary of 242 episodes. Anesth Analg. 2009;108(3):837–45.

63. Bampton PA, Reid DP, Johnson RD, Fitch RJ, Dent J. A comparison of transnasal and transoral oesophagogastroduodenoscopy. J Gastroenterol Hepatol. 1998;13(6):579–84.

64. Garcia RT, Cello JP, Nguyen MH, et al. Unsedated ultrathin EGD is well accepted when compared with conventional sedated EGD: a multicenter randomized trial. Gastroenterology. 2003;125(6): 1606–12.

65. Gorelick AB, Inadomi JM, Barnett JL. Unsedated small-caliber esophagogastroduodenoscopy (EGD): less expensive and less time-consuming than conventional EGD. J Clin Gastroenterol. 2001;33(3):210–4.

66. Peery AF, Hoppo T, Garman KS, et al. Feasibility, safety, acceptability, and yield of office-based, screening transnasal esophagoscopy (with video). Gastrointest Endosc. 2012;75(5):945–53.

Jonathan Pearl

Introduction

Since its inception over 40 years ago endoscopic retrograde cholagiopancreatography (ERCP) has evolved from a purely diagnostic study to predominantly a therapeutic intervention. Therapeutic ERCP has supplanted surgery for many biliary and pancreatic disease processes. The success of ERCP relies on a specialized team of endoscopists, nurses, and technicians. Its mastery requires additional training in advanced endoscopy, continuing practice of the technique, and dedication to continuing education in ERCP as the technology rapidly evolves.

Indications and Contraindications

ERCP is most commonly performed for biliary pathology (Table 19.1). Choledocholithiasis and postoperative bile duct leaks or biliary injuries are common indications for endoscopic cholangiography and biliary interventions. Bile duct strictures, both benign and malignant, can be diagnosed and treated with ERCP.

Endoscopic pancreatography is less frequently indicated compared to cholangiography. ERCP might be useful in the diagnosis of pancreatic adenocarcinoma. Treatment for pancreatic ascites or pancreatic pseudocyst can be accomplished with ERCP.

There are some additional conditions for which ERCP is sometimes useful. Sphincter of Oddi dysfunction can be assessed with ERCP and sphincter of Oddi manometry. Endoscopic sphincterotomy can be therapeutic in some cases of sphincter of Oddi dysfunction [1, 2]. Chronic pancreatitis may be improved with endoscopic removal of pancreatic duct stones or dilation of pancreatic duct strictures. Acute biliary pancreatitis is an occasional indication for ERCP when accompanied by worsening jaundice or cholangitis [3, 4].

Patients must be fit for moderate sedation or general anesthesia to undergo ERCP. Coagulation disorders should be corrected. The patient, or his or her representative, must comprehend the risks of ERCP and consent to the procedure.

ERCP can be difficult, but not impossible, in patients with previous upper gastrointestinal operations. Patients with prior Bilroth II anastamoses may require specialized equipment to cannulate the sphincter, and those with prior gastric bypass usually need an operative or interventional radiology gastrotomy to access the remnant stomach or biliopancreatic limb and, subsequently, the papilla.

Preparation for ERCP: Equipment, Personnel, and Patient Positioning

ERCP is best performed in an endoscopy room dedicated to ERCP (Fig. 19.1). The room should have the capacity to house a fluoroscopy machine (C-arm), endoscopy equipment, and monitors for both the endoscopic and radiologic images. The monitors are best positioned adjacent to each other in line with the endoscopist's natural stance. There should be ample room for anesthesia equipment and storage of the endoscopic accessories. Furthermore, there should be sufficient space for an endoscopist and an assistant to work.

A side viewing duodenoscope is used for ERCP. The typical scope has a diameter of 11 mm with working channels of

This chapter contains a video segment that can be found by accessing the following link: http://www.springerimages.com/videos/978-1-4614-6329-0.

J. Pearl, M.D. (✉)
Department of Surgery, Uniformed Services University, Bethesda, MD 20889, USA
e-mail: jpearlmd@yahoo.com

either 3.2 or 4.2 mm. A pediatric duodenoscope with a 2.0 mm working channel can be used in newborns and young children, but a standard duodenoscope is commonly used in children greater than 2 years old.

ERCP can be performed under conscious sedation or general anesthesia. Sedation is usually adequate with the exception of prior failed ERCP, patients with a history of narcotic use, or other conditions precluding the use of sedation [5, 6].

Continuous monitoring of pulse oximetry and heart rate, as well as intermittent blood pressure measurement, is standard. Supplemental oxygen is administered. Ready access to glucagon, atropine, and narcotic and benzodiazepine reversal agents should be assured. All team members should be certified in Advanced Cardiac Life Support.

Table 19.1 Indications for ERCP

Biliary pathology
Choledocholithiasis
Cholangitis
Bile duct stricture
Bile duct injury
Bile duct carcinoma
Pancreatic pathology
Chronic pancreatitis
Pancreatic ascites
Pancreatic pseudocyst
Acute biliary pancreatitis
Sphincter of Oddi dysfunction

The ERCP team consists of a nurse whose sole job is to administer sedation and monitor the patient. The endoscopist should have an assistant who is facile with the accessories required in ERCP. All team members should wear lead aprons and collars and personal protective equipment.

ERCP is best performed with patients in the prone position with the head turned toward the patient's right shoulder. The right arm may be positioned along the patient's right side or under the pillow that supports the patient's head. With the patient supine, the endoscopist stands at the patient's right shoulder and the C-arm is brought in from the patient's left. The assistant stands to the endoscopist's right with the accessories in close proximity.

Basic ERCP Technique (Video 19.1)

After the patient is adequately sedated the duodenoscope is advanced into the oropharynx and through the esophageal introitus. This is usually performed as a blind maneuver which is facilitated by angling the tip of the scope downward and asking the patient to swallow. Once the scope is felt entering the esophagus it is gently advanced through the length of the esophagus and into the stomach. The stomach is then gently inflated and the tip of the scope is angled downward to view the greater curvature of the stomach. The scope is then advanced toward the antrum.

Once past the incisura angularis the tip of the scope is further deflected downward and the pylorus is visualized. Because of the side-viewing configuration of the scope the

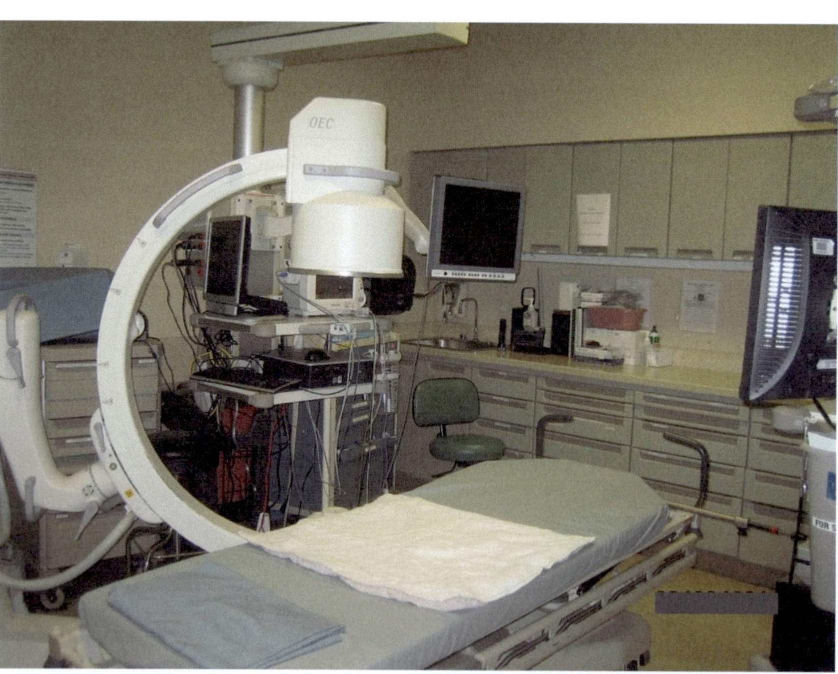

Fig. 19.1 Room setup for endoscopic retrograde cholangiopancreatography (ERCP). Picture-in-picture allows the combination of endoscopic and fluoroscopic images on one monitor

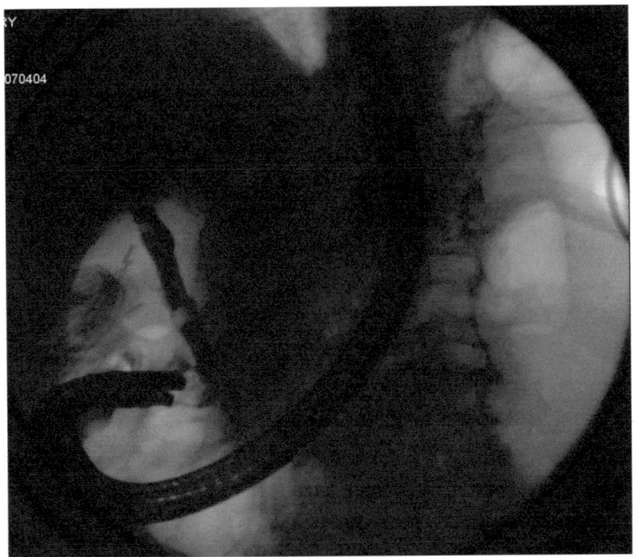

Fig. 19.2 Fluoroscopic image of the duodenoscope in the long position. This position may be used for difficult cannulations of the bile duct or, more commonly, for cannulation of the pancreatic duct

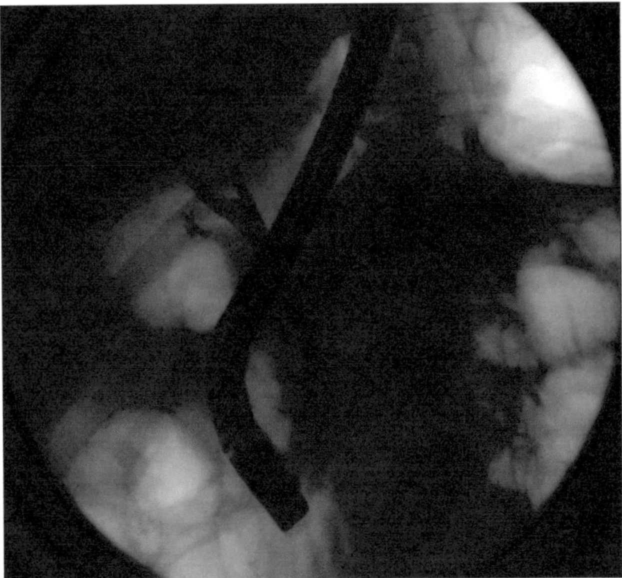

Fig. 19.3 Fluoroscopic image of the duodenoscope in the short position. The redundancy in the scope is removed to allow more responsiveness at its tip

pylorus cannot be traversed while directly visualized. The pylorus is initially placed in the center of the field. The tip is angled downward so that the pylorus appears to lie above the field of view, the so-called setting sun sign. The scope is then advanced into the duodenal bulb.

At this point the scope is angled upward and to the right and gently advanced into the second portion of the duodenum. This usually leaves the scope in the long position (Fig. 19.2) with the tip of the scope distal to the papilla and redundant scope present within the stomach. The scope is then withdrawn to place it into the short position (Fig. 19.3), thereby straightening the scope, and the papilla is located. The papilla is identified along the medial wall of the second portion of the duodenum. Additional landmarks for the papilla include a transverse fold of mucosa superior to its orifice or, sometimes, an adjacent diverticulum.

The papilla is ideally placed in the center of the visualized field (*en face*). This is accomplished with fine movements of the left–right and up–down dials. The endoscopist's left wrist may be gently torqued, and small changes in the position of the endoscopist's body may change the location of the papilla.

Selective cannulation of either the bile duct or pancreatic duct is the goal of ERCP cannulation. When in the *en face* position the bile duct is located at 11 o'clock and the pancreatic duct near 2 o'clock. The bile duct is best approached from below. The cannula is directed toward 11 o'clock. A fold of mucosa may need to be elevated and the cannula gently directed toward the bile duct. Excessive force should be avoided because this obscures the orifice with blood and leads to periampullary edema, both of which make cannulation more difficult.

Selective cannulation of the pancreatic duct may be performed in either the short or long position. The *en face* position usually provides access to the pancreatic duct, but the long position can be used in challenging cases. Many endoscopists find pancreatic cannulation simpler than selective biliary cannulation because the origin of the pancreatic duct is in line with the papillary orifice.

Once the cannula is inserted contrast may be injected to visualize the ducts or a wire may be advanced to provide access for other interventions. When the study is complete the cannula is removed and the scope is returned to the neutral position. It is gently withdrawn while suctioning air from the duodenum and stomach.

Difficult Cases

Some patients may find it difficult to swallow the scope while in the prone position. This can be overcome by supporting the patient in the left lateral decubitus position while the esophagus is intubated. The prone position also changes the orientation of the stomach compared to standard gastroscopy. The tip of the scope oftentimes is located in the fundus rather than directed toward the antrum and pylorus. This can be combated by suctioning air to decrease the distension of the stomach and angling the tip of the scope downward. Once the pylorus is located passage into the duodenum is usually feasible.

Locating the papilla may pose a challenge. In most cases this is the result of improper positioning of the scope. Fluoroscopic views can provide information regarding whether the tip of the scope is too proximal or distal in the duodenum. Once the proper short position is achieved some papillas remain obscured. Removing excess bubbles lining the mucosa with an anti-gas agent such as Simethicone may clarify its position. There are numerous additional cues to aid in the identification of a cryptic papilla [7]. Focal bile staining and the confluence of horizontal and vertical mucosa may direct the endoscopist to the papilla. The papilla may be located adjacent to a duodenal diverticulum or even within the lumen of the diverticulum.

Cannulation of the papilla may be difficult. Many endoscopists prefer a sphincterotome over a standard catheter for cannulation of the papilla [8]. The sphincterotome provides the ability to bow the tip of the instrument to align it with the course of the bile duct. The elevator on the duodenoscope can also direct the sphincterotome toward the 11 o'clock position. On occasion neither a cannula nor a sphincterotome provides access to the bile duct. In those cases a wire may be used for cannulation [9, 10]. The guidewire is placed through a cannula or a sphincterotome. It is then used to probe the papilla in the direction of the bile duct. Once the wire is advanced to the desired position under fluoroscopy the sphincterotome is advanced over it.

Cannulation is best performed with the papilla in the center of the field of view and in close proximity to the tip of the scope. Upward deflection of the tip of the scope can move it toward the papilla. Suctioning some of the air in the duodenum may also bring the papilla closer to the scope. If the papilla appears eccentric in the field of view gentle clockwise twisting of the endoscopist's wrist can bring it to a central location. The endoscopist may also subtly alter his or her positioning to change the field of view. In cases where smooth muscle contractions of the gut impede cannulation intravenous glucagon may be administered.

In some cases the pancreatic duct is easily cannulated but the bile duct is elusive. There are many techniques available to combat this. The scope may be advanced and the bile duct approached from below rather than *en face*. This may align the catheter with the direction of the bile duct. The double wire technique has also been described as a valuable adjunct in these cases [11, 12]. A wire may be left in the pancreatic duct followed by attempts to cannulate the bile duct (Fig. 19.4). The wire or pancreatic stent may occlude the pancreatic duct and direct the second wire to the bile duct. The pancreatic wire may also straighten the bile duct and facilitate its cannulation.

A sphincterotomy may be performed prior to accessing the bile duct with a wire or cannulation. This precut sphincterotomy can be used to access the duct in challenging cases [13, 14]. Precut sphincterotomy carries a significant risk of perforation and should be employed only when ERCP is imperative and other maneuvers have been attempted.

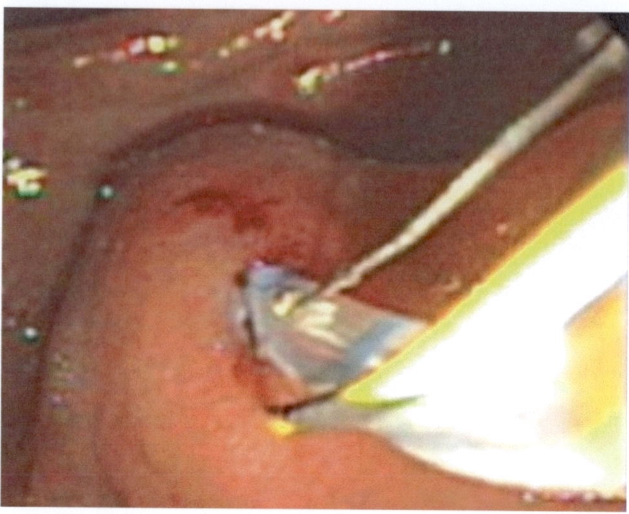

Fig. 19.4 Photograph of the double wire technique. A wire has been left in the pancreatic duct and a sphincterotome is used to cannulate the bile duct

Biliary Therapeutics

Biliary Sphincterotomy

Sphincterotomy of the bile duct is commonly performed for choledocholithiasis and bile duct leaks. Opening the sphincter provides easy access to the bile duct for complex interventions such as stenting and choledochoscopy.

Sphincterotomes are available in a variety of sizes and configurations. Most sphincterotomes have two or more lumens available for injection of contrast or passage of wires. The plastic catheter has 2–3 cm of exposed wire at its tip. The wire can be tightened or bowed to improve its contact with the papilla and sphincter. The external portion is attached to an electrosurgical unit.

After the bile duct is selectively cannulated a sphincterotomy can be performed. The sphincterotome is withdrawn so that approximately one-third of the wire lies within the papilla. The wire is then bowed to bring it into gentle apposition with the papilla. A blended current is then applied as the wire is directed toward the 11 o'clock position (Fig. 19.5).

The sphincterotomy is deemed adequate when the entire sphincter muscle complex has been incised (Fig. 19.6). The typical length of a sphincterotomy is 1 cm [15, 16]. Bile should flow freely through the sphincterotomy and an inflated 10 mm balloon should not deform as it passes into the duodenum.

The sphincterotomy should not extend beyond the impression of the common bile duct on the duodenum. This may be difficult to ascertain, so the transverse fold superior to the papilla can be used as another boundary. The sphincterotomy can be safely extended to the level of the transverse fold, but not beyond.

Stone Retrieval

Removal of stones from the common bile duct is indicated for choledocholithiasis (Fig. 19.7). Balloons and baskets are commonly employed for endoscopic stone retrieval.

The ease of stone removal depends on the extent of sphincterotomy and the size of the stones. Most stones less than 1 cm can be retrieved endoscopically. Larger stones may require alternate methods of removal to include lithotripsy or surgery.

An 8 Fr balloon can be passed over a wire above the common bile duct stones. The balloon can then be inflated up to 15 mm and dragged through the common duct into the duodenum. Stone extraction is best confirmed by visualizing the stone as it exits into the duodenum. It is normal for the balloon to encounter a bit of resistance at the distal common duct. Some of the air can be released from the balloon to diminish its diameter and aid its passage. Furthermore, deflecting the tip of the scope downward will help to pull the balloon and the stones into the duodenum (Fig. 19.8).

An alternate method of stone retrieval employs a wire basket. The collapsed basket is inserted into the common bile duct above the stone. It is opened and withdrawn until it engages the stone. The basket is then closed to capture the stone. The basket and stone are then withdrawn with the same maneuvers used in balloon extraction. A completion cholangiogram should be performed to confirm that all stones have been extracted.

Lithotripsy

Standard balloons and baskets are successful in retrieving more than 80 % of stones, regardless of size [17]. The addition

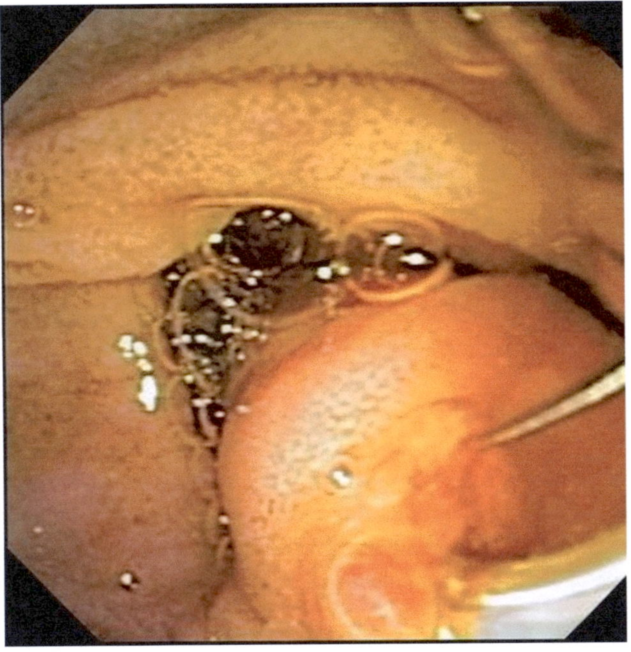

Fig. 19.5 Photograph of the initiation of a sphincterotomy. The wire is directed toward the 11 o'clock position in line with the bile duct

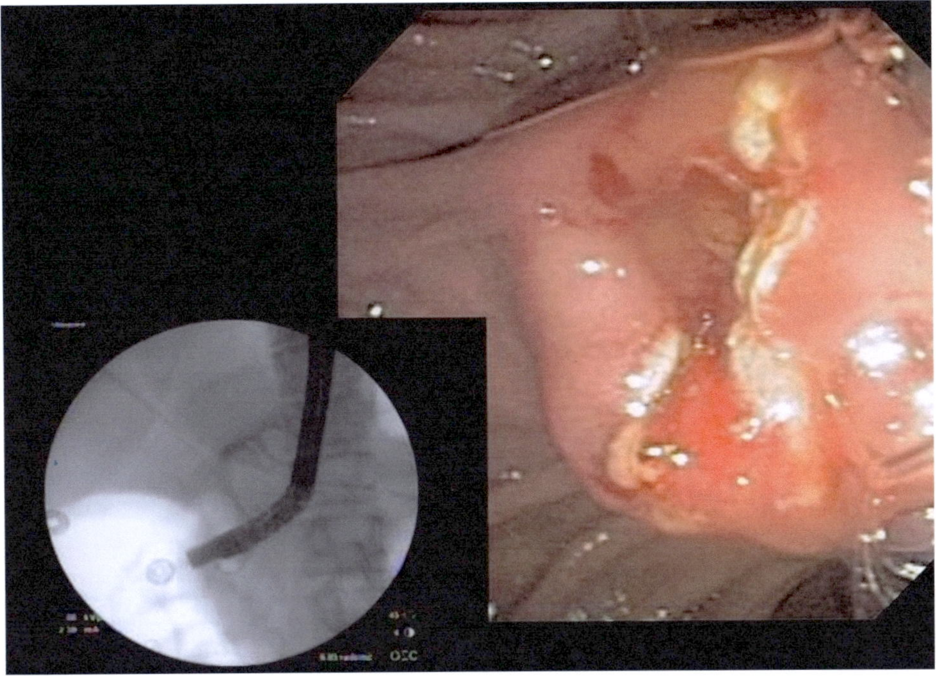

Fig. 19.6 Photograph of a completed sphincterotomy. The sphincterotomy was taken up to the level of the transverse fold

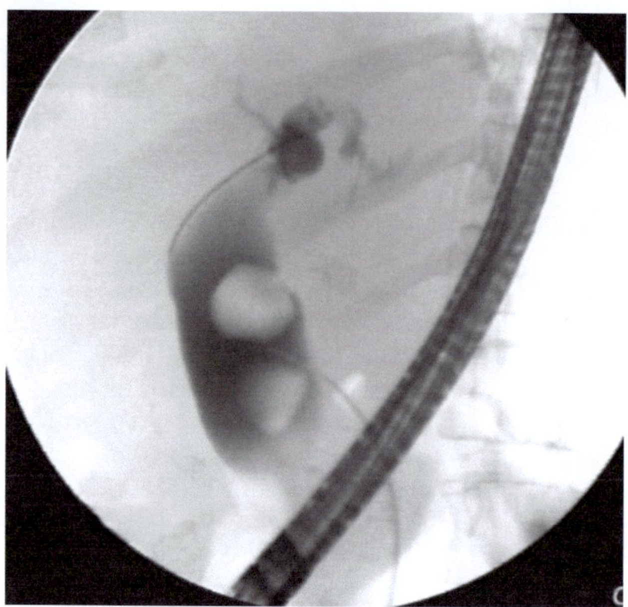

Fig. 19.7 Fluoroscopic image of large common bile duct stones

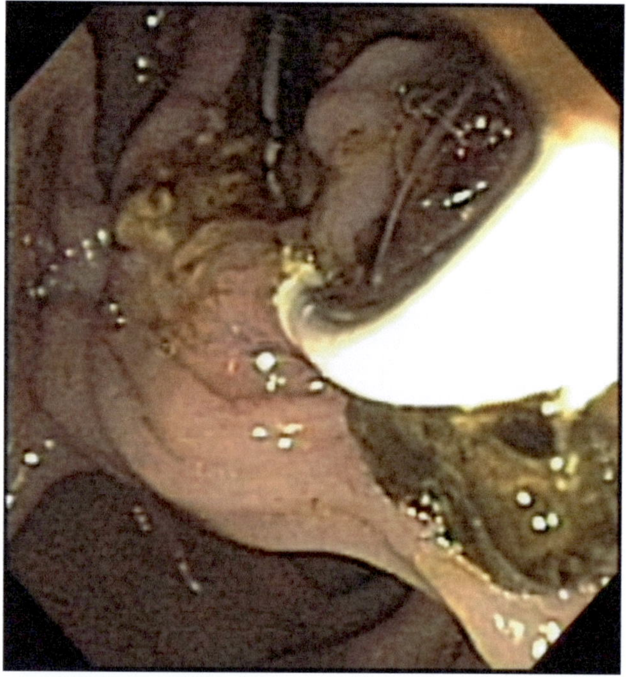

Fig. 19.8 Endoscopic image of stones being extracted into the duodenum

of mechanical lithotripsy improves the rate of endoscopic stone retrieval to greater than 90 % [18, 19]. Large stones with diameters above 15 mm can be difficult to remove by standard methods, especially if the sphincterotomy cannot be extended to match the size of the stones.

The simplest method of lithotripsy for extrahepatic bile duct stones is mechanical lithotripsy. The mechanical litho-

tripter consists of three parts: a basket, a metal sheath, and a handle. The basket is used to capture the large stone. The metal sheath is then advanced over the wire until it is adjacent to the stone. Once the sheath is in place the handle is used to slowly tighten the sheath against the stone, thereby fracturing the stone into smaller pieces.

The Soehendra lithotripter is used in cases of unanticipated stone and basket impaction. When this situation occurs, the handle of the basket is cut and the duodenoscope is removed. The metal sheath of the Soehendra lithotripter is advanced over the cut wires under fluoroscopic guidance up to the level of the stone. The cut wires are then threaded into the handle of the lithotripter. Basket impaction usually occurs when using a standard basket so the handle must be tightened slowly to avoid breaking the wires and exacerbating the complication.

Electrohydraulic lithotripsy relies on bathing the stones in fluid and creating a spark in the fluid [20, 21]. A shock wave of pressure is created from the spark, which serves to fragment a stone. Electrohydraulic lithotripsy is usually performed under direct vision using a choledochoscope. The lithotripsy probe is used in conjunction with a nasobiliary tube, which provides continuous irrigation. Electrohydraulic lithotripsy carries a significant risk of bile duct injury due to the use of intraductal electrical charges.

Laser Lithotripsy

Although infrequently performed, laser lithotripsy permits the safe disintegration of large bile duct stones without the requirement for cholangioscopic visualization. The Nd-YAG laser is inserted in close proximity to the stone [22]. The laser is applied while the stone is visualized using fluoroscopy. When the equipment is available laser lithotripsy can be a safe and effective method for fragmenting large bile duct stones.

Endoscopic Papillary Balloon Dilation

This method was recently developed as an alternative to sphincterotomy and stone extraction. Because the sphincter is not cut there is a lower risk of perforation and bleeding. In addition, the technique may be easier to perform compared to sphincterotomy in patients with altered or difficult anatomy (e.g., Bilroth II).

In papillary balloon dilation a large diameter balloon is inserted into the papilla. The balloon is then inflated up to 20 mm [23, 24]. The duration of dilation ranges from 30 s to 5 min [24]. After dilation is complete a standard stone extraction balloon is used to clear the common bile duct.

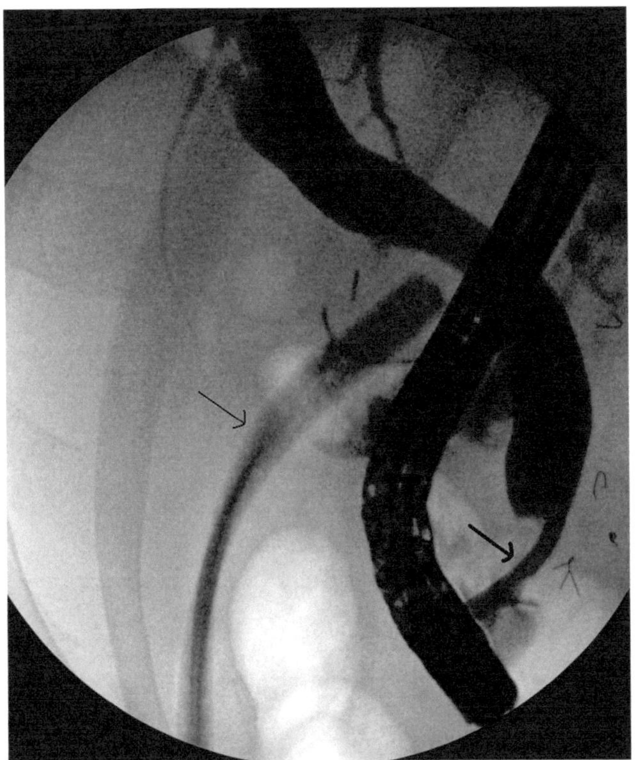

Fig. 19.9 Fluoroscopic image of a bile duct stent (*thick arrow*) in place. The stent was placed for a cystic duct stump leak. A closed-suction drain (*thin arrow*) had been placed at the time of operation

Balloon dilation of the papilla can also be used after endoscopic sphincterotomy for large stones as an alternative to lithotripsy [25]. After the sphincterotomy is complete the large diameter balloon can be used to stretch the orifice. There are many reports of the success of this technique in removing large stones and avoiding mechanical lithotripsy.

Stenting

Placing polyethylene stents in the common bile duct can be used to temporarily relieve biliary obstruction due to benign or malignant stricture. Stenting is also commonly employed to treat bile duct injuries and leaks (Fig. 19.9). Plastic stents may remain in place up to 3 months before the risk of occlusion necessitates their removal. Self-expanding metal stents are designed to remain in place permanently. These are used to palliate strictures in cases of inoperable malignancy.

The most common plastic stents are straight stents with flap anchoring systems. Biliary stents' outer diameters are 7, 10, or 11.5 Fr, and they vary in length from 5 to 15 cm. Double pigtail stents are rarely employed in the biliary system.

Stenting is performed after standard diagnostic ERCP. A sphincterotomy is not necessary but is often employed to ease the placement of the stent into the bile duct. A wire is left in the bile duct to guide placement of the stent. The stent is loaded onto an introducer system, which normally consists of an inner cannula and an outer pusher.

The stent is inserted through the working channel to the tip of the scope. The elevator is then used to direct the stent toward the bile duct. Raising and lowering the elevator while advancing the stent will direct it upward into the bile duct. The proximal extent of the stent should lie 1 cm above a stricture and approximately 1 cm of stent should rest in the lumen of the duodenum.

Short stents with a large diameter are best employed in cases of bile duct leak to equilibrate biliary and duodenal pressures. Longer stents may be required in stricture cases, depending on the location of the narrowing. Multiple stents can be placed in patients with chronic benign strictures. When multiple stents are used bile can flow within the stent lumen and in the interstices between the stents.

Dilation

Benign strictures of the biliary tree may respond to dilation with or without stenting. A through-the-scope balloon is generally used for biliary dilation. Balloons range from 4 to 8 mm in diameter and are up to 6 cm long.

After a diagnostic ERCP identifies the location of a stricture a wire is placed beyond it into the proximal biliary system. The balloon is then inserted over the wire under fluoroscopic guidance. The balloon is inflated with hydrostatic pressure using a solution of dilute contrast. A waist should appear on the balloon as dilation commences, and then the waist should disappear when the dilation is effectual.

Pancreatic Therapeutics

Although less commonly performed than biliary ERCP, pancreatic therapeutics can be effective at treating a variety of conditions. Acute and chronic pancreatitis, sphincter of Oddi dysfunction, and pancreatic pseudocysts are some of the conditions amenable to therapeutic pancreatic ERCP. Some endoscopists find pancreatic therapeutics more challenging that biliary therapeutics, likely because of the rarity with which they are performed.

Pancreatic Sphincterotomy

Division of the main pancreatic sphincter serves to relieve the pressure in the main pancreatic duct. Pancreatic sphincterotomy, with or without biliary sphincterotomy, has been shown to be effective in relieving the symptoms of sphincter of Oddi dysfunction [26]. Minor papilla sphincterotomy can be effective in relieving pancreatitis in some patients with pancreatic divisum [27]. There is no clearly defined role for pancreatic sphincterotomy in acute pancreatitis, but sphincterotomy may be performed in the treatment of some patients with chronic pancreatitis especially those with pancreatic duct stones [28, 29]. The sphincterotomy provides access to the pancreatic duct and allows removal of the stones. There may also be some utility in relieving the pressure in the distal pancreatic duct with respect to pain relief.

Pancreatic sphincterotomy is performed after diagnostic endoscopic pancreatography. A standard pull-type sphincterotome, as would be used for biliary sphincterotomy, may be employed. The sphincterotomy is inserted over a wire into the pancreatic duct and oriented toward 12 o'clock. The landmarks for complete sphincterotomy are not as well defined as biliary sphincterotomy. Most authors recommend cutting 5–10 mm in the 12 o'clock position [30, 31]. Another method for pancreatic sphincterotomy involves the placement of a stent in the duct. A needle knife can then be used to perform the sphincterotomy over the stent.

Stone Retrieval

The best candidates for pancreatic stone removal are those with chronic pancreatitis with main duct stones. Ductal strictures may impede stone removal and may require dilation to adequately clear the duct. Patients with a few small stones confined to the head of the pancreas can expect good pain relief with stone removal. The results are less salutary for those with stones larger than 10 mm, more than three stones, and associated stricture [32].

Stone removal is performed using standard baskets and balloons. A sphincterotomy is usually performed to facilitate passage of the stone into the duodenum. A tortuous pancreatic duct can make stone retrieval challenging, but wire guidance can facilitate the procedure.

Pancreatic Stenting

Placing stents in the pancreatic duct relieves the pressure at the sphincter and encourages flow of the pancreatic juice into the duodenum. This may be useful in cases of pancreatic pseudocyst where the connection between the main duct and the pseudocyst is confirmed. Pancreatic stenting may help relieve pain in some patients with chronic pancreatitis. Some endoscopists will use pancreatic stents to combat post-ERCP

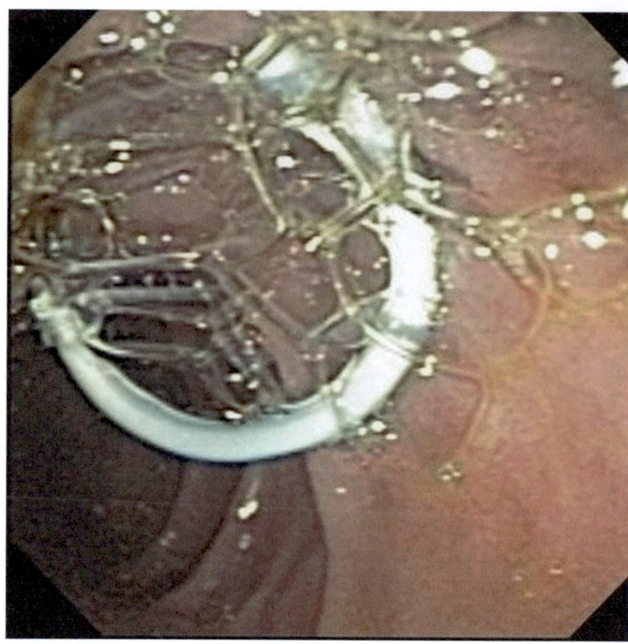

Fig. 19.10 Endoscopic picture of a pancreatic duct stent in place. The pigtail portion of the stent is visible within the duodenum

pancreatitis, especially after inadvertent manipulation of the pancreatic duct.

Pancreatic stents are usually longer and narrower than bile duct stents. The diameters range from 5 to 10 Fr. There are usually multiple side holes on the stents to accommodate pancreatic juice from the side branches of the duct. Most pancreatic stents have a pigtail on the duodenal side to prevent proximal migration into the duct (Fig. 19.10), and there may be a flap on the pancreatic end to anchor the stent in place.

Pancreatic stents are placed over a wire. The stents occlude fairly quickly with a biofilm similar to that which occludes biliary stents. When no anchor flap anchor is in place the stents have a tendency to migrate into the duodenum. Proximal migration into the pancreas is rare but can pose a challenge in removing the stent.

Dilation

Pancreatic duct strictures are amenable to balloon dilation. This can provide relief of pain in patients with chronic pancreatitis. Dilation of ductal strictures may also be required to remove pancreatic duct stones.

Pancreatic dilation is performed after diagnostic endoscopic pancreatogram. The stricture is identified and a wire is passed beyond it. A pancreatic sphincterotomy may or may not be performed. The balloon is then advanced to the level of the stricture and inflated. The hydrostatic balloon is then inflated under fluoroscopic guidance.

Complications of ERCP

ERCP is the riskiest of the common endoscopic procedures. The spectrum of complications has shifted from bleeding and perforation during ERCP's nascent period to a predominance of pancreatitis today. This shift in complications likely reflects refinements in technique and, perhaps, the fact that more ERCPs are being performed in high-risk patients.

Pancreatitis

Pancreatitis may occur in up to 7 % of patients undergoing ERCP [33, 34]. Almost all patients will have a mild elevation of the serum amylase and lipase after the procedure. Clinically significant pancreatitis is defined by elevation of the serum amylase to three times normal, significant pain, and requirement for admission to the hospital. The rate of pancreatitis is highest among patients with sphincter of Oddi dysfunction. ERCPs performed for stones and other common pathology carries a rate of significant pancreatitis of approximately 1 % [34, 35].

Certain technical factors dispose the patient to pancreatitis. Excessive manipulation of the pancreatic orifice will lead to edema and subsequent outflow obstruction. Forceful injection of contrast into the pancreatic duct, as evidenced by acinarization visualized on the radiograph, may lead to pancreatitis. It has often been surmised that sphincter of Oddi manometry causes pancreatitis, but most contemporary authors believe that the pancreatitis is from the sphincter dysfunction, rather than the manometry [26, 36].

Careful technique is the best means of avoiding pancreatitis. Gentle manipulation of the papilla is paramount for minimizing edema of the pancreatic orifice. Contrast should be injected into the pancreatic duct judiciously. Pharmacologic agents have not been shown to reduce the risk of post-ERCP pancreatitis [37–39], but stenting of the pancreatic duct in high-risk patients has shown some utility [40–42].

Pancreatitis is suspected after ERCP when patients present with epigastric pain. The differential diagnosis includes perforation. Laboratory studies and radiographs will usually pinpoint the diagnosis. Most patients with post-ERCP pancreatitis can be managed non-operatively with bowel rest and analgesia. On rare occasion the pancreatitis progresses to pancreatic necrosis and requires operative intervention.

Perforation

ERCP induced perforation may occur with the endoscope, with a wire or other accessory, or during sphincterotomy [36]. Endoscopic perforation is the least frequent but most

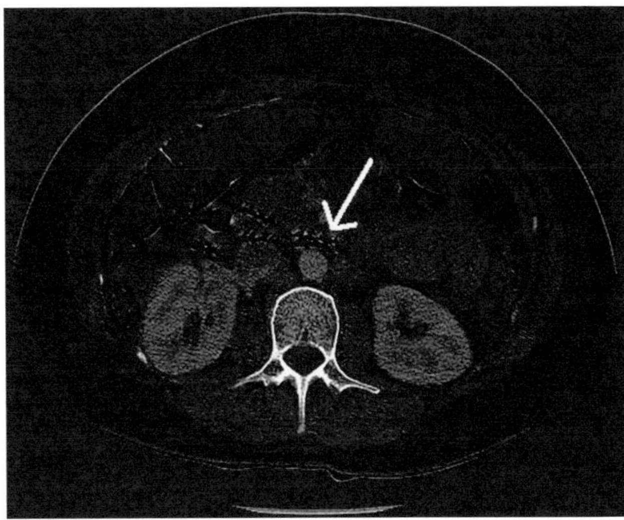

Fig. 19.11 CT scan of a patient with a retroperitoneal perforation after ERCP. There is copious air in the retroperitoneum surrounding the pancreas (*white arrow*)

serious. This can occur during introduction of the scope in the pharynx or during passage through the esophagus. The most common site of endoscopic perforation is the junction between the first and second portions of the duodenum. The lateral wall of the duodenum may be blown out because of forceful advancement of the scope. Because of the side-viewing nature of the duodenoscope a direct view in front of the scope's path is not present, and perforation may occur. Patients with strictures are also more susceptible to perforation.

Endoscopic perforation can be avoided by meticulous technique and recognition of predisposing factors. Scope manipulation in the oropharynx should be careful in elderly patients with Zencker's diverticula. The scope should be advance slowly without undue pressure in the esophagus. Passage from into the second portion of the duodenum can normally be accomplished by deflecting the tip of the scope upward and to the right. If this is not easily accomplished a forward-viewing scope might be useful to investigate for anatomic variants such are strictures.

Perforation of the medial duodenum into the retroperitoneum may occur during sphincterotomy. This can occur when biliary sphincterotomy is not in line with the intraduodenal bile duct or when the sphincterotomy is too long. A CT scan will show s significant amount of retroperitoneal air surrounding the pancreas and adjacent structures (Fig. 19.11).

Duodenal perforation due to sphincterotomy can be minimized by using judicious technique. When it does occur it should be promptly recognized. Most patients will recover without operation. Patients with pathology that requires intervention (e.g., choledocholithiasis and cholangitis) might require operation for the pathology. In those cases retroperitoneal drains should be placed and the pathology should be addressed. It is usually difficult or impossible to locate the duodenal perforation.

Wires or other instruments may puncture the duodenum or bile duct. This may be more common in patients with duodenal diverticula. When a small caliber accessory such as a wire traverses the duodenal wall it should be recognized and removed. There are usually no consequences to such an occurrence. Larger instruments that enter the retroperitoneum are best managed like a sphincterotomy-induced perforation.

Bleeding

Hemorrhage during ERCP occurs most commonly during sphincterotomy. Although most sphincterotomies bleed a bit, clinically significant bleeding occurs in only 0.5 % of cases [43]. The apex of the sphincterotomy is the most common location of hemorrhage, especially when the sphincterotomy deviates from the ideal course.

Significant bleeding should be managed endoscopically at its onset. Many techniques are available, but the endoscopist must remain cognizant of the impact on the pancreatic orifice with each technique. Balloon tamponnade or mechanical hemostasis with clips may stop bleeding without impinging on the pancreatic juice outflow. High-volume injection and electrocautery should be avoided unless other measures fail. A prophylactic pancreatic stent may be advisable in difficult cases.

When endoscopic hemostasis is not possible angiography is the next best option. Selective embolization of the bleeding vessel is possible in most cases. Operation is the last resort and may be difficult since the cut sphincter fails to hold sutures well.

Other Rare Complications

ERCP may induce an infection such as cholangitis or cholecystitis. These situations arise when adequate biliary drainage is not achieved, such as an occluded stent or impacted stone.

Stent and basket complications can occur. Both biliary and pancreatic stents can migrate proximally or become occluded. Extraction of migrated stents can usually be achieved with endoscopic instruments. Baskets may break during stone extraction and could require the Soehendra lithotripter for removal.

Patients may experience respiratory or cardiovascular compromise during ERCP. Significant deterioration of a patient's status requires that the procedure be suspended and the patient attended to.

Special Considerations

Variation from standard ERCP technique is required in some circumstances. Altered anatomy may preclude an antegrade approach to the papilla, or prior surgery may exclude the stomach from the path of the gastrointestinal tract. Difficulty accessing the papilla may also demand creative approaches to the biliary tree.

Bilroth II

Partial gastrectomy with Bilroth II reconstruction can be performed for gastric neoplasm or gastric ulcer. The afferent limb is in continuity with the biliary tree and can be accessed via the gastrojejunostomy. Because the papilla is approached from below, accessing the papilla is more challenging. Most endoscopists will use a therapeutic side-viewing duodenoscope for Bilroth II cases, although a forward-viewing scope may also be employed [44]. Cap-assisted ERCP using the forward viewing scope has also been shown to be effective in Bilroth II patients [45]. The orientation of the bile duct at the papilla is skewed because of the retrograde access. A specially designed sphincterotome is oriented to cut in the 5 o'clock position (rather than the standard 11 o'clock).

Gastric Bypass

As morbid obesity increases in the Western world so does bariatric surgery. Roux-en-Y gastric bypass involves construction of a long bilioenteric limb. Patients with gastric bypasses who require ERCP pose a challenge for accessing the papilla. Some endoscopists have had success with balloon enteroscopy [46, 47], but a more direct route is more commonly chosen.

More success has been achieved by accessing the remnant stomach and approaching the papilla from above [48]. The remnant stomach can be entered using laparoscopic or conventional gastrostomy or with percutaneous interventional radiology techniques. After the ERCP a tube gastrostomy can be left in place should additional procedures be necessary, or the gastrotomy may be closed.

Rendezvous

Selective cannulation of the bile duct is not possible in 1–5 % of cases. Difficult anatomy, impacted stones, or papillary stenosis may preclude cannulation. There are several alternatives to ERCP in these cases. One such method, the rendezvous technique, uses percutaneous transhepatic access to the biliary tree. Most commonly a percutaneous IR drain is placed into the biliary tree and across the papilla into the duodenum.

At a separate setting ERCP is performed. The side viewing duodenoscope is used. A wire is passed through the drain into the duodenum. The wire is grasped with a snare and brought through the channel of the scope. This provides access to the ducts and ERCP can then be performed in the standard fashion thereafter.

Pseudocyst

Pancreatic pseudocysts develop as a result of pancreatic duct disruption, usually due to pancreatitis or trauma. Symptomatic pseudocysts may require internal drainage. This may be accomplished in cases where the wall of the pseudocyst abuts the gastric or duodenal wall.

ERCP techniques can be useful for drainage of pancreatic pseudocysts. If the pseudocyst is seen bulging into the gastrointestinal lumen the cyst wall can be punctured directly with a needle knife. More commonly endoscopic ultrasound confirms the location of the pseudocyst and ensures the absence of intervening vascular structures. A needle is used to access the cyst under ultrasound guidance and a wire is passed into the cyst cavity. The connection between the pseudocyst and the visceral lumen is enlarged and multiple double pigtail drains are placed across the connection.

In selected cases endoscopic drainage of pancreatic pseudocysts is very successful. Some authors have also described debridement of pancreatic necrosis using similar techniques [49, 50]. The retroperitoneum is accessed through the stomach using ultrasound guidance. A scope is then passed into the retroperitoneum after enlarging the tract. Endoscopic snares and graspers can be used to debride dead tissue. Large caliber double pigtail drains are then left between the retroperitoneum and stomach. Effective treatment of pancreatic necrosis may require several sessions of debridement.

Summary

ERCP is an advanced endoscopic technique with utility in treating a wide range of biliary and pancreatic pathology. Most contemporary ERCP is reserved for therapy rather than diagnosis. Success of ERCP depends on careful patient selection, a team dedicated to performing the procedure, and meticulous technique. When post-procedure complications arise most can be managed using nonoperative methods.

References

1. Arguedas MR, Linder JD, Wilcox CM. Suspected sphincter of Oddi dysfunction type II: empirical biliary sphincterotomy or manometry-guided therapy? Endoscopy. 2004;36(2):174–8.
2. Bistritz L, Bain VG. Sphincter of Oddi dysfunction: managing the patient with chronic biliary pain. World J Gastroenterol. 2006;12(24):3793–802.
3. Moretti A, Papi C, Aratari A, et al. Is early endoscopic retrograde cholangiopancreatography useful in the management of acute biliary pancreatitis? A meta-analysis of randomized controlled trials. Dig Liver Dis. 2008;40(5):379–85.
4. van Santvoort HC, Besselink MG, de Vries AC, et al. Early endoscopic retrograde cholangiopancreatography in predicted severe acute biliary pancreatitis: a prospective multicenter study. Ann Surg. 2009;250(1):68–75.
5. Goulson DT, Fragneto RY. Anesthesia for gastrointestinal endoscopic procedures. Anesthesiol Clin. 2009;27(1):71–85.
6. Thomson A. Anaesthetic considerations during ERCP. Anaesth Intensive Care. 2007;35(2):302.
7. Carr-Locke DL. Biliary access during endoscopic retrograde cholangiopancreatography. Can J Gastroenterol. 2004;18(4):251–4.
8. Schwacha H, Allgaier HP, Deibert P, et al. A sphincterotome-based technique for selective transpapillary common bile duct cannulation. Gastrointest Endosc. 2000;52(3):387–91.
9. Shao LM, Chen QY, Cai JT. Role of wire-guided cannulation in the endoscopic retrograde cholangiopancreatography. Am J Gastroenterol. 2009;104(12):3110; author reply 3110–1.
10. Lee TH, Park do H, Park JY, et al. Can wire-guided cannulation prevent post-ERCP pancreatitis? A prospective randomized trial. Gastrointest Endosc. 2009;69(3 (Pt 1)):444–9.
11. Kramer RE, Azuaje RE, Martinez JM, Dunkin BJ. The double-wire technique as an aid to selective cannulation of the common bile duct during pediatric endoscopic retrograde cholangiopancreatography. J Pediatr Gastroenterol Nutr. 2007;45(4):438–42.
12. Gyokeres T, Duhl J, Varsanyi M, et al. Double guide wire placement for endoscopic pancreaticobiliary procedures. Endoscopy. 2003;35(1):95–6.
13. Deng DH, Zuo HM, Wang JF, et al. New precut sphincterotomy for endoscopic retrograde cholangiopancreatography in difficult biliary duct cannulation. World J Gastroenterol. 2007;13(32):4385–90.
14. Horiuchi A, Nakayama Y, Kajiyama M, Tanaka N. Effect of precut sphincterotomy on biliary cannulation based on the characteristics of the major duodenal papilla. Clin Gastroenterol Hepatol. 2007;5(9):1113–8.
15. Kim HJ, Choi HS, Park JH, et al. Factors influencing the technical difficulty of endoscopic clearance of bile duct stones. Gastrointest Endosc. 2007;66(6):1154–60.
16. Joyce AM, Kochman ML. Update on biliary endoscopy. Curr Opin Gastroenterol. 2005;21(3):354–8.
17. McHenry L, Lehman G. Difficult bile duct stones. Curr Treat Options Gastroenterol. 2006;9(2):123–32.
18. Akcakaya A, Ozkan OV, Bas G, et al. Mechanical lithotripsy and/or stenting in management of difficult common bile duct stones. Hepatobiliary Pancreat Dis Int. 2009;8(5):524–8.
19. Kratzer W, Mason RA, Grammer S, et al. Difficult bile duct stone recurrence after endoscopy and extracorporeal shockwave lithotripsy. Hepatogastroenterology. 1998;45(22):910–6.
20. Craigie JE, Adams DB, Byme TK, et al. Endoscopic electrohydraulic lithotripsy in the management of pancreatobiliary lithiasis. Surg Endosc. 1998;12(5):405–8.
21. Arya N, Nelles SE, Haber GB, et al. Electrohydraulic lithotripsy in 111 patients: a safe and effective therapy for difficult bile duct stones. Am J Gastroenterol. 2004;99(12):2330–4.

22. Neuhaus H, Zillinger C, Born P, et al. Randomized study of intracorporeal laser lithotripsy versus extracorporeal shock-wave lithotripsy for difficult bile duct stones. Gastrointest Endosc. 1998; 47(5):327–34.

23. Attam R, Freeman ML. Endoscopic papillary large balloon dilation for large common bile duct stones. J Hepatobiliary Pancreat Surg. 2009;16(5):618–23.

24. Tsujino T, Kawabe T, Isayama H, et al. Efficacy and safety of low-pressured and short-time dilation in endoscopic papillary balloon dilation for bile duct stone removal. J Gastroenterol Hepatol. 2008;23(6):867–71.

25. Bang S, Kim MH, Park JY, et al. Endoscopic papillary balloon dilation with large balloon after limited sphincterotomy for retrieval of choledocholithiasis. Yonsei Med J. 2006;47(6):805–10.

26. Elta GH. Sphincter of Oddi dysfunction and bile duct microlithiasis in acute idiopathic pancreatitis. World J Gastroenterol. 2008;14(7): 1023–6.

27. Madura II JA, Madura JA. Diagnosis and management of sphincter of Oddi dysfunction and pancreas divisum. Surg Clin North Am. 2007;87(6):1417–29, ix.

28. Cahen DL, Gouma DJ, Nio Y, et al. Endoscopic versus surgical drainage of the pancreatic duct in chronic pancreatitis. N Engl J Med. 2007;356(7):676–84.

29. Khanna S, Tandon RK. Endotherapy for pain in chronic pancreatitis. J Gastroenterol Hepatol. 2008;23(11):1649–56.

30. Halttunen J, Keranen I, Udd M, Kylanpaa L. Pancreatic sphincterotomy versus needle knife precut in difficult biliary cannulation. Surg Endosc. 2009;23(4):745–9.

31. Weber A, Roesch T, Pointner S, et al. Transpancreatic precut sphincterotomy for cannulation of inaccessible common bile duct: a safe and successful technique. Pancreas. 2008;36(2):187–91.

32. Sherman S, Lehman GA, Hawes RH, et al. Pancreatic ductal stones: frequency of successful endoscopic removal and improvement in symptoms. Gastrointest Endosc. 1991;37(5):511–7.

33. Cotton PB, Garrow DA, Gallagher J, Romagnuolo J. Risk factors for complications after ERCP: a multivariate analysis of 11,497 procedures over 12 years. Gastrointest Endosc. 2009;70(1):80–8.

34. Wang P, Li ZS, Liu F, et al. Risk factors for ERCP-related complications: a prospective multicenter study. Am J Gastroenterol. 2009;104(1):31–40.

35. Garcia-Cano J. The range of ERCP complications. Am J Gastroenterol. 2008;103(2):488–9; author reply 489–90.

36. Andriulli A, Loperfido S, Napolitano G, et al. Incidence rates of post-ERCP complications: a systematic survey of prospective studies. Am J Gastroenterol. 2007;102(8):1781–8.

37. Bai Y, Gao J, Zou DW, Li ZS. Prophylactic octreotide administration does not prevent post-endoscopic retrograde cholangiopancreatography pancreatitis: a meta-analysis of randomized controlled trials. Pancreas. 2008;37(3):241–6.

38. Bai Y, Gao J, Shi X, et al. Prophylactic corticosteroids do not prevent post-ERCP pancreatitis: a meta-analysis of randomized controlled trials. Pancreatology. 2008;8(4–5):504–9.

39. van Westerloo DJ, Rauws EA, Hommes D, et al. Pre-ERCP infusion of semapimod, a mitogen-activated protein kinases inhibitor, lowers post-ERCP hyperamylasemia but not pancreatitis incidence. Gastrointest Endosc. 2008;68(2):246–54.

40. Saad AM, Fogel EL, McHenry L, et al. Pancreatic duct stent placement prevents post-ERCP pancreatitis in patients with suspected sphincter of Oddi dysfunction but normal manometry results. Gastrointest Endosc. 2008;67(2):255–61.

41. Freeman ML. Pancreatic stents for prevention of post-endoscopic retrograde cholangiopancreatography pancreatitis. Clin Gastroenterol Hepatol. 2007;5(11):1354–65.

42. Chahal P, Baron TH, Petersen BT, et al. Pancreatic stent prophylaxis of post endoscopic retrograde cholangiopancreatography pancreatitis: spontaneous migration rates and clinical outcomes. Minerva Gastroenterol Dietol. 2007;53(3):225–30.

43. Christensen M, Matzen P, Schulze S, Rosenberg J. Complications of ERCP: a prospective study. Gastrointest Endosc. 2004;60(5): 721–31.

44. Swarnkar K, Stamatakis JD, Young WT. Diagnostic and therapeutic endoscopic retrograde cholangiopancreaticography after Billroth II gastrectomy—safe provision in a district general hospital. Ann R Coll Surg Engl. 2005;87(4):274–6.

45. Park CH, Lee WS, Joo YE, et al. Cap-assisted ERCP in patients with a Billroth II gastrectomy. Gastrointest Endosc. 2007;66(3): 612–5.

46. Dellon ES, Kohn GP, Morgan DR, Grimm IS. Endoscopic retrograde cholangiopancreatography with single-balloon enteroscopy is feasible in patients with a prior Roux-en-Y anastomosis. Dig Dis Sci. 2009;54(8):1798–803.

47. Emmett DS, Mallat DB. Double-balloon ERCP in patients who have undergone Roux-en-Y surgery: a case series. Gastrointest Endosc. 2007;66(5):1038–41.

48. Lopes TL, Clements RH, Wilcox CM. Laparoscopy-assisted ERCP: experience of a high-volume bariatric surgery center (with video). Gastrointest Endosc. 2009;70(6):1254–9.

49. Seifert H, Wehrmann T, Schmitt T, et al. Retroperitoneal endoscopic debridement for infected peripancreatic necrosis. Lancet. 2000;356(9230):653–5.

50. Gardner TB, Chahal P, Papachristou GI, et al. A comparison of direct endoscopic necrosectomy with transmural endoscopic drainage for the treatment of walled-off pancreatic necrosis. Gastrointest Endosc. 2009;69(6):1085–94.

Management of Endoscopic Complications

Jeremy Warren, David Hardy,
and Bruce MacFadyen Jr.

Introduction

Gastrointestinal (GI) endoscopy is an important tool for the diagnosis and treatment of a variety of gastrointestinal and biliopancreatic conditions. Over 60 million upper and lower endoscopies are performed annually [1]. Overall complications or adverse events from upper GI endoscopy are about 0.1 %, less than 3 % for colonoscopy, and 5–10 % for endoscopic retrograde cholangiopancreatography (ERCP) [2]. The vast majority of complications occur with therapeutic endoscopy, such as polypectomy, endoscopic mucosal resection (EMR), submucosal dissection (ESD), or sphincterotomy (ES).

The majority of General Surgeons perform at least some endoscopy, and for many surgeons, particularly in rural communities, endoscopy is a large part of their practice [3, 4]. For those who perform little or no endoscopy, they will still be called upon to manage some endoscopic complications. Enteric perforation is the most common complication requiring surgery, and can involve any part of the GI tract, depending on the endoscopic procedure performed. Severe, clinically significant bleeding as a result of endoscopy is rare, though occasionally requires surgical control. Mechanical failures of endoscopic instrumentation, such as stent migration, guidewire fracture, or impaction also potentially involve surgical treatment. This chapter reviews the potential complications of upper and lower GI endoscopy, the surgical decision making for each, and their treatment.

J. Warren, M.D. • D. Hardy, M.D.
Department of Surgery, Augusta State University and Georgia Health Sciences University, Augusta, GA, USA
e-mail: JWARREN@gru.edu

B. MacFadyen Jr., M.D. (⊠)
Department of Surgery, Medical College of Georgia,
Augusta, GA, USA
e-mail: bmacfadyen@georgiahealth.edu

Esophagogastroduodenoscopy

Esophagogastroduodenoscopy (EGD) is indicated in the evaluation and treatment of a wide range of conditions. The overall complication rate for upper GI endoscopy is very low, about 0.13 % [2], though this can be greater than 5 % for certain therapeutic interventions. Advanced interventions, such as dilation, EMR or ESD increase the likelihood of complications significantly. Esophageal, gastric, and duodenal perforations resulting from endoscopy often require surgical intervention, and it is critical for the surgeon to have knowledge of the surgical treatment of these complications, as well as potential alternatives to surgery.

Upper Endoscopy-Related Bleeding

Significant bleeding from diagnostic upper gastrointestinal (GI) endoscopy is an extremely rare complication. Thrombocytopenia, coagulopathy, and portal hypertension are potential risk factors, though the safety of endoscopy and biopsy has been demonstrated even in these patients. There is no evidence that the use of anticoagulants within the normal therapeutic range increases the risk of bleeding during therapeutic or diagnostic upper GI endoscopy. There is limited data on the safety of prescribing aspirin or nonsteroidal anti-inflammatory drugs (NSAIDs) use, though it is generally considered safe. However, the general consensus is that elective EGD should not be performed on fully anticoagulated patients, and caution should be exercised in patients with extreme thrombocytopenia (<20,000) or on antiplatelet therapy [2, 5]. Periprocedural management of anticoagulation and antiplatelet therapy is discussed in detail elsewhere in this text.

So called iatrogenic Mallory–Weiss tears occur in 0.07–0.49 % of upper GI endoscopies (Fig. 20.1). The majority is clinically benign and requires no treatment, though there are a handful of reports of endoscopic intervention for hemostasis [6]. Dilation of esophageal strictures, achalasia, malignancies, or pyloric outlet obstruction carries some risk of

J.M. Marks and B.J. Dunkin (eds.), *Principles of Flexible Endoscopy for Surgeons*,
DOI 10.1007/978-1-4614-6330-6_20, © Springer Science+Business Media New York 2013

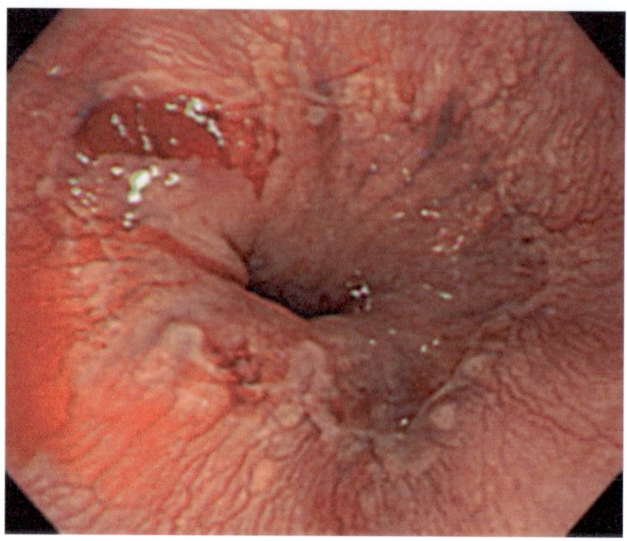

Fig. 20.1 Mallory–Weiss tear of the distal esophagus (with permission from [6], copyright 2009 @ John Wiley and Sons)

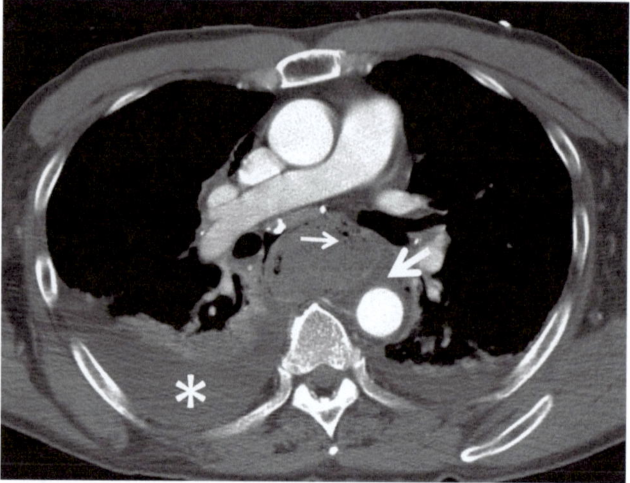

Fig. 20.2 CT thorax demonstrating esophageal perforation. Findings include pneumomediastinum (*small arrows*), pleural effusion (*asterisk*), and hemomediastinum (*large arrow*)

iatrogenic bleeding, but still occurs in less than 0.5 % of these procedures [7, 8]. Bleeding associated with EMR or ESD is much higher, occurring in about 5–13 % of cases [9, 10], and may present in a delayed fashion, even up to 8 weeks post-procedure. Clinically evident delayed bleeding follows a typical management algorithm, beginning with fluid resuscitation and transfusion as indicated, proton pump inhibitor therapy and emergent endoscopy for evaluation and hemostasis.

Surgical Management of Endoscopy-Related Hemorrhage

To the authors' knowledge there are no reports of surgical intervention required for EGD-related bleeding. With increasing utility of EMR and ESD there is certainly the potential for hemorrhage that cannot be controlled endoscopically. A combined surgical and endoscopic approach would be appropriate to localize the point of hemorrhage to allow surgical control. Surgical options would be similar to those for non-iatrogenic causes of UGI hemorrhage, including gastrotomy with suture ligation or cauterization, resection and reconstruction, or devascularization.

Alternatives to Surgical Management

Endoscopic hemostasis is the rule for iatrogenic UGI bleeding. Epinephrine injection, electrocautery, argon plasma coagulation (APC), and clips are commonly used in a variety of settings for hemostasis. These techniques are reviewed elsewhere in this text and are not discussed further here. In esophageal bleeding, placement of self-expanding metal stents is another alternative and has been used for bleeding esophageal varices refractory to standard techniques [11]. Angiographic

intervention is well described for non-iatrogenic bleeding and could be applied in these cases as well [12, 13].

Upper Endoscopy-Related Perforation

Perforation complicating EGD occurs in well less than 0.5 % of cases overall, with an overall mortality of 0.001 %. With therapeutic measures, such as dilation, EMR or ESD, or therapy for esophageal varices, this incidence can be as high as 5–15 %. Though overall mortality is low, complication specific mortality and morbidity remains about 25 and 50 %, and depends largely on the time to diagnosis and definitive treatment [2, 5, 14–16].

When recognized during endoscopy, EGD-related perforations are typically referred immediately for surgery, though are potentially treatable endoscopically. With delayed recognition, the location and mechanism of the injury, initial indication for the procedure, extent of the injury, and time from perforation influence the presentation. Gastric, duodenal and intraabdominal esophageal perforations present with abdominal or chest pain, vomiting, or peritonitis. Cervical esophageal perforations most often present with pain and subcutaneous emphysema, and dysphagia, dyspnea, or dysphonia may occur. Intrathoracic esophageal perforations present classically as Mackler's triad (vomiting, thoracic pain, emphysema), though this is present in less than a third of cases. Pleural effusion, dysphagia, and dyspnea are other common findings. Diagnosis can sometimes be confirmed with plain radiography, with findings of new pleural effusion, pneumothorax, pneumomediastinum, pneumoperitoneum, pneumoretroperitoneum, or subcutaneous emphysema. Contrast imaging with fluoroscopy can usually confirm the diagnosis, and computed tomography is virtually 100 % sensitive (Fig. 20.2). Repeat endoscopy was traditionally

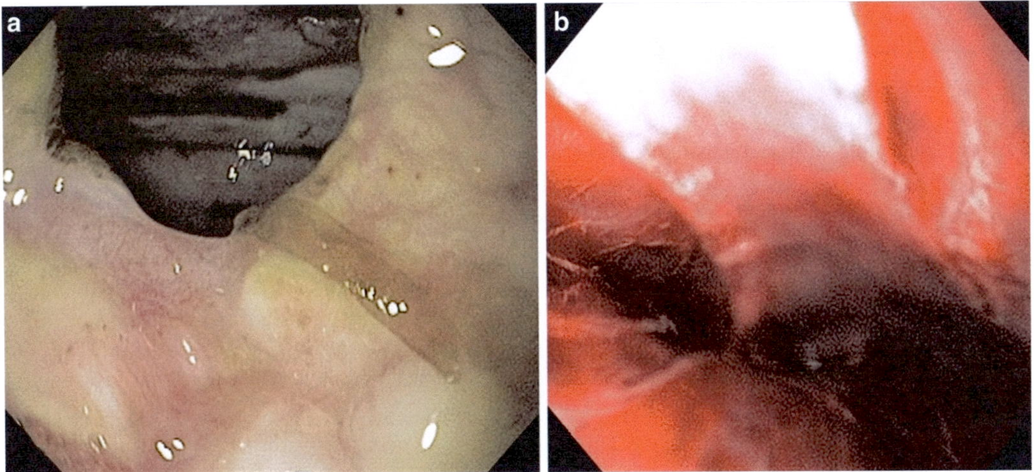

Fig. 20.3 (**a**) Distal esophageal perforation, (**b**) mid-esophageal perforation

discouraged for fear of worsening the injury, but is now recommended for diagnosis and possible treatment [16–18].

Esophageal Perforation

With the increasing utility of EGD, endoscopy-related perforation of the esophagus is now more common than spontaneous. Esophageal perforation accounts for over 50 % of EGD associated perforations (Fig. 20.3). Perforation during diagnostic procedures complicates only 0.03–0.1 % of cases, but the incidence rises with therapeutic intervention. Perforation complicates esophageal dilation in 0.5–7 %, sclerotherapy in up to 6 %, between 0.3 and 0.5 % of EMR, and up to 10 % of ESD [5, 14–19]. In the healthy esophagus, perforation is most common at Killian's triangle at the level of the cricopharyngeus and inferior pharyngeal constrictor, followed by other areas of relative thinning of the esophagus; the aortic arch, left bronchial indention and the esophagogastric junction. With therapeutic interventions, perforation most often occurs at the site of pathology [14–18]. There are no established guidelines for management of endoscopy-associated esophageal perforation. Treatment is individualized based on presentation, location and extent of injury, and endoscopist and surgeon experience. Outcome depends on the location of the perforation, etiology, the time from perforation to intervention, and the overall condition of the patient [14, 17, 20–23]. Cervical perforations fare the best, with mortality less than 10 %. Thoracic esophageal injuries carry the highest mortality due to rapid spread to the adjacent mediastinum and pleura [16]. Delayed presentation is associated with worse outcomes, with mortality rates increasing from 25 %, to more than 65 % with 24 h delay in diagnosis, and as high as 89 % if not diagnosed and treated in the first 48 h [14, 16, 18, 24–29]. There is newer data, however, suggesting that this difference may not be as great, and endoscopic perforations tend to fare better than spontaneous [16, 30, 31].

Surgical Management of Esophageal Perforation

Surgical indications for endoscopy-related perforations include clinical instability, sepsis, intraabdominal perforation, lack of medical contraindications to surgery, leak outside of the mediastinum, failure of medical and endoscopic management, and malignancy, obstruction, or stricture in the region of the perforation [14, 20, 29]. The goals of therapy are rapid source control by repair of the injury, debridement of nonviable tissue, drainage, and perioperative support [18]. When surgery is indicated, the surgeon must be familiar with the various approaches, techniques, and indications for each.

For cervical injuries, simple drainage is often adequate and can be approached via left cervicotomy. If the perforation is readily identified, a two-layer closure with absorbable suture, along with local drainage is preferred. Buttressing of the repair with surrounding healthy tissue is indicated for larger injuries with a high degree of contamination. Sternocleidomastoid, sternohyoid, sternothyroid, and pectoralis muscle flaps have all been described for reinforcement of cervical esophageal repairs [16, 18, 32]. For more extensive injuries with significant contamination and tissue necrosis, esophagostomy may be necessary.

Thoracic esophageal injuries tend to present with rapidly progressing mediastinal sepsis, and early source control is essential. Distal perforations may be approached via left thoracotomy or transhiatal via laparotomy. Mid-esophageal perforations are more easily approached via right thoracotomy, and this approach is also preferred if resection is planned. Identification of the perforation, debridement of nonviable tissue, complete closure of the injured mucosa, and drainage is essential to repair. A longitudinal esophagomyotomy is often required to fully delineate the mucosal injury. The mucosa is closed with absorbable suture, followed by repair of the muscular layer. Adjacent tissue reinforcement is often used due to the high rates of dehiscence. For thoracic esophageal injuries, pleura, pericardium, omentum, diaphragmatic or intercostal pedicle, and rhomboid or latissimus dorsi muscle flaps have all been described [16, 18]. Intercostal or pleural reinforcement at this level are the easiest to perform in the mid-esophagus. Wide local drainage with tube thoracostomy is necessary, and drainage of the esophagus is typically recommended as well, which can be accomplished with a nasogastric tube or a T-tube placed operatively at a level above the repair [16–18, 32]. Venting gastrostomy and feeding jejunostomy should also be considered.

Intraabdominal and distal thoracic esophageal perforations may be approached via laparotomy. Management principles are the same, with full exposure and closure of the mucosal injury, second layer repair of the muscular layer, with or without additional tissue buttressing. In this location, diaphragm or omental pedicle flap or gastric fundus reinforcement is most appropriate. Again, wide local drainage is indicated, and a feeding jejunostomy should be considered [16–18, 32].

Traditionally, delay in presentation more than 24 h was an indication for esophagectomy, though more recent evidence supports primary repair is still safe and should be considered [30, 31]. Esophagectomy with anastomosis is indicated for large injuries that cannot be closed without undue tension or excessive narrowing of the esophageal lumen, and in cases of severe mediastinal contamination, which is often the case with delayed presentation. It is also the preferred approach in cases of concomitant esophageal pathology, such as late stage achalasia, scleroderma, malignancy, or distal. Anastomosis should be performed in an uncontaminated field, often requiring a cervical anastomosis. Stomach, colon, and jejunum are all viable reconstructive options, which require thoracotomy and laparotomy or possibly transhiatal approach. Right thoracotomy is typically preferred to allow more complete esophageal exposure, mediastinal and pleural irrigation and drainage, and allow pleural decortication. The addition of a left cervicotomy enables anastomosis in the neck, which may improve outcomes if anastomotic leak occurs [16–18, 33–37].

In cases of extreme contamination and a clinically unstable patient, esophageal exclusion is another option. Suture or staple ligation of the esophagus above the level of injury, or cervical esophagostomy, along with wide local drainage and gastrostomy, has previously been advocated. This approach has fallen out of favor given the higher morbidity and mortality, need for reoperation to establish esophageal continuity and high rates of stricture at the site of injury, though is still appropriate approach in unstable patients who will not tolerate an extended operation [16–18]. Drainage of the mediastinum

alone is typically not effective in controlling sepsis, though the addition of a T-tube placed proximal to the site of injury may improve success by creating a controlled esophagocutaneous fistula. A T-tube may also be used to directly drain the perforation and may be accompanied by an omental buttress [17, 18, 32, 37]. Table 20.1 outlines the surgical options for esophageal perforation.

Alternatives to Surgical Management

Nonoperative treatment of esophageal perforations requires careful patient selection and close observation. Criteria for considering nonoperative management include early diagnosis, demonstration of a contained leak by contrast radiography, lack of other esophageal pathology and a clinically stable patient. This applies most often to cervical perforations, though combined with pleural drainage with tube thoracostomy, can be applied to select thoracic esophageal perforations [18, 24, 38, 39]. It is also appropriate for patients who present in a delayed fashion with minimal symptoms. This strategy includes broad spectrum antibiotics, *nil per os*, and mediastinal or pleural drainage when fluid collections are present. Nasogastric tube decompression should also be considered, but is not universally recommended [18].

Several endoscopic techniques have been described for the treatment of esophageal perforations (Fig. 20.4). Placement of a covered self-expanding metallic stent rapidly covers the area of perforation to prevent further contamination and provides a scaffold for mucosal healing (Fig. 20.5). Successful treatment is reported as high as 94 % with mortality less than 10 % [40, 41]. Pleural fluid collections still require tube thoracostomy, and surgery is still often needed for control of mediastinal and pleural contamination or pleural decortication to allow lung expansion. Stenting is less effective for long defects (>6 cm) and is generally not tolerated well in the cervical esophagus and should be avoided, particularly given the lower morbidity and mortality of operative intervention in the neck. Stent migration becomes a greater issue for very distal injuries and is typically not useful for intraabdominal esophageal perforations. Anchoring the stent to the mucosa with and endoclip can reduce migration and has been used successfully for distal perforations. Placement of endoclips for esophageal mucosal closure has also been reported with success [39, 42–44] and animal studies have demonstrated success with clips and endoscopic suturing techniques [45]. Fibrin glue injection into the submucosa has also been reported with success [17]. These techniques should be applied only in expert hands, and surgical consultation and close follow-up are strongly advised. Table 20.2 outlines the nonsurgical approach to esophageal perforations.

Table 20.1 Surgical options for endoscopy-related esophageal perforation

Surgical intervention	Indications	Contraindications
Primary repair	Early diagnosis with little or no mediastinal contamination Smaller perforations	Extensive mediastinal contamination Distal obstruction
Buttress (intercostal flap, pleural or pericardial flap, diaphragmatic pedicle, omental flap, adjacent neck musculature, gastric fundus)	May combine with any primary repair	If unable to repair primary defect Not necessary if esophagectomy performed Distal obstruction
Drainage only (T-tube, nasogastric tube, thoracostomy)	Perforation cannot be identified Cervical perforations Delayed presentation >24–48 h Surgeon inexperience ("damage control") Confirmed contained perforation by radiologic imaging	Early presentation of a reparable injury Distal obstruction Intraperitoneal perforation Uncontained perforation
Esophagostomy	Cervical perforations Proximal diversion (esophageal exclusion) for extensive injuries or extensive contamination	Intrathoracic or intraabdominal perforations
Esophagectomy with anastomosis	Extensive injury and mediastinal contamination not amenable to primary repair Obstruction due to malignancy or stricture Nonfunctional esophagus (e.g., scleroderma, advanced achalasia)	Surgeon inexperience with esophagectomy Minimal contamination or necrosis
Esophagectomy without anastomosis	Extensive injury and mediastinal contamination not amenable to primary repair *and* Surgeon inexperience with esophagectomy reconstruction ("damage control") Unstable patient	Primary repair or resection with anastomosis is always preferred
Jejunostomy	Esophageal exclusion Esophagectomy Extensive contamination with high risk for leak Surgeon judgment	Likely unnecessary for small iatrogenic perforations
Pleural decortication	Significant pleural contamination	Unnecessary for small injuries with minimal contamination

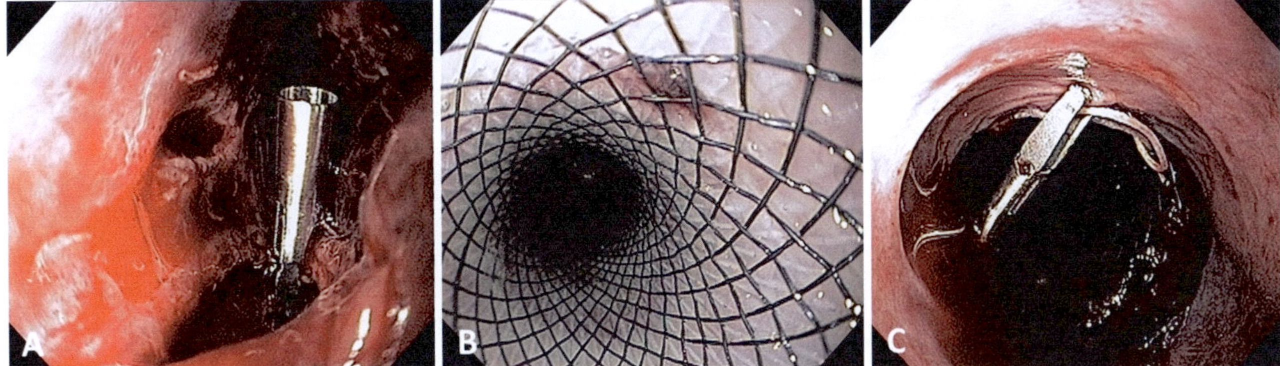

Fig. 20.4 Endoscopic management of esophageal perforation. (**a**) Attempted clipping of mid-esophageal perforation, (**b**) covered stent placement, (**c**) anchoring endoclip on the proximal stent

Gastroduodenal Perforation

Gastroduodenal perforation following EGD is rare, accounting for less than 5 % of upper endoscopy-related perforations. Altered anatomy from previous surgery, peptic stricture, duodenal diverticuli, and therapeutic interventions such as dilation, biopsy, EMR, or ESD account for most of these cases. Gastric perforation is reported in 0.5 % of EMR and 4–10 % of ESD procedures in the largest series [19]. Duodenal perforation accounts for up a third of all EGD-related perforations, with an overall incidence of only 0.01 % [15]. This is more common with ERCP, which is discussed later in this chapter.

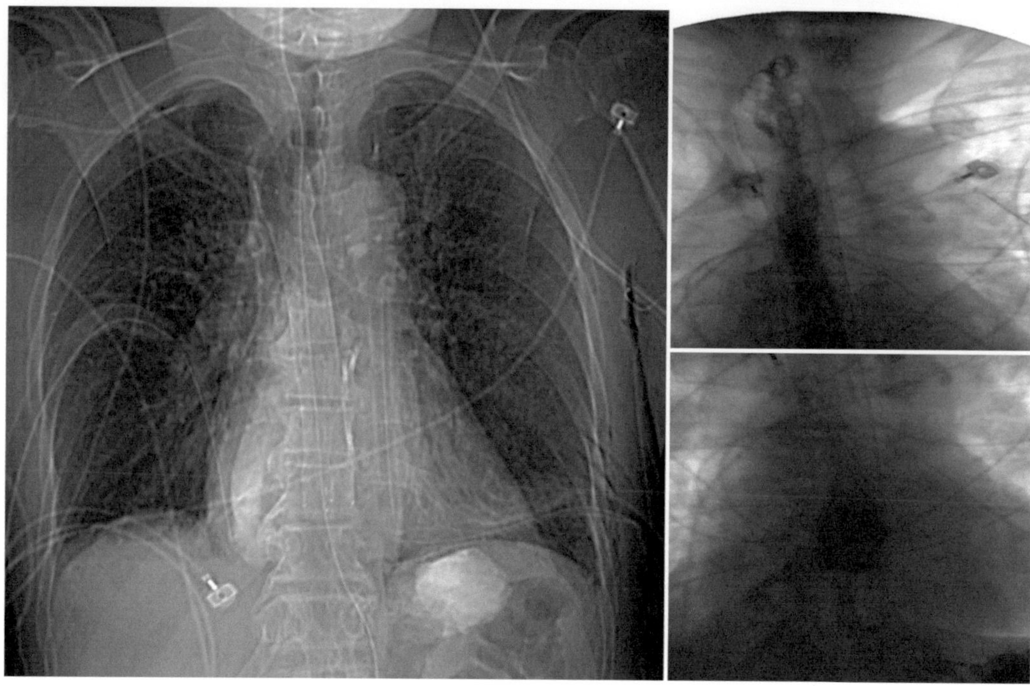

Fig. 20.5 (**a**) Esophageal stent placed for mid-esophageal perforation, (**b** and **c**) esophagram demonstrating stent coverage of the perforation

Table 20.2 Alternatives to surgery for endoscopy-related esophageal perforation

Procedure	Indications	Contraindications
Esophageal stenting	Early recognition Intrathoracic perforation Leak after primary repair Experienced endoscopist	Inexperienced endoscopist. Intraperitoneal perforation Large defects not completely covered by stent Inability to traverse injury
Drainage only	Perforation cannot be identified Cervical perforations Delayed presentation >24–48 h Surgeon inexperience ("damage control") Confirmed contained perforation by radiologic imaging	Early presentation of a reparable injury Distal obstruction Intraperitoneal perforation Uncontained perforation
Endoscopic clip or suturing	Immediately recognized injury Small defect Experienced endoscopist	Inexperienced endoscopist Large defect Delayed presentation

Surgical Management of Endoscopy-Related Gastroduodenal Perforations

Surgical management of duodenal perforations follows essentially the same algorithm as ERCP-related duodenal perforations, which are discussed in more detail later in this chapter. There are no published guidelines for surgical intervention of endoscopy-related gastric perforations. Reports of gastric perforations following EMR or ESD indicate that the majority of these can be managed without surgery. Several series mention a small percentage that requires surgery, but the specifics of surgical intervention are not recorded [9, 46–49]. Indications for surgery include endoscopically recognized perforation that cannot be closed endoscopically, clinical deterioration of the patient, and presence of pneumoperitoneum or pneumoretroperitoneum with associated fluid collection. If surgery is required, those injuries recognized early could be repaired primarily or with limited wedge resection. Debridement of any surrounding nonviable tissue should be performed to ensure efficacious repair. For large defects or significant contamination, resection and anastomosis may be required. An important consideration if surgery is required following ESD or EMR is the pathology of the lesion. Only 75–90 % of EMR and ESD resections are complete, and completeness of resection is made more difficult by bleeding or perforation [9, 19, 46]. In the case of incomplete resection, particularly of a proven or suspected malignancy, a wider margin of resection is necessary for both healing and treatment of the underlying pathology.

Alternatives to Surgical Management

Despite the intuitive need for surgery for gastric perforations, the vast majority is managed without surgery. Endoclip

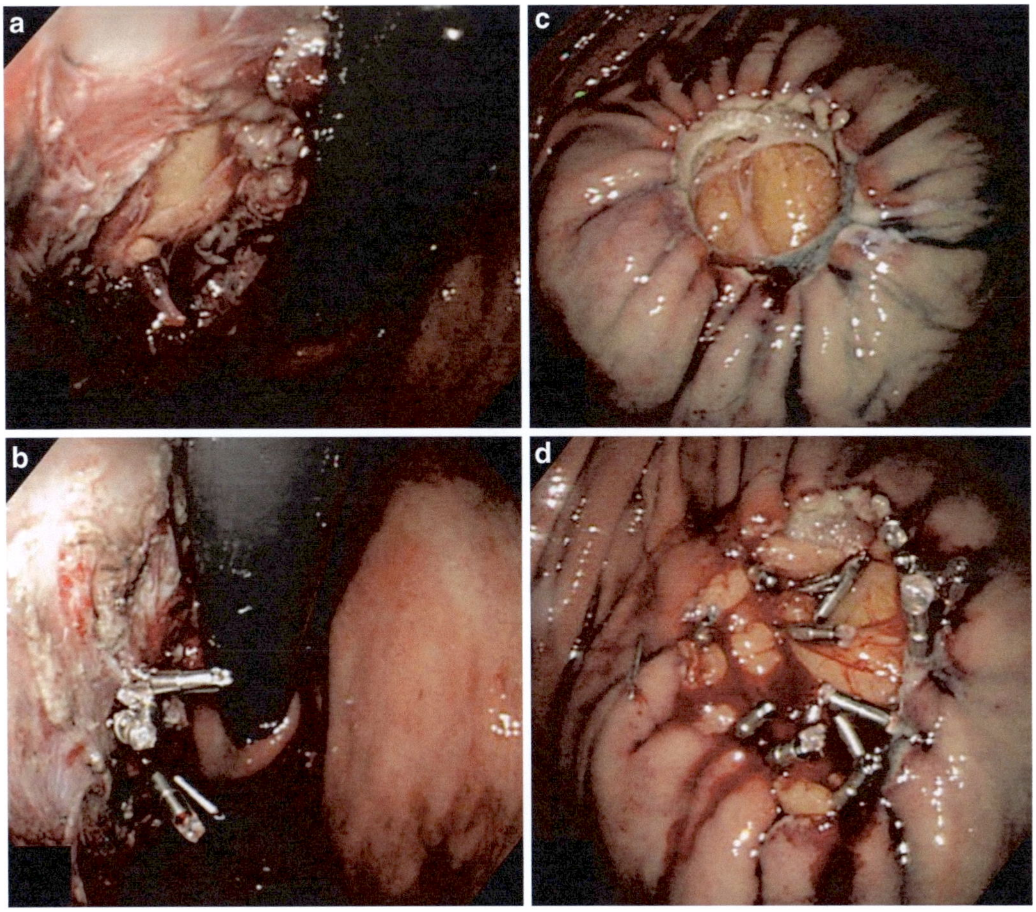

Fig. 20.6 Endoscopic closure of gastric perforation. (**a**) Gastric perforation after ESD, (**b**) closure with multiple endoscopic clips, (**c**) large gastric perforation after ESD, (**d**) omental patch closure using endoscopic clips (modified with permission from [49] (with video), copyright @ 2006 Elsevier)

closure is usually successful, with as many as 98 % of ESD and EMR-related perforations successfully closed with this technique. Even large perforations have been closed in this way by clipping the gastric wall to underlying omentum to create a patch (Fig. 20.6) [49]. It is important to recognize that standard endoclips provide mucosal reapproximation at best, and full thickness closure is not achieved. A newer device, the over the scope clip (OTSC), allows full thickness closure of GI perforations. This device has been applied to perforations and bleeding throughout the GI tract, including colorectal perforations up to 30 mm, GI fistulas, and bleeding. The OTSC applicator is integrated into the tip of the endoscope and deploys a bear-trap shaped, toothed nitinol clip that is able to penetrate deep enough to incorporate all layers of the intestinal wall (Fig. 20.7) [50, 51]. Microperforations resulting in pneumoperitoneum are typically managed expectantly, and intervention is not needed. Presence of pneumoperitoneum or pneumoretroperitoneum after ESD or EMR is seen with some frequency in asymptomatic patients. If free air is accompanied by a fluid collection, intervention is likely necessary, either percutaneous drainage, which is more appropriate for a delayed diagnosis, or surgical repair in the acute setting. Paracentesis for relief of tension pneumoperitoneum has been used effectively in several studies [46, 52, 53]. An algorithm for treatment of upper endoscopy-related perforations is shown in Fig. 20.8.

Colonoscopy

Endoscopy is widely used for diagnosis and treatment of a wide range of colorectal disease. Over 30 % of patients note some procedure-related gastrointestinal symptom, but true complications, such as perforation and hemorrhage, occur in less than 0.3 % of cases [5, 54–56]. Perforation is probably the most serious complication, primarily due to mechanical trauma to the sigmoid colon during diagnostic or therapeutic endoscopy. Perforation occurs in 0.03–0.07 % of cases [54, 57], and is the most common colonoscopy complication involving the surgeon. Perforation when EMR or ESD is performed is much higher, occurring in about 1 % of EMR cases and between 1 and 10 % after ESD [58, 59]. Bleeding,

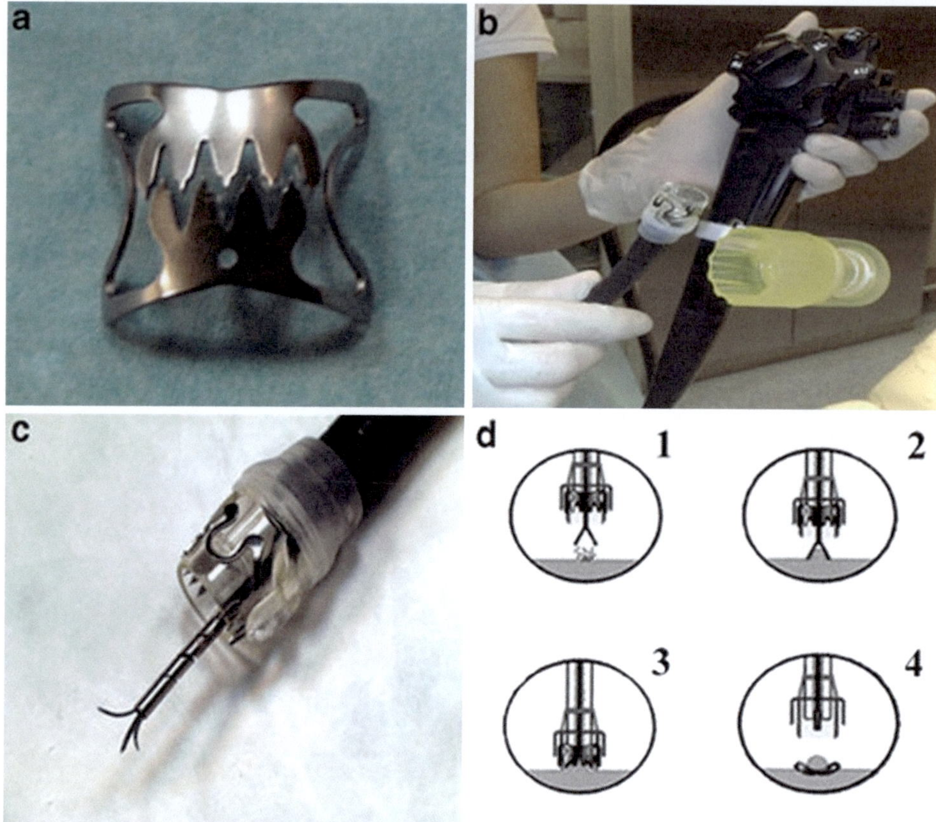

Fig. 20.7 The over-the-scope-clip system. (**a**) Nitinol clip, (**b**) OTSC system attached to the endoscope, (**c**) pre-installed OTSC to the tip of the endoscope, (**d**) schematic depiction of intestinal closure (modified with permission from [146], copyright @ 2012 Springer)

cardiopulmonary complications, post-polypectomy syndrome, transient bacteremia, or splenic injury are potential complications, though rarely, if ever, require surgery. Colonoscopy-specific mortality is extraordinarily rare, with only 7 deaths per 100,000 procedures [54].

Colonoscopy-Related Perforation

Though colonoscopy associated perforation is rare, mortality and morbidity are as high as 13 and 53 %, respectively [60]. Perforation occurs for three reasons: Mechanical perforation from direct endoscope or instrument trauma, pneumatic or barotrauma, or as a result of therapeutic intervention such as polypectomy, EMR or ESD, or use of electrosurgical devices. Pneumatic perforation occurs with excessive air insufflation, raising intraluminal pressure high enough to rupture the colon wall, which occurs most often in the cecum. It has been shown that a pressure of 169 mmHg is enough to cause cecal perforation [61]. Mechanical perforations tend to be linear and larger than nonmechanical injuries, and most often occur in the sigmoid colon. Therapeutic interventions more often result in small injuries isolated to the location of therapy. Rectosigmoid perforation due to scope trauma is most common, accounting for more than half of colonoscopy-related perforations, followed by cecal perforation, with descending colon perforations being the least common (Fig. 20.9) [57, 62–64].

Visualization of the viscera, inability to maintain insufflation, persistent or worsening abdominal distention despite intraluminal suction, and intraluminal bleeding in the absence of therapeutic intervention are all possible indicators of perforation [64]. However, the majority of perforations are not recognized during the procedure. Patients may present within the first hour post-procedure, or may be delayed as long as several days, though most present within 24 h [57, 62, 64]. If not recognized during colonoscopy, patients present with progressive abdominal pain, persistent abdominal distention, tachycardia, and fever. Post-procedure abdominal pain is common, reported in about 10 % of patients, and bloating is reported in 25 %, so a high index of suspicion is needed to ensure early diagnosis [54] Acute abdominal series is diagnostic in over 85 % of cases, and CT imaging demonstrating pneumoperitoneum or contrast extravasation is helpful if plain films are non-diagnostic [62]. As with other endoscopic perforations, the volume of pneumoperitoneum is not indicative of the size of the defect, but

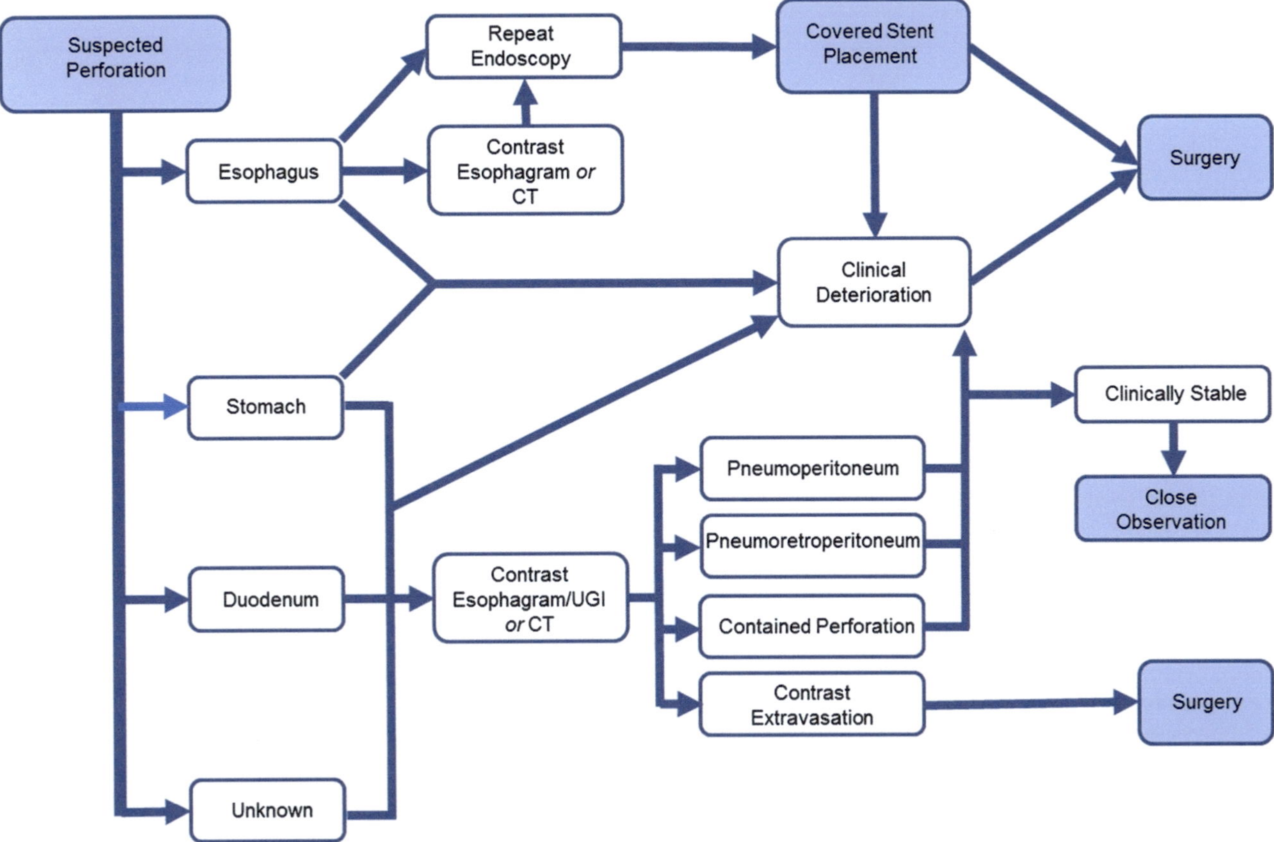

Fig. 20.8 Algorithm for management of suspected upper endoscopy-related perforation

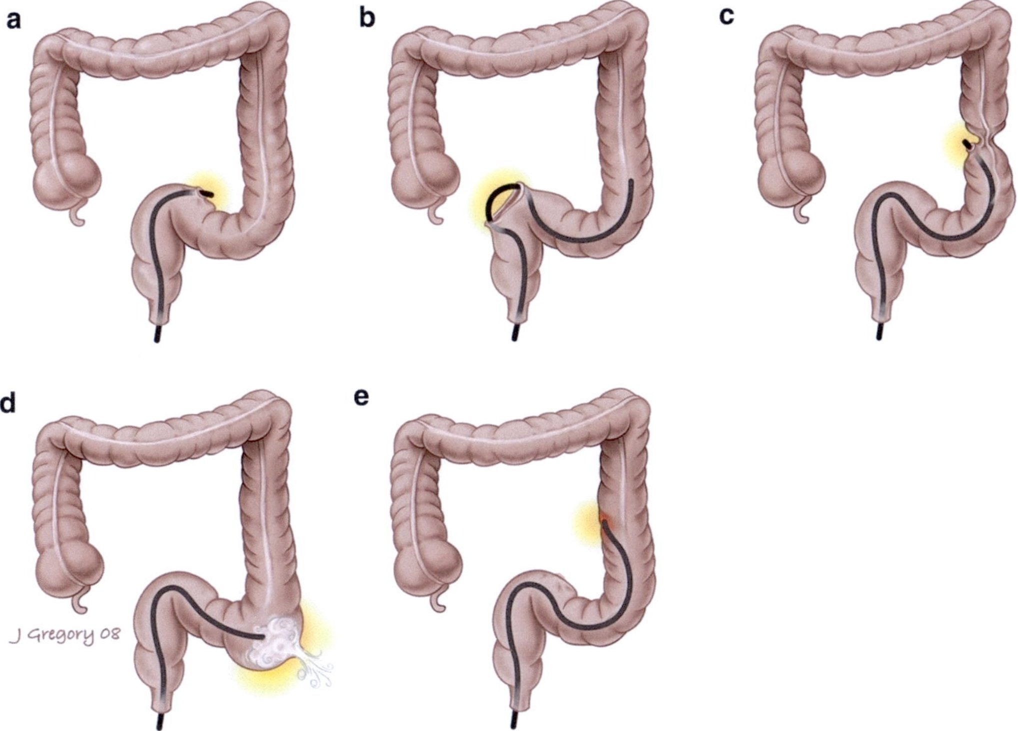

Fig. 20.9 Mechanisms of colonoscopy-related perforations. (**a**) Direct penetration of the colonoscope, (**b**) bowing of a loop, (**c**) at the site of pathology, (**d**) excessive insufflation, (**e**) direct injury during intervention, such as polypectomy or use of diathermy ([64], modified)

Table 20.3 Operative management of colonoscopy-related perforation

Author	Year	*n/#* Perforations	Successful nonoperative management	Primary repair	Repair with diversion	Resection with anastomosis	Resection, anastomosis and diversion	Resection and ostomy, nonrestorative	Mortality (%)
Korman [149]	2003	116,000/37	2 (7 %)	ns	ns	ns	ns	ns	0
Cobb [57]	2004	43,609/14	1 (7 %)	3 (21 %)	0	8 (57 %)	0	2 (14 %)	0
Luning [63]	2007	30,366/35	na	18 (56 %)	ns	8 (25 %)	ns	6 (19 %)	8.6
Iqbal [62]	2008	258,248/180	13 (7.9 %)	48 (29 %)	ns	55 (33 %)	16 (10 %)	46 (28 %)	7
Avgerinos [64]	2008	105,786/35	12 (34 %)	7 (20 %)[a]	ns	ns	ns	15 (43 %)[a]	3

[a]Operative intervention reported as "primary repair with or without protective ostomy" and "Hartmann's or other resection"

Table 20.4 Surgical options for colonoscopy-related perforation

Surgical intervention	Indications	Contraindications
Primary repair	Small perforation (<50 % colon circumference) Early diagnosis Mild intraabdominal contamination	Feculent peritonitis Large defects Distal obstruction Concomitant pathology requiring resection
Repair with defunctionalizing ostomy	Small perforation Mild to moderate contamination Concern for integrity of repair	Large defects Distal obstruction Concomitant pathology requiring resection
Resection and anastomosis	Large perforation Mild to moderate contamination	Hemodynamic instability Feculent peritonitis
Resection, anastomosis and defunctionalizing ostomy	Large perforation Mild to moderate contamination Concern for integrity of anastomosis	Hemodynamic instability Feculent peritonitis (relative)
Resection with non-restorative ostomy	Large perforation Feculent peritonitis Hemodynamic instability Increasing patient comorbidities Immune compromised patient	Excessively morbid for small perforations with minimal contamination that are recognized early

rather the amount of insufflated air. In the setting of polypectomy, particularly of multiple lesions, post-polypectomy electrosurgical syndrome may occur due to transmural thermal burn to the colon wall. This entity is important to recognize, as it may present clinically very similar to perforation, but without radiographic evidence of perforation, and does not require surgery [54].

Surgical Management of Colonoscopy-Related Perforations

Management of iatrogenic colon perforation requires surgery in 74–100 % of cases (Table 20.3) [62, 65]. The clinical presentation of the patient, their comorbid status, time to diagnosis, indication for colonoscopy, mechanism of perforation, and success of mechanical bowel preparation are all important factors in determining the most appropriate surgical approach. Laparotomy is used most often, though there are several series reporting safety and efficacy of laparoscopy in the treatment of iatrogenic colon perforations [65–67]. Regardless of the approach, the choice to repair, resect, anastomose, or divert depends on the location and extent of the injury, the time to diagnosis, the level of intraabdominal contamination, the indication for the colonoscopy, and the judgment of the operating surgeon. When diagnosed early, contamination is minimal and the injury is less than half the colon circumference, primary repair is appropriate. Larger injuries should be resected, and anastomosis is appropriate in stable patients with minimal contamination. If feculent or purulent peritonitis is present, which may be more likely in poorly prepped bowel, resection and diversion is more appropriate. This can be accomplished with an end colostomy and mucous fistula or Hartmann's pouch, or with a proximal diverting ileostomy if primary anastomosis is performed. Diversion is always the safe approach if there is concern for the integrity of the repair or anastomosis, in cases of significant contamination, or in clinically unstable patients. Delay in presentation greater than 24 h, poor quality bowel prep, and extensive injuries are more likely to develop feculent peritonitis and require diversion. Morbidity and mortality also increases with delayed diagnosis, with double the risk of death when presenting after more than 24 h [62]. However, evidence from experience with perforated diverticulitis suggests that anastomosis may be safe even in cases of purulent or feculent peritonitis, though defunctionalizing proximal stoma is recommended [65, 68, 69]. Table 20.4

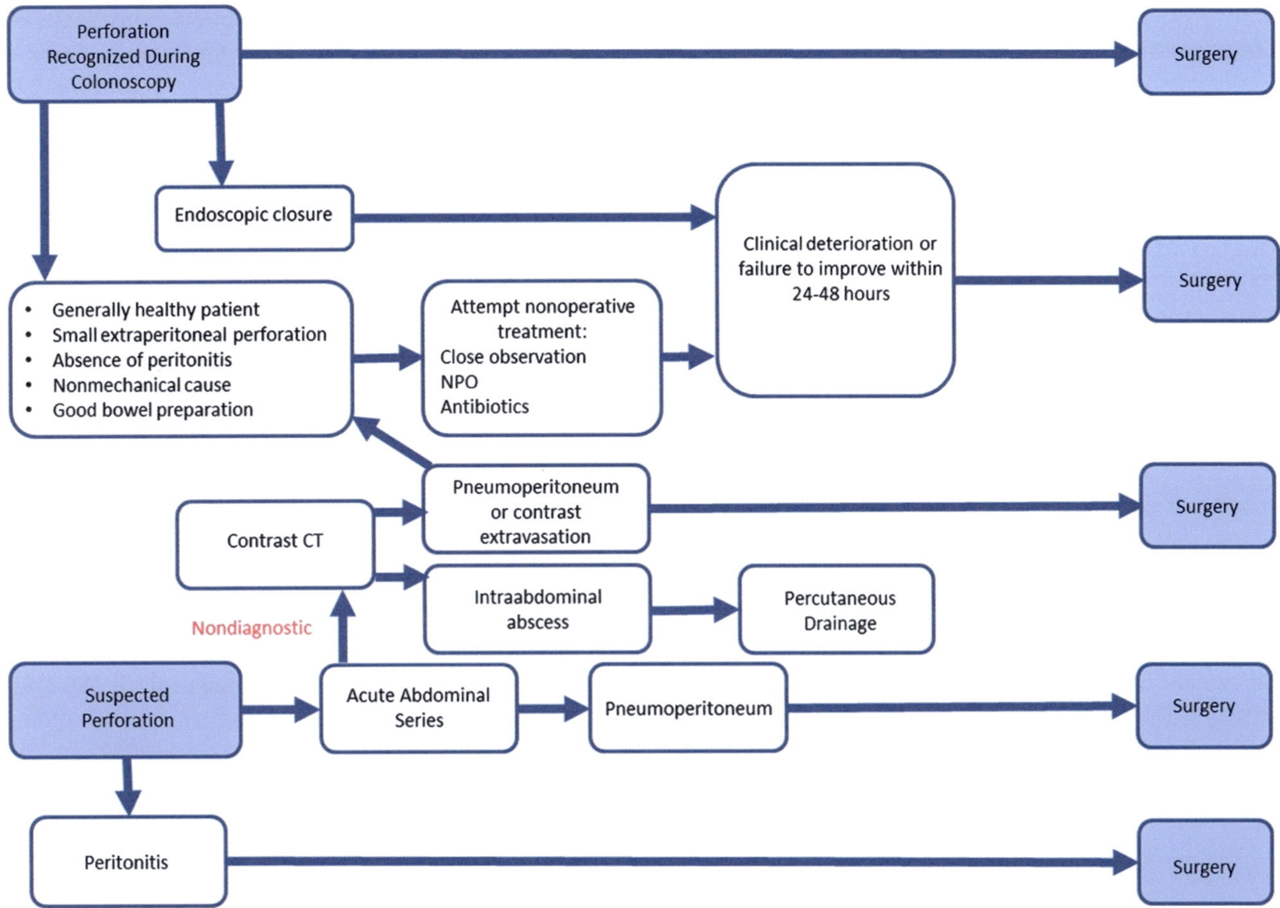

Fig. 20.10 Algorithm for management of suspected colonoscopy-related perforation

outlines the surgical options for patients with colonoscopy-related perforations.

Alternatives to Surgical Management

Clinically stable patients without peritonitis, in the absence of free intraabdominal perforation by radiography, may be treated expectantly in very select cases [62, 64, 70]. Small perforations presenting without peritonitis, patients presenting several days post-procedure with contained abscess, and extraperitoneal perforations often do not require surgery and can be managed with percutaneous drainage, antibiotics and bowel rest. Patients with perforation as a result of therapeutic intervention, such as polypectomy, are more likely able to have successful nonoperative management, probably because of increased early recognition and endoscopic intervention, and because perforations tend to be much smaller than with mechanical perforations [64, 65, 70]. Mechanical perforations are typically larger and linear in nature and nonoperative management is not recommended. If nonoperative management is attempted, patient must show clinical improvement within 24–48 h and be prepared for surgical intervention. The greatest risk of this

approach is the failure rate of 30–70 %. When surgery is delayed there is a much greater likelihood of requiring bowel resection and ostomy creation due to the higher degree of intraabdominal sepsis [65].

When recognized during the procedure, endoscopic closure of colonic perforations is possible with endoscopic clip placement. Endoclips can be applied anywhere in the colon and have are indicated for closure of small defects, typically 1 cm or less [59, 71]. There is good data from experience with EMR and ESD that this approach is successful in most cases [58, 59]. As with upper GI EMR/ESD perforation, tense pneumoperitoneum in the setting of a closed defect can be treated with needle decompression [58]. Clinical data on these techniques is currently limited to case reports and small case series, with significant support from animal studies [58, 59]. A newer device, the T-tag, has been used to successfully close large defects in animal models, but has not been reported in humans [72, 73]. The OTSC system has also been used for colonic perforations, with successful closure of up to 3 cm defects [50, 51]. Figure 20.10 shows the basic treatment algorithm for treatment of colonoscopy-related perforation.

Colonoscopy-Related Hemorrhage

Significant iatrogenic bleeding following colonoscopy is extremely rare, occurring most commonly during snare polypectomy or hot forceps biopsy. Incidence of bleeding is between 0.001 and 1.24 % following diagnostic colonoscopy. Bleeding with polypectomy occurs in 0.2–0.6 % of patients [54], and up to 12 % with EMR or ESD [58]. Patients on therapeutic anticoagulation or antiplatelet therapy have a higher risk of clinically significant bleeding after therapeutic colonoscopy [74, 75], though there is no definitive guideline for management of these medications, with great variability among physicians [76]. Caution should be used when considering elective colonoscopy in patients with severe thrombocytopenia and therapeutic anticoagulation or antiplatelet therapy [54].

When significant bleeding occurs following colonoscopy, the algorithm for treatment is similar to any lower GI bleed. Appropriate resuscitation and monitoring are the first priority, followed by localization and treatment when bleeding does not cease spontaneously. Repeat endoscopy with attempted endoscopic hemostasis should be attempted, and is successful in most cases [54, 58, 59]. Red blood cell (RBC) scintigraphy is helpful for confirming ongoing bleeding and roughly localizing the bleeding, and angiography can both diagnose and potentially treat ongoing post-colonoscopy bleeding.

Surgical Management of Colonoscopy-Related Hemorrhage

Surgical intervention is rarely needed for post-colonoscopy bleeding. Clinically evident bleeding, hemodynamic instability despite resuscitation, or failure of endoscopic or angiographic hemostasis is an indication for surgery. As with any other lower GI bleed, preoperative localization of the bleeding is essential to avoid unnecessarily excessive resection. Known site of polypectomy is helpful, and RBC scintigraphy or angiography may be used to localize the point of hemorrhage. Localized bleeding is treated with segmental or partial colectomy. It is important to consider coincident pathology if surgery becomes necessary, including additional resection and lymphadenectomy in the case of known or highly suspected malignancy, provided the patient is stable enough to tolerate the additional operative time. If bleeding is not able to be localized prior to surgery, subtotal colectomy may be required. Stoma creation may be necessary in hemodynamically unstable patients to avoid the higher risk of anastomotic leak in these patients. Alternatively, leaving the patient in discontinuity with a planned second operation is a good option for critically ill and unstable patients [54, 77, 78].

Alternatives to Surgery

Acute hemorrhage following polypectomy is often self-limited and ceases with resuscitation, correction of coagulopathy and transfusion. Repeat colonoscopy with endoscopic hemostasis is successful in controlling bleeding in most cases. If endoscopic techniques fail, angiography with selective embolization can achieve hemostasis in many cases [78, 79].

Colonoscopy-Related Splenic Injury

Though rare, splenic rupture due to colonoscopy has been reported and is likely to require surgery. Fewer than 50 cases have been reported, though it is potentially under recognized and under reported [80]. Hemodynamic instability, ongoing transfusion requirement, or evidence of grade IV or V splenic laceration are clear indications for splenectomy.

Endoscopic Retrograde Cholangiopancreatography

ERCP is an important modality in the evaluation and treatment of a variety of biliary, pancreatic, and ampullary conditions. Over 500,000 ERCPs are performed annually in the USA [81]. Complications occur in 5–10 % of patients undergoing ERCP, primarily related to therapeutic procedures [82–86]. Post-ERCP pancreatitis (PEP) is the most common complication, occurring in about 5–15 % of patients, followed by bleeding (0.3–2 %), biliary infection (1 %), perforation (<1 %), and cardiopulmonary complications (<1 %). Surgical management of ERCP-related complications is primarily related to duodenal perforation, though rarely may be required for intractable bleeding, complications of severe pancreatitis, or mechanical complications, such as basket impaction or guidewire fracture. Migration of biliary stents may present as obstruction or peritonitis, requiring surgical treatment. Severe and fatal complications are rare, occurring in less than 1 % of procedures [81, 87].

ERCP-Related Hemorrhage

Bleeding related to ERCP occurs almost exclusively in the setting of endoscopic sphincterotomy (ES) and complicates 0.3–2 % of procedures (Table 20.5). Immediate and delayed bleeding occurs with equal frequency, with delayed bleeding presenting up to several days to weeks after ERCP. Clinically significant bleeding is categorized as mild, moderate or severe based on clinical signs and symptoms and transfusion requirement, with severe bleeding occurring in only 0.1–0.5 % of cases [81, 88–90].

Surgical Management of ERCP-Related Hemorrhage

In the early experience with ERCP, bleeding requiring surgical intervention occurred in as many as 3 % of patients [90]. However, with the continued advances in technique, technology, and experience, surgical intervention is rarely needed. In pooled analysis of the largest recent series, surgery was reported in only 4 patients in over 25,000 procedures [82–84, 86, 91, 92]. There is no standard surgical approach, leaving the decision to the judgment and experience of the surgeon. Anatomically, the ampulla derives its blood supply from the gastroduodenal artery (GDA) and its branches, making ligation a good option for hemostasis [93, 94]. Direct control of hemorrhage at the papilla with suture ligation or cauterization is also successful. Of critical importance is the awareness of the ductal anatomy. Blind placement of sutures or excessive use of cautery could disrupt biliary and pancreatic ducts, leading to delayed stricture or acute pancreatitis [94]. The papilla can be approached via a longitudinal anterior duodenotomy, a supraduodenal gastrotomy, or a posterior distal duodenotomy [95, 96]. The risk of leak from duodenotomy repair, with risk of fistula development, must also be considered.

Alternatives to Surgical Management

The majority of ES bleeding is self-limited, though delayed bleeding can present days to weeks post-procedure.

Table 20.5 ERCP- and ES-related hemorrhage

Author	Year	n	Bleeding	Surgical intervention (n)	Mortality
Freeman [91]	1996	2,347	48 (2 %)	2	2 (0.08 %)[a]
Loperfido [83]	1998	2,769	21 (1.1 %)	2	2 (0.07 %)[b]
Masci [84]	2001	2,444	30 (1.2 %)	ns	0
Vandervoort [86]	2002	1,223	10 (0.8 %)	0	1 (0.08 %)[c]
Perini [150]	2005	2,711	96 (4.1 %)	0	0
Wang [92]	2009	3,178	46 (1.5 %)	ns	ns
Cotton [82]	2009	11,497	40 (0.3 %)	ns	0
Lukens [148]	2010	3,924	28 (0.7 %)	0	ns

[a]Neither patient underwent surgery
[b]Does not specify if death occurred in surgical patients
[c]Patient also had severe pancreatitis

Endoscopic management of post ES bleeding is effective in well over 90 % of cases [89, 90]. Initial treatment is epinephrine spray irrigation or submucosal injection. If injection alone is ineffective, use of electrosurgical coagulation [90], APC [90], balloon tamponade [97–99], or placement of endoscopic clips is often successful [90]. Fibrin glue application, placement of covered metallic stents, and alcohol injection have also been reported [99–101]. In the event of failed endoscopic hemostasis, angiography with selective embolization of the GDA or its branches is another alternative to surgery. There are only a handful of cases reported using this technique specifically for post-ES bleeding, though it is well established for the treatment of upper gastrointestinal hemorrhage in other settings [12, 13, 91, 102, 103].

ERCP-Related Perforation

The incidence of perforation during ERCP is well less than 1 % (Table 20.6) [82–84, 86, 91, 92, 104]. Both the severity and the management of ERCP-related perforations vary according to location and mechanism. Perforations are classified according to location, and the management of each type varies significantly (Fig. 20.11). The classification proposed by Stapfer et al. is used for this chapter [105]. Unique to ERCP is the possibility of biliopancreatic perforation from duct cannulation with guidewires, baskets or stents. These perforations occur are more likely to occur during technically difficult procedures, in patients with choledocholithiasis, biliary stricture or tumor due to increased use of guidewires and instrument manipulation. Overall mortality is low, only 0.2–0.5 %, but complication specific mortality is as high as 25 % for duodenal perforations.

Type II and III perforations are more often recognized during ERCP by extravasation of contrast or visualization of retroperitoneal free air. Post-procedure, any clinical signs of perforation should prompt immediate evaluation. Abdominal

Table 20.6 ERCP- and ES-related perforation

Author	Year	n	Overall	Type I	Type II	Type III	Surgical treatment	Mortality[a]
Freeman [91]	1996	2,347	11 (0.4 %)	8 (73 %)	ns	3 (27.3 %)	3 (27 %)	1 (9 %)
Loperfido [93]	1998	2,769	28 (1 %)	16 (57.1 %)	12 (42.9 %)	0	15 (53 %)	4 (14 %)
Howard [106]	1999	6,040	40 (0.6 %)	4 (10 %)	22 (55 %)	14 (35 %)	7 (17.5 %)[b]	2 (5 %)
Masci [84]	2001	2,444	16 (0.7 %)	2 (12 %)	14 (88 %)	0	7 (43 %)[b]	0
Vandervoort [86]	2002	1,223	1 (0.08 %)	ns	ns	ns	ns	0
Salminen [104]	2008	2,555	5 (0.2 %)	2 (40 %)	2 (40 %)	1 (20 %)	4 (80 %)[b]	1 (20 %)
Wang [92]	2009	3,178	7 (0.26 %)	ns	ns	ns	ns	ns
Cotton [82]	2009	11,497	16 (0.14 %)	12 (75 %)	4 (25 %)	0	11 (69 %)	1 (6.3 %)
Lukens [148]	2010	3,924	18 (0.5 %)	ns	ns	ns	ns	ns

Type I—perforation remote to the papilla; Type II—periampullary perforation (retroperitoneal); Type III—guidewire perforation of the bile duct
ns not specified
[a]Complication specific mortality
[b]Includes all patients with Type III perforations

Classification and Mechanism of ERCP-Related Perforations

Howard (1999)		Stapfer (2000)		Mechanism of Injury
Type III	Duodenal perforation remote from the papilla	Type I	Perforation of lateral duodenal wall (remote from papilla)	Direct scope trauma
Type II	Periampullary perforation	Type II	Periampullary perforation	Endoscopic sphincterotomy
Type I	Perforation of bile duct	Type III	Perforation of bile duct	Guidewire or other instrumentation
		Type IV	Retroperitoneal free air with no demonstrable perforation	Insufflation of compressed air during ERCP

Fig. 20.11 Classification and mechanism of ERCP-related perforations

pain is the most common presentation, which may be associated with fever, tachycardia, leukocytosis, or peritonitis. A high index of suspicion is needed, as up to a third of patients report abdominal pain following ES [106]. Patients with suspected perforation should undergo contrasted imaging with fluoroscopy or CT [107, 108]. Findings of large pneumoperitoneum or extravasation of contrast into the peritoneal cavity are clear indications for surgery [105]. The presence of a large amount of retroperitoneal free air is by CT imaging is concerning, but does not correlate with the degree of injury or the need for surgery. Up to 29 % of asymptomatic patients have pneumoretroperitoneum 24 h after ERCP. Similarly, pneumatosis may occur from submucosal air injection with misdirection of cannulation device, also without clinical significance [109–111]. Knudson et al. developed a scoring system to help guide the decision on who will need surgery. Clinical index (CI) scores are based on fever, tachycardia, leukocytosis, and guarding, with one point assigned for each. Patients with a CI score ≥ 3 underwent operative treatment 83 % of the time, versus only 11 % of patients with CI score ≤ 1 ($p < 0.001$, OR 40.0, 5.3–303.1 CI). Radiographic criteria were also evaluated, including free air, free fluid, retroperitoneal air, and retroperitoneal fluid. There was no statistically significant difference in patient undergoing operative versus nonoperative treatment base on these criteria [112, 113]. This system may have some utility in guiding treatment decisions, but should be used with caution, as it is a small study based on retrospective data, which limits its applicability.

The surgical approach depends on the location and size of the perforation, time to recognition of the injury, degree of peritoneal or retroperitoneal contamination, and surgeon judgment and experience. Key principles of surgical management include control of sepsis with washout and local drainage, repair of the injury with or without diversion, and appropriate perioperative resuscitation and support. Additional procedures, such as cholecystectomy, common duct exploration, or biliary or intestinal bypass, are sometimes necessary as well, depending on the initial indication for ERCP and the patients underlying condition. A recent review nicely summarizes the literature on the surgical management of ERCP-related perforations, highlighting the importance of individualization of surgical approach to the type, location and severity of the perforation, and consideration of any underlying disease [113]. Figure 20.12 and Table 20.7 outline the treatment algorithm and surgical options for ERCP-related perforations.

Surgical Management of Perforations Remote to the Papilla

Type I perforations occur most commonly at the lateral posterior duodenal wall, and usually not recognized at the time of ERCP because of the use of side viewing endoscopes (Fig. 20.13). Essentially all type I perforations require surgery. When recognized and treated early, primary repair of the enterotomy along with nasogastric drainage will likely be adequate. Repair should be done in two layers in a transverse fashion, with debridement of any devitalized tissue, and if possible, reinforced with an omental patch [113]. Closure of large perforations may be accomplished with jejunal serosal patch. Local closed suction drainage is recommended. There is one case reported of laparoscopic approach to a lateral retroperitoneal duodenal perforation closed successfully with intracorporeal repair and local drainage [114]. While use of laparoscopy is widespread, and each generation is increasingly facile with minimally invasive techniques, this approach should be used with caution, and only be attempted in cases of early recognition in expert hands.

In the case of delayed diagnosis, tissue is often inflamed and friable and the risk of anastomotic leak or dehiscence is high, potentially leading to enterocutaneous fistula or uncontrolled intraabdominal sepsis. Duodenal diversion with pyloric exclusion and gastrojejunostomy should be considered [105, 107, 115, 116]. Pyloric exclusion is performed with a non-cutting stapler across the pylorus, or suture closure

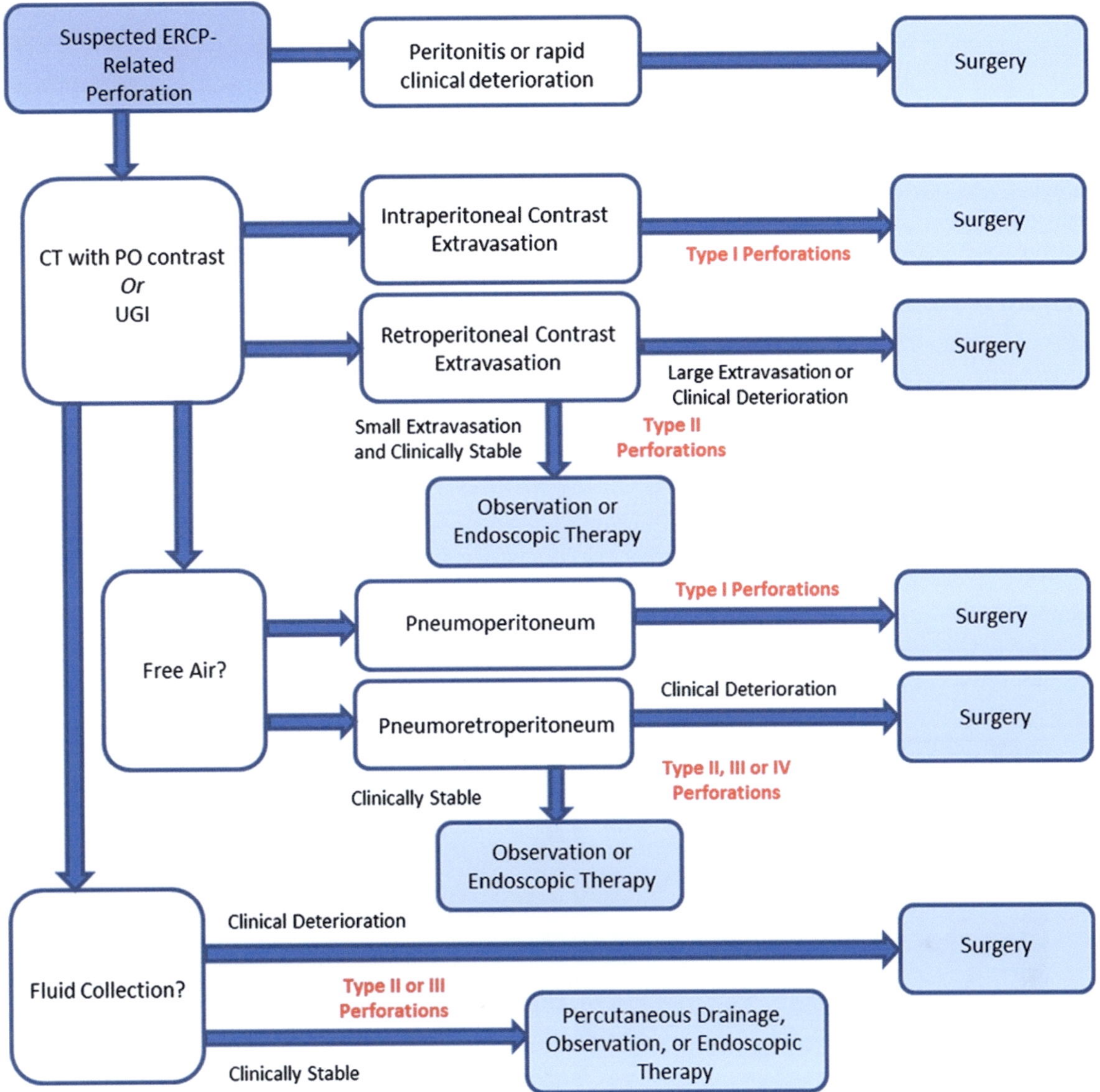

Fig. 20.12 Algorithm for operative intervention of suspected ERCP-related perforations

through an anterior gastrotomy. Pyloric closure will eventually break down and normal GI continuity is restored [113]. Drainage of the duodenum can be accomplished via lateral duodenostomy or a retrograde duodenostomy from a distal jejunal site. Retrograde duodenostomy may be safer in highly contaminated cases because the enterotomy created for its placement is well distal in healthy bowel. Consideration should be given to placement of enteral feeding access with a jejunostomy at the time of surgery as well.

If ERCP was initially performed for choledocholithiasis or cholangitis, or in cases with known cholelithiasis, concurrent cholecystectomy is recommended. Common bile duct exploration for clearance of choledocholithiasis and biliary diversion away from the site of injury may be indicated in the event of failed ERCP stone extraction or concomitant

bile duct injury. A T-tube should be placed for biliary drainage [105, 107, 112, 116]. Table 20.7 shows the various operations reported in the literature for type I perforations.

Periampullary Duodenal Perforations

Periampullary perforations are more often recognized at the time of ES. When recognized immediately, decompression with nasoenteric, nasobiliary, or internal biliary stents is typically employed, along with close observation for signs of progressive sepsis. As many as 85 % of these injuries can be managed expectantly without surgery. However, other studies show up to 30 % of these patients will later require surgery for clinical deterioration, making operative decision

Table 20.7 Surgical options for ERCP-related perforations

Surgical intervention	Indications	Contraindications
Simple repair	Immediate recognition with minimal contamination	Delayed recognition with significant contamination Large defect
Repair with omental patch	Adequate tissue for reinforcement	Significant contamination
Repair with pyloric exclusion and gastrojejunostomy	Delayed diagnosis with severe contamination Large injury	Unnecessary for small defects with minimal contamination that are recognized early
Cholecystectomy	ERCP done for gallstone disease Known cholelithiasis regardless of ERCP indication	No cholelithiasis
Common bile duct exploration	Common duct stones unable to be retrieved by ERCP Impacted instrumentation Type III injury	Unnecessary if stone disease not present or in the absence of type III injury
Transduodenal sphincteroplasty	Type II injury	Type I or III injuries
Drainage only	Retroperitoneal abscess Type II or III injury	Type I injury
Feeding jejunostomy	Severe sepsis with anticipated prolonged clinical course	Unnecessary for small defects with minimal contamination that are recognized early
Duodenal drainage (lateral or retrograde duodenostomy)	Type I injury Significant contamination with high risk of anastomotic dehiscence	Insufficient as only intervention
Laparoscopic approach	Early recognition of injury Diagnostic uncertainty (diagnostic laparoscopy)	Lack of surgical expertise in advanced laparoscopy

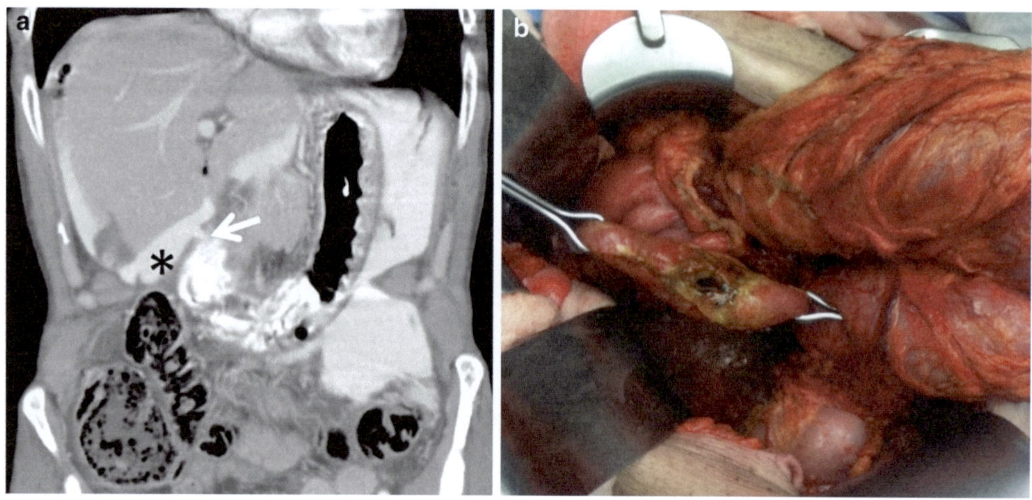

Fig. 20.13 Type I duodenal perforation. (**a**) CT image demonstrating duodenal perforation (*arrow*) with large contrast extravasation (*asterisk*) consistent with type I injury. (**b**) Operative image a lateral duodenal perforation

making difficult in this group [81, 105, 106, 108, 112]. Patients with delayed operative intervention, either due to delay in diagnosis or due to failed conservative therapy, have a prolonged hospital course and higher risk of mortality [105, 108, 112]. Extensive retroperitoneal contrast extravasation at the time of ERCP or on subsequent contrast imaging, or clinical deterioration of the patient are clear indications for surgery. Demonstration of extensive pneumoretroperitoneum is concerning, but does not necessarily correlate to the severity of the injury, rather is related to the quantity of air insufflated during endoscopy (Fig. 20.14) [109–111]. Significant fluid collection in conjunction with pneumoretroperitoneum, however, should prompt intervention with either surgery or percutaneous drainage [105, 107].

The best surgical approach to retroperitoneal duodenal perforations depends on the extent of injury, time to diagnosis, and degree of contamination. Simple retroperitoneal drainage may be sufficient in cases diagnosed early, and in stable patients with minimal contamination with small injuries, though this type of injury is more often able to be treated non-operatively. Repair of the perforation can be done through a transduodenal approach by direct repair or

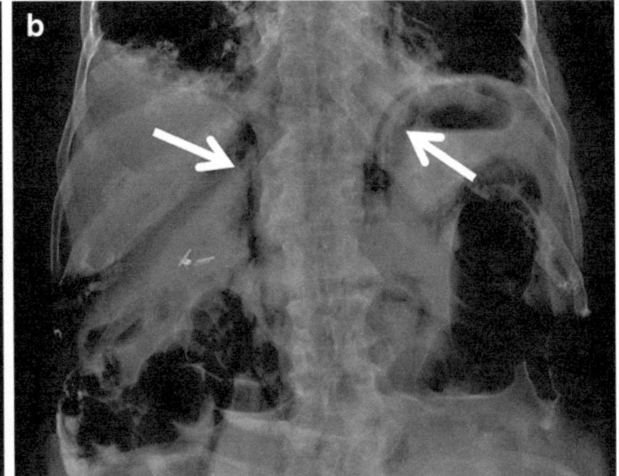

Fig. 20.14 Type II duodenal perforation. (**a**) CT demonstrating extensive retroperitoneal free air (*arrows*) with no extravasation of contrast from a periampullary perforation. (**b**) Plain film demonstrating pneumoretroperitoneum

sphincteroplasty using absorbable suture [113, 117]. A Fogarty catheter placed via the cystic or common bile duct, or a previously placed endoscopic biliary stent, can aid in locating the ampulla and guide position of the duodenotomy. Duodenal drainage, biliary drainage with a T-tube, pyloric exclusion, and gastrojejonostomy have commonly been employed as well, though are typically reserved for cases with significant contamination. Cholecystectomy and possible CBDE should also be performed at the time of surgery if cholelithiasis or choledocholithiasis was the indication for ERCP.

Bile Duct Perforations

Type III injuries are almost always diagnosed at the time of procedure by visualization of extravasated contrast from the bile duct [106, 108]. When diagnosis is delayed, patients will present with abdominal pain, fever, and leukocytosis, with radiographic findings of peritoneal or retroperitoneal fluid collection and free air [116]. The vast majority of these can be managed without surgery with percutaneous or endoscopic biliary drainage, along with percutaneous drainage of any fluid collections. Given the rarity of surgical intervention for these types of bile duct injuries, appropriate treatment is largely extrapolated from similar conditions, particularly CBD injury during cholecystectomy. Surgery may be required if the common duct is not able to be cleared endoscopically, or in the event of instrument impaction. A T-tube should be placed for common duct decompression and closed suction drains placed in the retroperitoneum for control of sepsis. Cholecystectomy should be performed as well [106, 116]. In the event of a large injury to the CBD precluding T-tube drainage, hepaticojejunostomy may be required. In this case, outcomes are significantly better when expert consultation is obtained and repair is done by an experienced surgeon. If immediate expertise is not available,

attempts at repair should not be made and placement of adequate large bore drains and transfer to a facility with expertise in this area is appropriate [118, 119].

Pneumoretroperitoneum in the Absence of Confirmed Perforation

Pneumoretroperitoneum with the absence of demonstrable perforation by endoscopy or radiographic imaging makes up type IV injuries. It is theorized that insufflation of compressed air used to maintain visualization ERCP causes this phenomenon. Pain may be presenting symptom, but many are asymptomatic. Up to 30 % of patients have pneumoretroperitoneum by CT imaging following ERCP with no correlation to the extent or location of the injury or the need for surgery [109–111]. No intervention is necessary, though patients should be monitored to ensure there is no clinical deterioration to indicate occult perforation [105].

Alternatives to Surgery

There are now several reports of endoscopic closure of iatrogenic perforations following ERCP, particularly for type II perforations [120–122]. There is a report of a large type I lateral duodenal perforation closed with endoloop and endoclip placement as well [123]. These cases were recognized during initial endoscopy and were small lesions, most are less than 1 cm. The OTSC has been applied to ERCP-related perforation of the jejunum in a patient with Billroth II anatomy, but has the potential to be used for more typical duodenal perforations [50, 51, 124]. Expertise in advanced endoscopy, as well as close post-procedure observation, is critical if this approach is attempted. Continued advancement in technology, particularly in the field of natural orifice

Table 20.8 Alternatives to surgery for ERCP-related perforations

Procedure	Indications	Contraindications
Endoscopic biliary stent	Type III injuries	Type I or II injuries
Percutaneous biliary stent	Type III injuries Biliary diversion in the event of anastomotic dehiscence after type I injury repair	Type II injuries
Percutaneous drainage	Contained fluid collections (any injury type) in stable patients	Clinically unstable patients
Endoscopic clipping	Small type I injuries (<1 cm) Type II injuries	Large type I injuries Endoscopist inexperience
Endoscopic suturing	Small type I injuries Type II injuries	Large type I injuries Endoscopist inexperience

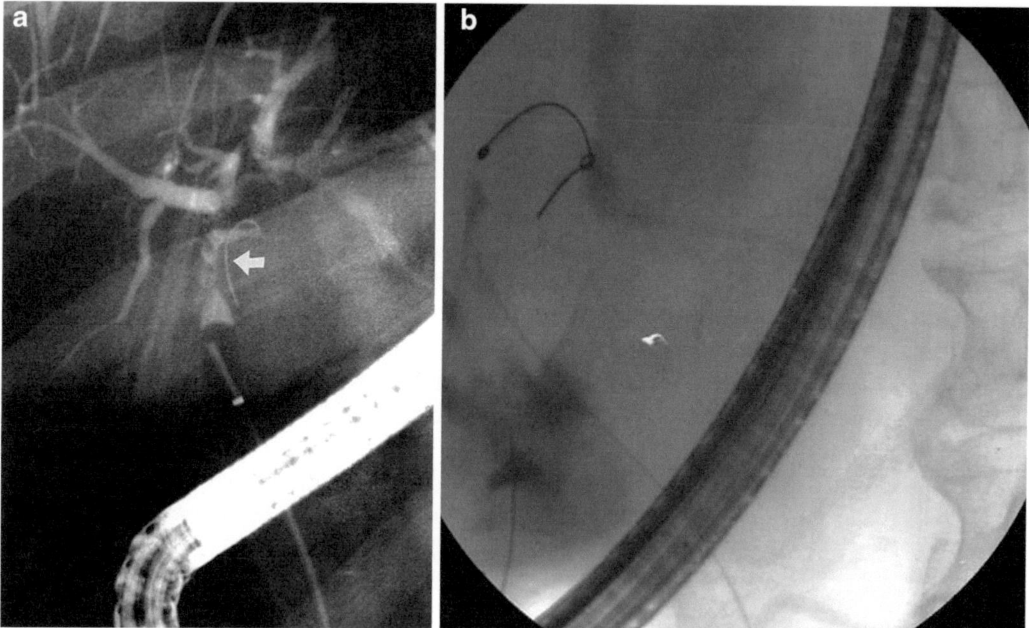

Fig. 20.15 (**a**) Fractured guidewire (with permission from [127], copyright 2006 @ Elsevier). (**b**) Knotted and fractured guidewire (with permission from [129], copyright 2006 @ Elsevier)

transluminal endoscopic surgery (NOTES) will certainly lead to new closure techniques and improved endoscopic suturing capability, which may eventually change this paradigm away from surgical management. For type III perforations, nonoperative treatment is the rule. Endoscopic biliary stenting, placement of nasobiliary drains, and gastric decompression are all commonly employed. Percutaneous drainage may be required if a significant perihepatic or retroperitoneal abscess develops [106, 125]. Table 20.8 outlines the nonsurgical options for treatment of ERCP-related perforations.

Knotting of guidewires while manipulating into position has also been reported [127–129]. Technological advances, particularly mechanical lithotripters, use of laser lithotripsy or extracorporeal shock-wave lithotripsy, have significantly decreased the incidence of basket impaction [130]. Wire or basket fracture may result from excess traction in attempts to remove the device, electrosurgical current applied across the wire, defects in the hydrophilic coating, or excessive torque applied while trying to manipulate the catheter tip into the desired position (Fig. 20.15) [127].

Instrument Complications

Biliopancreatic endoscopy and intervention carries the potential for malfunction, fracture, or retention of instrumentation. Some early series reported this incidence as high as 5.9 %, though more recent established incidence is well less than 1 % [83, 84, 92, 126]. This is most often basket or wire trapping during extraction of difficult common duct stones.

Surgical Management of Endoscopic Instrument Complications

Only a handful of surgical cases have been published for the treatment of instrument complications during ERCP. Extraction of the retained basket or wire can be done via duodenotomy or choledochotomy [131–134]. Biliary drainage with a T-tube should be used if common duct exploration is required. There is one report of laparoscopic retrieval of an impacted basket within the gallbladder by cholecystectomy [135]. Retrieval of impacted instru-ment could potentially be achieved with laparoscopic CBDE in experienced hands, though this has not been reported. There are no cases of guidewire fracture in which surgery was required, though the potential exists if the fragment cannot be retrieved [127]. Erosion of a retained guidewire fragment through the bile duct, pancreatic duct or intestine could potentially lead to abscess, fistula, pancreatitis, or peritonitis, but none of these potential complications have been reported.

Biliary stent migration is fairly common, occurring in up to 7 % of cases, and bowel obstruction biliary obstruction with cholangitis, abscess, perforation or enteroenteric fistula have all been reported. When distal stent migration is recognized early, it is often retrievable endoscopically. Even with more distal migration, spontaneous passage is the rule and surgery is rarely needed. In the event of complication, both open and laparoscopic approaches have been reported and the choice of operation depends on presentation, location, complication, and individual surgeon expertise. Control of sepsis, relief of obstruction, repair with or without diversion of enterotomies, and retrieval of the foreign body are critical to operative success [81, 136].

Alternatives to Surgery

Multiple endoscopic techniques have been described to free impacted stone and lithotripter baskets. Balloon dilation of the sphincter or lengthening of the sphincterotomy, mother–daughter biliary endoscopy, passage of a second basket adjacent to or proximal to the entrapped one, retrieval with toothed graspers, and percutaneous transhepatic retrieval have all been reported [126, 137–141]. More recently, use of mechanical, laser and extracorporeal shockwave lithotripters have been used to break apart large stones that are entrapped within a basket to allow retrieval [142, 143]. In the case of a

knotted and fractured guidewire, there are several reports of observation without intervention. Pruitt et al. report four cases of guidewire fracture due knot formation in the wire. In each case, no intervention was performed and no complications occurred [127]. In a single case of a retained portion of fractured guidewire resulting in cholangitis, repeat ERCP with retrieval of the fragment and drainage of the bile duct was successful [144].

ERCP-Related Biliary Infection

Acute cholecystitis and ascending cholangitis are recognized complications following ERCP (Table 20.9). Cholecystitis occurs in 0.1–0.5 % of cases, with cholangitis slightly more common, occurring in 0.3–1.4 % of cases. This may occur due to hydrostatic pressure into the biliary system during ERCP, failed stone extraction, incomplete or unsuccessful biliary drainage, or presence of malignant tumors. Biliary infections are also reported late complications from biliary stent placement, occurring in less than 1 % of cases [145, 146]. Treatment follows the same algorithm as non-iatrogenic biliary infection. Cholangitis is best treated with repeat ERCP with clearance of the bile duct or stent placement with subsequent cholecystectomy. Acute cholecystitis is best treated with cholecystectomy [81–84, 91, 92]. Pancreatitis is the most common complication of ERCP and ES, and severe pancreatitis can occur in this setting (Table 20.10). In cases of infected pancreatic necrosis,

Table 20.9 ERCP- and ES-related biliary infections

Author	Year	n	Cholecystitis	Cholangitis
Freeman [91]	1996	2,347	11 (0.5 %)	24 (1.0 %)
Loperfido [93]	1998	2,769	3 (0.1 %)	24 (0.9 %)
Masci [84]	2001	2,444	5 (0.2 %)	14 (0.6 %)
Vandervoort [86]	2002	1,223	3 (0.25 %)	9 (0.7 %)
Wang [92]	2009	3,178	6 (0.22 %)	38 (1.4 %)
Cotton [82]	2009	11,497	ns	38 (0.3 %)
Lukens [148]	2010	3,924	ns	16 (0.4 %)

Table 20.10 ERCP- and ES-related pancreatitis

Pancreatitis							
Author	Year	n	Overall	Mild	Moderate	Severe	Mortality[a]
Freeman [91]	1996	2,347	127 (5.4 %)	53 (41.7 %)	65 (51.2 %)	9 (7.1 %)	1 (0.8 %)
Loperfido [93]	1998	2,769	36 (1.3 %)	NA	NA	NA	1 (2.7 %)
Masci [84]	2001	2,444	44 (1.8 %)	41 (93.2 %)	0	3 (6.8 %)	0
Vandervoort [86]	2002	1,223	88 (7.2 %)	60 (68.2 %)	22 (25 %)	6 (6.8 %)	2 (2.3 %)
Cheng [147]	2006	1,115	168 (15.1 %)	112 (66.7 %)	45 (26.8 %)	11 (6.5 %)	NA
Wang [92]	2009	3,178	116 (4.3 %)	95 (81.9 %)	20 (17.2 %)	1 (0.9 %)	NA
Cotton [82]	2009	11,497	304 (2.6 %)	229 (75.3 %)	57 (18.8 %)	17 (5.6 %)	1 (0.3 %)
Lukens [148]	2010	3,924	38 (1 %)	NA	NA	NA	NA
Testoni [151]	2010	3,635	137 (3.8 %)	120 (87.6 %)	NA	17 (12.4 %)	5 (3.6 %)

NA not applicable

[a]Complication specific mortality

peripancreatic abscess, or pseudocyst formation, surgical or other interventional treatment may be required and follows the standard algorithm for each process.

Conclusion

Endoscopy is an important tool in the evaluation of gastrointestinal diseases, and advancing technology continues to push the boundaries of what this modality can accomplish. The surgeon must be familiar with the potential complications of diagnostic and therapeutic endoscopy. Given the overall rarity of complications that require surgery, familiarity with the published data and sound clinical judgment are key to successful patient outcomes.

References

1. National Center for Health Statistics. Health, United States, 2009, with special feature on medical technology. Hyattsville, MD: National Center for Health Statistics; 2010.
2. Eisen GM, Baron TH, Dominitz JA, Faigel DO, Goldstein JL, Johanson JF, et al. Complications of upper GI endoscopy. Gastrointest Endosc. 2002;55:784–93.
3. Valentine RJ, Jones A, Biester MS, Cogbill TH, Borman KR, Rhodes RS. General surgery workloads and practice patterns in the United States, 2007 and 2009. Ann Surg. 2011;254:520–6.
4. Nimeri AA, Hussein SA, Panzeter E, McNeill J, Gusz J, Chen PM, et al. The economic impact of incorporating flexible endoscopy into a community general surgery practice. Surg Endosc. 2005;19:702–4.
5. Silvis SE, Nebel O, Rogers G, Sugawa C, Mandelstam P. Endoscopic complications. Results of the 1974 American Society for Gastrointestinal Endoscopy survey. JAMA. 1976;235:928.
6. Shimoda R, Iwakiri R, Sakata H, Ogata S, Ootani H, Sakata Y, et al. Endoscopic hemostasis with metallic hemoclips for iatrogenic Mallory-Weiss tear caused by endoscopic examination. Dig Endosc. 2009;21:20–3.
7. Metman EH, Lagasse JP, d'Alteroche L, Picon L, Scotto B, Barieux JP. Risk factors for immediate complications after progressive pneumatic dilation for achalasia. Am J Gastroenterol. 1999; 94:1179–85.
8. Jung KW, Gundersen N, Kopacova J, Arora AS, Romero Y, Katzka D, et al. Occurrence of and risk factors for complications after endoscopic dilation in eosinophilic esophagitis. Gastrointest Endosc. 2011;73:15–21.
9. Park YM, Cho E, Kang HY, Kim JM. The effectiveness and safety of endoscopic subucosal dissection compared with endoscopic mucosal resection for early gastric cancer: a systemic review and metaanalysis. Surg Endosc. 2011;25:2666–77.
10. Tsuji Y, Ohata K, Ito T, Chiba H, Ohya T, Gunji T, et al. Risk factors for bleeding after endoscopic submucosal dissection for gastric lesions. World J Gastroenterol. 2010;16:2913–7.
11. Zehetner J, Shamiyeh A, Wayand W, Hubmann R. Results of a new method to stop acute bleeding from esophageal varices: implantation of a self-expanding stent. Surg Endosc. 2008;22:2149–52.
12. Loffroy R, Rao P, Ota S, De Lin M, Kwak BK, Geschwind JF. Embolization of acute nonvariceal upper gastrointestinal hemorrhage resistant to endoscopic treatment: results and predictors of recurrent bleeding. Cardiovasc Intervent Radiol. 2010;33: 1088–100.
13. Walker TG, Salazar GM, Waltman AC. Angiographic evaluation and management of acute gastrointestinal hemorrhage. World J Gastroenterol. 2012;18:1191–201.
14. Bhatia NL, Collins JM, Nguyen CC, Jaroszewski DE, Vikram HR, Charles JC. Esophageal perforation as a complication of esophagogastroduodenoscopy. J Hosp Med. 2008;3:256–62.
15. Merchea A, Cullinane DC, Sawyer MD, Iqbal CW, Baron TH, Wigle D, et al. Esophagogastroduodenoscopy-associated gastrointestinal perforations: a single center experience. Surgery. 2010;148:876–82.
16. Chirica M, Champault A, Dray X, Sulpice L, Munoz-Bongrand N, Sarfati E, et al. Esophageal perforations. J Visc Surg. 2010;147:e117–28.
17. Eroglu A, Turkyilmaz A, Aydin Y, Yekeler E, Karaoglanoglu N. Current management of esophageal perforation: 20 years experience. Dis Esophagus. 2009;22:374–80.
18. Brinster BA, Singhal S, Lawrence L, Marshall MB, Kaiser LR, Kucharczuk JC. Evolving options in the management of esophageal perforation. Ann Thorac Surg. 2004;77:1475–83.
19. Kantsevoy SV, Adler DG, Conway JD, Diehl DL, Farray FA, Kwon R, et al. Endoscopic mucosal resection and endoscopic submucosal dissection. Gastrointest Endosc. 2008;68:11–8.
20. Younes Z, Johnson DA. The spectrum of spontaneous and iatrogenic esophageal injury: perforations, Mallory-Weiss tears, and hematomas. J Clin Gastroenterol. 1999;29:306–17.
21. Siersema PD. Treatment of esophageal perforations and anastomotic leaks: the endoscopist is stepping into the arena. Gastrointest Endosc. 2005;61:897–900.
22. Bhatia P, Fortin D, Inculet RI, Malthaner RA. Current concepts in the management of esophageal perforations: a twenty-seven year Canadian experience. Ann Thorac Surg. 2011;92:209–15.
23. Wychulis AR, Fontana RS, Payne WS. Instrumental perforations of the esophagus. Dis Chest. 1969;55:184–9.
24. Bladergroen MR, Lowe JE, Postlethwait RW. Diagnosis and recommended management of esophageal perforation and rupture. Ann Thorac Surg. 1986;42:235–9.
25. Salo JA, Isolauri JO, Heikkila LJ, Markkula HT, Heikkinen LO, Kivilaakso EO, et al. Management of delayed esophageal perforation with mediastinal sepsis. Esophagectomy or primary repair? J Thorac Cardiovasc Surg. 1993;106:1088–91.
26. Kim-Deobald J, Kozarek RA. Esophageal perforation: an 8 year review of a multispecialty clinic's experience. Am J Gastroenterol. 1992;87:1112–9.
27. Sullivan M, Berry BE, Ferrante WA. The radiologist in the prevention and diagnosis of instrumental perforation of the esophagus. South Med J. 1974;67:830–6.
28. Michel L, Grillo HC, Malt RA. Operative and nonoperative management of esophageal perforations. Ann Surg. 1981;194:57–63.
29. Reeder LB, DeFilippi VJ, Ferguson MK. Current results of therapy for esophageal perforation. Am J Surg. 1995;169:615–7.
30. Whyte RI, Iannettoni MD, Orringer MB. Intrathoracicoesophageal perforation. The merit of primary repair. J Thorac Cardiovasc Surg. 1995;109:140–6.
31. Wright DC, Mathisen DJ, Wain JC, Moncure AC, Hilgenberg AD, Grillo HC. Reinforced primary repair of thoracic esophageal perforation. Ann Thorac Surg. 1995;60:245–9.
32. Bufkin BL, Miller JI, Mansour KA. Esophageal perforation: emphasis on management. Ann Thorac Surg. 1996;61:1447–52.
33. Orringer MB, Stirling MC. Esophagectomy for esophageal disruption. Ann Thorac Surg. 1990;49:35–42.
34. Iannettoni MD, Vlessis AA, Whyte RI, Orringer MB. Functional outcome after surgical treatment of esophageal perforation. Ann Thorac Surg. 1997;64:1606–9.
35. Altorjay A, Kiss J, Voros A, Sziranyi E. The role of esophagectomy in the management of esophageal perforations. Ann Thorac Surg. 1998;65:1433–6.

36. Matthews HR, Mitchell IM, McGuigan JA. Emergency subtotal oesophagectomy. Br J Surg. 1989;76:918–20.

37. Ochiai T, Hiranuma S, Takiguchi N, Maruyama M, Nagahama T, Kawano T, et al. Treatment strategy for Boerhaave's syndrome. Dis Esophagus. 2004;17:98–103.

38. Altorjay A, Kiss J, Voros A, Bohak A. Nonoperative management of esophageal perforations. Is it justified? Ann Surg. 1997;225:415–21.

39. Shaffer HA, Valenzuela G, Mittal RK. Esophageal perforation. A reassessment of the criteria for choosing medical or surgical therapy. Arch Intern Med. 1992;152:757–61.

40. Freeman RK, Ascioti AJ. Esophageal stent placement for the treatment of perforation, fistula, or anastomotic leak. Semin Thorac Cardiovasc Surg. 2011;23:154–8.

41. David EA, Kim MP, Blackmon SH. Esophageal salvage with removable covered self-expanding metal stents in the setting of intrathoracic esophageal leakage. Am J Surg. 2011; 202:796–801.

42. Rokszin R, Simonka Z, Paszt A, Szepes A, Kucsa K, Lazar G. Successful endoscopic clipping in the early treatment of spontaneous esophageal perforation. Surg Laparosc Endosc Percutan Tech. 2011;21:e311–2.

43. Voermans RP, Le Moine O, von Rentein D, Ponchon T, Giovannini M, Bruno M, et al. Efficacy of endoscopic closure of acute perforations of the gastrointestinal tract. Clin Gastroenterol Hepatol. 2012;10:603–8.

44. Fischer A, Schrag JH, Goos M, von Dobschuetz E, Hopt UT. Nonoperative treatment of four esophageal perforations with hemostatic clips. Dis Esophagus. 2007;20:444–8.

45. Fritscher-Ravens A, Hampe J, Grange P, Holland C, Olagbeye F, Milla P, et al. Clip closure versus endoscopic suturing versus thoracoscopic repair of an iatrogenic esophageal perforation: a randomized, comparative, long-term survival study in a porcine model (with videos). Gastrointest Endosc. 2010;72:1020–6.

46. Jeon SW, Jung MK, Kim SK, Cho KB, Park KS, Park CK, et al. Clinical outcomes for perforations during endoscopic submucosal dissection in patients with gastric lesions. Surg Endosc. 2010;24:911–6.

47. Hanaoka N, Uedo N, Ishihara R, Higashino K, Takeuchi Y, Inoue T, et al. Clinical features and outcomes of delayed perforation after endoscopic submucosal dissection for early gastric cancer. Endoscopy. 2010;42:1112–5.

48. Chung K, Lee JH, Lee SH, Kim SJ, Cho JY, Cho WY, et al. Therapeutic outcomes in 1000 cases of endoscopic submucosal dissection for early gastric neoplasms: Korean ESD study group multicenter study. Gastrointest Endosc. 2009;69:1228–35.

49. Minami S, Gotoda T, Ono H, Oda I, Hamanaka H. Complete endoscopic closure of gastric perforation by endoscopic resection of early gastric cancer using endoclips can prevent surgery (with video). Gastrointest Endosc. 2006;63:596–601.

50. Matthes K, Jung Y, Kato M, Gromski MA, Chuttani R. Efficacy of full-thickness GI perforation closure with a novel over-the-scope clip application device: an animal study. Gastrointest Endosc. 2011;74:1369–75.

51. Kirschniak A, Subotova N, Zieker D, Konigsrainer A, Dratt T. The over-the-scope clip for treatment of gastrointestinal bleeding, perforations, and fistulas. Surg Endosc. 2011;25:2901–5.

52. Fu K, Ishikawa T, Yamamoto T, Kaji Y. Paracentesis for successful treatment of tension pneumoperitoneum related to endoscopic submucosal dissection. Endoscopy. 2009;41 Suppl 2:E245.

53. Siboni S, Bona D, Abate E, Bonavina L. Tension pneumoperitoneum following endoscopic submucosal dissection of leiomyoma of the cardia. Endoscopy. 2010;42 Suppl 2:E152.

54. Fisher DA, Maple JT, Ben-Menachem T, Cash BD, Decker GA, Early DS, et al. Complications of colonoscopy. Gastrointest Endosc. 2011;74:745–52.

55. Levin TR, Zhao W, Conell C, Seeff LC, Manninen DL, Shapiro JA, et al. Complications of colonoscopy in an integrated health care delivery system. Ann Intern Med. 2006;145:880–6.

56. McDonnell WM, Loura F. Complications of colonoscopy. Ann Intern Med. 2007;147:212–3.

57. Cobb WS, Heniford BT, Signom LB, Hasan R, Simms C, Kercher KW, et al. Colonoscopic perforations: incidence, management, and outcomes. Am Surg. 2004;70:750–8.

58. Yoshida N, Yagi N, Naito Y, Yoshikawa T. Safe procedure in endoscopic submucosal dissection for colorectal tumors focused on preventing complications. World J Gastroenterol. 2010;16:1688–95.

59. Saito Y, Fukuzaw M, Matsuda T, Fukunaga S, Sakamoto T, Uraoka T, et al. Clinical outcome of endoscopic submucosal dissection versus endoscopic mucosal resection of large colorectal tumors as determined by curative resection. Surg Endosc. 2010;24:343–52.

60. Lohsiriwat V, Sujarittanakarn S, Akaraviputh T, Lertakyamanee N, Lohiriwat D, Kachinthorn U. Colonoscopic perforation: a report from the World Gastroenterology Organization endoscopy training center in Thailand. World J Gastroenterol. 2008;14:6722–5.

61. Kozarek RA, Earnest DL, Siverstein ME, Smith RA. Air-pressure induced colon injury during diagnostic colonoscopy. Gastroenterology. 1980;78:7–14.

62. Iqbal CW, Cullinane DC, Schiller HJ, Sawyer MD, Zietlow SP, Farley DR. Surgical management and outcomes of 165 colonoscopic perforations from a single institution. Arch Surg. 2008; 143:701–7.

63. Luning TH, Keemers-Gels ME, Barendregt WB, Tan AC, Rosman C. Colonoscopic perforations: a review of 30,366 patients. Surg Endosc. 2007;21:994–7.

64. Avgerinos DV, Llaguna OH, Lo AY, Leitman IM. Evolving management of colonoscopic perforations. J Gastrointest Surg. 2008;12:1783–9.

65. Lohsiriwat V. Colonoscopic perforation: incidence, risk factors, management and outcome. World J Gastroenterol. 2010;16:425–30.

66. Rotholtz NA, Laporte M, Lencinas S, Bun M, Canelas A, Mezzadri N. Laparoscopic approach to colonic perforation due to colonoscopy. World J Surg. 2010;34:1949–53.

67. Hansen AJ, Tessier DJ, Anderson ML, Schlinkert RT. Laparoscopic repair of colonoscopic perforations: indications and guidelines. J Gastrointest Surg. 2007;11:655–9.

68. Constantinides VA, Heriot A, Remzi F, Darzi A, Senapati A, Fazio V, et al. Operative strategies for diverticular peritonitis: a decision analysis between primary resection and anastomosis versus Hartmann's procedures. Ann Surg. 2007;245:94–103.

69. Brinda GA, Karas JR, Serventi A, Sokmen S, Amato A, Hydo L, et al. Primary anastomosis vs. norestorative resection for perforated diverticulits with peritonitis: a prematurely terminated randomized controlled trial. Colorectal Dis. 2012;14(11):1403–10.

70. Castellvi J, Pi R, Sueiras A, Vallet J, Bollo J, Tomas A, et al. Colonoscopic perforation: useful parameters for early diagnosis and conservative treatment. Int J Colorectal Dis. 2011;26:1183–90.

71. Raju GS, Pham B, Xiao SY, Brining D, Ahmed I. A pilot study of endoscopic closure of colonic perforations with endoclips in a swine model. Gastrointest Endosc. 2005;62:791–5.

72. Raju GS, Malhotra A, Ahmed I. Colonoscopic full-thickness resection of the colon in a porcine model as a prelude to endoscopic surgery of difficult colon polyps: a novel technique (with videos). Gastrointest Endosc. 2009;70:159–65.

73. Rieder E, Martinec DV, Dunst CM, Swanstrom LL. A novel technique for natural orifice endoscopic full-thickness colon wall resection: an experimental pilot study. J Am Coll Surg. 2011;13:422–9.

74. Singh M, Mehta N, Murthy UK, Kaul V, Arif A, Newman N. Postpolypectomy bleeding in patients undergoing colonoscopy on uninterrupted clopidogral therapy. Gastrointest Endosc. 2010;71:998–1005.

75. Johnson H. Management of major complications encountered with flexible colonoscopy. J Natl Med Assoc. 1993;85:916–20.

76. Lee SY, Tang SJ, Rockey DC, Weinstein D, Lara L, Sreenarasimhaiah J, et al. Managing anticoagulation and antiplatelet medications in GI endoscopy: a survey comparing the East and the West. Gastrointest Endosc. 2008;67:1076–81.

77. Sawheny MS, Salfiti N, Nelson DB, Lederle FA, Bond JH. Risk factors for severe delayed postpolypectomy bleeding. Endoscopy. 2008;40:115–9.

78. Sorbi D, Norton I, Conio M, Bald R, Zinsmeister A, Christopher J, et al. Postpolypectomy lower GI bleeding: descriptive analysis. Gastrointest Endosc. 2000;51:690–6.

79. Kuo WT, Lee DE, Saad WE, Patel N, Sahler LG, Waldman DL. Superselective microcoil embolization for the treatment of lower gastrointestinal hemorrhage. J Vasc Interv Radiol. 2003;14:1503–9.

80. Guerra JF, Fancisco IS, Pimentel F, Ibanez L. Splenic rupture following colonoscopy. World J Gastroenterol. 2008;14:6410–2.

81. Silviera ML, Seamon MJ, Porshinsky MP, Doraiswamy VA, Wang CF, Lorenzo M, et al. Complications related to endoscopic retrograde chalgiopancreatography: a comprehensive clinical review. J Gastrointestin Liver Dis. 2009;18:73–82.

82. Cotton PB, Garrow DA, Gallagher J, Romagnuolo J. Risk factors for complications after ERCP: a multivariate analysis of 11,497 procedures over 12 years. Gastrointest Endosc. 2009;70:80–8.

83. Loperfido S, Angelini G, Benedetti G, Chilovi F, Costan F, Berardinis F, et al. Major early complications from diagnostic and therapeutic ERCP: a prospective multicenter study. Gastrointest Endosc. 1998;48:1–10.

84. Masci E, Toti G, Mariani A, Curioni S, Lomazzi A, Dinelli M, et al. Complications of diagnostic and therapeutic ERCP: a prospective multicenter study. Am J Gastroenterol. 2001;96:417–23.

85. Jeurnink SM, Siersema PD, Steyerberg EW, Dees J, Poley JW, Haringsma J, et al. Predictors of complications after endoscopic retrograde cholangiopancreatography: a prognostic model for early discharge. Surg Endosc. 2011;25:2892–900.

86. Vandervoort J, Soetikno RM, Tham TC, Wong RC, Ferrari Jr AP, Montes H, et al. Risk factors for complications after performance of ERCP. Gastrointest Endosc. 2002;56:652–6.

87. Anderson MA, Fisher L, Jain R, Evans JA, Appalaneni V, Ben-Menachem T, et al. Complications of ERCP. Gastrointest Endosc. 2012;75:467–73.

88. Mellinger JD, Ponsky JL. Bleeding after endoscopic sphincterotomy as an underestimated entity. Surg Gynecol Obstet. 1991;172:465–9.

89. Wilcox CM, Canakis J, Monkemuller KE, Bondora AW, Geels W. Patterns of bleeding after endoscopic sphincterotomy, the subsequent risk of bleeding, and the role of epinephrine injection. Am J Gastroenterol. 2004;99:244–8.

90. Ferreira LEVVC, Baron TH. Post-sphincterotomy bleeding: who, what, when and how. Am J Gastroenterol. 2007;102:2850–8.

91. Freeman ML, Nelson DB, Sherman S, Haber GB, Herman ME, Dorsher PJ. Complications of endoscopic biliary sphincterotomy. N Engl J Med. 1996;335:909–18.

92. Wang P, Li ZS, Liu F, Ren X, Lu NH, Fan AN, et al. Risk factors for ERCP-related complications: a prospective multicenter study. Am J Gastroenterol. 2009;104:31–40.

93. Mirjalili SA, Stringer MD. The arterial supply of the major duodenal papilla and its relevance to endoscopic sphincterotomy. Endoscopy. 2011;43:307–11.

94. Sulkowski U, Kautz G, Nottberg H, Forster E. Surgical therapy of hemorrhage after endoscopic sphincterotomy (abstract only). Chirurg. 1996;67:26–31.

95. Jersek M, Vracko J. Sphincterotomy of Oddi's muscle through posterior distal duodenum: a modified technique with low morbidity and mortality. Hepatogastroenterology. 1996;43:377–80.

96. Makary MA, Elariny HA. Laparoscopic transduodenal sphincteroplasty. J Laparoendosc Adv Surg Tech A. 2006;16:629–32.

97. Itoi T, Yasuda I, Doi S, Mukai T, Kurihara T, Sofuni A. Endoscopic hemostasis using covered metallic stent placement for uncontrolled post endoscopic sphincterotomy bleeding. Endoscopy. 2011;43:369–72.

98. Shah JN, Marson F, Binmoeller KF. Temporary self-expandable metal stent placement of treatment of post-sphincterotomy bleeding. Gastrointest Endosc. 2010;72:1274–8.

99. Aslinia F, Hawkins L, Darwin P, Goldberg E. Temporary placement of a fully covered metal stent to tamponade bleeding from endoscopic papillary balloon dilation. Gastrointest Endosc. 2012;76(4):911–3.

100. Kim HJ, Kim MH, Kim DI, Lee HJ, Myung SJ, Yoo KS, et al. Endoscopic hemostasis in sphincterotomy-induced hemorrhage: its efficacy and safety. Endoscopy. 1999;31:431–6.

101. Mutignani M, Seerden T, Tringali A, Feisal D, Perri V, Familiary P, et al. Endoscopic hemostasis with fibrin glue for refractory postsphincterotomy bleeding. Gastrointest Endosc. 2010;71:856–60.

102. Saeed M, Kadir S, Kaufman SL, Murray RR, Milligan F, Cotton PB. Bleeding following endoscopic sphincterotomy: angiographic management by transcatheter embolization. Gastrointest Endosc. 1989;35:300–3.

103. Mohan B, Sidhu SS, Goyal O, Goyal P, Wander GS. Embolotherapy in massive post sphincterotomy bleed. J Assoc Physicians India. 2010;58:47–8.

104. Salminen P, Laine S, Gullichsen R. Severe and fatal complications after ERCP: analysis of 2555 procedures in a single experienced center. Surg Endosc. 2008;22:1965–70.

105. Stapfer M, Selby R, Stain SC, Katkhouda N, Parekh D, Jabbour N, et al. Management of duodenal perforation after endoscopic retrograde cholangiopancreatography and sphincterotomy. Ann Surg. 2000;232:191–8.

106. Howard TJ, Tan T, Lehman GA, Sherman S, Madura JA, Fogel E, et al. Classification and management of perforations complicating endoscopic sphincterotomy. Surgery. 1999;126:658–65.

107. Krishna RP, Singh RK, Behari A, Kumar A, Saxena R, Kapoor VK. Post-endoscopic retrograde cholangiopancreatography perforation managed by surgery or percutaneous drainage. Surg Today. 2011;41:660–6.

108. Wu HM, Dixon E, May GR, Sutherland FR. Management of perforation after endoscopic retrograde cholangiopancreatography (ERCP): a population-based review. HPB (oxford). 2006;8:393–9.

109. Assalia A, Suissa A, Ilivitzki A, Mahajna A, Yassin K, Hashmonai M, et al. Validity of clinical criteria in the management of endoscopic retrograde cholangiopancreatography-related duodenal perforations. Arch Surg. 2007;142:1059–64.

110. Genzlinger JL, McPhee MS, Risher JK, Jacob KM, Helzberg JH. Significance of retroperitoneal air after endoscopic retrograde cholangiopancreatography with sphincteroitomy. Am J Gastroenterol. 1999;94:1267–70.

111. Pannu HK, Fishman EK. Complications of endoscopic retrograde cholangiopancreatography: spectrum of abnormalities demonstrated with CT. Radiographics. 2001;21:1441–53.

112. Knudson K, Raiburn CD, McIntyre RC, Shaw RJ, Chen YK, Brown WR, et al. Management of duodenal and pancreaticobiliary perforations associated with periampullary endoscopic procedures. Am J Surg. 2008;196:975–82.

113. Machado NO. Management of duodenal perforation post-endoscopic retrograde cholangiopancreatography. When and whom to operate and what factors determine the outcome? A review article. JOP. 2012;13:18–25.

114. Palanivelu C, Jategaonkar PA, Rangarajan M, Anand NV, Senthilnathan P. Laparoscopic management of a retroperitoneal

duodenal perforation following ERCP for periampullary cancer. JSLS. 2008;12:399–402.

115. Avgerinos DV, Llaguna OH, Lo AY, Voli J, Leitman IM. Management of endoscopic retrograde cholangiopacreatography related duodenal perforations. Surg Endosc. 2009;23:833–8.

116. Preetha M, Chung YF, Chan WH, Ong HS, Chow PK, Wong WK, et al. Surgical management of endoscopic retrograde cholangiopancreatography related perforations. ANZ J Surg. 2003;73:1011–4.

117. Sarli L, Porrini C, Costi R, Regina G, Violi V, Ferro M, et al. Operative treatment of periampullary retroperitoneal perforation complicating endoscopic sphincterotomy. Surgery. 2007;142:26–32.

118. Connor S, Garden OJ. Bile duct injury in the era of laparoscopic cholecystectomy. Br J Surg. 2006;93:158–68.

119. Flum DR, Cheadle A, Prela C, Dellinger EP, Chan L. Bile duct injury during cholecystectomy and survival in Medicare beneficiaries. JAMA. 2003;290:2168–73.

120. Kaneko T, Akamatsu T, Shimodaira K, Ueno T, Gotoh A, Mukawa K, et al. Nonsurgical treatment of duodenal perforation by endoscopic repair using a clipping device. Gastrointest Endosc. 1999;50:410–3.

121. Rerknimitr R, Aekpongpaisit S, Kullavanijaya P. Use of endoclips to close sphincterotomy-related perforation. Endoscopy. 2008;40 Suppl 2:E169.

122. Baron TH, Gostout CH, Herman L. Hemoclip repair of a sphincterotomy-induced duodenal perforation. Gastrointest Endosc. 2000;52:566–8.

123. Nakagawa Y, Nagai T, Soma W, Okawara H, Nakashima H, Tasaki T, et al. Endoscopic closure of a large ERCP-related lateral duodenal perforation by using endoloops and endoclips. Gastrointest Endosc. 2010;72:216–7.

124. Buffoli F, Grassia R, Iiritano E, Bianchi G, Dizioli P, Staiano T. Endoscopic "retroperitoneal fatpexy" of a large ERCP-related jejunal perforation by using a new over-the-scope cliop device in a Billroth II anatomy (with video). Gastrointest Endosc. 2012;75:1115–7.

125. Fatima J, Baron TH, Topazian MD, Houghton SG, Iqbal CW, Ott BJ, et al. Pancreaticobiliary and duodenal perforations after periampullary endoscopic procedures. Arch Surg. 2007;142:448–55.

126. Katsinelos P, Fasoulas K, Beltsis A, Chatzimavroudis G, Zavos C, Terzoudis S, et al. Large-balloon dilation of the biliary orifice for the management of basket impaction: a case series of 6 patients. Gastrointest Endosc. 2011;73:1298–301.

127. Pruitt A, Shutz SM, Baron T, McClendon D, Lang KA. Fractured hydrophilic guidewire during ERCP: a case series. Gastrointest Endosc. 1998;48:77–80.

128. Bhasin DK, Poddar U, Wig JD. Knot formation in a floppy-tipped guidewire in the common bile duct: an unusual complication of ERCP. Endoscopy. 2000;32:S17.

129. Gross G, Kiker D. Intraductal knot formation in a guidewire during ERCP. Gastrointest Endosc. 2006;64:815–6.

130. Katanuma A, Maguchi H, Osanai M, Takahashi K. Endoscopic treatment of difficult common bile duct stones. Dig Endosc. 2010;22:S90–7.

131. Fukino N, Oida T, Kawasaki A, Mimatsu K, Kuboi Y, Kano H, et al. Impaction of a lithotripsy basket during endoscopic lithotomy of a common bile duct stone. World J Gastroenterol. 2010;16:2832–4.

132. Cid JA, Lobo DN. Impacted biliary basket. Gastrointest Endosc. 2005;61:110–1.

133. Payne WG, Norman JG, Pinkas H. Endoscopic basket impaction. Am Surg. 1995;61:464–7.

134. Mustard R, Mackenzie R, Jamieson C, Haber GB. Surgical complications of endoscopic sphincterotomy. Can J Surg. 1984;27:215–7.

135. Ng WT, Yiu MK, Lee K. Impaction of a stone basket in the gallbladder with laparoscopic rescue. Gastrointest Endosc. 1993;39:217–8.

136. Diller R, Senninger N, Kautz G, Tubergen D. Stent migration necessitating surgical intervention. Surg Endosc. 2003;17:1802–7.

137. Borgaonkar M. Impacted biliary basket. Gastrointest Endosc. 2005;62:474.

138. Ryozawa S, Iwano H, Taba K, Senyo M, Sakaida I. Successful retrieval of an impacted mechanical lithotripsy basket: a case report. Dig Endosc. 2010;S1:S111–3.

139. Tanaka K, Yasuda K, Uno K, Kawabata H, Kawamura T, Morikawa S. Case report: trouble-shooting for difficult cases of common bile duct stones with endoscopic treatment. Dig Endosc. 2010;S1:S114–7.

140. Ranjeev P, Goh KI. Retrieval of an impacted Dormia basket and stone in situ using a novel method. Gastrointest Endosc. 2000;51:504–6.

141. Kwon JH, Lee JK, Lee JH, Lee YS. Percutaneous transhepatic release of an impacted lithotripter basket and its fractured traction wire using a goose-neck snare: a case report. Korean J Radiol. 2011;12:247–51.

142. Schutz SM, Chinea C, Friedrichs P. Successful endoscopic removal of a severed, impacted Dormia basket. Am J Gastroenterol. 1997;92:679–81.

143. Attila T, May GR, Kortan P. Nonsurgical management of an impacted mechanical lithotripter with fractured traction wires: endoscopic intracorporeal electrohydraulic shock wave lithotripsy followed by extra-endoscopic mechanical lithotripsy. Can J Gastroenterol. 2008;22:699–702.

144. Fry LC, Linder JD, Monkemuller KE. Cholangitis as a result of hydrophilic guidewire fracture. Gastrointest Endosc. 2002;56: 943–4.

145. Gomez-Oliva C, Guamer-Argent C, Concepcion M, Jiminez FJ, Rodriguez S, Gonzalez-Huix F, et al. Partially covered self-expanding metal stent for unresectable malignant extrahepatic biliary obstruction: results of a large prospective series. Surg Endosc. 2012;26:222–9.

146. Galizia G, Napolitano V, Castellano P, Pinto M, Zamboli A, Schettino P, et al. The over the scope clip system is effective in the treatment of chronic esophagejejunal anastomotic leakage. J Gastrointest Surg. 2012;16(8):1585–9.

147. Cheng CL, Sherman S, Watkins JL, Barnett J, Freeman M, Geenen J, et al. Risk factors for post-ERCP pancreatitis: a prospective multicenter study. Am J Gastroenterol. 2006;101(1):139–47.

148. Lukens FJ, Howell DA, Upender S, Sheth SG, Jafri SM. ERCP in the very elderly: outcomes among patients older than eighty. Dig Dis Sci. 2010;55(3):847–51.

149. Korman LY, Overholt BF, Box T, Winker CK. Perforation during colonoscopy in endoscopic ambulatory surgical centers. Gastrointest Endosc. 2003;58(4):554–7.

150. Perini RF, Sadurski R, Cotton PB, Patel RS, Hawes RH, Cunningham JT. Post-sphincterotomy bleeding after the introduction of microprocessor-controlled electrosurgery: does the new technology make the difference? Gastrointest Endosc. 2005;61(1):53–7.

151. Testoni PA, Vailati C, Giussani A, Notaristefano C, Mariani A. ERCP-induced and non-ERCP-induced acute pancreatitis: two distinct clinical entities with different outcomes in mild and severe form? Dig Liver Dis. 2010;42(8):567–70.

Photodocumentation of Endoscopic Findings

Bruce Schirmer and Lane Ritter

Introduction

The ability to document endoscopic findings is markedly different in the twenty-first century than it was in the twentieth century during the early days of flexible endoscopy. Early flexible endoscopes transmitted images through fiber-optic bundles, with images dependent on the light transmission through these bundles. Early endoscopes also had no ability to transmit the image from the endoscope itself to another interface or location. The endoscopist viewed the image through the viewing end of the endoscope itself. "Teaching attachments" were soon developed so another individual could also view the image by attaching a device with a side-directed fiber-optic channel for dual viewing.

During the fiber-optic era of endoscopes, the only potential for photo documentation of endoscopic findings was to actually attach a camera with an adapter that fit over the end of the endoscope. Figure 21.1 shows such a typical photodocumentation of an endoscopic finding using this technology. The captured images were quite small, being limited by the aperture of viewing of the endoscope. In addition, in order to capture an image, the camera had to be inserted on the end of the scope, a photograph taken, and the camera detached before any further progress of the examination could occur. Technicians needed to document which pictures of the roll of film were for which patient, and for which finding. Photo documentation to the medical record was dependent on the time lag for the development of the roll of film in the camera, then the processing and subsequent pasting of the picture in the paper medical file of the patient. Due to these limitations of the ease and cost of obtaining photo documentation of endoscopic findings, there was a definite negative incentive to the endoscopist to document any

findings other than those felt particularly crucial and definitive for any endoscopic procedure. Normal findings were rarely documented.

In addition to the limitations of the imaging capacity of photo documentation of pathology in that era, there was by default a decrease in the accuracy of diagnosis as well. Documentation of endoscopic findings was left to the discretion and decision of usually only one endoscopist. Subjectivity therefore almost certainly decreased accuracy in those days. The difficulty and expense of documenting findings also was relevant to the accuracy of the documented findings of any individual examination. In summary, the process, even if appropriately done and for the correct image capture and documentation, was a tedious and laborious process.

Once fiber-optic technology was replaced by the videochip, the ability to capture digital information in photographic or video form became significantly easier, cost-effective, and commonplace. Understanding the capacity of videochip technology requires the understanding of some basic definitions of images captured by the videochip itself.

The first step in the process of recording an image with a videoendoscope still involves the illumination of the field with a fiber-optic light source. Then the surface reflectance is captured and the image is magnified as specified by the software of the system. Computer videochip conversion of the reflected light from the image to an electronic signal is the next key step in the process. This conversion from light to electronic signaling allows computerization, quantification, analysis and storage of the signal using digital systems. The electronic signal can be transmitted to a monitor where the image can be projected.

Videoendoscopy involved the conversion of an analogue image to a digital image. An analogue image is essentially a continuous signal, which must be transduced or converted by an analogue-to-digital device. A device in the computerized processing of an analogue image, called a frame grabber, or capture board, converts each analogue image into a video image which is composed of digital forms of the image. In order to replicate the analogue image, digital technology

B. Schirmer, M.D. (✉) • L. Ritter, M.D.
Department of Surgery, University of Virginia Health System,
Charlottesville, VA, USA
e-mail: bs@virginia.edu

J.M. Marks and B.J. Dunkin (eds.), *Principles of Flexible Endoscopy for Surgeons*,
DOI 10.1007/978-1-4614-6330-6_21, © Springer Science+Business Media New York 2013

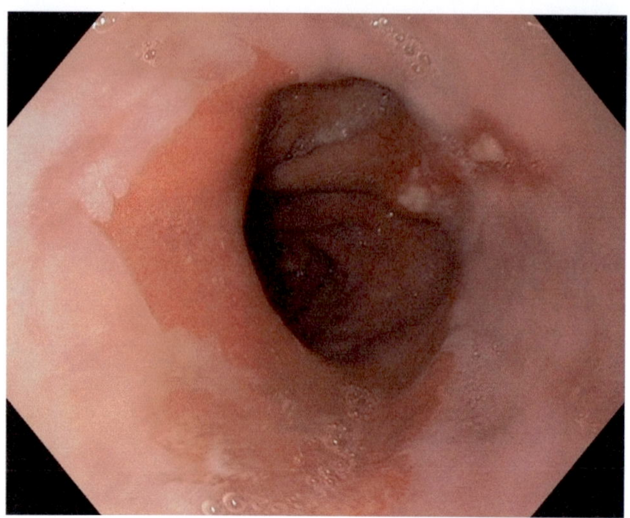

Fig. 21.1 Videoendoscopic view of the distal esophagus in a patient. The changes of Barrett's esophagus are evident

captures the data points at evenly spaced intervals and converts these data points to individual light capturing units called pixels to record the image findings. The density of the pixels, the color recording digitization and capture capacity, and the compressibility of an image all play important roles in the process of converting an analogue to a digital image.

Pixel density (sampling density) is the number of pixels/unit area into which an image is divided by the frame grabber. Higher pixel density equates to greater image resolution. Digital images are defined by their pixel density. A $1{,}024 \times 768$ (XGA resolution) image has an image that is 1,024 pixels wide by 768 pixels high. Lower density pixel images may not "zoom" well due to granularity of the image when enlarged. Similarly, images, which have a pixel resolution greater than the capacity for the viewing equipment, result in images with higher computer storage requirements but no improvement in imaging capacity due to the limitations of the monitor or viewing system.

Digitization of color requires an understanding of the methods by which color can be recorded in digital or analogue systems. Colors that are imaged by a videoendoscope are continuous variables, and must be digitally recorded into a digital equivalent. There are three systems to convert analogue to digital color. Each has some application with respect to endoscopy, depending on the image recorded and by what method [1].

The RGB color system breaks color images down into the various contributions of green blue, and red. Each of the three colors has a scale from 0 to 255. All three colors at 255 yields a white image, while all three colors at 0 yields a black image.

The HSB system of color describes color in one axis and incorporates several aspects of that color. HSB stands for *Hue*, *Saturation*, and *Brightness*. The *Hue* is the wavelength of the light transmitted from an object, or the position on the color wheel. Saturation is the density of the color (0 being no color and 100 being full strength). Brightness of the color reflects just that: at 0 % a color is black and at 100 % it is fully light.

A final system to categorize color for photo documentation involves the use of four primary colors, cyan, magenta, yellow, and black. Thus, this system is designated as the CMYB system. It is largely used for printing color documents, with elements of each of the four colors used to reproduce a color image seen on a screen. Figure 21.1 shows a typical recorded image of the distal esophagus, with Barrett's esophagus present, that incorporates the color elements to reproduce the color image seen on the screen.

Trimodal Imaging

Recent advances in the ability to image surface vasculature of the gastrointestinal tract have conferred increased ability to detect vascular abnormalities, angiogenesis, and other traits of abnormal mucosal properties during endoscopic examinations. The three modalities used for these purposes include autofluorescence imaging, as well as the combined modalities of magnifying endoscopy and narrow band imaging. These modalities allow much more detailed viewing of the vascular pattern of neoplastic and pre-neoplastic lesions of the gastrointestinal tract. While they are also now used to image many other areas of the body, including the biliary system and other digestive areas, we will focus on their role in assessing lesions of the alimentary tract.

Early vascular changes in pre-neoplastic lesions of the gastrointestinal tract mucosa may not be easily detected by standard white light endoscopy. Endoscopic autofluorescence imaging (AFI) produces tissue images that are based on the tissue's own natural fluorescence pattern generated from light waves of excitation frequency shining on the tissue's endogenous fluorophores (such as nicotinamide, porphyrins, flavin, etc.). Early tumors will impart a different pattern from imaging by excitation light than will normal tissue, allowing the differences to be appreciated by recording differences in the tissue fluorescence properties [2].

Short wavelength light, which excites the fluorophores in the mucosal tissues, causes these tissues to take on a green color pattern if normal, a dark green pattern for blood vessels, and a magenta color for dysplastic or early neoplastic tissue. AFI is excellent at detecting abnormalities in tissues, having a very high sensitivity for detecting abnormal lesions. However, AFI also has been shown to have a significant incidence of identifying false positive lesions as well, and so its specificity is not high [3].

Magnification endoscopy with narrow band imaging (ME-NBI), on the other hand, takes advantage of enhanced visualization of the mucosal vasculature through the increased penetration of the mucosal surface to the submucosal vascular pattern and surface texture to pick up early lesions based on

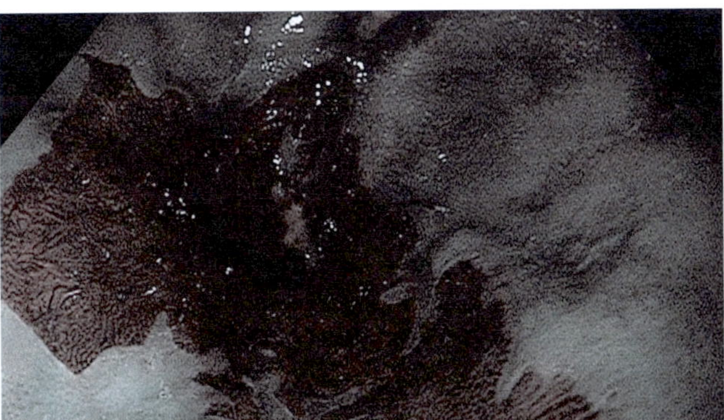

Fig. 21.2 The distal esophagus in a patient with Barrett's esophagus using the NBI technique. The NBI technique allows visualization of the vasculature of the lesion, which in this case showed no signs of dysplasia

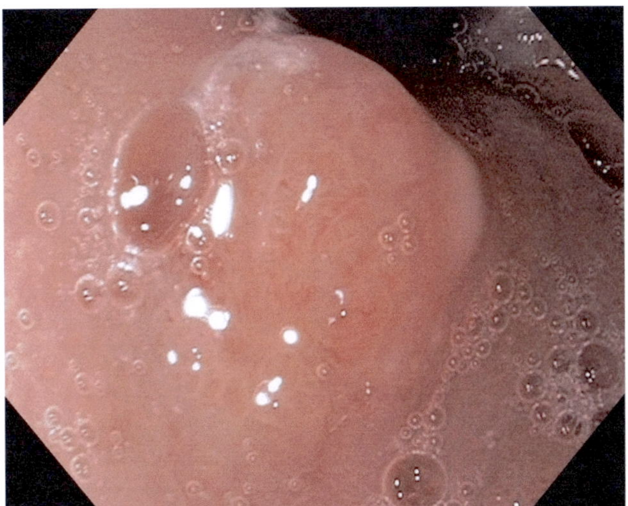

Fig. 21.3 A patient with nodular Barrett's esophagus on videoendoscopic imaging

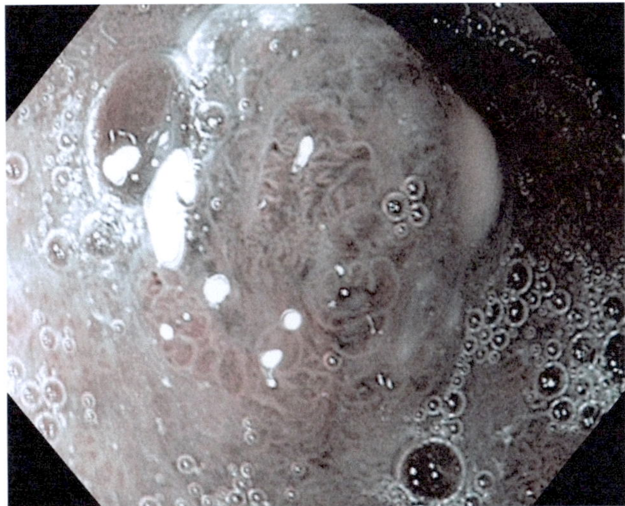

Fig. 21.4 The same patient's nodular area viewed using the NBI technique. Here the abnormality of the vasculature pattern is obvious and biopsy confirmed dysplasia

the differences in these surface and vascular properties between normal and dysplastic or early neoplastic tissue. When combined with AFI, it can improve the diagnostic accuracy of the examination considerably, by detecting abnormal patterns in the mucosal vasculature that are apparent with the use of this combined technique. The NBI technique involves using narrow band-pass filters for the light that limit its passage to two narrow bandwidths of light. These widths are for blue (415 nm) and green (540 nm) light waves. These wavelengths also correspond to the optimal absorption wavelengths for hemoglobin. Thus, the 415 nm wavelength light causes the hemoglobin to appear brown, while the 540 nm wavelength causes it to appear cyan. The resulting brown and magenta images seen with the magnification technique allow for much easier identification of early neoplastic lesions by the endoscopist. Figure 21.2 shows an image obtained using the NBI technique of a patient with Barrett's esophagus and no dysplasia [4].

One diagnostic area where NBI has proven particularly effective and useful is in the assessment of dysplasia in Barrett's esophagus.

Using a basic classification system based on appearance of mucosa and surface vessels with ME-NBI, most endoscopists can improve their ability to detect and biopsy abnormal esophageal tissue involved in the stages of this disease process. Figure 21.3 shows a typical endoscopic view of a patient with a nodular Barrett's esophagus lesion. The normal color of the videoendoscopic image is not nearly as helpful for determining whether abnormal vasculature is present or the dysplastic potential of the lesion. Figure 21.4 shows the same nodule using an NBI technique. The distinctively abnormal vasculature (compared to Fig. 21.2 above) is evident on this view of the nodule, which was confirmed by biopsy to by dysplastic.

NBI requires magnification to detect lesions in the stomach, due to the larger and darker lumen of the stomach itself. Early gastric cancers show a distinctive light blue hue on the edges of the mucosal surfaces with ME-NBI [5].

Storage of Images

The ability to capture increasingly larger and more complex digital images leads to the issue of the ability to store these images. In today's typical endoscopic examination room, computers with image capture cards and network capabilities permit the images seen during an endoscopic examination to be routinely captured, stored, printed, and transmitted. Most endoscopic images are currently in the VGA realm (usually 320×240 but up to 640×400 pixels) though SVGA (800×600 pixels resolution) images may soon be the industry standard within a few years if imaging technology improves as expected.

The higher density of digital information for modern imaging makes it essential that they be compressed for storage and transmission. The formula for compression is given as the ratio of the size of the original file divided by the size of the compressed file. For most color images, compression ratios of up to 20:1 do not result in very much informational detail loss. Compression of color images is considerably better than that of black and white images, since the human eye detects brightness differences much more accurately than color hue differences. Compression of a black and white file of 5:1 is the usual limit beyond which the image suffers deterioration of detail.

Pixel density determines file size. A VGA range 24 bit color picture would be calculated by multiplying the width and length of the image in pixels then multiplying by 24. This calculation yields a typical 900 kilobyte size for a standard endoscopic image. Having higher density or larger file sizes is only appropriate when all the components of the system can handle such file size. Current computers screens, for example, are usually only able to handle files in the VGA range. Thus, although the chip in most endoscopic cameras is now capable of recording images in the SVGA range, doing so will not improve the image seen on a standard computer screen.

Image Transmission

Image files these days are typically transmitted electronically in certain file formats. The most common of these is the JPEG file. The Joint Photographic Experts Group (JPEG) is a file format capable of image transfer on the Internet. Other file formats available for Internet transmission include the GIF (Graphical Interchange Format) and PNG (Portable Network Graphics). JPEG files have the advantage of maintaining 24 color bit images during transmission, whereas GIF images deteriorate slightly during transmission. PNG is the most recent format for image transmission in terms of image transfer capability properties.

Once again, it is imperative that images be compressed in order to allow reasonably rapid transmission using today's electronic software capacity.

Recommended Image Recording for Procedures

It is recommended that for certain studies, images of the key anatomic mucosal and anatomic structures be recorded.

The most important images are from key pathologic findings, which are discovered during the endoscopic procedure. The number and type of images that are felt to be necessary to document pathologic findings will vary from examination to examination and from endoscopist to endoscopist. Potentially malignant lesions may require one or two standard images if they are polyps, ulcers, or other manifestations with clearly abnormal configuration. Alternatively, several pictures may be needed using special recording imagery such as magnification endoscopy with narrow band imaging (ME-NBI) if recording slightly abnormal areas of the distal esophagus for a survey of progression of Barrett's esophagus. Certain anatomic areas being investigated as part of the reason for the examination should be documented. For example, the size of a recurrent hiatal hernia in a patient with recurrent GERD after surgery who is being considered as a possible candidate for reoperative therapy should have multiple images of the gastroesophageal junction recorded as part of the examination.

The recording of normal findings is variable based on the preference of the endoscopist and the nature of the examination. Many endoscopists prefer to document the typical anatomic findings in the cecum to document achieving reaching this part of the colon on a routine screening colonoscopy. Follow-up examinations for benign diseases such as ulcers with the observation of complete healing should also be documented.

Standardization of which images should be recorded for which examinations is still far from uniform or complete. Suffice it to say that the documented text and images from an endoscopic procedure should leave little doubt when reviewed by other clinician's minds as to what was seen, where it was seen, and any other relevant information documented regarding information needed for further therapy.

Image Terminology

While there is still no real standard for which images should be recorded for endoscopic examinations, there is no absolute standard for the terminology used to describe normal and abnormal findings on an endoscopic examination. Language which attempts to make such descriptions standard had now been developed by organizations such as the American Society of Gastrointestinal Endoscopy (ASGE) and its European counterpart (ESGE). A minimal standard terminology (MST) for endoscopy has been developed [6]. This terminology is designed to cover most of the terms needed for typical endoscopic practice. There are lists of terms in the MST system, although these terms were designed more for developing uniformity among software companies working in the field of digital imaging than for the individual endoscopist.

Standardization of Image Recording

The major endoscopic societies (ASGE and ESGE) have developed recommended guidelines for image documentation during normal and abnormal examinations [7]. These guidelines are particularly important where imaging and biopsy combine to monitor diseases with potential malignancy, such as Barrett's esophagus [8]. Standards for imaging have not been as large a focus of recent reviews of quality in endoscopic performance. Instead, frequency of procedure, following appropriate indications for performing endoscopic procedures, quality metrics such as polyp eradication, and complication rates of procedures have been more highly emphasized and have more significant ramifications in terms of quality than do number and type of endoscopic images performed per procedure. It is safe to state, however, that improved imaging capability has made obtaining images, including video, more routine in standard practice over the past decade.

While standards and recommendations may be present, recent literature suggests that gastroenterologists do not routinely use imaging as part of the documentation of their endoscopies. One study showed that 56 % of surveyed gastroenterologists do not routinely use pictures to document completion of colonoscopy. When shown pictures of the cecum or another area, identification was only 51 % specific and 89 % sensitive in terms of correct identification. This article also points out that a single pair of photographs alone may not be sensitive or specific enough to be reliable for documentation [9].

Video Imaging

With the advent of electronic databases being standard for most hospitals and practices now, the ability to routinely use video imaging as documentation of endoscopic findings becomes much more practical. The limitation of video is that it requires a computer and computer screen and an electronic system by which to view it, whereas single image pictures could be documented in paper or print form. The latter, however, are more commonly being preserved in electronic file form in the electronic medical record as well.

Video imaging has distinct advantages in terms of recording therapeutic procedures, as well as recording physiologic phenomenon such as gastric peristalsis or colonic peristalsis. Routine endoscopic examinations, however, do not normally require the extra cost and information storage capacity needed for the video file.

Video file storage and recording is a dynamic field that is rapidly improving and evolving. The standard for endoscopic videos, the MPEG file, will likely be replaced by improved image file storage file systems in the future, as video is the cutting edge of medical imaging documentation in many areas besides endoscopy, and has now become a standard part of many journal articles in fields such as endoscopy. Video compression software is also evolving rapidly, making storage and transmission of larger video files feasible for the individual medical record. Video compression can often be done at a higher ration than is possible for individual photographs or images.

A relative balance between the appropriateness of documentation and the increasing technical requirements and informational storage space continues to be an evolving process in much of medicine, including endoscopy. Overall, however, the process is clearly evolving to one where there is increased capacity for the use of video and photo documentation of important endoscopic findings, and that those findings can now be more easily transferred between institutions and systems for better information exchange about patients. Clinical practice patterns are likely to follow the ease of electronic documentation to the overall increase of photo and video documentation of endoscopic imaging in the years ahead. The option of focused specialized imaging such as trimodal imaging give the endoscopist even further options for documentation of the key elements of an endoscopic examination, and render improved diagnostic accuracy in the treatment of gastrointestinal diseases.

Actual Measurements During Endoscopy

Endoscopists are expected to document the size of lesions; sometimes in length (Barrett's mucosal changes), width (gastric ulcers), or in three dimensions (colonic polyps). The measurements that we document have a direct impact on clinical treatment, surveillance, and sometimes the decision for operative intervention. The problem is that exact quantitative measurements during endoscopic exams are notoriously inaccurate.

The innate problem is in the instrumentation itself. The standard wide-angle lenses within our endoscopes create a fair amount of image distortion [10, 11]. The periphery of the field is compressed compared to the center. This so-called barrel distortion is more pronounced the farther the scope is from the object in question. Various methods of measurement have been used by endoscopists; from directly comparing a lesion to an object of known size that has been introduced into the visual field to applying advanced image processing to endoscopic photographs [10, 12–14].

As an illustration, Morales et al. [12] demonstrated that colonoscopists consistently *over*estimated the size of polyps by using the "open biopsy forceps" technique, wherein a forceps with a known diameter of 8 mm were placed onto the polyps in vivo and used to estimate size. 74 % of polyps

Table 21.1 Prague C & M classification of Barrett's esophagus

Identify the gastroesophageal junction (tops of gastric folds) (be certain to recognize presence of hiatal hernia). Measure this distance from incisors [scope insertion measurement to that depth (i.e., 38 cm)]
Look for displacement of squamocolumnar junction above gastroesophageal junction
Measure location of most proximal circumferential extent of suspected columnar metaplasia (Barrett's involvement) (i.e., 35 cm)
Measure depth of maximum extension of islands of Barrett's esophagus proximally (i.e., 30 cm)
Subtract the depth of circumferential and maximal extents from the depth at the gastroesophageal junction (i.e., 38–35 C=3 cm 38–30 M=8 cm)
Prague classification would be C3 and M7

measured in this manner endoscopically were actually smaller on the post-polypectomy measurements performed by pathologists. In 2010, Moug et al. [15] reported a pattern of endoscopic *under*estimation in their series of colon polyp measurements. Both studies ultimately recommend that surveillance strategies for colonic polyps should be based on documented pathology specimen size and not on endoscopic estimations.

The evidence for endoscopic accuracy in measuring the length of Barrett's esophagus is not much better. Even in ideal conditions using a training model of an esophagus, both fellows and practicing gastroenterologists overestimated the length of Barrett's epithelium 47 % of the time and underestimated in 37 % in one study [16]. Even the serial measurements made on the same model by the same endoscopist demonstrated considerable variability. Endoscopists are asked to evaluate for regression of Barrett's after patients are placed on aggressive anti-reflux treatment, it has been found that the change in length between consecutive measurements must be greater than 1.6 cm to overcome the inter- and intra-observer range of variability [17].

The current standard classification for measuring the extent and length of Barrett's esophagus was first agreed upon in a meeting held in Prague in 2004 by an international working group dedicated to the topic. The published report on the Prague CM classification has now become the standard by which Barrett's esophagus is measured for purposes of assessment for treatment, especially with RFA ablation [18]. The steps of reporting the CM classification of Barrett's are given in Table 21.1.

There currently are not any reliable solutions to address the problem of endoscopic inaccuracy of measurements. Using endoscopes with 1 cm incremental markings may be more useful than the standard 5 cm. Advanced image processing programs have been created to provide more precise measurements of endoscopic images but these are certainly not widely available in practice [10, 14].

What is important in practice as surgical endoscopists is to maintain awareness of how our crude methods of endoscopic measurements are interpreted. When there is alternative means to measure a lesion, such as grossly after resection or by computer analysis for example, that value should be deferred to in use for clinical decision-making. Of course, efforts to hone one's endoscopic skills are important as there is some evidence that experience begets accuracy although even this is somewhat disputed [17]. Maintaining continuity of care and performing consecutive studies on the same patient takes away the added variability that comes from multiple proceduralists [17, 18]. Lastly, one must remain humble and avoid using our measurements to create a false sense of security in our patients' clinical courses.

Vienna Classification of Barrett's Esophagus

The term Barrett's esophagus refers to the change from normal squamous epithelium of the distal esophagus to columnar epithelium that is undergoing intestinal metaplasia. It is most often caused by chronic exposure to gastric contents caused by gastroesophageal reflux disease. Barrett's esophagus follows a predictable progression of cellular changes from intestinal metaplasia to dysplasia to carcinoma. Current upper endoscopy screening recommendations as published by the American College of Gastroenterology are shown in Table 21.2 [19].

To the surgical endoscopist, the diagnosis and surveillance of Barrett's esophagus has obvious important interventional implications. Not only is the appropriate surveillance schedule crucial in monitoring this premalignant condition in its predictable progression of neoplastic changes, but timely pathologic diagnosis offers the opportunity to perform less morbid interventions such as local endoscopic resection. Having an active, collegial relationship with gastrointestinal pathologists and having the willingness to become versed in the histologic diagnosis of Barrett's will provide the best multidisciplinary care for one's patients.

Accurate pathologic diagnosis and documentation in Barrett's esophagus is vital to determining appropriate surveillance and intervention. Prior to an international consensus conference in 1998, there was a significant difference in the interpretation of gastrointestinal neoplastic lesions between pathologists within the international arena [20, 21]. The histology in question included lesions of the esophagus, stomach, colon, and rectum. The two main classification schemas at the time were often referred to as the Western and the Japanese systems. The Japanese based their histologic interpretation more on cytologic and architectural changes when distinguishing between dysplasia and carcinoma [20–22]. The Western contingent had a tendency to rely more heavily

Table 21.2 Guidelines for surveillance of Barrett's esophagus [19]

Dysplasia	Documentation	Follow-up
None	Two EGDs with biopsy within 1 year	Endoscopy every 3 years
Low grade	Highest grade on repeat	1 year interval until no dysplasia×2
	EGD with biopsies within 6 months	
	Expert pathologist confirmation	
High grade	Mucosal irregularity	Endoscopic resection
	Repeat EGD with biopsies to rule out adenocarcinoma within 3 months	Continued 3-month surveillance or intervention based on results and patient
	Expert pathologist confirmation	

Table 21.3 Inflammatory Bowel Disease Dysplasia Morphology Study Group classification [23]

Negative
Normal mucosa
Inactive colitis
Active colitis
Indefinite
Probably negative (probably inflammatory)
Unknown
Probably positive (probably dysplastic)
Positive
Low-grade dysplasia
High-grade dysplasia

Table 21.4 Revised Vienna classification of gastrointestinal epithelial neoplasia [26]

	Pathologic diagnosis	Clinical recommendation
Category 1	Negative for neoplasia	Optional surveillance
Category 2	Indefinite for neoplasia	Surveillance
Category 3	Mucosal low-grade neoplasia	Endoscopic treatment or surveillance
Category 4	Mucosal high-grade neoplasia	Endoscopic or surgical local treatment
	1. High-grade adenoma/dysplasia	
	2. Noninvasive carcinoma	
	3. Suspicious for invasive carcinoma	
	4. Intramucosal carcinoma	
Category 5	Submucosal invasion of neoplasia (carcinoma invading the submucosa or beyond)	Surgical treatment

on the depth of cellular invasion, or breach of the lamina propria (submucosa in colorectal tissue), in diagnosing carcinoma and has its roots in the system devised by the inflammatory bowel disease morphology study group in 1983 (Table 21.3) [23]. This classification system has been more broadly applied to dysplastic changes anywhere within the gastrointestinal tract.

There was a call for international uniformity in nomenclature so that there could be improved interpretation of cancer research across borders. There was also hope for a classification system that could be better applied to surveillance, intervention, and ultimately, clinical outcomes. Hence, the Vienna Classification of gastrointestinal epithelial neoplasia was formulated by a consensus panel in 1998 following a workshop in Vienna, Austria [24]. Note the use of "noninvasive neoplasia" instead of "dysplasia." Of particular utility in this scheme is its ability to make an allowance for borderline pathology in the grouping anointed as Category 4, as this was the group that accounted for the largest discrepancy between pathologists. This would help eliminate the over- or under-diagnosis of carcinoma that occurs if pathologists are forced to label a biopsy specimen as either "benign" or "malignant." As an illustration, the agreement between leading Western and Japanese pathologists in the diagnosis of carcinoma in esophageal specimens prior to the Vienna Classification only reached 14 % during slide interpretation exercises at the workshop. After the development of the new system, the agreement in this slide interpretation significantly improved to 62 % [24]. Soon thereafter, there was the realization that these categories, as defined, did not accurately correlate with the categories of treatment modalities for Barrett's esophagus and other gastrointestinal neoplasms. Therefore, the Vienna classification was revised in 2000 to better provide a schema of histologic categories that could be directly matched to the recommended treatment modality for each said category along the progression of neoplastic changes (Table 21.4) [25, 26].

Several subsequent studies have verified the reproducibility of the revised Vienna Classification [27–29]. Despite this, the widespread use of the Vienna system in the West remains somewhat limited [21]. It is imperative to recognize that the Vienna classification was developed as an effort to reduce discrepancies, simplify nomenclature, and aid in intercountry communication about gastrointestinal dysplasia [19, 30]. It certainly does not eliminate all the problems in the histologic characterization of Barrett's esophagus. It is important for the surgical endoscopist to recognize and have a working understanding of the various schemas so that one can apply them appropriately to diagnostic and literature interpretation.

Correct Grade of Hemorrhoids

Hemorrhoids arise from submucosal blood vessels in the anal canal. Vessels which are located distal to the dentate line give rise to external hemorrhoids. External hemorrhoids are covered with skin or epidermis, and have exquisite sensitivity due to this fact. They are normally small (<1–1.5 cm) but may enlarge, especially if combined with an adjacent internal hemorrhoid into a larger combined complex hemorrhoid. Most often, however, external hemorrhoids remain separate as they arise from separate vascular plexuses and are not aligned with the typical internal hemorrhoidal plexuses. The latter, located just above the dentate line, are traditionally described as being in the 1 o'clock (right anterior), 5 o'clock (right posterior), and 9 o'clock (left lateral) positions around the anal canal when viewed with the patient in the prone jackknife position.

Internal hemorrhoids are classified according to grades, based on size and characteristics. Table 21.5 lists the four grades of internal hemorrhoids based on these characteristics [31]. The major characteristic that distinguishes the official grade of a hemorrhoid is its degree of prolapse. Grade 1 hemorrhoids are small and never prolapse. Diagnosis of grade 1 hemorrhoids is therefore only possible through endoscopic means. Hemorrhoids which are Grade 2 or higher have some degree of prolapse, though Grade 2 hemorrhoids can only be seen to prolapse with the forceful contraction of the rectal musculature in the process of defecation. Hemorrhoids which are Grade 3 and 4 are more easily diagnosed by examination, where they are either intermittently or constantly present.

Treatment of hemorrhoids is grade-related. Grade 1 hemorrhoids rarely require any treatment other than conservative measures of changing diet, avoiding dehydration, and avoiding excessive straining at defecation. Grade 1 hemorrhoids may occasionally be treated with outpatient office-based procedures if they are causing annoying minor hemorrhage.

Grade 2 hemorrhoids are generally amenable to a variety of office-based treatments, including rubber band ligation, injection, or infrared photocoagulation. Treatment is based on symptoms frequency and severity and lack of response to standard conservative measures as described above. Grade 3 hemorrhoids are also most often amenable to office-based therapy as well. However, larger hemorrhoids, especially if they have an external skin component, may not be amenable to ligation or other treatments where epidermal skin pain precludes such treatment. Grade 4 and larger grade 3 hemorrhoids require operative therapy. Resectional therapy is performed using several techniques, with resection of the hemorrhoidal plexus being the common theme. Standard excisional therapy has now also been joined by stapled hemorrhoidectomy as a possible alternative for many cases of grade 3 of 4 hemorrhoids [32].

External hemorrhoids rarely need excision or surgical treatment unless they become acutely thrombosed. In such cases, evacuation of the clot from within the hemorrhoid will provide immediate and significant relief for the patient. Such procedures may be usually performed under local anesthesia in the office setting [33, 34].

Table 21.5 Grade classification of internal hemorrhoids

Grade	Characteristic
1	Small sized hemorrhoid with NO prolapsed
2	Medium sized hemorrhoid that prolapses with defecation and spontaneously reduces
3	Medium to larger sized hemorrhoid that prolapses with defecation and must be manually reduced (but does reduce)
4	Medium to larger sized hemorrhoid that is chronically prolapsed and cannot be reduced

References

1. Connor MJ, Sharma P. Chromoendoscopy and magnification endoscopy for diagnosing esophageal cancer and dysplasia. Thorac Surg Clin. 2004;14:87–94.
2. Filip M, Iordache S, Saftiou A, Ciurea T. Autofluorescence imaging and magnification endoscopy. World J Gastroenterol. 2011;17:9–14.
3. Okhawa A, Miwa H, Namihisa A, et al. Diagnostic performance of light-induced fluorescence endoscopy for gastric neoplasms. Endoscopy. 2004;36:515–21.
4. Singh R, Anagnostopoulos GK, Yao K, et al. Narrow-band imaging with magnification in Barrett's esophagus: validation of a simplified grading system of mucosal morphology patterns against histology. Endoscopy. 2008;40:457–63.
5. Uedo N, Ishedo N, Ishihara R, Iishi H, et al. A new method of diagnosing gastric intestinal metaplasia: narrow-band imaging with magnifying endoscopy. Endoscopy. 2006;38:819–24.
6. Delvaux M, Korman LY, Armengol-Miro JR, Crespi M, Cass O, Hagenmuller F, et al. The minimal standard terminology for digestive endoscopy: introduction to structured reporting. Int J Med Inform. 1998;48(1–3):217–25.
7. Rey JF, Lambert R. ESGE recommendations for quality control in gastrointestinal endoscopy: guidelines for image documentation in upper and lower GI endoscopy. Endoscopy. 2001;33(10):901–3.
8. Sampliner RE. Updated guidelines for the diagnosis, surveillance, and therapy of Barrett's esophagus. Am J Gastroenterol. 2002;97: 1888–95.
9. Thuraisingam AI, Brown JL, Anderson JT. What are the sensitivity and specificity of endoscopic photographs in determining completion of colonoscopy? Results from an online questionnaire. Eur J Gastroenterol Hepatol. 2008;20:567–71.
10. Vakil N. Measurement of lesions by endoscopy: an overview. Endoscopy. 1995;27:695–7.
11. Margulies C, Krevsky B, Catalano MF. How accurate are endoscopic measurements of size? Gastrointest Endosc. 1994;40: 174–7.
12. Morales TG, Sampliner RE, Garewal HS, et al. The difference in colon polyp size before and after removal. Gastrointest Endosc. 1996;43:25–8.
13. Rikimaru T. New method of endoscopic measurement. Lancet. 1990;335:672–3.

14. Vakil N, Smith W, Bourgeois K, et al. Endoscopic measurement of lesion size: improved accuracy with image processing. Gastrointest Endosc. 1994;40:178–83.
15. Moug SJ, Vernall N, Saldanha J, et al. Endoscopists' estimation of size should not determine surveillance of colonic polyps. Colorectal Dis. 2010;12:646–50.
16. Guda NM, Partington S, Vakil N. Inter- and intra-observer variability in the measurement of length at endoscopy: implications for the measurement of Barrett's esophagus. Gastrointest Endosc. 2004;59:655–8.
17. Dekel R, Wakelin DE, Wendel C, et al. Progression or regression of Barrett's esophagus—is it all in the eye of the beholder? Am J Gastroenterol. 2003;98:2612–5.
18. Sharma P, Dent J, Armstrong D, et al. The development and validation of an endoscopic grading system for Barrett's esophagus: The Prague C & M criteria. Gastroenterology. 2006;131:1392–9.
19. Padda S, Ramirez FC. Accuracy in the diagnosis of short-segment Barrett's esophagus: the role of endoscopic experience. Gastrointest Endosc. 2001;54:605–8.
20. Wang KK, Sampliner RE, Practice Parameters Committee of the American College of Gastroenterology. Updated guidelines 2008 for the diagnosis, surveillance and therapy of Barrett's esophagus. Am J Gastroenterol. 2008;103:788–97.
21. Schlemper RJ, Itabashi M, Kato Y, et al. Differences in diagnostic criteria for gastric carcinoma between Japanese and Western pathologists. Lancet. 1997;349:1725–9.
22. Odze RD. Diagnosis and grading of dysplasia in Barrett's oesophagus. J Clin Pathol. 2006;59:1029–38.
23. Schlemper RJ, Kato Y, Stolte M. Review of histological classifications of gastrointestinal epithelial neoplasia: differences in diagnosis of early carcinomas between Japanese and Western pathologists. J Gastroenterol. 2001;36:445–56.
24. Riddell RH, Goldman H, Ransohoff DF, et al. Dysplasia in inflammatory bowel disease: standardized classification with provisional clinical applications. Hum Pathol. 1983;14:931–68.
25. Schlemper RJ, Riddell RH, Kato Y, et al. The Vienna classification of gastrointestinal epithelial neoplasia. Gut. 2000;47:251–5.
26. Schlemper RJ, Kato Y, Stolte M. Diagnostic criteria for gastrointestinal carcinomas in Japan and Western countries: proposal for a new classification system of gastrointestinal epithelial neoplasia. J Gastroenterol Hepatol. 2000;15:G49–57.
27. Dixon MF. Gastrointestinal epithelial neoplasia: Vienna revisited. Gut. 2002;51:130–1.
28. Schlemper RJ, Iwashita A. Classification of gastrointestinal epithelial neoplasia. Curr Diag Pathol. 2004;10:128–39.
29. Kaye PV, Haider SA, Ilyas M, et al. Barrett's dysplasia and the Vienna classification: reproducibility, prediction or progression and impact on consensus reporting and p53 immunohistochemistry. Histopathology. 2009;54:699–712.
30. Stolte M. The new Vienna classification of epithelial neoplasia of the gastrointestinal tract: advantages and disadvantages. Virchows Arch. 2003;442:99–106.
31. Jass JR. Vienna consensus criteria for pathological diagnosis. In: Fujita R, Jass JR, Kaminishi M, Schlemper RJ, editors. Early cancer of the gastrointestinal tract. Tokyo: Springer; 2006. p. 135–40.
32. Brill AI, Fleshman Jr JW, Ramshaw BJ, et al. Weighing the evidence: benefits and risks. J Family Pract. 2005;54(suppl):5–18.
33. Cataldo P, Ellis CN, Gregoryck S, et al. Practice parameters for the management of hemorrhoids (revised). Dis Colon Rectum. 2005;48:189–94.
34. American Society of Colon & Rectal Surgeons. Hemorrhoids http://www.fascrs.org. Accessed 16 Jul 2012.

Future of Endoscopy

Eric Hungness and Ezra Teitelbaum

Introduction

Since the advent and wide spread adoption of laparoscopic cholecystectomy in the late 1980s, the field of gastrointestinal (GI) surgery has continually evolved towards less invasive techniques. Laparoscopy has been used to perform almost every intra-abdominal operation and has replaced the open approach as "standard-of-care" for many procedures. Concurrently, endoscopy has been increasingly adopted to assist in laparoscopic and open abdominal surgery. Applications are as wide-ranging as evaluation of the myotomy during laparoscopic Heller, combined endoscopic and surgical techniques for placement of percutaneous endoscopic gastrostomy (PEG) tubes, and intra-operative lesion identification during gastric or colon resection.

This utilization of endoscopy by GI surgeons has coincided with the development of more advanced intraluminal procedures by gastroenterologists. These endoscopic interventions incorporate "surgical" techniques such as retraction, dissection of tissue planes, hemostasis, and respect for oncologic principles. More than ever before, the boundaries between the fields of GI surgery and gastroenterology are blurred, and physicians in both specialties must incorporate methods from the other. The evolution of natural orifice transluminal endoscopic surgery (NOTES) is a logical culmination of this hybridization. Whether or not NOTES becomes widely adopted, there is no doubt that endoscopy will play an increasingly substantial role in the armamentarium of future surgeons. The following procedures are examples of such emerging techniques in the field of surgical endoscopy.

Endoluminal Techniques

Endoscopic Repair of Perforations

Background

Since the 1970s, flexible endoscopy has played a central role in the diagnosis and treatment of gastric and colonic lesions. Colonoscopy is now a mainstay of preventative healthcare and polypectomy during routine screening has been linked to a decrease in the incidence of colorectal adenocarcinoma [1]. Although rare, iatrogenic perforations during diagnostic and therapeutic colonoscopies result in significant morbidity and even mortality. As techniques for resection of benign lesions become more advanced and aggressive, iatrogenic perforations could become more frequent. Currently, management of such perforations often involves surgery and may require bowel resection and anastomosis. Reliable techniques for repairing these perforations endoscopically would significantly reduce their associated morbidity and allow for increased endoscopist confidence when performing difficult polypectomies.

Repair of Perforations

The first repair of a large iatrogenic colon perforation using endoscopic clips was reported in 1997 [2]. Recently several retrospective reviews have described series of such repairs [3, 4]. At the time of colonoscopy, perforations are defined as either "evident" with endoscopic visualization of intraperitoneal tissues or "suspected" based on a suspicious mucosal injury without visible intraperitoneal structures. An endoscopic repair can be attempted for either category of perforation and is

E. Hungness, M.D. (✉) • E. Teitelbaum, M.D.
Department of Surgery, Northwestern University,
Chicago, IL, USA
e-mail: ehungnes@nmh.org

J.M. Marks and B.J. Dunkin (eds.), *Principles of Flexible Endoscopy for Surgeons*,
DOI 10.1007/978-1-4614-6330-6_22, © Springer Science+Business Media New York 2013

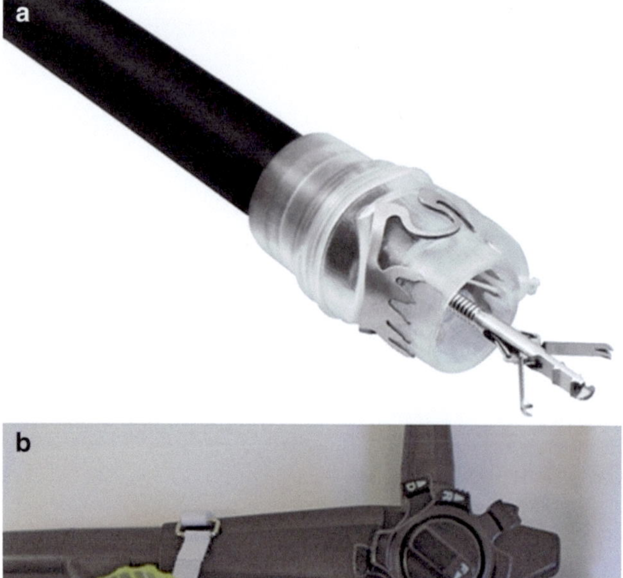

Fig. 22.1 (a) The over-the-scope-clip (OTSC) deployed on a standard endoscope with Twin Grasper endoscopic instrument. (b) Scope-mounted OSTC hand-wheel control" mechanism (Copyright Ovesco Endoscopy, Germany). With permission from Ovesco Endoscopy AG [5]

best performed immediately at the time of perforation. Patients with perforations discovered post-endoscopy are probably best managed operatively, or conservatively if signs of peritonitis are absent. Endoscopic repair should also not be attempted in the presence of an inadequate bowel prep or for perforations greater than 2 cm in diameter.

The defect is first visually inspected and insufflation is changed to CO_2 to speed post-procedure absorption of pneumoperitoneum. A Veress needle can be inserted transabdominally to release the pneumoperitoneum if the patient develops signs of abdominal compartment syndrome. Endoscopic clips are first placed at both corners of the defect to facilitate approximation of the perforation edges. Subsequent clips are then applied working from the corners toward the center of the defect until closure is complete.

Another technique uses the over-the-scope-clip (OTSC) system to close the perforation (Ovesco Endoscopy, Germany) [5]. OTSC deploys a nitinol clip that is preloaded onto a transparent plastic cap mounted on the tip of the endoscope (Fig. 22.1). OTSC clips come in three sizes, designed

to close defects of 9, 10, and 11 mm respectively. First, an endoscopic grasper or suction is used to pull the defect edges into the OTSC cap. Once fixed within the cap, the clip is deployed by a thread attached to a hand-wheel on the scope controls. Regardless of the method of closure, patients should be kept NPO post-procedure with administration of broad-spectrum IV antibiotics. Patients who subsequently develop evidence of peritonitis require either laparoscopic or open operative exploration. In recent series only 42–71 % of perforations were able to be repaired endoscopically, so surgical "back-up" must be available at all times [4, 5].

Repair of Anastomotic Leaks

Another application for endoscopic repair of luminal defects is in the management of anastomotic leakage. This potentially devastating complication results in significant morbidity and mortality and usually requires reoperation and often resection with recreation of the anastomosis or creation of a stoma for diversion. An endoscopic repair could potentially eliminate the need for morbid reoperations or prolonged courses of parenteral nutrition in cases of enteral fistulas resulting from leaks.

Hampe et al. have described a method for repair of an anastomotic leak following gastrectomy and esophagojejunostomy [6]. An upper endoscopy is first performed and endoscopic ultrasound is used to identify any adjacent abscess cavity resulting from the leak. The abscess is then irrigated and drained using an ERCP catheter. The edges of the defect are inspected and if they do not appear ischemic, an endoscopic closure may be attempted.

Repair is accomplished using the Tissue Apposition System (TAS) (Ethicon Endo-Surgery, Cincinnati, OH). TAS is an endoscopic suturing system that has been used in NOTES procedures to close visceral defects. A small metal bar or "T-tag" with attached suture is mounted onto a loading system, which consists of a needle passed through the endoscope's working channel (Fig. 22.2). The needle is used to puncture the bowel lumen adjacent to the defect and the T-tag is deployed through the needle onto the far side of the bowel wall. A second T-tag is then placed on the opposite side of the defect. The paired sutures are drawn taught to bring the T-tags together and close the defect. A tubular "knot-tying" element is then passed over the sutures and tightened to secure the T-tags in place. Paired T-tags are placed sequentially until the entire length of the defect is closed.

Care must be taken when placing the T-tags, as the "inline" nature of the endoscopic needle limits visualization of structures behind the bowel wall that is being punctured. This is evidenced in an animal study by Raju et al. in which T-tags were inadvertently placed into the bladder and adjacent colon during colotomy closure [7]. Some authors have

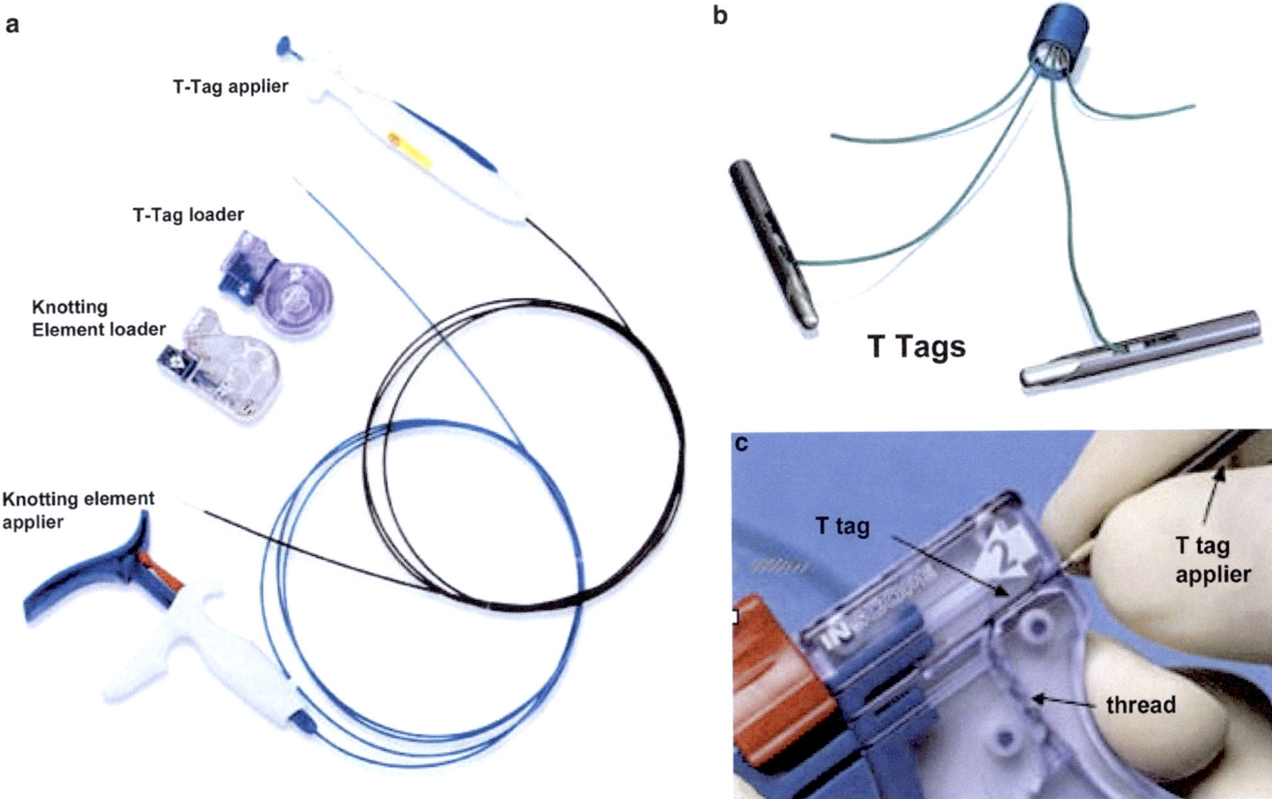

Fig. 22.2 (**a**) The tissue apposition system (TAS). (**b**) T-tags. (**c**) T-tag loader. Reprinted from [8], copyright 2010, with permission from Elsevier

discouraged use of the TAS for visceral defect closure without concurrent laparoscopic visualization [8]. Postoperatively, an X-ray or fluoroscopy study with contrast can be obtained to confirm closure of the leakage prior to initiation of diet.

Several other endoscopic suturing devices have recently been developed for use in combination with standard flexible endoscopes. These devices have the potential to be used to repair both iatrogenic perforations and anastomotic leaks. The fact that they are adaptable to standard endoscopes may ease their transition into more widespread clinical use by surgeons already skilled in traditional upper endoscopic interventions.

One such device, the EndoCinch suturing system (C.R. Bard, Murray Hill, NJ), is able to deploy suture through tissue in parallel with the endoscope and was originally developed to perform gastric cardia plication as an endoscopic treatment for gastroesophageal reflux. The EndoCinch applies suction to the target tissue for stabilization and a needle within the device places the suture across it. After another bite is taken, the tissue is approximated using a knotting element, similar to the one employed by the TAS. Fernandez-Esparrach et al. used this system in order to close gastro-gastric fistulas occurring after Roux-en-Y gastric bypass [9]. Although closure of the tract was achieved initially in 90 % of cases, the majority of those patients (65 %) presented

with fistula recurrence at a mean interval of 177 days, highlighting the difficult and chronic nature of such fistulas. However, despite such a high failure rate, initial treatment with an endoscopic suturing technique may still have a clinical role, given the high morbidity associated with reoperative laparoscopic bariatric surgery.

Several other similar suturing devices have also been recently introduced. The g-Prox system (USGI Medical, San Clemente, CA) combines the elements of a large tissue grasper and needle suture-passer into a single flexible endoscopic instrument. This enables tissue to be approximated prior to suture placement, allowing the surgeon to visualize what the configuration of the plicated tissue will be before committing to suturing. Another device, the OverStitch (Apollo Endosurgery, Austin, TX) most closely replicates the action of suturing with a curved needle during laparoscopic or open surgery. OverStitch is also mounted on a standard endoscope and contains an oscillating needle driver, which allows for placement of either interrupted or running suture configurations without the need to reload the device after each suture pass. Further laboratory and clinical investigation is needed to compare devices, and to define clinical criteria for which perforations and fistulas may be amenable to a purely endoscopic repair.

Full Thickness Resections

Background

As endoscopic techniques continue to evolve, lesions of the stomach and colon that would have been previously deemed "unresectable" endoscopically can now be managed without surgical intervention. Endoscopic mucosal resection (EMR) has been utilized to remove benign and early-stage malignant gastric lesions. Endoscopic submucosal dissection (ESD) allows for endoscopic "en bloc" resection of larger mucosal, as well as some submucosal and intra-muscular lesions. In the lower GI tract, techniques for the resection of larger and sessile adenomatous polyps have been refined. Hybrid procedures involving laparoscopic visualization and assistance have enhanced the safety and feasibility of these procedures. However, completely endoscopic full thickness resection for either gastric or colonic lesions remains in the early stages of development, largely limited to animal experiments. Important issues that need to be addressed going forward include the following: enteric spillage and contamination, the security of defect closures, visualization and tissue manipulation problems, and the oncologic ramifications of endoscopic resection.

Full Thickness Resection of the Stomach

Building on their experience with EMR and ESD, Zhou et al. have performed a series of completely endoscopic full thickness resections of gastric submucosal tumors using the following technique [10]. Preoperatively, patients undergo a diagnostic upper endoscopy with endoscopic ultrasound, confirming a submucosal lesion originating from the muscularis propria. A CT scan is also obtained and the mass must be less than 5 cm in diameter. The resection procedure is performed under general anesthesia with endotracheal intubation. A standard single or dual channel endoscope fitted with a transparent dissecting cap is used. A solution of 100 ml of saline, 1 ml indigo carmine, and 1 ml of epinephrine is injected in dots circumferentially around the lesion to mark it and assist in developing a submucosal dissection plane. The mucosa is then incised circumferentially using needle-knife cautery. At this point, the entire mucosal and submucosal area overlying the lesion can be removed with a snare to achieve better visualization. Endoscopic submucosal dissection techniques are then used to dissect circumferentially down to the muscle layer.

A decision is then made as to whether the lesion is superficial enough to be dissected free without the need for an en bloc full thickness resection. If full thickness resection is required, then the muscularis propria and serosa are carefully divided with hook cautery to enter the peritoneal cavity. It is important to repeat an evacuation of gastric contents prior to this step to avoid spillage and the potential for chemical peritonitis. If a dual channel endoscope is being used, a grasper can be inserted through the non-working channel to secure the lesion prior to freeing it completely from the surrounding stomach wall. Once a full thickness defect in the stomach wall is created, scope insufflation will cause pneumoperitoneum and potentially an abdominal compartment syndrome. If this occurs, a Veress needle can be inserted transabdominally to release the pneumoperitoneum.

Once the lesion has been excised, endoscopic clips are used to close the gastric defect (Fig. 22.3). If the defect is narrow, the clips can be applied sequentially starting at the edges and moving towards the center. If the edges will not approximate to a distance smaller than the maximum clip width, suction can be used to hold the margins together and enable clipping. If this technique is unsuccessful, omentum can be grasped and clipped circumferentially to the edges of the defect to form a modified Graham patch. Alternatively, the procedure can be converted to laparoscopy and the gastrotomy closed with suture.

To avoid an open gastric defect while still achieving a full thickness resection, Wang et al. use an alternative technique [11]. Once the mucosa and submucosa is incised, a nylon loop is placed around the mass and tightened to create a stalk-like effect. A snare is then used to resect the lesion superficial to the position of the loop. Clips are additionally applied to secure the closure. This technique may help reduce intra-peritoneal escape of both insufflation gas and gastric contents.

Another endoscopic procedure for resection of a full thickness segment of stomach wall employs a more "conventional" linear stapling technique. Kaehler et al. described the use of the flexible endoscopic powered stapling platform SurgAssist (Power Medical Interventions, Langhorne, PA) in order to essentially perform an "inside-out" gastric wedge resection using entirely intraluminal instrumentation in a human cadaver model (of note, Power Medical Interventions has since been acquired by Covidien, and the SurgAssist stapler is no longer commercially available) [12]. First, the SurgAssist stapler is passed down the esophagus and into the stomach under direct endoscopic visualization. In a porcine model, the diameter of the esophagus and lower esophageal sphincter prohibited the passage of both the stapler and gastroscope concurrently, highlighting the spatial constraints inherent to this method. As such techniques are transitioned to clinical use, it will be imperative that trauma or perforation of the esophagus is avoided when multiple endoscopic instruments are used in combination.

Once the stapler is safely introduced into the stomach, the target lesion is identified and retracted toward the scope using an endoscopic grasper. This retraction causes an invagination of the stomach wall, allowing the stapler to be passed around the base of the lesion. The stapler is fired via an electronically powered mechanism to create a full thickness wedge resection of up to 4 × 4 cm of gastric tissue. One should be cautioned that when using this and

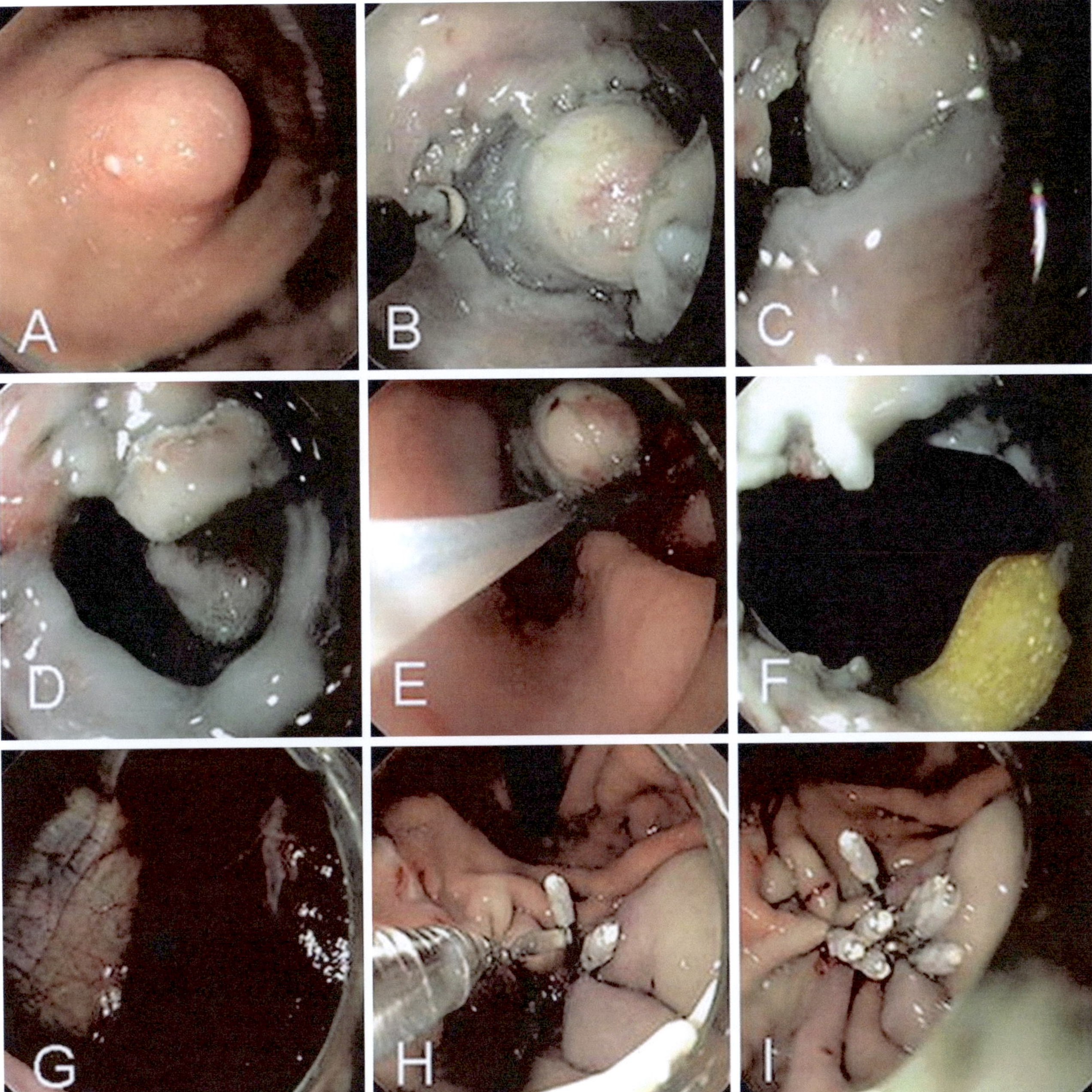

Fig. 22.3 Sequence of gastric tumor resection: (**a**) Endoscopic view of the submucosal tumor. (**b**) Circumferential dissection to the muscularis propria. (**c**) Initial muscular and serosal division. (**d**) Partially completed division. (**e**) Tumor removal with a snare. (**f**) The gastric defect after resection. (**g**) Diaphragm and liver visualized through the defect. (**h**) Defect closure with clips. (**i**) View of the final closure. With permission from [10], copyright 2011 Springer Verlag

other intraluminal techniques, just because the peritoneal cavity is not entered does not mean that its structures are not at risk for injury. On postoperative necropsy, Kaehler and colleagues discovered that omentum had been trapped and transected within the gastric staple-line in one case. The authors postulated that endoscopic ultrasound could potentially be used to ensure that no intra-abdominal contents are caught within the stapler jaws prior to firing, a method that requires further investigation [12].

Full Thickness Resection of the Colon

Transanal endoscopic microsurgery (TEM) has been used for almost 20 years to perform full thickness resections for benign and early-stage cancerous rectal masses. While evolving techniques and laparoscopic assistance have allowed for the safe removal of larger and flatter colonic lesions, full thickness colon resections have yet to be performed entirely endoscopically in humans. Concern for enteric spillage and oncologic compromise play an even larger role in the setting of the colon.

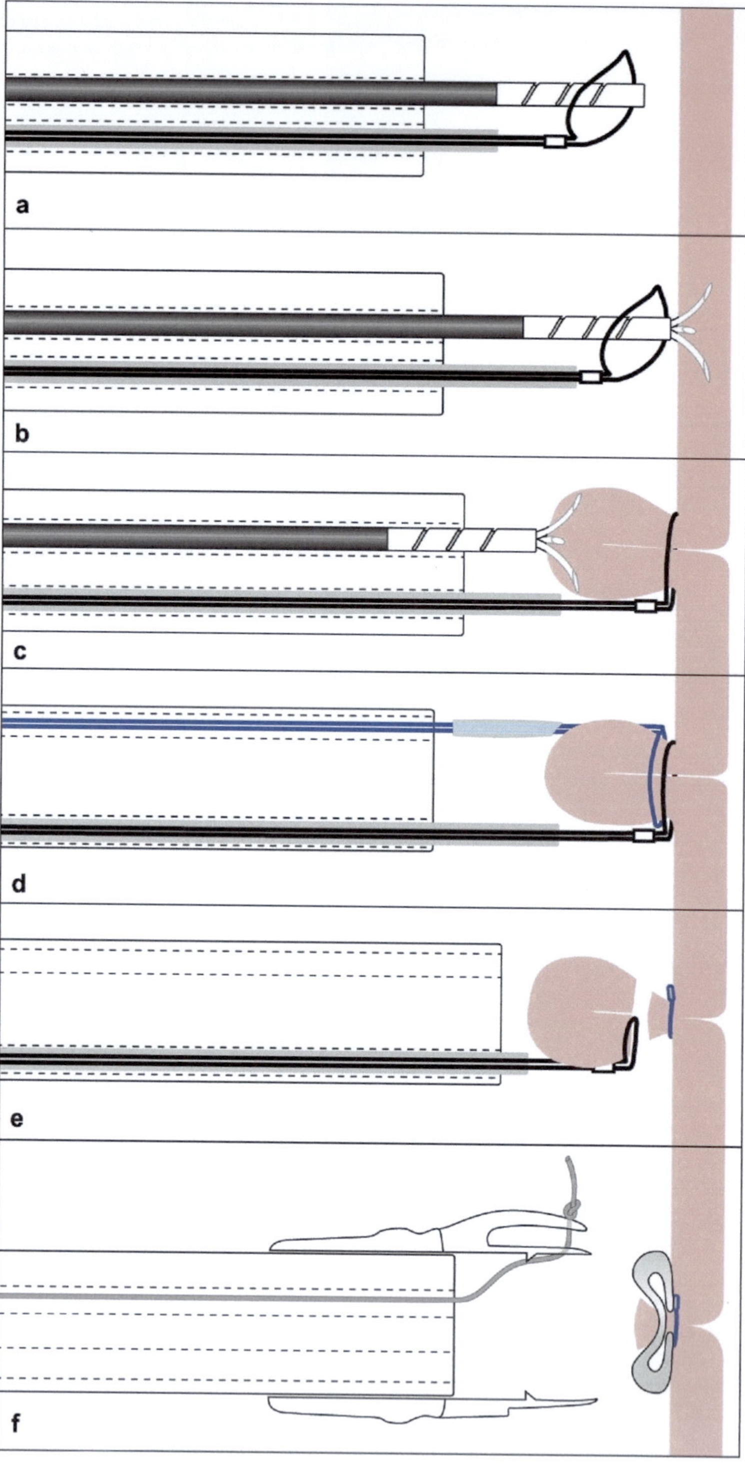

Fig. 22.4 Sequence of full thickness colon resection: (**a** and **b**) The tissue anchor is passed through the snare and deployed into the colonic wall. (**c**) The tissue anchor is partially withdrawn and the snare closed at the base of the lesion. (**d**) An endoloop is secured. (**e**) The lesion is resected with the snare. (**f**) An over-the-scope-clip is applied to secure the closure. Reprinted from [13], copyright 2010, with permission from Elsevier

While several animal experiments have yielded promising results, they have also shed light on potential pitfalls.

In one animal study a dual channel endoscope was used to visualize the lesion and introduce a tissue anchor (Ovesco Endoscopy, Germany) [13]. This tissue anchor deploys three needle-like prongs at its tip in order to grasp and retract the target lesion. A snare is then deployed through the second scope channel and seated around the base of the now pedunculated lesion. At this point the mass can be resected with snare cautery. Alternatively a suture loop can be placed deep to the snare in order to seal the defect prior to resection. Over-the-scope clips are then used to close the defect or secure the edges of the suture closure (Fig. 22.4). However, several complications occurred using this technique including inadequate closure, luminal obstruction, and injury to adjacent bowel by both the tissue anchor and closure clips.

Another method tested in an animal model involves initial circumferential resection with a grasper and needle cautery in a "lift-and-cut" technique [7]. This leads to an open defect and pneumoperitoneum necessitating transabdominal needle decompression. Closure is then achieved with the TAS system.

An alternative technique allows for full thickness colon resection without the creation of an open defect [14]. In this method TAS T-tags are first placed circumferentially around the lesion. The T-tag sutures are used to pull the lesion into an over-the-scope-clip that is then fired to secure the "base" of the now pedunculated tissue. A cautery snare is used to resect the lesion above the level of the clip. Despite solving the problem of an open colon defect, this method still requires blind placement of T-tags. Also, pre-resection clip placement limits the size of lesions that can be treated using the technique, as evidenced by an average resection diameter of 22 mm in the study.

Intraluminal Anastomoses

Background

NOTES and advanced endoscopic techniques have been used increasingly in the diagnosis and palliation of advanced GI malignancies. Transgastric peritonoscopy may be able to effectively stage intra-abdominal cancers with reduced morbidity and endoscopic stent placement has been established as a modality for palliation of inoperable obstructing cancers. Furthering this concept, an endoscopically performed bowel anastomosis might achieve more durable GI flow or be used when stenting is technically impossible. Several groups have explored techniques to accomplish such an anastomosis in animal models. Other potential applications could lie in NOTES bariatric surgery or bowel resections.

Transluminal Gastrojejunostomy

In a porcine model Simopoulos et al. performed gastrojejunostomies using the following technique [15]. A double channel endoscopic is used and the anterior gastric wall indentified by external abdominal palpation. A gastrotomy is made in the anterior gastric wall with a needle-knife and a guidewire is fed through the defect. A dilating balloon is then used to enlarge the gastrotomy and the scope is advanced into the peritoneal cavity behind the still-inflated balloon. A Veress needle may be needed at this point to reduce pneumoperitoneum.

Once intra-peritoneal, the segment of jejunum for anastomosis is identified. This bowel is grasped with an endoscopic forceps that has been passed through an open snare introduced through the second scope-channel. The forceps is then used to pull the bowel into the snare, which is closed to secure the loop. The scope and bowel are then withdrawn

together into the stomach. Endoscopic clips are used to fasten the jejunum to the edges of the gastrotomy defect. The needle-knife is again used to open the intra-gastric serosa of the jejunal loop. A second row of clips is then applied to circumferentially to seal the cut edges of the stomach and small bowel, thus creating an anastomosis.

Intraluminal Magnetic Gastrojejunostomy

The use of pressure necrosis to create a bowel anastomosis was first described in 1892 by John Murphy [16]. His "Murphy button" consisted of circular pieces of metal sutured within two ends of bowel. When brought together, the two pieces created an area of pressure necrosis over the section of bowel wall between them. The serosal edges surrounding the rings sealed, thus creating a "suture-less" anastomosis. Several devices have since been developed based on this concept but none have gained wide-spread usage. One such technique involves the use of paired circular magnets to create the area of pressure necrosis without any additional attachment to the bowel wall. This concept lends itself to endoscopic use as no intraluminal suturing is required.

Myers et al. used this magnetic technique to create a completely endoscopic gastrojejunostomy in an animal model, without intra-operative entrance into the peritoneal cavity [17]. An upper endoscopy is performed and a guidewire is passed into the jejunum under direct visualization. The scope is then removed, and a ring-shaped magnet is passed over the wire and the scope reinserted. The scope is then used to push the magnet into a position chosen for the distal (jejunal) limb of the anastomosis. A balloon can be passed over the guidewire and inflated within the ring of the magnet to fix it in place and assist in manipulation. Once the magnet is in the correct jejunal location, a large external magnet is placed over the anterior abdominal wall to hold it in position.

A second ring magnet is then inserted into the stomach in the same "over the wire" fashion and a second external magnet is used to fix its position as well. The two external magnets are then brought together to affix the internal ring magnets and create an area of pressure necrosis between them. This step is visualized endoscopically from the stomach. Diana et. al. added the use of an external magnetic tracking system to this technique to guide alignment of the two internal magnets [18].

At necropsy 1 week post-operatively, all of the placed rings in the original experiment had formed a leak-free anastomosis. The rings were all within the stomach or at the anastomotic site, facilitating easy endoscopic removal. However, the procedure failed in one animal because the distal magnetic ring would not fit through the pylorus. This technique solves the problems of intraperitoneal contamination and endoscopic suturing difficulties in creating enteric anastomoses. It has the potential to become a key tool as endoscopic GI operations become increasingly complex.

Transluminal Techniques

Overview of NOTES

Background

The first human NOTES procedure was a transgastric appendectomy, performed by Rao et al. in 2005 [19]. The same year, the Society of American Gastrointestinal and Endoscopic Surgeons (SAGES) formed the Natural Orifice Surgery Consortium for Assessment and Research (NOSCAR), an organization tasked to guide NOTES research and ensure its safe introduction into clinical practice. NOSCAR published the results of their initial meeting, termed the "white paper," in which anticipated barriers to implementation of NOTES in clinical practice were described [20]. These obstacles were: peritoneal access, gastric (or other visceral defect) closure, prevention of infection, suturing and anastomotic devices, development of a multitasking platform, management of intraperitoneal complications and hemorrhage, physiologic untoward events caused by NOTES, and NOTES training. Also emphasized were the importance of a multidisciplinary team that had trained on animal or cadaver models and the supewrvision of all human trials under IRB approval. Since this initial NOSCAR meeting, significant technical advances have been achieved and clinical implementation has progressed, most notably in Brazil and Germany. A NOTES approach has been utilized in operations as varied as cholecystectomy, appendectomy, esophageal myotomy, nephrectomy, partial gastrectomy, sigmoidectomy, partial hepatectomy, hernia repair, and splenectomy [21]. While the safety of NOTES access, closure and cholecystectomy has been shown in fairly large series, evidence as to clinical benefits over a laparoscopic approach is lacking. Going forward, the most significant clinical impact of the NOTES approach may lie in esophageal and colorectal applications, some of which are currently under investigation.

NOTES Cholecystectomy

NOTES cholecystectomy has been performed in humans using a number of different techniques. Both transgastric and transvaginal access have been used, although the transvaginal approach is much more prevalent. This is due to increased ease of access, visualization, tissue manipulation, and closure. With a transgastric approach a flexible endoscope is used, whereas in transvaginal cholecystectomy either a flexible or rigid scope can be employed. A review of the NOTES literature in 2010 found that of all reported transvaginal NOTES cholecystectomies, a rigid endoscope was used in 64 % of cases [21]. While "pure" NOTES cholecystectomies (in which no laparoscopic ports are utilized) have been performed, the vast majority of cases have used a

"hybrid" technique with one or more transabdominal trocars for assistance in retraction, dissection and/or visualization.

The International Prospective Multicenter Trial on Clinical NOTES (IMTN) is a registry of NOTES operations performed at 16 centers in 9 countries. They reported a series of 240 transvaginal cholecystectomies and described four unique methods for performing the procedure (Fig. 22.5) [22].

1. *"Pure NOTES" with dual flexible endoscopes*: The patient is placed in lithotomy position and topical iodopovidone or chlorhexidine solution is used for vaginal disinfection, in addition to prophylactic IV antibiotics. A Sims speculum and two lateral vaginal wall retractors are positioned for access and the cervix is grasped and retracted anteriorly. The posterior vaginal fornix is then opened under direct visualization to enter the peritoneal cavity.

   Two flexible endoscopes (one single and one dual-channel) are then inserted through the posterior colpotomy. A laparoscopic insufflator is used through the single-channel scope to maintain pneumoperitoneum. This scope retracts the gallbladder with an endoscopic grasper. The dual-channel endoscope is then used to perform the dissection of the triangle of Calot. A combination of hot-biopsy forceps, polypectomy snare and endoscopic hook cautery are used. Once the dissection is completed, endoscopic clips are applied to the cystic duct and artery and they are divided with endoscopic scissors. The gallbladder is dissected off the liver bed using a polypectomy snare cautery and is then grasped with the snare and extracted through the colpotomy. The pneumoperitoneum is evacuated and the colpotomy is closed directly with absorbable suture.

2. *"Pure NOTES" with multichannel port*: In this technique, patient preparation and transvaginal access are carried out in an identical fashion. Once the posterior colpotomy is made, a multichannel port is inserted through it. This port allows for passage of a flexible endoscope and laparoscopic instruments, as well as connection of tubing for CO_2 insufflation. A reticulating grasper is used for retraction of the gallbladder and the flexible endoscope is used for visualization and dissection. Once dissection is complete, the cystic duct and artery are clipped using a laparoscopic clip applier. The endoscope is used to divide these structures and dissect the gallbladder off the liver bed. Gallbladder extraction and direct colpotomy closure are performed as in the prior method.

3. *"Hybrid NOTES" with both transabdominal and transvaginal visualization*: Some centers relied on traditional laparoscopic visualization to ensure safety during access and dissection. In these procedures, a laparoscope is first inserted transabdominally using standard techniques. Posterior vaginal access is then created with both direct and laparoscopic visualization. Dissection proceeds as described previously using a flexible endoscope inserted transvaginally. The addition a rigid laparoscope to assist

Fig. 22.5 Instrument positions for four methods of NOTES transvaginal cholecystectomy: (**a**) "Pure NOTES" with dual flexible endoscopes. (**b**) "Pure NOTES" with multichannel port. (**c**) "Hybrid NOTES" with both transabdominal and transvaginal visualization. (**d**) "Hybrid NOTES" using minilaparoscopic instruments. Reprinted from [22], with permission from SAGE Publications, copyright 2010 SAGE Publications

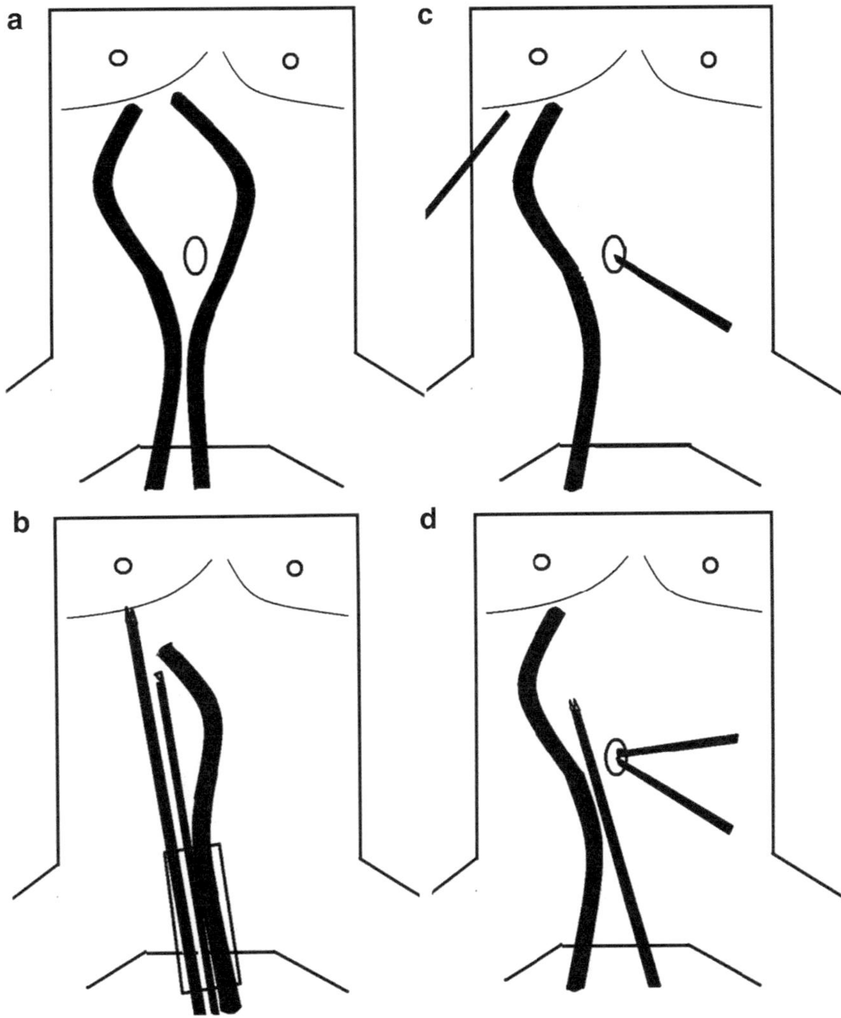

in visualization is helpful in maintaining orientation and defining anatomic landmarks. The authors noted that this technique resulted in faster operative times. Additional laparoscopic ports can be inserted to assist with retraction and dissection. The gallbladder is removed transvaginally and a direct closure of the colpotomy is performed.

4. *"Hybrid NOTES" using minilaparoscopic instruments*: This technique relies on laparoscopic instrumentation with transvaginal endoscopic visualization. A Veress needle is first inserted to insufflate the abdomen in order to displace the small bowel. Subsequently a posterior colpotomy is performed under direct visualization as described previously. A flexible endoscope is inserted transvaginally and provides visualization for the remainder of the case. Under retroflexed view, a 10 mm trocar is inserted through the posterior vaginal fornix alongside the endoscope. Two 3 mm trocars are then inserted transabdominally through the umbilicus. Three millimeter minilaparoscopic instruments are used for gallbladder

retraction and dissection is performed with the flexible endoscope. Clips are placed on the cystic duct and artery with a standard laparoscopic clip-applier inserted through the 10 mm transvaginal trocar. The gallbladder is extracted with a laparoscopic grasper inserted through this trocar and the vaginal wall is closed under direct visualization.

The German NOTES Registry (GNR) has reported the largest series to-date of 488 hybrid transvaginal cholecystectomies [23]. The vast majority of these were performed using the following method. A 5 mm laparoscopic trocar is first placed through the umbilicus and a laparoscope inserted. A 10 and 5 mm trocar are then placed through the posterior vaginal fornix under laparoscopic guidance. Visualization is then switched to a *rigid* 45° laparoscope placed through the 10 mm transvaginal trocar. A laparoscopic grasper retracts the gallbladder through the 5 mm transvaginal trocar. Dissection, clipping and cutting are all performed with instrumentation passed through the umbilical trocar in a fashion identical to standard laparoscopic cholecystectomy.

The gallbladder is removed transvaginally and the colpotomies closed directly.

The IMTN and GNR studies reported 6.9 and 3.3 % complication rates respectively with no mortalities. In the IMTN study, five cases of intra-operative hemorrhage were reported. One was treated with endoscopic clipping and four with laparoscopically placed clips. One case of gastric perforation resulted from dense adhesions between the stomach and gallbladder. Two cases of biliary leak occurred, although neither from a common bile duct or hepatic duct injury. The GNR study reported two rectal injuries and four bladder injuries related to transvaginal trocar placement and instrumentation. One pelvic abscess occurred that required laparoscopic drainage and two cases of minor post-operative vaginal bleeding occurred that did not require intervention.

Neither registry compared clinical outcomes with standard laparoscopy. However, a separate case-matched study evaluated 108 pairs of laparoscopic and hybrid transvaginal NOTES cholecystectomies [24]. There were longer operative times in the NOTES group, with no difference in post-operative analgesic usage, hospital length of stay, time off work, or complications. A multicenter randomized controlled trial organized by NOSCAR is currently underway comparing outcomes between NOTES and standard laparoscopic cholecystectomies.

Potential Applications

A criticism levied against the NOTES approach for cholecystectomy and other intra-abdominal operations is that it creates an "unnecessary" visceral defect with associated potential for morbidity. In the case of hybrid NOTES procedures that require laparoscopic ports, the risk of this additional enteral access site may not be eclipsed by benefits of reduced pain and convalescence. Recent NOTES applications have focused on procedures in which the planned visceral access point is prerequisite to the operation or those that can be performed in a "pure" NOTES fashion. Peroral endoscopic myotomy and transanal rectosigmoidectomy are two examples of such novel operations. In addition, for more advanced intraluminal surgery to become technically feasible, a new generation of operating endoscopes will be needed. These will be able to provide triangulation of instrumentation with multiple degrees of freedom of movement, more powerful retraction, and more precise dissection capabilities. Several such platforms are currently under development.

Per-Oral Endoscopic Myotomy

Per-Oral Endoscopic Myotomy (POEM) was first performed in humans as a treatment for achalasia by Haru Inoue, who published his initial results in 2010 [25]. POEM achieves a completely endoscopic myotomy of the inner circular muscle layer above and below the lower esophageal sphincter (LES), while sparing the longitudinal muscle fibers.

Preoperative work-up includes upper GI X-rays, high-resolution manometry and upper endoscopy to exclude causes of pseudo-achalasia.

For the procedure, the patient is placed under general anesthesia with endotracheal intubation in a supine position. An upper endoscopy is performed and the distance from incisors to esophagogastric junction (EGJ) is measured. A submucosal injection with a saline and indigo carmine solution is made in the anterior esophagus at a distance approximately 13 cm proximal to the EGJ. This injection serves to develop a submucosal plane, as well as maintain anterior orientation for dissection. After injection, a 2 cm longitudinal incision in the anterior esophageal mucosa is made with a needle-knife. The opening can be dilated with an endoscopic balloon to facilitate scope entry. Endoscopic submucosal dissection techniques using spray electrocautery are then used to create a submucosal tunnel down the length of the distal esophagus and 3 cm past the EGJ onto the stomach. At the LES, the esophageal layers are tighter and dissection can be more difficult.

The scope is then withdrawn partially and dissection of the inner circular muscle layer is begun approximately 3 cm distal to the mucosal entry. A triangle-tip cautery is used to hook, lift and then divide individual muscle fibers. The myotomy is advanced to 2 cm past the EGJ. At this point the scope is withdrawn from the tunnel and the compliance of the LES is observed. A retroflexed view is used to confirm that the myotomy has been extended into the stomach. Once the myotomy is complete, the tunnel is irrigated with antibiotic solution and the mucosal opening is closed with a series of endoscopic clips (Fig. 22.6).

Post-operatively the patient is kept NPO and an upper GI series is obtained on post-operative day one to rule out esophageal leak. Liquid diet is then initiated and maintained for 2 weeks.

Transanal Rectosigmoidectomy

Recently the TEM platform has been used to perform transanal rectosigmoidectomies with little or no laparoscopic assistance in laboratory models [26, 27]. An appealing aspect of this technique is that the NOTES rectotomy is incorporated into the eventual colorectal anastomosis, eliminating concerns over the security of an additional visceral closure.

The first human operation was recently reported by Sylla et al. using the following method for treatment of a rectal adenocarcinoma [28, 29]. The patient is placed in lithotomy position and a standard anal retractor is first inserted. Under direct visualization, a purse-string suture is placed approximately 4 cm from the anal verge to close the rectal lumen. The TEM proctoscope is then inserted and the rectal mucosa is divided just distal to the purse-string closure. Full-thickness rectal dissection is then begun posteriorly to enter the avascular presacral plane using TEM instrumentation for retraction

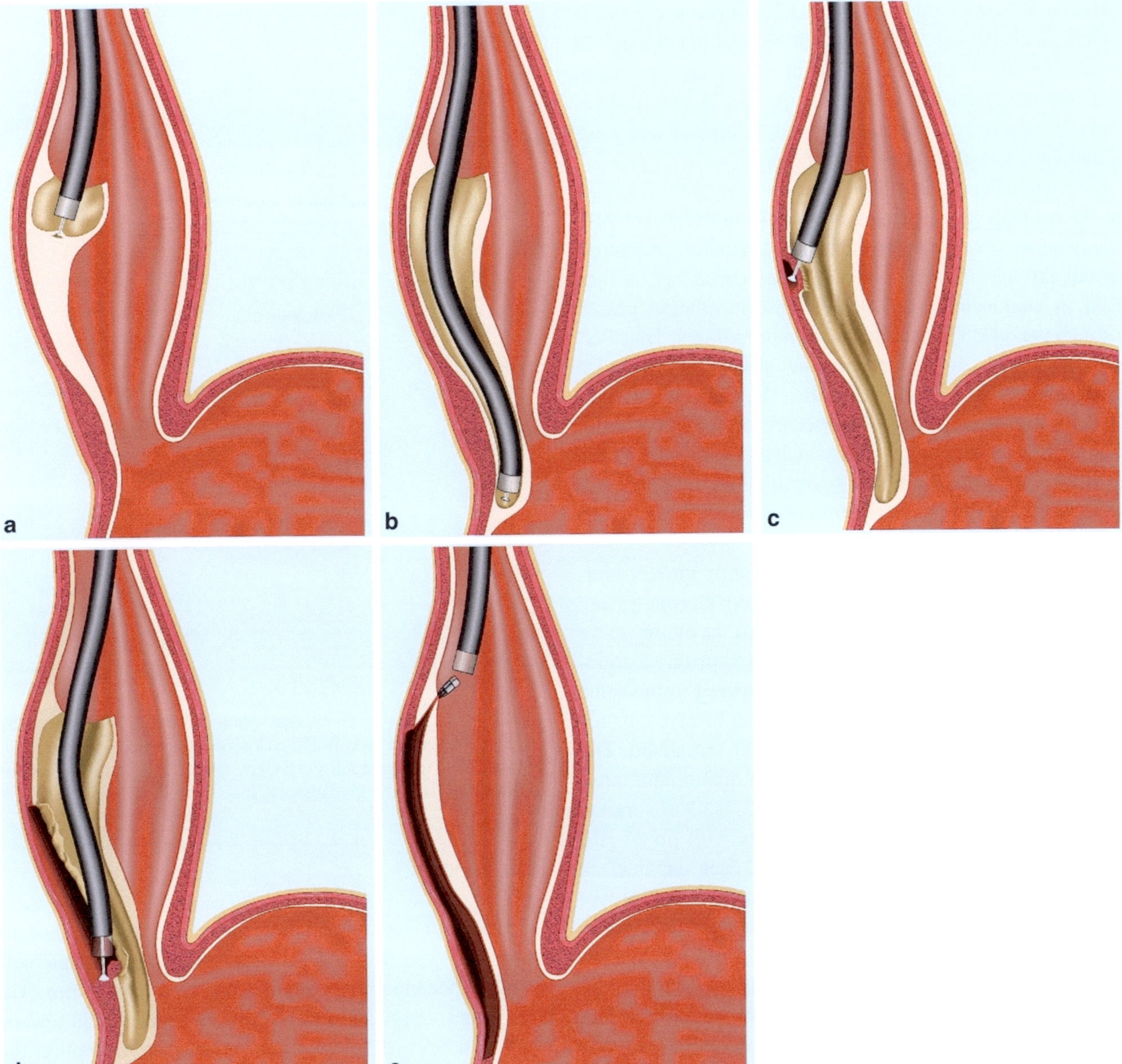

Fig. 22.6 Sequence for POEM: (**a**) Entry into the submucosal space. (**b**) Dissection of a submucosal tunnel. (**c** and **d**) Division of the circular muscle fibers. (**e**) Closure of the mucosal defect with clips. From [25], copyright 2010 George Thieme Verlag, with permission from George Thieme Verlag, Stuttgart

and a laparoscopic energy device for cautery. Bilateral medial and then anterior dissection follow in order to create a circumferential total mesorectal excision.

Once the peritoneal cavity is entered, the rectal specimen is reflected upwards to allow for sigmoid dissection. At this point, laparoscopic trocars can be added to aid with retraction and dissection. Vascular control and division is accomplished with an endoscopic GIA stapler passed through the TEM platform. Once the rectosigmoid is completely mobilized, the TEM proctoscope is removed and the specimen is delivered transanally. Proximal bowel division is performed externally with a GIA stapler. A hand-sewn anastomosis is then performed under direct visualization. Alternatively an anvil can be placed in the proximal colon end and an EEA stapler used to create the anastomosis.

Future Endoscopic Platforms

Although endoscopic techniques have continually evolved since the first colonoscopic polypectomies, the scopes themselves have for the most part remained rooted in the same technology. New instrumentation has developed to overcome technical challenges such as suturing and retraction but severe limitations in terms of lateral instrument movement and complex tissue manipulation still exist. A new generation of endoscopes is currently under development and seeks to address some of these insufficiencies.

The TransPort (USGI Medical, San Clemente, CA) is a newly available flexible endoscopic platform with four working channels [29]. Visualization is via a standard endoscope passed through the main channel. This endoscope is then used in conjunction with flexible instrumentation passed through the other channels to perform procedures. TransPort is able to "lock" in a flexed orientation and thus allow for more stable dissection and retraction. The platform has been used for transgastric NOTES procedures in the upper abdomen such as cholecystectomy, in which a partially retroflexed working view is necessary. However, it is limited by the use of standard endoscopes and instrumentation with their inherent insufficiencies.

Two novel endoscopic platforms currently under development, the Anubis (Karl Storz, Tutlingen, Germany) and EndoSamurai (Olympus, Tokyo, Japan), seek to solve some of the current problems regarding instrument triangulation and dexterity [30]. Anubis is steered in the same manner as a standard endoscope but has a bivalve capsule tip that opens after the target structure is visualized. The "wings" of this open tip each displace an instrument laterally, allowing for triangulation (Fig. 22.7). The surgeon operates specialized flexible instruments with pistol-grip controls through these lateral channels, each capable six degrees of movement. An assistant controls scope movement and flexion, as well as a standard endoscopic instrument through a third centrally positioned working channel. EndoSamurai provides similar instrument triangulation by means of two articulating arms at the scope's tip. A key difference is that the EndoSamurai's lateral instruments are controlled by a floor-stand interface that replicates the handle controls and movements of laparoscopic instruments. In a bench-top experiment, the EndoSamurai was used to successfully place and tie standard sutures in an "intra-corporeal" fashion [31].

Future endoscopic procedural challenges will likely require the incorporation of robotic end-effectors to apply more powerful lateral retraction forces and quicker, more precise, instrument movement. The clinical success of the DaVinci platform (Intuitive Medical, Sunnyvale, CA) provides optimism for such development but miniaturization of robotic instruments to fit the tip of an endoscope creates significant design challenges. Such systems are in the infancy of development and wide-spread clinical application of a robotic endoscopic platform is likely a bit further off on the horizon.

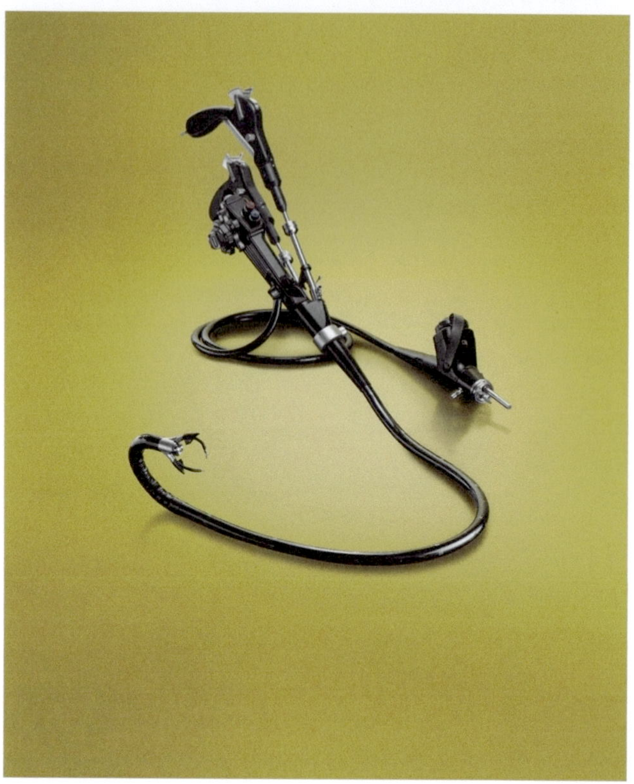

Fig. 22.7 The Anubis endoscopic platform under development by Karl Storz. Inset is a view of the endoscope tip, which opens to allow for instrument triangulation [29]. Copyright 2011 Photo Courtesy of KARL STORZ Endoscopy-America, Inc

Conclusions

As endoscopic instrumentation and platforms continue to evolve, the spectrum of their potential applications will expand exponentially. Recent development has occurred via three routes: application of existing instrumentation toward new procedures, development of novel instrumentation for use with standard endoscopes, and development of entirely new flexible endoscopic operating platforms. While the later avenue will take the longest to develop (with no systems commercially available to-date), advances based on the first two have already enabled significant progress over the last several years. For example, the POEM procedure is performed using only standard and preexisting endoscopic instrumentation. By simply applying the principles and instruments used in other endoscopic procedures such as ESD, an entirely novel treatment modality for achalasia was devised, one that may end up supplanting laparoscopic Heller myotomy as the standard-of-care.

Innumerate possibilities for similar innovation and adaptable exist. While envisioned as an intra-abdominal platform, investigations into thoracic applications of a NOTES approach have recently gained momentum. Procedures such as transesophageal lymph node biopsy offer the potential to reduce morbidity by eliminating cervical or thoracic incisions completely. While these and other advanced endoscopic procedures on the close horizon offer the potential to improve clinical outcomes, the research grounds on which they are based must remain firm in order to maintain patient safety as the utmost priority. Under the direction of the NOSCAR and other surgical societies, investigation into novel NOTES procedures has thus far followed a incremental path from laboratory study to IRB-guided and approved clinical trials. As public demand for these procedures increases, surgeons must resist pressure to apply them prematurely outside of a strictly controlled research setting, before adequate evidence of their safety and benefit over existing treatment modalities exists.

Undoubtedly, in the near future surgeons will be able to more effectively utilize the endoscope as a tool to assist in laparoscopic surgery, as well as to perform "surgical" procedures endoluminally. Rather than being viewed as an "experimental" procedure, NOTES has the potential to become integrated into standard surgical practice. NOTES techniques may come to be seen simply as an extension of endoscopy and as a compliment to, rather than a replacement of, laparoscopic GI surgery.

References

1. Winawer SJ, Zauber AG, Ho MN, O'Brien MJ, Gottlieb LS, Sternberg SS, et al. Prevention of colorectal cancer by colonoscopic polypectomy. The National Polyp Study Workgroup. N Engl J Med. 1993;329:1977–81.
2. Yoshikane H, Hidano H, Sakakibara A, Ayakawa T, Mori S, Kawashima H, et al. Endoscopic repair by clipping of iatrogenic colonic perforation. Gastrointest Endosc. 1997;46:464–6.
3. Yang DH, Byeon JS, Lee KH, Yoon SM, Kim KJ, Ye BD, et al. Is endoscopic closure with clips effective for both diagnostic and therapeutic colonoscopy-associated bowel perforation? Surg Endosc. 2010;24:1177–85.
4. Jovanovic I, Zimmermann L, Fry LC, Monkemuller K. Feasibility of endoscopic closure of an iatrogenic colon perforation occurring during colonoscopy. Gastrointest Endosc. 2011;73:550–5.
5. Seebach L, Bauerfeind P, Gubler C. "Sparing the surgeon": clinical experience with over-the-scope clips for gastrointestinal perforation. Endoscopy. 2010;42:1108–11.
6. Hampe J, Schniewind B, Both M, Fritscher-Ravens A. Use of a NOTES closure device for full-thickness suturing of a postoperative anastomotic esophageal leakage. Endoscopy. 2010;42:595–8.
7. Raju GS, Malhotra A, Ahmed I. Colonoscopic full-thickness resection of the colon in a porcine model as a prelude to endoscopic surgery of difficult colon polyps: a novel technique (with videos). Gastrointest Endosc. 2009;70:159–65.
8. Agrawal D, Chak A, Champagne BJ, Marks JM, Delaney CP. Endoscopic mucosal resection with full-thickness closure for difficult polyps: a prospective clinical trial. Gastrointest Endosc. 2010;71:1082–8.
9. Fernandez-Esparrach G, Lautz DB, Thompson CC. Endoscopic repair of gastrogastric fistula after Roux-en-Y gastric bypass: a less-invasive approach. Surg Obes Relat Dis. 2010;6:282–8.
10. Zhou PH, Yao LQ, Qin XY, Cai MY, Xu MD, Zhong YS, et al. Endoscopic full-thickness resection without laparoscopic assistance for gastric submucosal tumors originated from the muscularis propria. Surg Endosc. 2011;25(9):2926–31.
11. Wang L, Ren W, Fan CQ, Li YH, Zhang X, Yu J, et al. Full-thickness endoscopic resection of nonintracavitary gastric stromal tumors: a novel approach. Surg Endosc. 2011;25:641–7.
12. Kaehler GF, Langner C, Suchan KL, Freudenberg S, Post S. Endoscopic full-thickness resection of the stomach: an experimental approach. Surg Endosc. 2006;20:519–21.
13. von Renteln D, Schmidt A, Vassiliou MC, Rudolph HU, Caca K. Endoscopic full-thickness resection and defect closure in the colon. Gastrointest Endosc. 2010;71:1267–73.
14. Rieder E, Martinec DV, Dunst CM, Swanstrom LL. A novel technique for natural orifice endoscopic full-thickness colon wall resection: an experimental pilot study. J Am Coll Surg. 2011;213(3):422–9.
15. Simopoulos C, Kouklakis G, Zezos P, Ypsilantis P, Botaitis S, Tsalikidis C, et al. Peroral transgastric endoscopic procedures in pigs: feasibility, survival, questionings, and pitfalls. Surg Endosc. 2009;23:394–402.
16. Murphy J. Cholecysto-intestinal, gastrointestinal, enterointestinal anastomosis and approximation without sutures (original research). Med Rec. 1892;42:665–76.
17. Myers C, Yellen B, Evans J, DeMaria E, Pryor A. Using external magnet guidance and endoscopically placed magnets to create suture-free gastro-enteral anastomoses. Surg Endosc. 2010;24:1104–9.
18. Diana M, Wall J, Perretta S, Dallemagne B, Gonzales KD, Harrison MR, et al. Totally endoscopic magnetic enteral bypass by external guided Rendez-Vous technique. Surg Innov. 2011;18(4):317–20.
19. Rao GV, Reddy DN, Banerjee R. NOTES: human experience. Gastrointest Endosc Clin N Am. 2008;18:361–70; x.
20. Rattner D, Kalloo A. ASGE/SAGES Working Group on Natural Orifice Translumenal endoscopic surgery. October 2005. Surg Endosc. 2006;20:329–33.
21. Auyang ED, Santos BF, Enter DH, Hungness ES, Soper NJ. Natural orifice translumenal endoscopic surgery (NOTES(®)): a technical review. Surg Endosc. 2011;25(10):3135–48.
22. Zorron R, Palanivelu C, Galvao Neto MP, Ramos A, Salinas G, Burghardt J, et al. International multicenter trial on clinical natural orifice surgery—NOTES IMTN study: preliminary results of 362 patients. Surg Innov. 2010;17:142–58.
23. Lehmann KS, Ritz JP, Wibmer A, Gellert K, Zornig C, Burghardt J, et al. The German registry for natural orifice translumenal endoscopic surgery: report of the first 551 patients. Ann Surg. 2010;252:263–70.
24. Zornig C, Siemssen L, Emmermann A, Alm M, von Waldenfels HA, Felixmuller C, et al. NOTES cholecystectomy: matched-pair analysis comparing the transvaginal hybrid and conventional laparoscopic techniques in a series of 216 patients. Surg Endosc. 2011;25:1822–6.
25. Inoue H, Minami H, Kobayashi Y, Sato Y, Kaga M, Suzuki M, et al. Peroral endoscopic myotomy (POEM) for esophageal achalasia. Endoscopy. 2010;42:265–71.
26. Rieder E, Spaun GO, Khajanchee YS, Martinec DV, Arnold BN, Smith Sehdev AE, et al. A natural orifice transrectal approach for oncologic resection of the rectosigmoid: an experimental study and comparison with conventional laparoscopy. Surg Endosc. 2011;25(10):3357–63.
27. Sylla P, Sohn DK, Cizginer S, Konuk Y, Turner BG, Gee DW, et al. Survival study of natural orifice translumenal endoscopic surgery for rectosigmoid resection using transanal endoscopic microsurgery with or without transgastric endoscopic assistance in a swine model. Surg Endosc. 2010;24:2022–30.
28. Sylla P, Rattner DW, Delgado S, Lacy AM. NOTES transanal rectal cancer resection using transanal endoscopic microsurgery and laparoscopic assistance. Surg Endosc. 2010;24:1205–10.

29. Santos BF, Hungness ES. Natural orifice translumenal endoscopic surgery: progress in humans since white paper. World J Gastroenterol. 2011;17:1655–65.
30. Swanstrom LL. NOTES: platform development for a paradigm shift in flexible endoscopy. Gastroenterology. 2011;140:1150–4.e1.
31. Spaun GO, Zheng B, Swanstrom LL. A multitasking platform for natural orifice translumenal endoscopic surgery (NOTES): a benchtop comparison of a new device for flexible endoscopic surgery and a standard dual-channel endoscope. Surg Endosc. 2009;23(12):2720–7.

Index

J.M. Marks and B.J. Dunkin (eds.), *Principles of Flexible Endoscopy for Surgeons*,
DOI 10.1007/978-1-4614-6330-6, © Springer Science+Business Media New York 2013